Research of Pathogenesis and Novel Therapeutics in Arthritis 3.0

Research of Pathogenesis and Novel Therapeutics in Arthritis 3.0

Editor

Chih-Hsin Tang

MDPI • Basel • Beijing • Wuhan • Barcelona • Belgrade • Manchester • Tokyo • Cluj • Tianjin

Editor
Chih-Hsin Tang
China Medical University
Taichung
Taiwan

Editorial Office
MDPI
St. Alban-Anlage 66
4052 Basel, Switzerland

This is a reprint of articles from the Special Issue published online in the open access journal *International Journal of Molecular Sciences* (ISSN 1422-0067) (available at: https://www.mdpi.com/journal/ijms/special_issues/arthritis_3).

For citation purposes, cite each article independently as indicated on the article page online and as indicated below:

LastName, A.A.; LastName, B.B.; LastName, C.C. Article Title. *Journal Name* **Year**, *Volume Number*, Page Range.

ISBN 978-3-0365-8084-5 (Hbk)
ISBN 978-3-0365-8085-2 (PDF)

Contents

About the Editor

Chih-Hsin Tang

Professor Chih-Hsin Tang served as a faculty in the Department of Pharmacology, Faculty of Medicine, China Medical University, after completing his doctoral and postdoctoral training in the Institute of Pharmacology, National Taiwan University, in 2006. He was promoted to professor in 2012 and became the Director of the Institute of Basic Medicine in 2013. Since 2016-2023, he has served as the R&D Dean of the Research and Development Department. The research mainly focuses on skeletal system diseases, including osteoporosis, arthritis, and bone cancer, etc., in order to develop novel molecular targets and find drugs with therapeutic potential. He has overseen more than 430 related academic papers, owns 3 domestic and foreign patents, and has achieved an Academic Career H index of 57, according Web of Science. These research results have received the "Taiwan Pharmacological Association Young Scholar Award", the "Professor Chen-Yuan Lee Young Scholar Award for Medical Research", the "China Medical University Outstanding Research Teacher Award", the "National Science Council Da-Yu Wu Memorial Award", the "Santa Cruz 2011 July Award", the "Ten Outstanding Young Scholars" award, the "China Medical University Young Research Talents Deep Cultivation Program Award", the "TaJen University of Science and Technology Outstanding Alumni" award, the "Ministry of Science and Technology Outstanding Young Scholar Research Program Award", and the "Outstanding Research Award of the Pharmacological Society in Taiwan". He also listed among the "World's Top 2% Scientists 2020 (Scopus)", "World's Top 2% Scientists 2021 (Scopus)", Best Scientists in the Medicine field around the world (Research.com 2022), and the Best Scientists in the Medicine field and the Biology and Biochemistry field around the world (Research.com 2023).

International Journal of *Molecular Sciences*

Editorial

Research of Pathogenesis and Novel Therapeutics in Arthritis 3.0

Chih-Hsin Tang [1,2,3,4]

1 Department of Pharmacology, School of Medicine, China Medical University, Taichung 404333, Taiwan; chtang@mail.cmu.edu.tw; Tel.: +886-2205-2121 (ext. 7726); Fax: +886-4-2233-3641
2 Chinese Medicine Research Center, China Medical University, Taichung 404333, Taiwan
3 Department of Biotechnology, College of Health Science, Asia University, Taichung 400354, Taiwan
4 Department of Medical Research, China Medical University Hsinchu Hospital, Hsinchu 30272, Taiwan

Arthritis has a high prevalence globally and includes over 100 types, the most common of which are rheumatoid arthritis (RA), osteoarthritis (OA), psoriatic arthritis (PsA), and inflammatory arthritis. All types of arthritis share common features of the disease, including monocyte infiltration, inflammation, synovial swelling, pannus formation, stiffness in the joints, and articular cartilage destruction. The exact etiology of arthritis remains unclear, and no cure exists as of yet. Anti-inflammatory drugs (NSAIDs and corticosteroids) are commonly used in the treatment of arthritis. However, these drugs are associated with significant side effects, such as gastric bleeding and an increased risk for heart attack and other cardiovascular problems. It is therefore crucial that we continue to research the pathogenesis of arthritis and seek to discover novel modes of therapy.

Our call for papers for this Special Issue attracted several articles, all of which underwent rigorous peer review. A total of 18 papers (13 research papers and 5 reviews) satisfied the inclusion criteria for publication in this Special Issue. The research papers cover cellular, preclinical, and clinical investigations. The reviews discuss aspects of treatment with hyaluronic acid, corticosteroids, and platelet-rich plasma in patients with temporomandibular joint OA, the potential of a novel micro-immunotherapy medicine that uses ultra-low doses of proinflammatory cytokines as well as other immune factors in an attempt to restore bodily homeostasis in patients with RA, a discussion of vascular endothelial growth factor (VEGF) biology and its potential as a therapeutic target in rheumatic diseases, and lastly, a summary of current insights into the involvement of the CCN family in RA and OA, accompanied by evidence in support of the targeting of CCN proteins in these diseases. All of these papers are discussed below.

(i) Cellular investigations. Sohn and colleagues describe how the synthesis of adenosine by human RA or OA synoviocytes is crucial to anti- or pro-inflammatory effects mediated by adenosine receptor subtypes A2A and A2B in response to interleukin (IL)-6, IL-10, and tumor necrosis factor (TNF) [1]. The researchers suggest how this function may be exploited to serve as a future therapeutic strategy in RA or OA [1]. Immunofluorescence analysis of immunophenotypes of different cell populations in knee synovial tissue samples obtained from healthy controls or patients with early or advanced knee OA helps to elucidate the pathophysiology of this disease, according to Ostojic and colleagues [2]. They found that macrophages appear to be the most active cells in early OA through the nuclear factor-κB (NF-κB) production of inflammatory factors (inducible nitric oxide synthase [iNOS] and matrix metalloproteinase-9 [MMP-9]) in the intima, whereas, in advanced OA, NF-κB is mostly expressed by leukocytes in the synovial subintima (stroma) [2]. Ostojic and colleagues suggest that it may be worth blocking macrophageal and leukocyte NF-κB expression to slow the disease behavior of OA [2]. The other research group indicates that cytokines released in complete Freund's adjuvant (CFA)-induced arthritis in ICR mice as well as the regulation of blood levels of cytokines by two peptides of the innate immunity

Citation: Tang, C.-H. Research of Pathogenesis and Novel Therapeutics in Arthritis 3.0. *Int. J. Mol. Sci.* **2023**, *24*, 10166. https://doi.org/10.3390/ijms241210166

Received: 29 May 2023
Accepted: 30 May 2023
Published: 15 June 2023

protein Tag7 (PGLYRP1) capable of blocking the activation of the TNFR1 receptor [3]. The Taiwanese research group also demonstrates that IL-17 promotes vascular cell adhesion molecule 1 (VCAM-1) production in human OA synovial fibroblasts (OASFs) and subsequently increases monocyte adhesion by reducing miR-5701 expression through the PKC-α and JNK signaling cascades, which may help with the design of more effective OA treatments [4].

(ii) Preclinical investigations. Makalish and colleagues describe how treatment with the antisense oligonucleotide Cytos-11 effectively inhibits TNF-α gene expression in a rat model of RA, with results that are comparable to those from other studies using adalimumab treatment in rats with RA [5]. Makalish and colleagues detail reductions in joint inflammation and pannus development, reduced lymphocytic infiltration of joint tissues, and decreases in peripheral blood concentrations of TNF-α [5]. Sykora and colleagues describe how administering intraperitoneal injections of high-dose unconjugated bilirubin significantly improved the clinical course of disease in rats with adjuvant-induced arthritis [6]. These researchers acknowledge that while murine models of arthritis have many limitations with regard to human RA, the specific effects of unconjugated bilirubin administration in this experimental model of arthritis may be relevant for further RA pharmacotherapy investigations [6]. In experiments involving mice with collagen-induced arthritis (CIA), administration of the natural flavone kurarinone has shown promise as a potentially beneficial adjunct treatment option for RA, according to Tang and colleagues [7]. In particular, kurarinone inhibited pathogenic Th1 and Th17 cell differentiation and exerted antioxidative activity, which contributed to the amelioration of arthritis in the CIA mice [7]. Experimental investigations conducted by Vita and colleagues indicate that berberine may have a role as a prophylactic supplement for RA [8]. They report that in mice with CIA, berberine markedly delayed the onset of arthritic symptom onset, apparently by suppressing T cell populations [8]. Vita and colleagues call for future investigations that examine the effects of berberine on the immune system under normal physiological conditions [8]. The research team from Canada used two metrological properties of two performance-based outcome measures including Effort Path (Path) and Stairs Assay Compliance (Stairs) for feline OA [9]. The results suggest that both are promising performance-based outcome measures to better diagnose and manage feline OA pain [9]. Using the inhibitory peptide sequence IA9 of triggering receptors expressed on myeloid cells (TREMs) are a family of activating immune receptors that regulate the inflammatory response, diminished release of proinflammatory cytokines, and dramatically suppressed joint inflammation and damage in CIA mice [10].

(iii) Clinical investigations. Investigations into serum levels of brain-derived neurotrophic factor (BDNF) have found significantly increased levels in patients with RA, as opposed to low serum levels in RA patients with anxiety, but not depression, or who were using biologic therapy, report Lai and colleagues [11]. They call for further study into the effect of elevated serum BDNF levels in patients with RA or other systemic autoimmune diseases, such as primary Sjögren's syndrome [11]. In another study, which analyzed the distribution patterns of iNOS, MMP-9, and the anti-apoptotic protein BCL-2 in the hip synovial tissue of patients with OA, the results suggest that iNOS, MMP-9, and BCL-2 expression regulates hip OA [12]. Korchynskyi and colleagues describe a potential glycosylation site at the asparagine-14 residue within human monocyte chemoattractant protein-1 (MCP-1) revealing lower expression levels in mammalian expression systems [13]. The glycosylation-mediated recombinant chemokine stabilization allows the production of citrullinated MCP-1, which can be effectively used to calibrate crucial assays in RA [13].

Reviews. The five reviews in this Special Issue begin with a systematic review conducted by Derwich et al., regarding the current evidence on the mechanisms of action and the efficacy of hyaluronic acid (HA), corticosteroids (CS), and platelet-rich plasma (PRP) in the treatment of patients aged $\geq$ 16 years with temporomandibular joint (TMJ) OA [14]. The researchers conclude that the evidence is inconclusive; it does not definitively clarify whether such methods of treatment are more beneficial than arthrocentesis alone for patients diagnosed with TMJ OA [14]. The second systematic review and meta-analysis, registered on PROSPERO (CRD42021279368), shows a weak efficacy of collagen and a very marked non-effect of chondroitin-glucosamine nutraceuticals, which recommends that the latter products should no longer be recommended for pain management in canine and feline OA [15]. The other review describes the use of micro-immunotherapy medicine in RA, a holistic therapeutic approach that employs ultra-low doses of IL-1β, IL-2, and TNF-α, as well as other immune factors, to restore bodily homeostasis [16]. Jacques and colleagues summarize the evidence showing how micro-immunotherapy treatment is associated with fewer adverse effects than the currently available single-target approaches designed to inhibit RA inflammation [16]. Van Le and colleagues have reviewed the evidence on VEGF biology and its function in rheumatic diseases, the contribution of VEGF bioavailability in the pathogenesis of rheumatic diseases, and the potential implications of therapeutic approaches targeting VEGF for these diseases [17]. The last review in this Special Issue is by MacDonald and colleagues, who discuss the involvement of the CCN family in the inflammatory pathologies of RA and OA, as well as the potential of the CCN proteins as therapeutic targets in these diseases [18].

Our hope is that this Special Issue will encourage more research into the pathogenesis of arthritis that ultimately leads to new therapeutic strategies.

Funding: This work was supported by a grant from the Ministry of Science and Technology of Taiwan (MOST-110-2320-B-039-022-MY3).

Conflicts of Interest: The author declares no conflict of interest.

References

1. Sohn, R.; Junker, M.; Meurer, A.; Zaucke, F.; Straub, R.H.; Jenei-Lanzl, Z. Anti-inflammatory effects of endogenously released adenosine in synovial cells of osteoarthritis and rheumatoid arthritis patients. *Int. J. Mol. Sci.* **2021**, *22*, 8956. [CrossRef] [PubMed]
2. Ostojic, M.; Zevrnja, A.; Vukojevic, K.; Soljic, V. Immunofluorescence analysis of nf-kb and inos expression in different cell populations during early and advanced knee osteoarthritis. *Int. J. Mol. Sci.* **2021**, *22*, 6461. [CrossRef] [PubMed]
3. Telegin, G.B.; Chernov, A.S.; Minakov, A.N.; Balmasova, I.P.; Romanova, E.A.; Sharapova, T.N.; Sashchenko, L.P.; Yashin, D.V. Short peptides of innate immunity protein tag7 inhibit the production of cytokines in cfa-induced arthritis. *Int. J. Mol. Sci.* **2022**, *23*, 12435. [CrossRef] [PubMed]
4. Wu, T.-J.; Chang, S.L.-Y.; Lin, C.-Y.; Lai, C.-Y.; He, X.-Y.; Tsai, C.-H.; Ko, C.-Y.; Fong, Y.-C.; Su, C.-M.; Tang, C.-H. Il-17 facilitates vcam-1 production and monocyte adhesion in osteoarthritis synovial fibroblasts by suppressing mir-5701 synthesis. *Int. J. Mol. Sci.* **2022**, *23*, 6804. [CrossRef] [PubMed]
5. Makalish, T.P.; Golovkin, I.O.; Oberemok, V.V.; Laikova, K.V.; Temirova, Z.Z.; Serdyukova, O.A.; Novikov, I.A.; Rosovskyi, R.A.; Gordienko, A.I.; Zyablitskaya, E.Y.; et al. Anti-rheumatic effect of antisense oligonucleotide cytos-11 targeting tnf-alpha expression. *Int. J. Mol. Sci.* **2021**, *22*, 1022. [CrossRef] [PubMed]
6. Sykora, T.; Babal, P.; Mikus-Kuracinova, K.; Drafi, F.; Ponist, S.; Dvorakova, M.; Janega, P.; Bauerova, K. Hyperbilirubinemia maintained by chronic supplementation of unconjugated bilirubin improves the clinical course of experimental autoimmune arthritis. *Int. J. Mol. Sci.* **2021**, *22*, 8662. [CrossRef] [PubMed]
7. Tang, K.T.; Lin, C.C.; Lin, S.C.; Wang, J.H.; Tsai, S.W. Kurarinone attenuates collagen-induced arthritis in mice by inhibiting th1/th17 cell responses and oxidative stress. *Int. J. Mol. Sci.* **2021**, *22*, 4002. [CrossRef] [PubMed]
8. Vita, A.A.; Aljobaily, H.; Lyons, D.O.; Pullen, N.A. Berberine delays onset of collagen-induced arthritis through t cell suppression. *Int. J. Mol. Sci.* **2021**, *22*, 3522. [CrossRef] [PubMed]
9. Delsart, A.; Moreau, M.; Otis, C.; Frezier, M.; Drag, M.; Pelletier, J.-P.; Martel-Pelletier, J.; Lussier, B.; del Castillo, J.; Troncy, E. Development of two innovative performance-based objective measures in feline osteoarthritis: Their reliability and responsiveness to firocoxib analgesic treatment. *Int. J. Mol. Sci.* **2022**, *23*, 11780. [CrossRef] [PubMed]
10. Sigalov, A.B. Inhibition of trem-2 markedly suppresses joint inflammation and damage in experimental arthritis. *Int. J. Mol. Sci.* **2022**, *23*, 8857. [CrossRef] [PubMed]
11. Lai, N.S.; Yu, H.C.; Huang Tseng, H.Y.; Hsu, C.W.; Huang, H.B.; Lu, M.C. Increased serum levels of brain-derived neurotrophic factor contribute to inflammatory responses in patients with rheumatoid arthritis. *Int. J. Mol. Sci.* **2021**, *22*, 1841. [CrossRef] [PubMed]
12. Caric, D.; Tomas, S.Z.; Filipovic, N.; Soljic, V.; Benzon, B.; Glumac, S.; Rakovac, I.; Vukojevic, K. Expression pattern of inos, bcl-2 and mmp-9 in the hip synovium tissue of patients with osteoarthritis. *Int. J. Mol. Sci.* **2021**, *22*, 1489. [CrossRef] [PubMed]
13. Korchynskyi, O.; Yoshida, K.; Korchynska, N.; Czarnik-Kwaśniak, J.; Tak, P.P.; Pruijn, G.J.M.; Isozaki, T.; Ruth, J.H.; Campbell, P.L.; Amin, M.A.; et al. Mammalian glycosylation patterns protect citrullinated chemokine mcp-1/ccl2 from partial degradation. *Int. J. Mol. Sci.* **2023**, *24*, 1862. [CrossRef] [PubMed]

14. Derwich, M.; Mitus-Kenig, M.; Pawlowska, E. Mechanisms of action and efficacy of hyaluronic acid, corticosteroids and platelet-rich plasma in the treatment of temporomandibular joint osteoarthritis-a systematic review. *Int. J. Mol. Sci.* **2021**, *22*, 7405. [CrossRef] [PubMed]
15. Barbeau-Gregoire, M.; Otis, C.; Cournoyer, A.; Moreau, M.; Lussier, B.; Troncy, E. A 2022 systematic review and meta-analysis of enriched therapeutic diets and nutraceuticals in canine and feline osteoarthritis. *Int. J. Mol. Sci.* **2022**, *23*, 384. [CrossRef] [PubMed]
16. Jacques, C.; Floris, I.; Lejeune, B. Ultra-low dose cytokines in rheumatoid arthritis, three birds with one stone as the rationale of the 2larth® micro-immunotherapy treatment. *Int. J. Mol. Sci.* **2021**, *22*, 6717. [CrossRef] [PubMed]
17. Le, T.H.V.; Kwon, S.M. Vascular endothelial growth factor biology and its potential as a therapeutic target in rheumatic diseases. *Int. J. Mol. Sci.* **2021**, *22*, 5387. [CrossRef] [PubMed]
18. MacDonald, I.J.; Huang, C.C.; Liu, S.C.; Lin, Y.Y.; Tang, C.H. Targeting ccn proteins in rheumatoid arthritis and osteoarthritis. *Int. J. Mol. Sci.* **2021**, *22*, 4340. [CrossRef] [PubMed]

International Journal of *Molecular Sciences*

MDPI

Article

Mammalian Glycosylation Patterns Protect Citrullinated Chemokine MCP-1/CCL2 from Partial Degradation

Olexandr Korchynskyi [1,2,3,4,*,†], Ken Yoshida [5,6,†], Nataliia Korchynska [4], Justyna Czarnik-Kwaśniak [1], Paul P. Tak [7,8], Ger J. M. Pruijn [9], Takeo Isozaki [5], Jeffrey H. Ruth [5], Phillip L. Campbell [5], M. Asif Amin [5] and Alisa E. Koch [5]

1 Department of Human Immunology and Centre for Innovative Biomedical Research, Medical Faculty, University of Rzeszow, 1a Warzywna St., 35-310 Rzeszów, Poland
2 Department of Clinical Immunology and Rheumatology, Academic Medical Center/University of Amsterdam, 1105 AZ Amsterdam, The Netherlands
3 Department of Molecular Immunology, Palladin Institute of Biochemistry, National Academy of Sciences of Ukraine, 01054 Kyiv, Ukraine
4 Department of Public Development and Health, S. Gzhytskyi National University of Veterinary Medicine and Biotechnologies, 79010 Lviv, Ukraine
5 Division of Rheumatology, University of Michigan Medical School, Ann Arbor, MI 48109, USA
6 Division of Rheumatology, Department of Internal Medicine, the Jikei University School of Medicine, Tokyo 105-8461, Japan
7 Department of Internal Medicine, University of Cambridge, Cambridge CB2 1TN, UK
8 Candel Therapeutics, Needham, MA 02494, USA
9 Department of Biomolecular Chemistry, Institute for Molecules and Materials, Radboud University, 6525 AJ Nijmegen, The Netherlands
* Correspondence: olexkor@hotmail.com
† These authors contributed equally to this work.

Abstract: Monocyte chemoattractant protein-1 (MCP-1/CCL2) is a potent chemotactic agent for monocytes, primarily produced by macrophages and endothelial cells. Significantly elevated levels of MCP-1/CCL2 were found in synovial fluids of patients with rheumatoid arthritis (RA), compared to osteoarthritis or other arthritis patients. Several studies suggested an important role for MCP-1 in the massive inflammation at the damaged joint, in part due to its chemotactic and angiogenic effects. It is a known fact that the post-translational modifications (PTMs) of proteins have a significant impact on their properties. In mammals, arginine residues within proteins can be converted into citrulline by peptidylarginine deiminase (PAD) enzymes. Anti-citrullinated protein antibodies (ACPA), recognizing these PTMs, have become a hallmark for rheumatoid arthritis (RA) and other autoimmune diseases and are important in diagnostics and prognosis. In previous studies, we found that citrullination converts the neutrophil attracting chemokine neutrophil-activating peptide 78 (ENA-78) into a potent macrophage chemoattractant. Here we report that both commercially available and recombinant bacterially produced MCP-1/CCL2 are rapidly (partially) degraded upon in vitro citrullination. However, properly glycosylated MCP-1/CCL2 produced by mammalian cells is protected against degradation during efficient citrullination. Site-directed mutagenesis of the potential glycosylation site at the asparagine-14 residue within human MCP-1 revealed lower expression levels in mammalian expression systems. The glycosylation-mediated recombinant chemokine stabilization allows the production of citrullinated MCP-1/CCL2, which can be effectively used to calibrate crucial assays, such as modified ELISAs.

Keywords: monocyte chemoattractant protein-1; post-translational modifications; glycosylation; citrullination; peptidylarginine deiminase; partial degradation

Citation: Korchynskyi, O.; Yoshida, K.; Korchynska, N.; Czarnik-Kwaśniak, J.; Tak, P.P.; Pruijn, G.J.M.; Isozaki, T.; Ruth, J.H.; Campbell, P.L.; Amin, M.A.; et al. Mammalian Glycosylation Patterns Protect Citrullinated Chemokine MCP-1/CCL2 from Partial Degradation. *Int. J. Mol. Sci.* **2023**, *24*, 1862. https://doi.org/10.3390/ijms24031862

Academic Editor: Chih-Hsin Tang

Received: 13 December 2022
Accepted: 11 January 2023
Published: 18 January 2023

1. Introduction

Chemokines are members of the chemoattractant cytokines with molecular weights from 8 to 12 kDa, divided into four subfamilies (C, CC, CXC and CX3C), based on the position and spacing of their N-terminal cysteine residues [1–3]. These cytokines have a unique ability to recruit and activate monocytes, neutrophils and lymphocytes [4]. The monocyte chemoattractant proteins (MCPs) constitute an important group within the CC-chemokine sub-family. Five MCPs have been named and classified: MCP-1/CCL2, MCP-2/CCL8, MCP-3/CCL7, MCP-4/CCL13 and MCP-5/CCL12.

In humans, MCP-1/CCL2 was the first described and is the best characterized to date. The *CCL2* gene is located on chromosome 17 and encodes a 13 kDa protein composed of 76 amino acids [4,5]. MCP-1/CCL2 is produced by different cell types, including macrophages, dendritic cells and endothelial cells. MCP-1/CCL2 is well known for its activities in the immune context: it exerts chemotactic activity for several cell types, such as monocytes, T lymphocytes, NK cells, basophils and induces directed leukocyte motility. The chemokine stimulates the migration of T cells to infected or damaged sites [6,7]. MCP-1/CCL2 was found in the synovium of patients with rheumatoid arthritis (RA), gout, traumatic arthritis, atherosclerosis, multiple sclerosis and various cancers [8,9]. Several studies have shown increased levels of MCP-1/CCL2 in synovial tissue and fluids, as well as in the sera and plasma of RA patients versus osteoarthritis or other arthritis patients [10,11].

The post-translational citrullination modification of proteins is based on the enzymatic conversion (deimination) of arginine (Arg) to citrulline (Cit). Such conversion leads to very minor changes in the molecular mass of the MCP-1/CCL2 protein, but causes loss of a positive charge [12,13]. This post-translational conversion into citrulline is catalysed by peptidylarginine deiminases (PADs). In mammals, five isotypes have been described: PAD1-4 and PAD6. PAD enzymes are generally found in the cytoplasm of various cell types, except for PAD4 which can translocate to the nucleus [14,15]. Protein citrullination occurs during the physiological 'maturation' of the skin, while its aberrant increase is linked to various diseases, including cancer, lupus, multiple sclerosis, and, as mentioned, RA. This last disorder constitutes an autoimmune disorder with a high morbidity, often leading to the progressive destruction of the joints, resulting in pain and stiffness. Rheumatic joints are rich with pro-inflammatory cytokines, including tumor necrosis factor-α (TNF-α), interleukin 1 and 6, granulocyte-macrophage colony-stimulating factor and chemokines, such as interleukin-8 [16]. Nowadays, anti-citrullinated peptide antibodies (ACPAs) are considered a hallmark of the disease and routinely used to diagnose it [17].

Glycosylation represents another well-known, highly heterogeneous, post-translational modification of proteins, involved in folding, protease protection and protein-protein contact. N-linked glycosylation refers to the co-translational attachment of sugars to the nitrogen atom of asparagine residues, concentrated on the exterior of mature proteins. During maturation, it also contributes to protein folding. O-glycosylation of proteins is a post-translational event that takes place subsequently to N-glycosylation and protein folding. It refers to the O-linked attachment of sugars to serine and threonine, and, to a lesser extent, hydroxyproline and hydroxylysine. Human and mouse CC chemokines may be glycosylated. MCP-1/CCL2 is expressed as an 8 kDa protein which contains a short N-terminal secretion signal. During processing, this signal peptide is removed, thus allowing the N-terminal glutamate residue to be cyclised to pyroglutamate. MCP-1/CCL2 also contains two consensus glycosylation sequences, one for N-glycosylation in the N-terminal region (asparagine residue at position 14 in mature MCP-1/CCL2 protein and another for O-glycosylation). Ruggiero et al. suggested the possibility that the majority of human and mouse MCP-1/CCL2 remains unprotected against proteases because of inefficient glycosylation [3,18,19].

Recombinant human MCP-1/CCL2 has been expressed in many different expression systems, such as *Escherichia coli*, the methylotrophic yeast *Komagataella* (previously referred to as *Pichia) pastoris*, COS-1 fibroblast-like cells (derived from monkey kidney tissue), or insect cells [3]. Depending on the type of the expression system used, differences in protein activity were observed. For example, if *E. coli* is used for expression, the recombinant human MCP-1/CCL2 is unstable, but active, and similar observations were made after expression in insect cells or *K.pastoris* [3]. In all the cases, protein stability remains an issue.

The main goal of our study is to establish an efficient procedure for the preparation of stable citrullinated chemokine MCP-1/CCL2, which would be highly useful for different research applications. In light of a fact that we detected a quick loss of bacterially produced MCP-1 upon in vitro citrullination, we surmised that citrullinated chemokines can be stabilized and protected from quick degradation by other post-translational modifications in mammalian cells.

2. Results

The main goal of our work was to generate a standard procedure to prepare stable citrullinated MCP-1/CCL2 chemokine suitable for research applications. We amplified the sequences encoding full length and mature versions of MCP-1/CCL2 from cDNA prepared from IL-1β-treated primary synovial fibroblasts derived from RA patients. A mature version equivalent to completely processed MCP-1/CCL2, was cloned into a frame with a C-terminal 6xHis-tag into pET19b bacterial expression vector that allows expression of the insert in bacterial cells.

Commercially available recombinant MCP-1/CCL2 from two different suppliers (Peprotech, United Kingdom and R&D Systems, Minneapolis, MN, USA) as well as self-made bacterially produced MCP-1/CCL2 were citrullinated in vitro using recombinant human PAD2, PAD4 or rabbit PAD2. Reaction products were analyzed by SDS-PAGE with subsequent colloidal Coomassie staining (Figure 1a) or western blotting (Figure 1b).

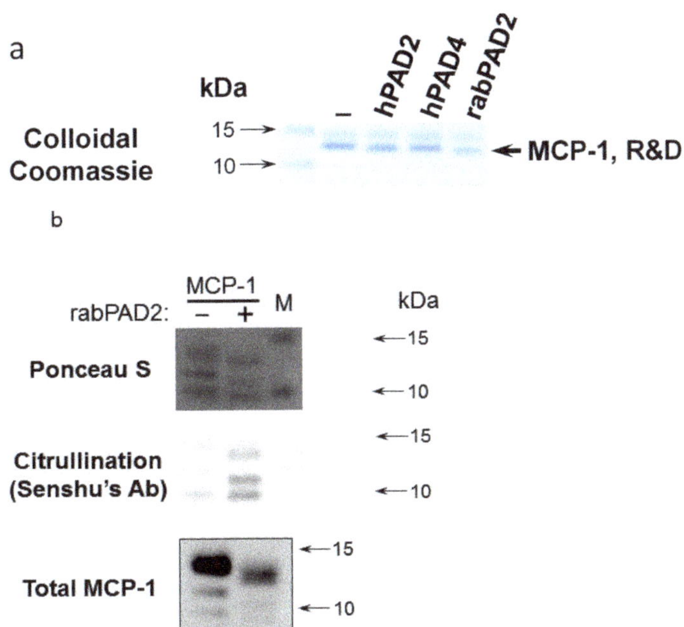

Figure 1. In vitro citrullination of bacterially produced chemokines leads to their partial degradation. (**a**) Colloidal Coomassie stained SDS-PAGE analysis of the MCP-1/CCL2 products of in vitro citrullination. In vitro citrullination of commercially available recombinant MCP-1/CCL2 and self-made

bacterially produced MCP-1/CCL2 performed with recombinant human PAD2 and PAD4 or rabbit PAD2, respectively. Colloidal Coomassie stained MCP-1 bands are shown while recombinant humanPAD2/4 or rabbit PAD2 (Sigma Aldrich/Merck, Waltham, MA, USA) were added to reactions into the quantities below the Colloidal Coomassie sensitivity limits and cannot be visualized. (**b**) Immunoblot analysis of bacterially produced MCP-1/CCL2 upon an in vitro citrullination reaction. Self-made full-length bacterially produced MCP-1/CCL2 was citrullinated in vitro with rabbit PAD2 and resolved on SDS-PAGE, stained with Ponceau S. detection of total MCP-1/CCL2 and modified citrullines with Senshu's antibody that recognizes that modified citrullines were made according to Senshu's protocol [20]. Results shown are a representative of three or more repetitive experiments.

Overall, we failed to detect robust citrullination of MCP-1/CCL2. First, we found that both self-made bacterially produced MCP-1/CCL2 and commercially available bacterially-produced recombinant MCP-1/CCL2 from two different producers (Peprotech, United Kingdom and R&D Systems, Minneapolis, MN, USA.) were quickly degraded during the in vitro citrullination; see a representative example in Figure 1b.

Therefore, the 6xHis-tagged version of MCP-1/CCL2 chemokine cDNA was further re-cloned into mammalian pcDEF expression vector, in an order to confer a high expression level of MCP-1/CCL2 chemokine. The mammalian expression vector was transfected into HEK 293T cells using a PEI reagent. The cellular lysate with glycosylated mature MCP-1/CCL2 was collected and purified with ProBond nickel beads and gradually eluted with 50, 100, 150 and 200 mM imidazole. Both the pre-protein and its mature version contain four arginine residues at the positions corresponding to 18, 24, 29 and 30 in the mature protein (Figure 2a). The diagnostic 1-Da mass shift occurring upon citrullination of MCP-1/CCL2, was identified by mass spectrometry at the peptide that contains Arg-18 of the mature protein (Figure 2b). In spite of the presence of three more arginine residues at the positions 24, 29 and 30 within the mature MCP-1 protein (Figure 2a), we failed to detect citrullination at those residues using a mass-spectrometry.

a

MKVSAALLCL LLIAATFIPQ GLA-

QPDAINAPVT CCYNFTN®KI SVQ®LASY®® ITSSKCPKEA VIFKTIVAKE ICADPKQKWV QDSMDHLDKQ TQTPKT

b

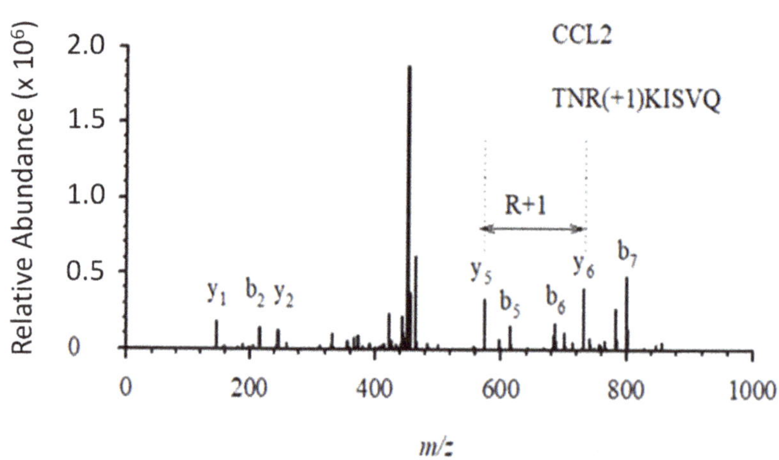

Figure 2. Mass-spectrometry verification of successful in vitro citrullination of MCP-1/CCL2. (**a**) Amino acid sequence of MCP-1/CCL2 (mature form of the protein spans residues 24–99). The first

row shows 23 amino acid-long signaling peptide and the second row–mature protein of 76 residues. All arginine residues are highlighted with circles. The boxed areas show the peptide that contains the citrullinated arginine residues that were detected. (**b**) Annotated tandem mass spectrometry (MS/MS) fragmentation spectrum for the citrullinated MCP1/CCL2 peptide, showing the citrullinated arginine residue at position 3 of the studied peptide (R45). The MS/MS fragmentation data were annotated using Expert System (Max Planck Institute of Biochemistry). The precursor ion was observed with a mass error of 1 part per million, and the error for the fragment ions was 0.02 daltons.

The quality and quantity of in vitro citrullinated *E. coli* expressed recombinant protein purchased from R&D systems (Figure 3a) was compared with the self-made recombinant protein produced in HEK293T cells (Figure 3b) using an ELISA specific for this protein. Interestingly, upon successful citrullination (Figures 1 and 2) all of the preparations (two commercially produced ones and multiple aliquots of self-made prep) of bacterially produced chemokines appeared to be very unstable: we were able to detect some random remains of recombinant proteins in such preps, exclusively immediately after the in vitro citrullination reaction. All of the citrullinated bacterial proteins were undetectable upon storage under −70 °C. A suitability of the mammalian cells-produced chemokine standards was confirmed with a high coefficient of determination (R^2 = 0.99386, Figure 3b) versus the low R squared value for the bacterially produced chemokine (R^2 = 0.70629, Figure 3a). Thus, we have shown that in vitro citrullinated mammalian cell-produced (Figure 3b), but not the bacterially produced MCP-1/CCL2 chemokine (Figure 3a) can be efficiently used as the good quality standards in ELISA.

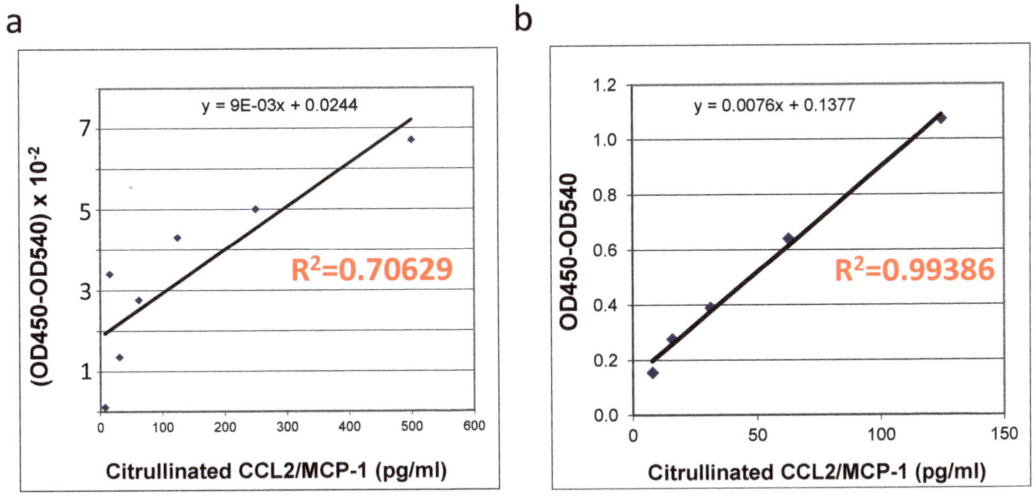

Figure 3. Detection of citrullinated recombinant human MCP-1/CCL2. Standard curves of citrullinated recombinant human MCP-1/CCL2 were set up using enzyme-linked immunosorbent assay in duplicate (**a**) standard curve of citrullinated *E. coli* produced recombinant human MCP-1/CCL2 chemokine (R&D Systems), (**b**) standard curve for citrullinated MCP-1/CCL2 chemokine produced by and purified from human HEK 293T cells. Absorbance at 450 nm is shown. Coefficients of determination R^2 are indicated in red on the relevant plots. Results shown are a representative of three or more repetitive experiments.

In silico analysis of MCP-1 reveals a potential glycosylation site at the asparagine residue at position 14 (N-14, Figure 4a). To confirm the importance of glycosylation at this mentioned residue, we performed a site-directed mutagenesis aiming to convert asparagine into a chemically very similar glutamine residue, which still cannot serve as a docking site for glycosylation. A western blot analysis revealed both wild type and mutant recombinant proteins hMCP-1/CCL2 (Figure 4b). At the same time, the expression level of N14Q mutant hMCP-1/CCL2 protein was significantly lower than of wild-type protein. As expected, the glycosylation slightly shifted a recombinant wild-type protein (for around 2 kDa), in a comparison with bacterially produced chemokine (Figure 4b). To compare the stability of wild-type and N14Q mutant recombinant hMCP-1/CCL2 upon their citrullination, we performed a citrullination of different MCP-1 protein versions with recombinant human PAD2/3/4 enzymes overexpressed and produced into HEK293T cell (Figure 4b). Similarly to the described above results (Figure 1), a hPAD2/3/4 led to the destruction of bacterially produced hMCP-1/CCL2. In the case of PAD2 and PAD4, such destruction was practically complete, while for PAD3 it was partial (Figure 4b). The mammalian cell-produced recombinant hMCP-1/CCL2 was successfully detected upon treatment with all three PAD enzymes, albeit at slightly lower levels, than the protein untreated with PAD (Figure 4b).

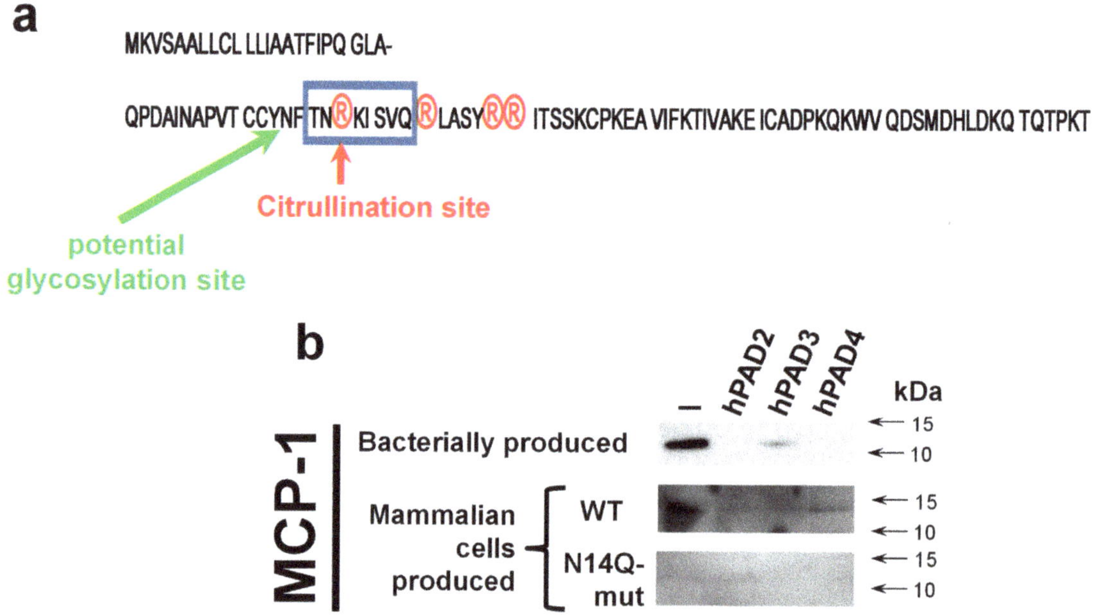

Figure 4. Site-directed mutagenesis of potential glycosylation site at asparagine-14 in mammalian cell-produced MCP-1 significantly destabilizes recombinant human MCP-1/CCL2. (**a**) Amino acid sequence of MCP-1/CCL2 with indicated positions of predicted N-glycosylation and citrullination site confirmed by a mass-spectrometry. (**b**) Immunoblot analysis of bacterially versus mammalian cell-produced MCP-1/CCL2 upon an in vitro citrullination reaction. Bacterially produced wild-type MCP-1/CCL2 or HEK293T cell-produced wild-type and N14Q mutant version of chemokine were incubated with EDTA-free proteinase inhibitor cocktail supplemented cellular lysates prepared from the control (vehicle-transfected) or indicated hPAD enzyme-transfected HEK293T cells. Citrullination reactions that were performed directly within cellular lysates essentially as published before [21]. Recombinant chemokine was concentrated with immunoprecipitation and resolved on 10–18% polyacrylamide gradient SDS-PAGE. Results shown are a representative of three experiments.

3. Discussion

It is well known that post-translational modifications affect the chemical and biological properties of proteins. For example, glycosylation modulates the specific biological and biochemical activities of some cytokines [22], including chemokines. MCP-1/CCL2, MCP-3/CCL7 and HCC-1 have been demonstrated to be glycosylated in vivo [19]. MCP-1/CCL2 is one of the first identified chemokines, which can be detected in both glycosylated and non-glycosylated forms [23]. Rutledge et al., 1995 have shown that glycosylated MCP-1/CCL2 was two- to threefold less chemotactic for monocytes and THP-1 cells than non-glycosylated MCP-1/CCL2 [22]. In the case of CCL5 and CCL11 chemokines, there were no differences in in vitro eosinophil chemotactic activity between glycosylated and non-glycosylated forms [24]. Dong et al. used insect cells to produce recombinant XCL1 chemokine. In their chemotaxis assays performed with primary $CD4^+$ T cells, recombinant, glycosylated, the XCL1 chemokine was more potent when compared to the non-glycosylated form and it was a more effective inhibitor of T cell proliferation [19]. In our current study, we are demonstrating that the glycosylation process strongly stabilizes citrullinated MCP-1/CCL2 and protects it against gradual degradation, which occurs with a bacterially (*E. coli)* produced purified recombinant protein. It can be inferred that glycosylation of the CC-class chemokine MCP-1/CCL2, as well as of other chemokines (in our studies validated for CCL3/MIP-1α) protects the molecules against proteases. In turn, recombinant mouse CCL2 expressed in CHO cells, is highly glycosylated at the C-terminus with mainly O-linked sugars and this glycosylation is not essential for chemotaxis induction [18]. Through O-glycosylation, the different molecular masses of MCP-1/CCL2 were shown, which additionally contributed to the chemotactic potency reduction [25].

Currently, there are different systems for the expression of recombinant proteins. By using the yeast *Komagataella* (earlier referred to as *Pichia*) *pastoris* expression system Ruggiero et al., 2003 have shown that human recombinant MCP-1/CCL2 glycosylated in yeast was 4–20 times less active in a chemotactic assay in vitro, compared to non-glycosylated *E. coli* expression system [3]. In the current study, we have also presented a tool for MCP-1/CCL2 chemokine expression in mammalian HEK 293T cells. In our model, we found that glycosylation dramatically stabilizes the chemokine and only mammalian properly glycosylated CCL2/MCP-1 can be efficiently used for in vitro citrullination reactions. Our data are still insufficient to draw clear conclusions, if such instability of bacterially produced chemokines upon their citrullination in vitro, is an intrinsic feature of this and other chemokines. Even highly purified commercial chemokines or PAD2 enzyme preparations potentially still can have some undetectable contamination with proteinases. Most likely, only artificial synthesis of the citrullinated versus non-citrullinated protein could provide such an answer.

PAD enzymes specificity were the subject of previous studies. We compared the sequence of human MCP-1/CCL2 with proposed optimal sites for human PAD2 and PAD4 enzymes [21]. However, neither neighboring amino acid residues of successfully citrullinated arginine at position 18 (Figure 2), nor for arginine residues at positions 24, 29 and 30 shared any significant similarity to the predicted optimal recognition site for both human PAD2 or PAD4 [21].

Most of the detailed studies devoted to MCP-1/CCL2 glycosylation were performed with the murine protein [26, 27}. Their results show a much more heavily glycosylated protein of 25–30 kDa [26,27], than 12–14 kDa 6His-tagged protein in our studies (Figures 1 and 4). Such results suggest multiple sites of additional O-linked glycosylation in murine MCP-1/CCL2, than we saw for human protein (Figure 4b). However, studies performed with recombinant human MCP-1/CCL2 [28] revealed a protein product of size comparable with a protein in our studies (Figure 4b). In addition, the study of Needham et al., 1996 [28} suggests the presence of both glycosylated and nonglycosylated forms of recombinant human protein upon its production in mammalian expression systems. Such potential partial presence of a nonglycosylated protein form in our recombinant human MCP-1/CCL2 can explain why we also lost some portion of the recombinant HEK293 cell produced protein upon its citrullination by PAD enzymes in vitro (Figure 4b). At the same time, our data suggest the crucial importance of N-glycosylation at asparagine-14 for the stability of recombinant citrullinated MCP-1 (Figure 4b).

4. Materials and Methods

4.1. Reagents

Rabbit PAD2 was purchased from Sigma-Aldrich/Merck (Utrecht, The Netherlands). Recombinant MCP-1/CCL2 duo-kit (ELISA) and monoclonal mouse antibody specific for MCP-1/CCL2 were purchased from R&D Systems (Minneapolis, MN, USA). pET19b vector was purchased from Novagen/Merck-Millipore (Utrecht, The Netherlands). pDEF vector was kindly provided by Dr. Goldman.

4.2. Cell Culture

The studies were performed using immortalized human embryonic kidney 293T cells (HEK 293T) purchased from the American Type Culture Collection (ATCC; Bethesda, MD, USA). The cells were cultured in Dulbecco's Modified Eagle's Medium (DMEM; Biowest, Nuaillé, France), supplemented with 10% (*v*/*v*) fetal bovine serum (FBS; Biowest, Nuaillé, France) and 1% (*v*/*v*) penicillin/streptomycin (Biowest, Nuaillé, France). Cells were routinely split twice a week, when ~80% confluency was reached. The culture was maintained in a humidified atmosphere of 95% air and 5% CO_2 at 37 °C.

4.3. MCP-1/CCL2 cDNA Cloning

Full-length MCP-1/CCL2 complementary DNA (cDNA) was prepared from total mRNA isolated from primary synovial fibroblasts derived from a patient with RA. Tissue samples were obtained after approval by the AMC Institutional Review Board and provision of informed consent by the subjects. The cDNA fragments encoding mature protein were PCR-amplified with the following primers (forward and reverse, respectively): 5′-TAATCCATGGGA-CAGCCAGATGCAATCCAATGCC-3′ and 5′-TAAGAATTCTCAGTGA TGGTGATG-GTGATGAGTCTTCGGAGTTTGGGTTTG-3′. We incorporated a *Nco*I restriction site in the forward primer and an endogeneous stop codon with six preceding codons encoding histidines and the *Eco*RI restriction site in the reverse primer. All sequences were verified using BigDye Terminator sequencing (Life Technology/Thermo Fisher Scientific, Waltham, MA, USA). The 77 amino acid long mature version of MCP-1/CCL2 was cloned in frame with C-terminal 6xHis-tag into a pET19b expression vector which allows to express the insert in bacteria. For optimization of expression in mammalian cells, the insert containing a C-terminus 6xHis-tag was later re-cloned into a pcDEF expression vector [1,29].

4.4. Transformation of *E. coli* BL21 and Purification of Recombinant Human MCP-1/CCL2

The BL21-Rosetta (Novagen\Merck, Berlington, MA, USA) strain of *E. coli* was used for the transformation with bacterial expression vector pET19b to produce MCP-1/CCL2 chemokine. A single colony of bacteria cells was grown in 2 L of LB medium at 37 °C until reaching 0.6 at OD_{600}, 1mM IPTG was then added to induce the protein expression for 6 h, at 30 °C. Following the induction, cells were harvested by centrifugation and resuspended into the ice-cold buffer consisting of: 150 mL 50mM sodium phosphate (pH8.0), 300 mM NaCl, 10 mM imidazole, 1 mM β-mercapto-ethanol, 10 µM leupeptin, 10 µM pepstatin, 10 µM aprotinin and 10 µM phenylmethylsulfonyl fluoride (PMSF, Sigma-Aldrich\Merck, Berlington, MA, USA). The suspension was sonicated on wet ice with 10 × 1s-long pulses at maximal energy and target protein from the extracts was collected and purified using ProBond nickel beads (Life Technologies/Thermo Fisher Scientific, Waltham, MA, USA), as described below.

4.5. Transfection of HEK 293T Cells and Purification of Recombinant Human MCP-1/CCL2

HEK 293T were seeded at 50% confluency in 15 cm Petri dishes. Next, the cells were transfected with the pDEF vector expressing 6xHis-tagged MCP-1/CCL2. Transfection was carried out using transfection reagent polyethylenimine (PEI; Polysciences Inc., Warrington, PA, USA) following the manufacturer's protocol. Following transfection (5–6 h), culture medium was replaced with fresh complete medium. Then, 48 h after transfection, the cells were lysed with lysing buffer containing 1% Triton X-100, 150 mL 50mM sodium phosphate (pH8.0), 300 mM NaCl, 10 mM imidazole, 1mM β-mercaptoethanol, as well as 10 μM leupeptin, 10μM pepstatin, 10 μM aprotinin and 10 μM PMSF. The 6xHis-tagged MCP-1/CCL2 from HEK 293T cell lysates was purified upon immobilization on ProBond nickel beads (Life Technologies, Carlsbad, CA, USA), rinsed with 10 mM imidazole added to the same lysis buffer and eluted gradually with 50 mM, 100 mM, 150 mM and 200 mM imidazole. The quality and quantity of the expressed recombinant MCP-1/CCL2 was assessed with the DuoSet ELISA kit (R&D Systems, Minneapolis, MN, USA), specific for this chemokine and with colloidal Coomassie staining after the sodium dodecyl sulfate-polyacrylamide gel electrophoresis (SDS-PAGE) resolution [1].

4.6. *In Vitro Citrullination of MCP-1/CCL2*

Then, the concentration of purified MCP-1/CCL2 was measured, 100 microliters of purified recombinant human chemokine (~100 ng/mL) was incubated with 0.5 units of rabbit skeletal muscle PAD (Sigma-Aldrich\Merck, Berlington, MA, USA) in 40 mM Tris-HCl, pH 7.6, 10 mM calcium chloride and 2.5 mM dithiothreitol for 2 h at 37 °C. Deimination was stopped with 25 mM EDTA. The diagnostic 1-Da mass shift occurring upon citrullination was identified by liquid chromatography tandem mass spectrometry (MS Bioworks, Ann Arbor, MI, USA) [1].

4.7. *Site-Directed Mutagenesis*

The targeted change of a glycosylation site at asparagine 14 into a glutamine was performed with a Quik-change method (Stratagene, La Jolla, CA, USA) essentially as before [29], using forward CTGCTGTTAT-cAa-TTCACCAATAG and reverse CTATTGGTGAA-tTg-ATAACAGCAG primers. The success of mutagenesis was confirmed with a sequencing of resulting plasmids.

4.8. *Western Blotting*

Western blotting was performed as described previously [20]. A monoclonal mouse antibody specific for human MCP-1/CCL2 (BioLegend, San Diego, CA, USA) was used at a dilution of 1:1000. The procedure for citrulline modification was described before [1,20]. Rabbit polyclonal antibody against modified citrulline [20] was used at a dilution of 1:1000. Secondary horseradish peroxidase-conjugated goat anti-rabbit IgG antibody (Amersham-Pharmacia\Merck, Berlington, MA, USA) was used in a 10^4-fold dilution. Detection was performed by enhanced chemoluminescence (ECL; Thermo Fisher Scientific, Waltham, MA, USA). To increase the quality of the western blot detection for 293T cell produced recombinant hMCP-1, an immunoprecipitation with anti- human MCP-1/CCL2 antibody was performed.

4.9. *Detection of Recombinant Human MCP-1/CCL2 by a Modified Enzyme-Linked Immunosorbent Assay (ELISA)*

The anti-modified citrulline ELISA-based method uses a commercial ELISA kit developed for the detection of total chemokines in a combination with Senshu's antibody that recognizes the modified citrullines. Briefly, ninety-six-well plates (Thermo Fisher Scientific, Waltham, MA, USA) were coated overnight at room temperature (RT) with a mouse anti-human MCP-1/CCL2 antibodies (R&D Systems, Minneapolis, MN, USA). Following each step, the plates were washed with phosphate buffered saline (PBS) which contained 0.05% of Tween20. The plates were then blocked with 1% bovine serum albumin (BSA) in PBS for 1 h at RT and incubated with samples or standards for 2 h at RT. Citrullinated recombinant human MCP-1/CCL2 and native–noncitrullinated recombinant human MCP-1/CCL2 purified from the transformed *E. coli* BL21 and transfected HEK 293T cells were used as standards and negative controls, respectively, for the ELISA. The samples were crosslinked on the plate with 1% glutaraldehyde in PBS for 30 min at RT [1].

The plates were then incubated with 0.2 mM Tris-HCl (pH 7.8) for 30 min at RT to block the crosslinking. Subsequently, the plates were incubated overnight at 37 °C in a citrulline-modification solution consisting of 2 parts of solution A that contained 0.0025% (*w*/*v*) iron (III) chloride, 4.6 M sulfuric acid and 3.0 M phosphoric acid; 1 part of solution B that contained 1% diacetylmonoxime, 0.5% antipyrine and 1M acetic acid; and 1 part of water [1,21]. Next, the plates were incubated for 2 h at RT with rabbit anti-modified citrulline antibodies (Merck-Millipore/Sigma-Aldrich, USA), diluted 1:2500 in PBS containing 1% BSA. The plates were then incubated for 2 h at RT with horseradish peroxidase (HRP)-conjugated swine anti-rabbit IgG (Dako/Agilent, Santa Clara, CA, USA), diluted 1:1,000 in PBS containing 1% BSA. Biotin-Tyramide Reagent (PerkinElmer, Waltham, MA, USA), diluted 1:1000 in 0.05 M tris-base (pH 8.5), was added, followed by HRP-conjugated streptavidin [1]. The classic colour reaction detection was performed, according to the manufacturer´s protocol.

4.10. Statistical Analysis

All quantitative experiments were repeated at least three times in duplicate. Concentration determinations and data plotting were performed in Microsoft Excel. The coefficient of determination R^2 was calculated on the free web calculator EasyCalculations.com website (https://www.easycalculation.com/statistics/r-squared.php (accessed on 7 December 2022 at 1.22 a.m)).

5. Conclusions

Glycosylation is lacking in bacterially-produced proteins but is present in mammalian cells stabilized citrullinated MCP-1/CCL2. This process protects the chemokine against rapid partial degradation. Moreover, properly glycosylated MCP-1/CCL2 produced by mammalian cells can be further citrullinated in vitro and efficiently used as a standard in citrullination-specific ELISAs, as well as in further biological investigations.

Author Contributions: Conceptualization: O.K.; methodology: O.K., K.Y., J.H.R., G.J.M.P. and A.E.K.; validation: O.K., K.Y., N.K., P.L.C., J.H.R. and A.E.K.; formal analysis, O.K., K.Y., J.C.-K.; and J.H.R.; investigation: O.K., K.Y., N.K., P.L.C., T.I., M.A.A., J.H.R. and A.E.K.; resources, O.K., G.J.M.P., J.H.R., P.P.T. and A.E.K.; data curation, O.K., K.Y. and J.H.R.; writing—original draft preparation: O.K. and J.C.-K.; writing—review and editing: O.K., K.Y., N.K., J.C.-K., J.H.R., G.J.M.P., T.I., P.L.C., M.A.A., P.P.T. and A.E.K.; visualization: O.K., K.Y. and J.H.R.; supervision: O.K. and A.E.K.; project administration: O.K.; funding acquisition: O.K., P.P.T. and A.E.K. All authors have read and agreed to the published version of the manuscript.

Funding: The study was performed with support of the National Science Centre, Poland (Project No 2016/23/B/NZ5/02627).

Institutional Review Board Statement: The study was conducted according to the guidelines of the Declaration of Helsinki, and approved by the Institutional Ethics Committee Review Board of Academic Medical Centre, University of Amsterdam (protocol METC # 07/079 approved 16 April 2010).

Informed Consent Statement: Informed consent was obtained from all subjects involved in the study.

Data Availability Statement: Representative research data demonstrated into the manuscript, any data not shown can be provided upon special request.

Acknowledgments: We are grateful to Tetsuo Senshu for generous providing us with anti-modified citrulline antibody.

Conflicts of Interest: The authors declare no conflict of interest.

References

1. Yoshida, K.; Korchynskyi, O.; Tak, P.-P.; Isozaki, T.; Ruth, J.H.; Campbell, P.L.; Baeten, D.L.; Gerlag, D.M.; Amin, M.A.; Koch, A.E. Citrullination of epithelial neutrophil-activating peptide 78/CXCL5 results in conversion from a non-monocyte-recruiting chemokine to a monocyte-recruiting chemokine. *Arthritis Rheumatol.* **2014**, *66*, 2716–2727. [CrossRef] [PubMed]
2. Nasser, M.W.; Elbaz, M.; Ahirwar, D.K.; Ganju, R.K. Conditioning solid tumor microenvironment through inflammatory chemokines and S100 family proteins. *Cancer Lett.* **2015**, *365*, 11–22. [CrossRef] [PubMed]
3. Ruggiero, P.; Flati, S.; Di Cioccio, V.; Maurizi, G.; Macchia, G.; Facchin, A.; Anacardio, R.; Maras, A.; Lucarelli, M.; Boraschi, D. Glycosylation enhances functional stability of the chemotactic cytokine CCL2. *Eur. Cytokine Netw.* **2003**, *14*, 91–96. [PubMed]
4. Bose, S.; Cho, J. Role of chemokine CCL2 and its receptor CCR2 in neurodegenerative diseases. *Arch. Pharm. Res.* **2013**, *36*, 1039–1050. [CrossRef]
5. Conductier, G.; Blondeau, N.; Guyon, A.; Nahon, J.-L.; Rovère, C. The role of monocyte chemoattractant protein MCP-1/CCL2 in neuroinflammatory diseases. *J. Neuroimmunol.* **2010**, *224*, 93–100. [CrossRef]
6. Soria, G.; Ben-Baruch, A. The inflammatory chemokines CCL2 and CCL5 in breast cancer. *Cancer Lett.* **2008**, *267*, 271–285. [CrossRef]
7. Salcedo, R.; Ponce, M.L.; Young, H.A.; Wasserman, K.; Ward, J.M.; Kleinman, H.K.; Oppenheim, J.J.; Murphy, W.J. Human endothelial cells express CCR2 and respond to MCP-1: Direct role of MCP-1 in angiogenesis and tumor progression. *Blood* **2000**, *96*, 34–40. [CrossRef]
8. Harigai, M.; Hara, M.; Yoshimura, T.; Leonard, E.J.; Inoue, K.; Kashiwazaki, S. Monocyte chemoattractant protein-1 (MCP E J-1) in inflammatory joint diseases and its involvement in the cytokine network of rheumatoid synovium. *Clin. Immunol. Immunopathol.* **1993**, *69*, 83–91. [CrossRef]
9. Chen, C.-Y.; Fuh, L.J.; Huang, C.C.; Hsu, C.-J.; Su, C.M.; Liu, S.-C.; Lin, Y.M.; Tang, C.-H. Enhancement of CCL2 expression and monocyte migration by CCN1 in osteoblasts through inhibiting miR-518a-5p: Implication of rheumatoid arthritis therapy. *Sci. Rep. NPJ* **2017**, *7*, 421. [CrossRef]
10. Koch, A.E.; Kunkel, S.L.; Harlow, L.A.; Johnson, B.; Evanoff, H.L.; Haines, G.K.; Burdick, M.D.; Pope, R.M.; Strieter, R.M. Enhanced production of monocyte chemoattractant protein-1 in rheumatoid arthritis. *J. Clin. Investig.* **1992**, *90*, 772–779. [CrossRef]
11. Koch, A.E. Chemokines and their receptors in rheumatoid arthritis future targets? *Arthritis Rheum.* **2005**, *52*, 710–721. [CrossRef] [PubMed]
12. György, B.; Tóth, E.; Tarcsa, E.; Falus, A.; Buzás, E. Citrullination: A posttranslational modification in health and disease. *Int. J. Biochem. Cell Biol.* **2006**, *38*, 1662–1677. [CrossRef] [PubMed]
13. Van Venrooij, W.J.; Pruijn, G.J.M. Citrullination: A small change for a protein with great consequences for rheumatoid arthritis. *Arthritis Res.* **2000**, *2*, 249–251. [CrossRef] [PubMed]
14. Mangat, P.; Wegner, N.; Venables, P.J.; Potempa, J. Bacterial and human peptidylarginine deiminases: Targets for inhibiting the autoimmune response in rheumatoid arthritis? *Arthritis Res. Ther.* **2010**, *12*, 209. [CrossRef]
15. Vossenaar, E.R.; Zendman, A.J.; van Venrooij, W.J.; Pruijn, G.J. PAD, a growing family of citrullinating enzymes: Genes, features and involvement in disease. *BioEssays* **2003**, *25*, 1106–1118. [CrossRef]
16. Feldmann, M.; Brennan, F.M.; Maini, R.N. Role of cytokines in rheumatoid arthritis. *Annu. Rev. Immunol.* **1996**, *14*, 397–440. [CrossRef]
17. Tilvawala, R.; Nguyen, S.H.; Maurais, A.J.; Nemmara, V.V.; Nagar, M.; Salinger, A.J.; Nagpal, S.; Weerapana, E.; Thompson, P.R. The Rheumatoid Arthritis-Associated Citrullinome. *Cell Chem. Biol.* **2018**, *25*, 691–704. [CrossRef]
18. Proost, P.; Struyf, S.; Van Damme, J.; Fiten, P.; Ugarte-Berzal, E.; Opdenakker, G. Chemokine isoforms and processing in inflammation and immunity. *J. Autoimmun.* **2017**, *85*, 45–57. [CrossRef]
19. Dong, C.; Chua, A.; Ganguly, B.; Krensky, A.M.; Clayberger, C. Glycosylated recombinant human XCL1/lymphotactin exhibits enhanced biologic activity. *J. Immunol. Methods* **2005**, *302*, 136–144. [CrossRef]
20. Senshu, T.; Akiyama, K.; Kan, S.; Asaga, H.; Ishigami, A.; Manabe, M. Detection of deiminated proteins in rat skin: Probing with a monospecific antibody after modification of citrulline residues. *J. Investig. Dermatol.* **1995**, *105*, 163–169. [CrossRef]
21. Assohou-Luty, C.; Raijmakers, R.; Benckhuijsen, W.E.; Stammen-Vogelzangs, J.; de Ru, A.; van Veelen, P.A.; Franken, K.L.; Drijfhout, J.W.; Pruijn, G.J. The human peptidylarginine deiminases type 2 and type 4 have distinct substrate specificities. *Biochim. Biophys. Acta* **2014**, *1844*, 829–836. [CrossRef] [PubMed]
22. Rutledge, B.J.; Rayburn, H.; Rosenberg, R.; North, R.J.; Gladue, R.P.; Corless, C.L.; Rollins, B.J. High level monocyte chemoattractant protein-1 expression in transgenic mice increases their susceptibility to intracellular pathogens. *J. Immunol.* **1995**, *155*, 4838–4843. [CrossRef] [PubMed]
23. Mortier, A.; Gouwy, M.; Van Damme, J.; Proost, P. Effect of posttranslational processing on the in vitro and in vivo activity of chemokines. *Exp. Cell Res.* **2011**, *317*, 642–654. [CrossRef] [PubMed]
24. Oran, P.E.; Sherma, N.D.; Borges, C.R.; Jarvis, J.W.; Nelson, R.W. Intrapersonal and populational heterogeneity of the chemokine RANTES. *Clin. Chem.* **2010**, *56*, 1432–1441. [CrossRef] [PubMed]
25. Taghavi, Y.; Hassanshahi, G.; Kounis, N.G.; Koniari, I.; Khorramdelazad, H. Monocyte chemoattractant protein-1 (MCP-1/CCL2) in diabetic retinopathy: Latest evidence and clinical considerations. *J. Cell Commun. Signal* **2019**, *13*, 451–462. [CrossRef]

26. Ernst, C.A.; Zhang, Y.J.; Hancock, P.R.; Rutledge, B.J.; Corless, C.L.; Rollins, B.J. Biochemical and biologic characterization of murine monocyte chemoattractant protein-1. Identification of two functional domains. *J. Immunol.* **1994**, *152*, 3541–3549. [CrossRef] [PubMed]
27. Liu, Z.G.; Chen, W.F.; Van Damme, J. 30 kD MCP-1 protein produced by mouse thymic epithelial cell line MTEC1. *Shi Yan Sheng Wu Xue Bao* **1998**, *31*, 245–250. [PubMed]
28. Needham, M.; Barratt, D.; Cerillo, G.; Green, I.; Warburton, H.; Anderson, M.; Sturgess, N.; Rollins, B.; Reilly, C.; Hollis, M. High level expression of human MCP-1 using the LCR/MEL expression system. *Protein Expr. Purif.* **1996**, *7*, 173–182. [CrossRef]
29. Korchynskyi, O.; ten Dijke, P. Identification and functional characterization of distinct critically important bone morphogenetic protein-specific response elements in the Id1 promoter. *J. Biol. Chem.* **2002**, *277*, 4883–4891. [CrossRef]

International Journal of
Molecular Sciences

MDPI

Article

Short Peptides of Innate Immunity Protein Tag7 Inhibit the Production of Cytokines in CFA-Induced Arthritis

Georgii B. Telegin [1,*], Aleksandr S. Chernov [1], Alexey N. Minakov [1], Irina P. Balmasova [2], Elena A. Romanova [3], Tatiana N. Sharapova [3], Lidia P. Sashchenko [3] and Denis V. Yashin [3]

1 Institute of Bioorganic Chemistry (RAS), 117997 Moscow, Russia
2 Moscow State University of Medicine and Dentistry, 127473 Moscow, Russia
3 Institute of Gene Biology (RAS), 119334 Moscow, Russia
* Correspondence: telegin@bibch.ru

Abstract: The pathogenesis of autoimmune arthritis is a hot topic in current research. The main focus of this work was to study cytokines released in CFA-induced arthritis in ICR mice as well as the regulation of blood levels of cytokines by two peptides of the innate immunity protein Tag7 (PGLYRP1) capable of blocking the activation of the TNFR1 receptor. Arthritis was induced by local periarticular single-dose injections of 40 μL of complete Freund's adjuvant (CFA) into the left ankle joints of mice. The levels of chemokines and cytokines in plasma were measured using a Bio-Plex Pro Mouse Cytokine Kit at 3, 10, and 21 days after arthritis induction. Tag7 peptides were shown to decrease the blood levels of the pro-inflammatory cytokines IL-6, TNF, and IL-1β. Administration of peptides also decreased the levels of chemokines MGSA/CXCL1, MIP-2α/CXCL2, ENA78/CXCL5, MIG/CXCL9, IP-10/CXCL10, MCP-1/CCL2, and RANTES/CCL5. Furthermore, a decrease in the levels of cytokines IL7, G-CSF, and M-CSF was demonstrated. Addition of the studied peptides strongly affected IFN-γ concentration. We believe that a decrease in the levels of cytokine IFN-γ was associated with a therapeutic effect of Tag7 peptides manifested in alleviation of the destruction of cartilage and bone tissues in the CFA-induced arthritis.

Keywords: mice; CFA; inflammation; arthritis; TNFα; Tag7; 17.1 and 17.1a peptides

Citation: Telegin, G.B.; Chernov, A.S.; Minakov, A.N.; Balmasova, I.P.; Romanova, E.A.; Sharapova, T.N.; Sashchenko, L.P.; Yashin, D.V. Short Peptides of Innate Immunity Protein Tag7 Inhibit the Production of Cytokines in CFA-Induced Arthritis. *Int. J. Mol. Sci.* **2022**, *23*, 12435. https://doi.org/10.3390/ijms232012435

Academic Editor: Chih-Hsin Tang

Received: 28 July 2022
Accepted: 13 October 2022
Published: 17 October 2022

1. Introduction

The study of the pathogenesis of autoimmune arthritides, including rheumatoid arthritis, is mostly based on experimental animal models. Cytokines play a key role in the pathogenesis of rheumatoid arthritis. They are present in the complex process of disease initiation and orchestrate the common phenotype of persistent synovial hyperplasia, immune cell infiltration, and joint destruction that ensues [1]. Most commonly, the pool of cytokines at the first stage of disease is formed in the setting of inflammatory processes [2].

Pro-inflammatory cytokines are involved in the development of these inflammatory processes. Cytokines IL-1β, IL-6, and TNF often play a key role [3]. IL-6 is one of the principal mediators of the acute phase of inflammation. It stimulates the proliferation and differentiation of B and T cells as well as leukopoesis [4]. Cytokine IL-1β is produced by cells in an inactive form as part of the intracellular molecular complex, inflammasome, and is activated after release from the cell during apoptosis [5]. At subsequent stages, cytokines of several different groups are involved in the development of pathological processes. An important role in the development of chronic inflammation is played by the colony-stimulating factors (CSF), such as macrophage CSF (M-CSF) and granulocyte CSF (G-CSF), which maintain proliferation and activation of the main cells of an immune system producing pro-inflammatory cytokines. It has been shown that, in mice with arthritis, G-CSF levels are increased both in the serum and inflamed extremities, and that a G-CSF blockage results in a significant decrease in the severity of arthritis and reduction in blood neutrophil counts [6,7].

To date, it has been shown that osteoclasts play an important role in the development of articular bone erosion in adjuvant-induced arthritis, and M-CSF is recognized as a key factor responsible for survival and proliferation of the osteoclast progenitor cells [8,9]. An important role in the proliferation of immune cells is played by IFN-γ, which triggers the activation of natural killer (NK) cells and lymphocytes [10]. The depletion of the non-activated lymphocyte pool results in a production of growth factors and chemokines stimulating the migration of new cells to a site of autoimmune response and their consequent proliferation [11]. The resulting pathological immune response is dependent on the balance between activating cytokines and anti-inflammatory cytokines. Among the latter, IL-10 and IL-4 play an important role [12]. IL-4 takes part in the launch of humoral immune responses, contributing to the differentiation of naive helper T cells into Th2. Upon the IL-4-mediated activation, Th2 subsequently produce additional IL-4. Experiments have shown that, in collagen-induced arthritis, IL-4 suppresses the production of IL-17 [13], thus reducing the intensity of inflammatory response.

A particular role in the progress of autoimmune arthritis is played by TNF [14]. This cytokine has been well studied, and it was demonstrated that, in addition to its ability to induce the production of other cytokines, it possesses other activities, including an ability to directly induce programmed cell death [15]. TNF exerts its activity by binding to a specific TNFR1 receptor. We have shown previously that the innate immunity protein Tag7 is able to bind directly to a TNF receptor, the TNFR1 protein, and to inhibit signaling through this receptor [16]. The mammalian gene encoding Tag7 was initially discovered at our institute. Subsequently, it was also discovered in insects and named PGRP-S (PGLYRP1). [17,18]. In insects, the protein encoded by this gene plays an important role in the immune response because it directly binds to peptidoglycans on the bacterial wall and, via interaction with the Spätzle protein, transmits a signal directly to the Toll receptor [19]. In mammals, there are several Toll receptors that interact directly with various types of pathogens, including peptidoglycans; however, the Tag7 protein retains its important function of activating the immune system [20].

We have shown that the Tag7 protein is involved in the activation of TREM-1 receptor that serves as an enhancer of the pro-inflammatory In review Running Title 3 signal induced by Toll receptors [21]. Accordingly, in mammals, Tag7 also serves as a co-activator of the cascade of immune reactions induced through the Toll receptor. We have identified a site in Tag7 that is responsible for binding to TNFR1 and have isolated a receptor-binding peptide [22,23]. This peptide, 17.1, and its truncated variant, 17.1a, have the potential to inhibit cytotoxic signal transmission through the TNFR1 receptor [23]. Recently, it has been shown that administration of peptide 17.1 to mice with the CFA-induced experimental arthritis has a protective effect against cartilage and bone destruction [24,25].

This work was aimed at identification of cytokines that are involved in pathological processes in the CFA-induced arthritis and what are the effects of the 17.1 peptide (TNFR1 inhibitor) and its truncated variant, 17.1a, on the levels of these cytokines.

2. Results

2.1. Pro-Inflammatory Cytokines

We used a mouse model of adjuvant-induced arthritis, and at early time-points of the experiment, levels of "classical" pro-inflammatory cytokines, such as IL-1β, IL-6, and TNF, were measured. The levels of these cytokines in the serum of experimental animals against the controls (intact animals) are shown in Figure 1 (see Supplementary Materials Tables S1–S5) at the time-points from the start of the study.

From the provided results, it can be seen that CFA administration results in an increase in the levels of three pro-inflammatory cytokines (IL-1β, IL-6, and TNF). An increase in IL-6 levels was the most pronounced. Without any treatment, the levels of this cytokine reached their peak values (3.5 times above baseline) by study day 10, after which they decreased but still remained about two times higher than the control values. With Norocarp, this increase declined during the entire follow-up period. The study peptides 17.1 and

17.1a (the truncated variant) exerted inhibitory activity on day 21, and on days 10 and 21, respectively. TNF was the second most elevated cytokine. With CFA treatment, serum levels of this cytokine also reached their peak values (two times above the baseline) by day 10. An increase in TNF levels by day 10 was inhibited by the addition of both Norocarp and the studied peptide 17.1a. On day 21, the TNF level returns to subnormal. IL-1β is produced by cells in an inactive form and is activated when released during apoptosis [5]. From this point of view, an analysis of the effects of these peptides on IL-1β levels warrants investigation of the mechanisms of their action and their relation to apoptosis.

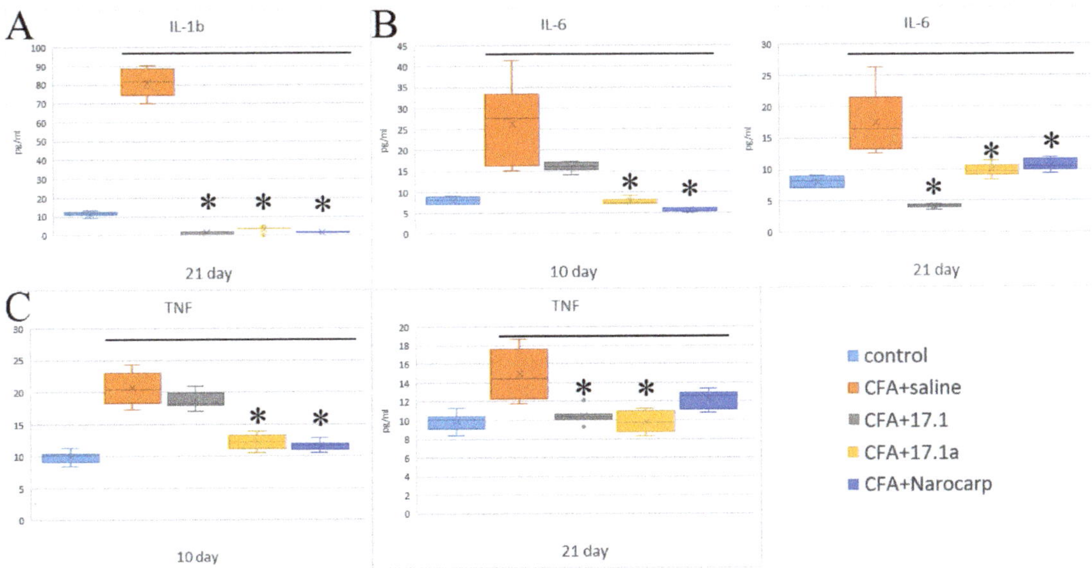

Figure 1. Changes in the level of pro-inflammatory cytokines ((**A**) IL-1b; (**B**) IL-6; (**C**) TNF) in the plasma 145 of mice after CFA-induced arthritis. (Control—control animals without CFA injection, CFA—animals with induced via CFA arthritis, + saline—animals were treated by phosphate buffered saline [PBS], +17.1a, +17.1, +Norocarp—animals were treated by a specified agent; $n = 7$ for each group). (p-value: * < 0.05).

The IL-1β levels demonstrate a rather high increase (by 5.4-fold) on day 21, which suggests a significant activation of apoptosis during this period. All tested agents demonstrated a statistically significant reduction in IL-1β levels, with peptide 17.1a and Norocarp achieving reduction on day 21, and peptide 17.1 on days 10 and 21. The levels of IL-1α and IL-17A did not change in the setting of CFA-induced arthritis.

2.2. Chemokines

When analyzing the results of measuring chemokines in the serum of animals exposed to different agents, all chemokines were divided into two groups according to their structure and mechanism of action on the cells of immune system. The first group consisted of CXCL chemokines with an effect on neutrophilic granulocytes and lymphocytes, while the second group consisted of CCL chemokines having effects on monocytes, lymphocytes, eosinophils, and basophils. The first group included the following chemokines: MGSA/CXCL1 (peptide with melanoma growth stimulatory activity), MIP-2α/CXCL2 (macrophage inflammatory protein 2α), ENA78/CXCL5 (epithelial cell-derived neutrophil-activating protein-78), MIG/CXCL9 (monokine induced by gamma interferon), and IP-10/CXCL10 (interferon gamma inducible protein 10) (Figure 2) (see Supplementary Materials Tables S1–S5).

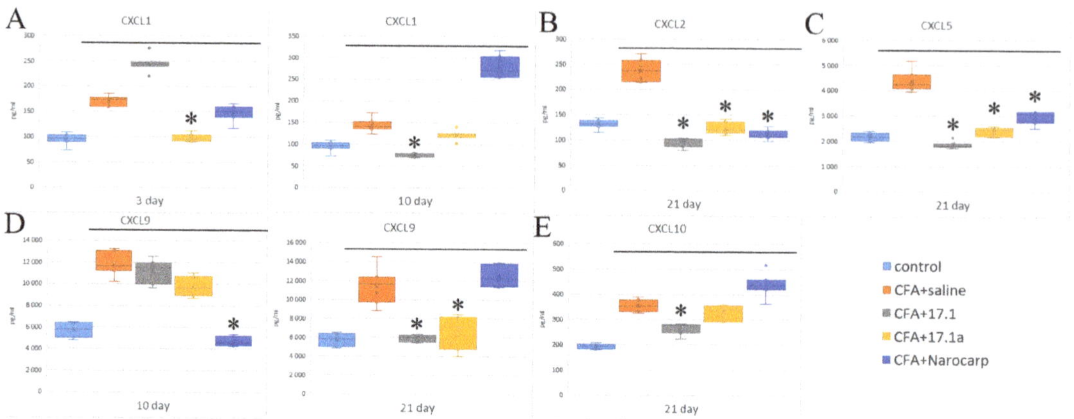

Figure 2. Changes in the level of chemokines ((**A**) CXCL1; (**B**) CXCL2; (**C**) CXCL5; (**D**) CXCL9; (**E**) CXCL10) in the plasma of mice after CFA-induced arthritis. (Control—control animals without CFA injection, CFA—animals with induced via CFA arthritis, +saline—animals were treated by phosphate buffered saline (PBS), +17.1a, +17.1, +Norocarp—animals were treated by a specified agent, $n = 7$ for each group). (p-value: * < 0.05).

Among the CXCL chemokines, IP-10/CXCL10 demonstrated the highest degree of deviation from the controls in all groups of animals, with levels increased above the controls. Without exposure to any agents in the setting of mouse experimental arthritis, the levels of this cytokine were increased 2.2-fold already on day 3, and stayed close to this level over the next 3 weeks. In the mice treated with Norocarp, the levels of this cytokine were decreased by day 10, whereas in mice treated with both study peptides, its levels were decreased by day 21. MGSA/CXCL1 is the second chemokine of this group, the levels of which were the most increased after treatment with these agents. Without exposure to any agents, the levels of this chemokine were increased 1.8-fold already on day 3, after which they steadily decreased, reaching the control values by day 21. Norocarp caused a decrease in the levels of this chemokine on day 10. Peptide 17.1a reduced the levels of CXCL1 on days 3 and 10, while peptide 17.1 reduced them only on day 10. In the setting of this experiment, the levels of MIG/CXCL9 were moderately increased (1.3- to 1.7- fold) over the entire period of the experiment. Norocarp reduced the levels of this chemokine on day 10, peptide 17.1a on days 10 and 21, and peptide 17.1 only on day 21. Under the effect of CFA, the levels of MIP-2α/CXCL2 were increased on day 21; however, this increase was suppressed by all tested agents. The levels of ENA-78/CXCL5 were also increased on day 21, and this increase was suppressed by all tested agents. The second group of chemokines included MCP-1/CCL2 (monocyte chemoattractant protein-1) and RANTES/CCL5 (regulated upon activation, normal T cell expressed and secreted). The time course of serum levels of these chemokines in the setting of adjuvant-induced arthritis in different groups is shown in Figure 3 (see Supplementary Materials Tables S1–S5).

Chemokines of this group play a particularly important role in adjuvant-induced arthritis in animals [26,27]. The levels of MCP-1/CCL2 on day 3 were the highest in untreated animals (5.8-fold above control) and in animals treated with peptide 17.1 (5.4-fold); the least pronounced increase (3.1-fold) was observed in animals treated with peptide 17.1a. Starting from day 10, the levels of this cytokine sharply decreased in all groups, except in mice treated with Norocarp, in which, on the contrary, an 8.7-fold increase in the levels of MCP-1/CCL2 was observed. The inhibitory effect was apparent only for peptide 17.1a, while peptide 17.1 and Norocarp exerted no therapeutic effect. The levels of RANTES/CCL5 demonstrated a rather high increase on day 10, while in mice treated with peptides 17.1 and 17.1a, they remained in a range close to the control values. Treatment with Norocarp reduced the levels of this cytokine only on day 21. The levels of chemokines MCP-1/227 CCL2, MIP-1α/CCL3, MIP-1β/CCL4, and eotaxin/CCL11 did not change by treatment with the tested peptides.

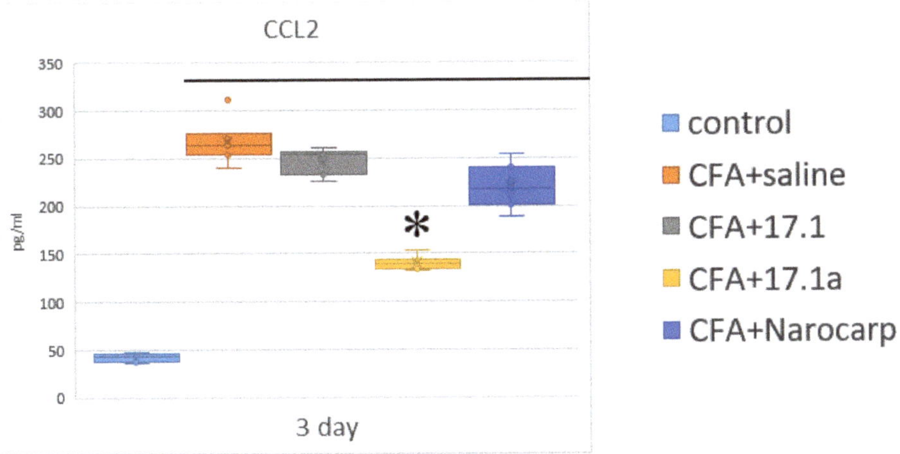

Figure 3. Changes in the level of CCL2 chemokine (CCL2) in the plasma of mice after CFA212 induced arthritis. (Control—control animals without CFA injection, CFA—animals with induced via CFA arthritis, +saline—animals were treated by phosphate buffered saline (PBS), +17.1a, +17.1, +Norocarp—animals were treated by a specified agent, $n = 7$ for each group). (p-value: * < 0.05).

2.3. Hematopoietic Cytokines and Growth Factors

Another group of cytokines involved in the regulation of hematopoiesis consists of cytokines that function as colony-stimulating and growth factors (Figure 4) (see Supplementary Materials Tables S1–S5). They include IL-7, granulocyte colony-stimulating factor (G-CSF), and macrophage colony-stimulating factor (M234-CSF). The levels of these factors measured during the experiment are summarized in Figure 4. In the group of mice with adjuvant-induced arthritis without exposure to any agents, lymphopoetin IL-7 demonstrated the highest degree of deviation from controls, with a 2.5-fold increase by day 10 and subsequent decrease to control values. Treatment with all agents resulted in a decrease in IL-7 levels, which was statistically significant for peptide 17.1a and, in particular, peptide 17.1.

Our studies on the mouse model of adjuvant-induced arthritis have shown that G-CSF levels were above the baseline during the entire period of study. Norocarp and 17.1a peptide resulted in a decrease in cytokine levels by day 10 and by day 21, respectively. M-CSF levels were increased by day 21; however, this increase was suppressed by all agents tested. The levels of IL-3, IL-5, IL-9, and LIF, as well as those of GM-CSF and VEGF, did not increase in the setting of CFA-induced arthritis.

2.4. Cytokines of the Effector Phase of Immune Response

The measured levels of cytokines that induce cellular (cytotoxic) immune reactions, such as IFN-γ inducing cellular (cytotoxic) immune response and IL-4 involved in the induction of humoral immune response, in the setting of experiments are shown in Figure 5 (see Supplementary Materials Tables S1–S5). The levels of IFN-γ, one of the core components of the effector phase of cellular response in autoimmune diseases, progressively increased during the entire study period. The most pronounced suppression of this increase by all agents was observed on day 10.

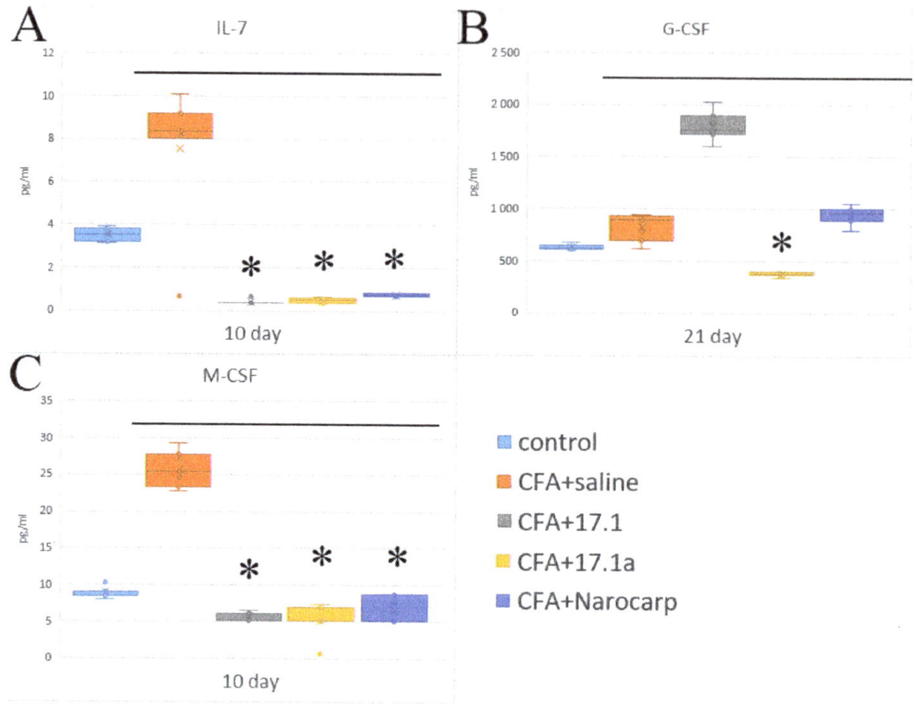

Figure 4. Changes in the level of hematopoietic cytokines ((**A**) IL-7) and growth factors ((**B**) G-CSF; ((**C**) M-CSF) in the plasma of mice after CFA-induced arthritis. (Control—control animals without CFA injection, CFA—animals with induced via CFA arthritis, +saline—animals were treated by phosphate buffered saline (PBS), +17.1a, +17.1, +Norocarp—animals were treated by a specified agent, $n = 7$ for each group). (p-value: * < 0.05).

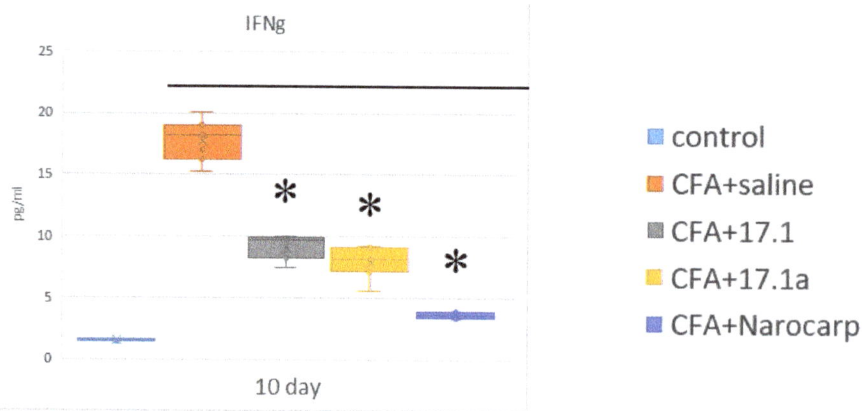

Figure 5. Changes of the level of cytokines in the effector phase of immune response (IFN-γ) in the plasma of mice after CFA-induced arthritis. (Control—control animals without CFA injection, CFA—animals with induced via CFA arthritis, +saline—animals were treated by phosphate buffered saline (PBS), +17.1a, +17.1, +Norocarp—animals were treated by a specified agent, $n = 7$ for each group). (p-value: * < 0.05).

IL-4 demonstrated an increase on days 10 and 21 of the study, but the level of this cytokine stays rather low. Peptide 17.1a and Norocarp demonstrated an inhibitory effect in both study periods. The levels of IL-2, IL-12p40, IL-12p70, and IL-15, as well as those of IL-10 and IL-13, did not increase in the setting of CFA-induced arthritis.

3. Discussion

The results obtained in this study permit drawing the following conclusions:

(1) Under the effect of CFA, there is an increase in the levels of all pro-inflammatory cytokines, such as IL-1β, IL-6, and TNF, all chemokines tested (except CCL11), and IFN-γ, as well as IL-7, G-CSF, and M-CSF.

(2) Peptide 17.1 and its truncated variant 17.1a caused a decrease in the levels of above-mentioned cytokines and chemokines, which was most pronounced by days 10 and 21. In our previous work, we have shown that administration of peptide 17.1 may reduce the effect of CFA-induced arthritis on mouse cartilage and bone tissue [24].

In the experiments conducted in that work, a protective effect of peptide 17.1 was most pronounced on day 21. In this work, we used blood samples from the mice from our previous work, so that we had the possibility to connect the clinical picture of our previous data, namely a strong reduction in inflammatory symptoms and a very strong reduction in damage to cartilage and bone tissue in the CFA-induced arthritis, to the concentrations of broad spectra of cytokines and chemokines. In this work, we have also demonstrated that peptides 17.1 and 17.1a exert the most pronounced effects on the levels of expressed cytokines and chemokines by days 21 and 10 of the study, respectively.

Earlier, we have also shown that peptide 17.1 could inhibit the production of cytokines IL-1β, IL-6, TNF, and IFN-γ expressed by human blood cells ex vivo upon induction with lipopolysaccharide. The results of the study described here confirm that the levels of pro-inflammatory cytokines IL-1β, IL-6, and TNF, as well as those of IFN-γ, an immune response initiator, that were increased upon induction by CFA are reduced after administration of peptides 17.1 and 17.1a. The list of CFA-induced cytokines, the levels of which are suppressed by administration of peptide 17.1 and its truncated variant 17.1a, has been expanded during this study. The expanded list includes chemokines CXCL1, CXCL2, CXCL5, CXCL9, CXCL10, as well as CCL2 and CCL5. IP-10/CXCL10 is known to be secreted upon induction with IFN-γ by neutrophils, eosinophils, monocytes, epithelial and endothelial cells, and stromal cells, as well as keratinocytes; this chemokine acts as a ligand of the CXCR3 receptor expressed by activated T and B cells, NK cells, dendritic cells, and macrophages. IP-10/CXCL10 triggers chemotaxis, apoptosis, and inhibition of cell growth and angiostasis [28]; thus, they are decreasing the intensity of the cellular immune response, which should be considered as a quite beneficial effect in autoimmune arthritides that usually undergo a cellular type of development [29]. MGSA/CXCL1 is produced by macrophages, neutrophils, epithelial cells, or Th17 cells, and its expression could be induced by IL-1, TNF, or IL-17. MGSA/CXCL1 acts as a chemoattractant for neutrophils or other non-hematopoietic cells, recruiting them to the site of damage or infection, and plays an important role in the regulation of immune and inflammatory reactions [30]. MIG/CXCL9 activity is manifested in response to IFN-γ and realized via the attraction of cytotoxic T-lymphocytes (CTL), NK cells, NK T cells, and macrophages [31].

Chemokine MIP-2α/CXCL2 is produced by mast cells and macrophages, induces the attraction of neutrophils, and often acts synergistically with MGSA/CXCL1 [32]. MIP-1α/CCL3 and RANTES/CCL5 demonstrated high constitutive expression on macrophages in adjuvant-induced arthritis, which correlated with the expression of CCR2 (MCP-1/CCL2 receptor) by macrophages and was proved to play an important role in maintaining inflammatory changes in the joints. At the same time, RANTES/CCL5 may act through another receptor, CCR3, the expression of which is suppressed in this experimental model [31]. In the clinical setting, a high degree of concordance has been demonstrated between the status of oxidative stress in rheumatoid arthritis and the levels of MIP-1β/CCL4 and MCP-1/CCL-2 [33].

In the study conducted here, we have also demonstrated a protective effect of the tested peptides against an increase in the levels of cytokines IL-7, G-CSF, and M-CSF. Observations made in our work suggest that peptides 17.1 and 17.1a prevent the transmittance of the TNF signal via the TNFR1 receptor [22,23], and exert inhibitory effects, reducing an increase in the levels of pro-inflammatory cytokines and those of the cytokines that initiate autoimmune responses. This activity may be one of the mechanisms accounting for their protective effect against the destruction of bone and cartilage tissue in the CFA-induced arthritis. The second mechanism may consist of direct inhibition of TNF-induced cell death, which is indirectly evidenced by a significant increase in the levels of IL-1β on day 21 and suppression of this increase by both peptides tested. We have noticed that both peptides significantly reduced the levels of IFN-γ, which are dramatically 26-fold increased during induction of arthritis. It is known that the choice of arthritis model is of paramount importance for studying the mechanisms of immune reactions as emphasized in current literature reviews devoted to this topic [9]. Currently, the most recognized are the models of arthritis induced by adjuvant [34], serum transfer [35], and tumor necrosis factor [36]. We have used a model where intra-articular changes were caused by a non-specific agent, complete Freund's adjuvant. In this setting, reactions with preferential involvement of innate immune cells are likely to prevail. As emphasized in one recent work devoted to this topic, in this model, IFN-γ may play a key role in the extension of arthritis at the early stage. This cytokine produced by T-helper cells, CD4+, was involved in the induction of pro-inflammatory cytokines (TNF and Il-1β) and reprogramming the vascular network, which resulted in changes in vascular permeability, thus permitting autoantibodies to enter the target tissues [37].

With regard to our data, the pathogenetic role of IFN-γ was most apparent on day 10 of the experiment, with the degree of change being higher than for any other cytokine. In a group of mice not exposed to any additional agent, the levels of IFN-γ demonstrated a 3-fold increase on day 3 already, and, by day 10, they reached a peak value that was 8.8 times above the control values. By day 21 of the experiment, the levels of this cytokine decreased but still remained elevated (3.9-fold above control values). In other words, it is reasonable to believe that IFN-γ is one of the key players in the adjuvant-induced arthritis. Moreover, as mentioned earlier, all three agents significantly suppressed this predominant effect (in particular, peptide 17.1a).

The prevalence of rheumatoid arthritis is 0.5–1%, with a female:male ratio of 3:1 [38,39]. In the literature, this is explained by gender differences in the biological and molecular mechanisms underlying the pathogenesis of pain in arthritis [40,41]. At the same time, morphological differences in the development of CFA-induced arthritis in male and female mice are rather weakly expressed [42]. In our study, we present the results of using peptides 17.1 and 17.1a in the CFA-induced arthritis model in male ICR mice only. The use of female mice may produce different results because there are gender differences in rheumatoid arthritis [41,43].

4. Materials and Methods

4.1. Animals

Male ICR mice with an average weight (±SEM) 39.3 ± 1.65 g were used. All animals were housed under standard conditions for laboratory animals as specified by BIBC, RAS (the Unique Research Unit Bio-Model of the BIBCh, RAS; the Bioresource Collection—Collection of SPF Laboratory Rodents for Fundamental, Biomedical and Pharmacological, contract No. 075-15-2021-1067), which has an international accreditation from AAALACi. All experiments and manipulations were approved by the institutional animal care and use committee (IACUC protocol No. 713/20 from 06/08/20).

4.2. Experimental Groups

The animals were randomly assigned to five treatment groups with five animals in each group (n = 7): Group 1, control, intact animals; Group 2, induction of arthritis in animals that received intravenous injection of 100 μL of physiological saline; Group 3, induction of arthritis in animals that received peptide 17.1a (intravenous injection of 120 μg in 100 μL of physiological saline); Group 4, induction of arthritis in animals that received Norocarp (intravenous injection of 150 μg carprofen); and Group 5, induction of arthritis in animals that received peptide 17.1 (intravenous injection of 120 μg in 100 μL of physiological saline). The animals were followed up for 3, 10, and 21 days.

4.3. CFA-Induced Arthritis Model

Induction of arthritis was performed by a single injection of 40 μL complete Freund's adjuvant (CFA) into the left ankle joint according to a method described earlier [22]. The study peptides and reference agents were intravenously injected 24 h after the induction of inflammation.

4.4. The Assay of Chemokines and Cytokines

The levels of chemokines and cytokines in mouse plasma were measured using Bio-Plex Pro Mouse Cytokine Panel 33-Plex kit (Bio-Rad, Hercules, California, USA). Blood was collected individually from the retro-orbital sinus at 3, 10, and 21 days after arthritis induction, into EDTA tubes to obtain plasma. Plasma samples diluted at 1:3 (50 μL) were incubated with magnetic capture beads, washed, and then incubated with the detecting antibodies and SA-PE. Data were obtained using a Luminex 200 analyzer and analyzed using xPONENT software, v.4.3. (Saluggia, Italy).

4.5. Peptides

The peptide synthesis was performed on an automated peptide synthesizer, Gilson Quad-Z. Purification of peptides was performed on a preparative chromatography system, HPLC Gilson, consisting of a gradient pump (322), detector (155), and a fraction collector (GX 271) under the control of Trilution® software (v.4). Analysis of purity was performed on a chromatograph (Thermo Accela UPLC) with an ion trap mass spectrometer detector (Thermo Finnigan LCQ Deca XP Plus). The following chemicals were used: a block-copolymer carrier, Tentagel HL, with the terminal amino group modified with carboxy-trityl linker (Tentagel-TRT), Fmoc-protected amino acids (Iris Biotech), 4-methylpiperidine and collidine (Acros Organics), HATU (Sigma-Aldrich), and trifluoracetic acid (Solvay).

4.6. Statistical Analysis

Data were analyzed using Statistica software (StatSoft®, v.12.6). The results are presented as mean ±SD. Statistically significant differences were determined using *t*-tests. A value of $p < 0.05$ was considered to be statistically significant, compared with the CFA+saline group. The plate-specific intra-assay coefficient of variation (CV) for each marker was calculated as follows: (standard deviation (SD) of the duplicate values/mean of the duplicate values) ×100 (see Supplementary Materials Tables S1).

5. Conclusions

Thus, it should be acknowledged that all three agents (peptides 17.1a and 17.1, as well as Norocarp) exhibit some immunomodulatory activity, which is most potent in the peptide 17.1a. This activity is mainly manifested in the prevention of a high increase in the levels of a key cytokine, IFN-γ. Furthermore, as was shown in the final stages of the study, this agent does not produce some adverse effects typical for this model: it does not result in a diagnostically meaningful decrease in lymphopoetins and IL-10 with its immunosuppressive and anti-inflammatory effects and does not cause an increase in the levels of IL-17A and TNF, which are the main signs of a chronic process.

Supplementary Materials: The following supporting information can be downloaded at: https://www.mdpi.com/article/10.3390/ijms232012435/s1.

Author Contributions: Conceptualization, G.B.T., L.P.S. and D.V.Y.; Methodology, T.N.S., G.B.T. and A.S.C.; Software, D.V.Y.; Validation, L.P.S. and D.V.Y.; Formal Analysis, I.P.B., L.P.S. and D.V.Y.; Investigation, E.A.R., T.N.S., G.B.T., A.N.M., A.S.C., L.P.S. and D.V.Y.; Resources, G.B.T. and D.V.Y..; Data Curation, A.S.C., L.P.S. and D.V.Y.; Writing—Original Draft Preparation, L.P.S. and D.V.Y.; Writing—Review and Editing, L.P.S. and D.V.Y.; Supervision, L.P.S. and G.B.T.; Project Administration, L.P.S. and D.V.Y.; Funding Acquisition, L.P.S. and G.B.T. All authors have read and agreed to the published version of the manuscript.

Funding: This work was supported by the Ministry of Science and Higher Education of the Russian Federation, contract No. 075-15-2021-1067. The Bioresource Collection—Collection of SPF Laboratory Rodents for Fundamental, Biomedical, and Pharmacological Studies.

Institutional Review Board Statement: The animal study was reviewed and approved by all experiments, and manipulations were approved by the institutional animal care and use committee (IACUC protocol No. 713/20 from 6 August 2020).

Informed Consent Statement: Not applicable.

Data Availability Statement: Not applicable.

Conflicts of Interest: The authors declare that the research was conducted in the absence of any commercial or financial relationships that could be construed as a potential conflict of interest.

References

1. Ridgley, L.A.; Anderson, A.E.; Pratt, A.G. What Are the Dominant Cytokines in Early 383 Rheumatoid Arthritis? *Curr. Opin. Rheumatol.* **2018**, *30*, 207–214. [CrossRef] [PubMed]
2. Kondo, N.; Kuroda, T.; Kobayashi, D. Cytokine Networks in the Pathogenesis of Rheumatoid Arthritis. *Int. J. Mol. Sci.* **2021**, *22*, 10922. [CrossRef]
3. Mateen, S.; Zafar, A.; Moin, S.; Khan, A.Q.; Zubair, S. Understanding the Role of Cytokines in the Pathogenesis of Rheumatoid Arthritis. *Clin. Chim. Acta Int. J. Clin. Chem.* **2016**, *455*, 161–171. [CrossRef] [PubMed]
4. Srivastava, S.; Rasool, M. Underpinning IL-6 Biology and Emphasizing Selective JAK Blockade as the Potential Alternate Therapeutic Intervention for Rheumatoid Arthritis. *Life Sci.* **2022**, *298*, 120516. [CrossRef] [PubMed]
5. Malik, A.; Kanneganti, T.D. Function and Regulation of IL-1α in Inflammatory Diseases and 394 Cancer. *Immunol. Rev.* **2018**, *281*, 124–137. [CrossRef]
6. Hamilton, J.A.; Achuthan, A. Colony Stimulating Factors and Myeloid Cell Biology in Health and Disease. *Trends Immunol.* **2013**, *34*, 81–89. [CrossRef]
7. Crotti, C.; Agape, E.; Becciolini, A.; Biggioggero, M.; Favalli, E.G. Targeting Granulocyte-Monocyte Colony-Stimulating Factor Signaling in Rheumatoid Arthritis: Future Prospects. *Drugs* **2019**, *79*, 1741–1755. [CrossRef]
8. Christensen, A.D.; Haase, C.; Cook, A.D.; Hamilton, J.A. Granulocyte Colony-Stimulating Factor (G-CSF) Plays an Important Role in Immune Complex-Mediated Arthritis. *Eur. J. Immunol.* **2016**, *46*, 1235–1245. [CrossRef]
9. Alves, C.H.; Farrell, E.; Vis, M.; Colin, E.M.; Lubberts, E. Animal Models of Bone Loss in Inflammatory Arthritis: From Cytokines in the Bench to Novel Treatments for Bone Loss in the Bedside-a Comprehensive Review. *Clin. Rev. Allergy Immunol.* **2016**, *51*, 27–47. [CrossRef]
10. van Hamburg, J.P.; Tas, S.W. Molecular Mechanisms Underpinning T Helper 17 Cell Heterogeneity and Functions in Rheumatoid Arthritis. *J. Autoimmun.* **2018**, *87*, 69–81. [CrossRef]
11. Maciejewska Rodrigues, H.; Jüngel, A.; Gay, R.E.; Gay, S. Innate Immunity, Epigenetics and Autoimmunity in Rheumatoid Arthritis. *Mol. Immunol.* **2009**, *47*, 12–18. [CrossRef] [PubMed]
12. Troshina, E.A. The role of cytokines in the processes of adaptive integration of immune and neuroendocrine reactions of the human body. *Probl. Endokrinol.* **2021**, *67*, 4–9. [CrossRef] [PubMed]
13. Sandoghchian Shotorbani, S.; Zhang, Y.; Baidoo, S.E.; Xu, H.; Ahmadi, M. IL-4 Can Inhibit IL-17 Production in Collagen Induced Arthritis. *Iran. J. Immunol.* **2011**, *8*, 209–217. [PubMed]
14. Kruglov, A.; Drutskaya, M.; Schlienz, D.; Gorshkova, E.; Kurz, K.; Morawietz, L.; Nedospasov, S. Contrasting Contributions of TNF from Distinct Cellular Sources in Arthritis. *Ann. Rheum. Dis.* **2020**, *79*, 1453–1459. [CrossRef]
15. Kalliolias, G.D.; Ivashkiv, L.B. TNF Biology, Pathogenic Mechanisms and Emerging Therapeutic Strategies. *Nat. Rev. Rheumatol.* **2016**, *12*, 49–62. [CrossRef]
16. Yashin, D.V.; Ivanova, O.K.; Soshnikova, N.V.; Sheludchenkov, A.A.; Romanova, E.A.; Dukhanina, E.A.; Tonevitsky, A.G.; Gnuchev, N.V.; Gabibov, A.G.; Georgiev, G.P.; et al. Tag7 (PGLYRP1) in Complex with Hsp70 Induces Alternative Cytotoxic Processes in Tumor Cells via TNFR1 Receptor. *J. Biol. Chem.* **2015**, *290*, 21724–21731. [CrossRef]

17. Kang, D.; Liu, G.; Lundström, A.; Gelius, E.; Steiner, H. A Peptidoglycan Recognition Protein in Innate Immunity Conserved from Insects to Humans. *Proc. Natl. Acad. Sci. USA* **1998**, *95*, 10078–10082. [CrossRef]
18. Kustikova, O.S.; Kiselev, S.L.; Borodulina, O.R.; Senin, V.M.; Afanas'eva, A.V.; Kabishev, A.A. Cloning of the Tag7 gene expressed in metastatic mouse tumors. *Genetika* **1996**, *32*, 621–628.
19. Michel, T.; Reichhart, J.M.; Hoffmann, J.A.; Royet, J. Drosophila Toll Is Activated by Gram-Positive Bacteria through a Circulating Peptidoglycan Recognition Protein. *Nature* **2001**, *414*, 756–759. [CrossRef]
20. Dziarski, R.; Gupta, D. Mammalian PGRPs: Novel Antibacterial Proteins. *Cell. Microbiol.* **2006**, *8*, 1059–1069. [CrossRef]
21. Sharapova, T.N.; Ivanova, O.K.; Soshnikova, N.V.; Romanova, E.A.; Sashchenko, L.P.; Yashin, D.V. Innate Immunity Protein Tag7 Induces 3 Distinct Populations of Cytotoxic Cells That Use Different Mechanisms to Exhibit Their Antitumor Activity on Human Leukocyte Antigen-Deficient Cancer Cells. *J. Innate Immun.* **2017**, *9*, 598–608. [CrossRef] [PubMed]
22. Romanova, E.A.; Sharapova, T.N.; Telegin, G.B.; Minakov, A.N.; Chernov, A.S.; Ivanova, O.K.; Bychkov, M.L.; Sashchenko, L.P.; Yashin, D.V. A 12-Mer Peptide of Tag7 (PGLYRP1) Forms a Cytotoxic Complex with Hsp70 and Inhibits TNF-Alpha Induced Cell Death. *Cells* **2020**, *9*, 488. [CrossRef] [PubMed]
23. Telegin, G.B.; Chernov, A.S.; Kazakov, V.A.; Romanova, E.A.; Sharapova, T.N.; Yashin, D.V.; Gabibov, A.G.; Sashchenko, L.P. A 8-Mer Peptide of PGLYRP1/Tag7 Innate Immunity Protein Binds to TNFR1 Receptor and Inhibits TNFα-Induced Cytotoxic Effect and Inflammation. *Front. Immunol.* **2021**, *12*, 622471. [CrossRef] [PubMed]
24. Sharapova, T.N.; Romanova, E.A.; Chernov, A.S.; Minakov, A.N.; Kazakov, V.A.; Kudriaeva, A.A.; Belogurov, A.A.; Ivanova, O.K.; Gabibov, A.G.; Telegin, G.B.; et al. Protein PGLYRP1/Tag7 Peptides Decrease the Proinflammatory Response in Human Blood Cells and Mouse Model of Diffuse Alveolar Damage of Lung through Blockage of the TREM-1 and TNFR1 Receptors. *Int. J. Mol. Sci.* **2021**, *22*, 11213. [CrossRef] [PubMed]
25. Telegin, G.B.; Chernov, A.S.; Konovalov, N.A.; Belogurov, A.A.; Balmasova, I.P.; Gabibov, A.G. Cytokine Profile as a Marker of Cell Damage and Immune Dysfunction after Spinal Cord Injury. *Acta Nat.* **2020**, *12*, 92–101. [CrossRef] [PubMed]
26. Berke, M.S.; Fensholdt, L.K.D.; Hestehave, S.; Kalliokoski, O.; Abelson, K.S.P. Effects of buprenorphine on model development in an adjuvant-induced monoarthritis rat model. *PLoS ONE* **2022**, *17*, e0260356. [CrossRef]
27. Abdel Jaleel, G.A.; Azab, S.S.; El-Bakly, W.M.; Hassan, A. Methyl palmitate attenuates adjuvant induced arthritis in rats by decrease of CD68 synovial macrophages. *Biomed. Pharmacother.* **2021**, *137*, 111347. [CrossRef]
28. Liu, M.; Guo, S.; Hibbert, J.M.; Jain, V.; Singh, N.; Wilson, N.O.; Stiles, J.K. CXCL10/IP-10 in Infectious Diseases Pathogenesis and Potential Therapeutic Implications. *Cytokine Growth Factor Rev.* **2011**, *22*, 121–130. [CrossRef]
29. Woodell-May, J.E.; Sommerfeld, S.D. Role of Inflammation and the Immune System in the Progression of Osteoarthritis. *J. Orthop. Res. Off. Publ. Orthop. Res. Soc.* **2020**, *38*, 253–257. [CrossRef]
30. De Filippo, K.; Dudeck, A.; Hasenberg, M.; Nye, E.; van Rooijen, N.; Hartmann, K.; Gunzer, M.; Roers, A.; Hogg, N. Mast Cell and Macrophage Chemokines CXCL1/CXCL2 Control the Early Stage of Neutrophil Recruitment during Tissue Inflammation. *Blood* **2013**, *121*, 4930–4937. [CrossRef]
31. Schoenborn, J.R.; Wilson, C.B. Regulation of Interferon-Gamma During Innate and Adaptive Immune Responses. *Adv. Immunol.* **2007**, *96*, 41–101. [PubMed]
32. Haas, C.S.; Martinez, R.J.; Attia, N.; Haines, G.K.; Campbell, P.L.; Koch, A.E. Chemokine Receptor Expression in Rat Adjuvant-Induced Arthritis. *Arthritis Rheum.* **2005**, *52*, 3718–3730. [CrossRef] [PubMed]
33. Shah, D.; Wanchu, A.; Bhatnagar, A. Interaction Between Oxidative Stress and Chemokines: Possible Pathogenic Role in Systemic Lupus Erythematosus and Rheumatoid Arthritis. *Immunobiology* **2011**, *216*, 1010–1017. [CrossRef] [PubMed]
34. Kong, Y.Y.; Feige, U.; Sarosi, I.; Bolon, B.; Tafuri, A.; Morony, S.; Capparelli, C.; Li, J.; Elliott, R.; McCabe, S.; et al. Activated T Cells Regulate Bone Loss and Joint Destruction in Adjuvant Arthritis through Osteoprotegerin Ligand. *Nature* **1999**, *402*, 304–309. [CrossRef] [PubMed]
35. Pettit, A.R.; Ji, H.; von Stechow, D.; Müller, R.; Goldring, S.R.; Choi, Y.; Benoist, C.; Gravallese, E.M. TRANCE/RANKL Knockout Mice Are Protected from Bone Erosion in a Serum Transfer Model of Arthritis. *Am. J. Pathol.* **2001**, *159*, 1689–1699. [CrossRef]
36. Binder, N.B.; Puchner, A.; Niederreiter, B.; Hayer, S.; Leiss, H.; Blüml, S.; Kreindl, R.; Smolen, J.S.; Redlich, K. Tumor Necrosis Factor-Inhibiting Therapy Preferentially Targets Bone Destruction but Not Synovial Inflammation in a Tumor Necrosis Factor-Driven Model of Rheumatoid Arthritis. *Arthritis Rheum.* **2013**, *65*, 608–617. [CrossRef]
37. Ma, H.; Xu, M.; Song, Y.; Zhang, T.; Yin, H.; Yin, S. Interferon-γ Facilitated Adjuvant-Induced Arthritis at Early Stage. *Scand. J. Immunol.* **2019**, *89*, e12757. [CrossRef]
38. Intriago, M.; Maldonado, G.; Cárdenas, J.; Ríos, C. Clinical Characteristics in Patients with Rheumatoid Arthritis: Differences between Genders. *Sci. World J.* **2019**, *2019*, 8103812. [CrossRef]
39. Almoallim, H.; Al Saleh, J.; Badsha, H.; Ahmed, H.M.; Habjoka, S.; Menassa, J.A.; El-Garf, A.A. Review of the Prevalence and Unmet Needs in the Management of Rheumatoid Arthritis in Africa and the Middle East. *Rheumatol Ther.* **2021**, *8*, 1–16. [CrossRef]
40. Kim, J.R.; Kim, H.A. Molecular Mechanisms of Sex-Related Differences in Arthritis and Associated Pain. *Int. J. Mol. Sci.* **2020**, *21*, 7938. [CrossRef]

41. Yu, C.; Liu, C.; Jiang, J.; Li, H.; Chen, J.; Chen, T.; Zhan, X. Gender Differences in Rheumatoid Arthritis: Interleukin-4 Plays an Important Role. *J. Immunol. Res.* **2020**, *2020*, 4121524. [CrossRef] [PubMed]
42. Liu, L.; Karagoz, H.; Herneisey, M.; Zor, F.; Komatsu, T.; Loftus, S.; Janjic, B.M.; Gorantla, V.S.; Janjic, J.M. Sex Differences Revealed in a Mouse CFA Inflammation Model with Macrophage Targeted Nanotheranostics. *Theranostics* **2020**, *10*, 1694–1707. [CrossRef] [PubMed]
43. Zhang, C. Flare-up of cytokines in rheumatoid arthritis and their role in triggering depression: Shared common function and their possible applications in treatment (Review). *Biomed. Rep.* **2021**, *14*, 16. [CrossRef] [PubMed]

International Journal of *Molecular Sciences*

MDPI

Article

Development of Two Innovative Performance-Based Objective Measures in Feline Osteoarthritis: Their Reliability and Responsiveness to Firocoxib Analgesic Treatment

Aliénor Delsart [1], Maxim Moreau [1,2], Colombe Otis [1], Marilyn Frezier [1], Marlene Drag [3], Jean-Pierre Pelletier [2], Johanne Martel-Pelletier [2], Bertrand Lussier [1,2], Jérôme del Castillo [1] and Eric Troncy [1,2,*]

1 Groupe de Recherche en Pharmacologie Animale du Québec (GREPAQ), Department of Biomedical Sciences, Faculty of Veterinary Medicine, Université de Montréal, St.-Hyacinthe, QC J2S 2M2, Canada
2 Osteoarthritis Research Unit, University of Montreal Hospital Research Center (CRCHUM), Montréal, QC H2X 0A9, Canada
3 Boehringer Ingelheim Animal Health, Fulton, MO 65251, USA
* Correspondence: eric.troncy@umontreal.ca

Abstract: The metrological properties of two performance-based outcome measures of feline osteoarthritis (OA), namely Effort Path (Path) and Stairs Assay Compliance (Stairs), were tested. Cats naturally affected by OA (n = 32) were randomly distributed into four groups (A: 0.40, B: 0.25, C: 0.15, or D: 0.00 mg firocoxib/kg bodyweight) and assessed during baseline, treatment, and recovery periods. For Path, from an elevated walking platform, the cats landed on a pressure-sensitive mattress and jumped up onto a second elevated platform. Analysis included velocity, time to completion, peak vertical force (PVF), and vertical impulse. For Stairs, the number of steps and time to completion were recorded for 16 steps up and down in a 4 min period. Reliability was moderate to very good for Path and poor to good for Stairs. Different normalization methods are described in the manuscript. The placebo group remained stable within-time in Path, whereas treated cats trotted faster on the ramp ($p < 0.0001$), improved their PVF ($p < 0.018$) and completed the task quicker ($p = 0.003$). The percentage of cats completing the Stairs finish line was higher under treatment ($p < 0.036$), with huge effect size, the placebo group results being stable within-time. Both are promising performance-based outcome measures to better diagnose and manage feline OA pain.

Keywords: feline; osteoarthritis; firocoxib; gait analysis; stairs; performance

Citation: Delsart, A.; Moreau, M.; Otis, C.; Frezier, M.; Drag, M.; Pelletier, J.-P.; Martel-Pelletier, J.; Lussier, B.; del Castillo, J.; Troncy, E. Development of Two Innovative Performance-Based Objective Measures in Feline Osteoarthritis: Their Reliability and Responsiveness to Firocoxib Analgesic Treatment. *Int. J. Mol. Sci.* **2022**, *23*, 11780. https://doi.org/10.3390/ijms231911780

Academic Editor: Chih-Hsin Tang

Received: 1 August 2022
Accepted: 26 September 2022
Published: 4 October 2022

1. Introduction

An outcome measure is the result of a test critical to understanding an individual's status and progress over time. Hence, according to evidence-based medicine, outcome measures are imperative: they provide credible justification for therapeutic purposes only if they are reliable (unchanged measurement upon test and retest or across different assessors), able to demonstrate similar values across a range of individuals and eventually sensitive/responsive enough to an intervention, if any.

Among existing outcomes measurement, performance-based measures are known to evaluate how an individual performs on specific tasks, including how the task was approached [1]. As in humans [2], such clinical endpoints are of an utmost importance for veterinary medicine, particularly with the challenge that represents the detection of joint pain or disability in companion animals affected by osteoarthritis (OA). In OA cats, performance-based outcome measures are obtained through disease-specific questionnaires, or the so-called clinical metrology instruments, in which functional impairments are assessed by the owners (or veterinarians) [3–5]. Complementary to those subjective questionnaires, mobility or activity can be monitored in an objective manner by accelerometer-based devices [6,7]. In addition, valuable contributions to veterinary literature have been made based upon the objective analysis of ground reaction forces [4,8,9] (also called podobarometric gait analysis) in cats moving across a pressure-sensitive mattress. Performance-based outcome measures provide an overview of the cat's overall functioning. Central sensitization may develop during OA disease progression. In addition to performance-based outcome measure, quantitative sensory tests are static or dynamic research tools that could be used to characterize the somatosensory profile of OA cats [10]. As there is no gold standard to evaluate the domains of joint pain and disability in cats with OA, there is, therefore, a fertile ground for the development of novel, reliable, and sensitive to treatment outcome measures.

Firocoxib, a COX-2 specific non-steroidal anti-inflammatory drug is commonly used to manage canine and equine OA pain (Previcox® or Equioxx®; Boehringer Ingelheim Animal Health). Its treatment effect was mostly measured using physical examination and pain scale but also objective podobarometric (force plate) gait analysis [11,12]. Some studies investigated the use of coxibs to manage OA feline pain, but no veterinary non-steroidal anti-inflammatory drugs are currently approved in North America for the safe, long-term control of OA pain in cats [13,14]. One explanation for this delay could be the lack of objective outcome measures in the feline OA pain domain. With this thought in mind, the purpose of this study was to present the Effort Path (Path) and Stairs Assay Compliance (Stairs), two novel assessments of functional impairment in geriatric cats with OA. The aim of this study was to determine to what extent the proposed performance-based outcome measures provide reliable, homogeneous results among OA cats and their sensitivity to discriminate a dose-dependent response to an analgesic COX-2 specific treatment.

The following hypotheses will be challenged: (1) the moderate dispersion of data within successive trials (for Path) and good reliability (as mirrored by close agreement between baseline acquisition sessions) will be observed for a given animal subjected to Path and Stairs. Despite such reliability, it is assumed that the recorded outcomes will still be heterogeneous among the whole population sample. Therefore, we raised, as a second hypothesis: (2) that the uniformity of the results among cats will be improved after having normalized the data according to morphometric measurements (i.e., height, length), body weight, as well as walking velocity and time to task completion for Path. The third hypothesis concerned the sensitivity to OA therapeutics; (3) using the normalized data, Path and Stairs will be sensitive enough to discriminate a treatment effect.

2. Results

2.1. *Effort Path*

At the first Baseline acquisition session, cats had a mean bodyweight of 4.8 kg (3.4–6.8, Min–Max). Before jumping down, cats travelled the walking ramp at a velocity of 1.4 m/s (0.2–2.7). The coefficient of dispersion for this first outcome measure was 13.9% between trials, while it was more than twice as high (33.2%) between individuals. Outcomes recorded using the pressure-sensitive mattress are summarized in Table 1. When the cats hit the mattress, the peak vertical force (PVF) produced by each thoracic limb was higher than the mean bodyweight of the cats, reaching values higher by 123%. The inter-trials coefficients of dispersion were less than 10% for PVF and vertical impulse (VI), while they were grossly twice as high between individuals. As shown in Table 1, the values of the right and left thoracic limbs were summated for the PVF and VI outcomes, which resulted in a decrease in the dispersion of the data.

After having hit the pressure-sensitive mattress, cats get prepared to jump on the second ramp. The time necessary to perform this task, the time to completion, was considered as frames. On average, cats required 50 (25–236) frames to get off the mattress and to jump on to the second elevated ramp. The inter-trial and inter-animal coefficients of dispersion for this outcome were 12.4% and 53.5%, respectively.

The pelvic PVF produced to leave the mattress had higher coefficient of dispersion values compared to the jumping down but remained less than 20%. However, VI was the outcome with the highest coefficient of dispersion, being more than 30%. The PVF required to lift the cat was higher than its body weight, reaching values near 158%.

Table 1. Effort Path values of the first Baseline acquisition session.

	Jumping down (Thoracic Limbs)			Jumping up (Pelvic Limbs)		
Peak Vertical Force (kg)	**Right**	**Left**	**Sum of Thoracic Limbs**	**Right**	**Left**	**Sum of Pelvic Limbs**
Mean of 3 trials (Min–Max)	5.8 (3.5–8.7)	6.0 (3.1–8.7)	11.8 (6.6–15.8)	7.5 (3.7–13.4)	7.7 (3.2–12.3)	15.3 (7.7–24.0)
Coefficient of dispersion						
Inter-trials	6.9%	6.4%	**4.9%**	13.5%	10.6%	**10.2%**
Inter-individual	13.0%	14.4%	**12.3%**	19.3%	17.9%	18.5%
Vertical impulse (kg*s)						
Mean of 3 trials (Min–Max)	0.5 (0.3–0.8)	0.5 (0.3–1.5)	1.0 (0.7–2.2)	0.8 (0.4–6.1)	0.8 (0.2–5.1)	1.6 (0.8–11.2)
Coefficient of dispersion						
Inter-trials	8.7%	9.0%	**5.9%**	13.7%	14.6%	**12.3%**
Inter-individual	16.9%	19.5%	16.9%	37.4%	30.9%	33.1%

The peak vertical force and vertical impulse are summarized for thoracic and pelvic limbs. The coefficient of dispersion was presented to resume the dispersion of the data.

The vertical forces recorded for the second Baseline acquisition session as well as their spread were comparable to those obtained for the first session. The concordance of the PVF data between the first and the second Baseline acquisition sessions is presented in Figure 1. For the thoracic PVF (sum), the Spearman's ϱ was 0.80 with a coefficient of determination (R^2) of 0.72. The dispersion of the data was slightly higher for pelvic PVF (sum) compared to thoracic PVF values corresponding to a Spearman's ϱ of 0.79 and a R^2 of 0.67. Using intraclass coefficient correlation (ICC) index, the reliability between the acquisition sessions were as follows: values of 0.82 (95% confidence interval (CI_{95}) 0.66–0.91) and 0.55 (CI_{95} 0.25–0.75) for the thoracic and pelvic PVF values, respectively. For thoracic and pelvic VI (sum), the ICC index was 0.67 (CI_{95} 0.36–0.83) and 0.63 (CI_{95} 0.35–0.81), respectively.

As an attempt to limit the dispersion of the data recorded on the pressure-sensitive mattress, selected variables (i.e., height, length, and body weight of the cat as well as velocity and time to completion) were used to normalize the PVF and VI (sum) values.

Table 2 presents raw as well as normalized, thoracic, or pelvic PVF and VI data, after having combined values of both Baseline acquisition sessions. For the PVF generated when the thoracic limbs hit the mattress, normalization by the height (ground to shoulders) of the cats reached the lowest data dispersion. For the pelvic PVF and VI, normalization by the body weight led to the lowest data dispersion.

Normalized data were used to determine a treatment effect. The placebo group was stable over time according to the univariate analysis ($p > 0.114$). A significant within-time change for the pooled treatment group was reported for the velocity on the ramp ($p < 0.001$), the time to task completion ($p = 0.003$), thoracic PVF ($p = 0.004$), pelvic PVF ($p = 0.018$), and thoracic VI ($p = 0.002$).

Cats in the pooled treatment group trotted faster on the ramp and spent less time passing the mattress at timepoints Day 15 (treatment period) and Day 24 (first recovery timepoint; Recov-1) compared to their Baseline ($p < 0.038$). Their velocity was higher on the platform at the first (Day 24) compared to Recov-2 (Day 36) timepoint ($p = 0.016$) whereas they tended to spend less time on the mattress compared to placebo group ($p = 0.058$) at Recov-1. By comparing the different dose-groups, group B had a higher platform velocity at Recov-1 compared to Baseline ($p < 0.001$) and even to Treatment ($p < 0.001$) periods. Group B showed a significant ($p = 0.004$) decrease in velocity between both recovery timepoints (see Figure 2 for the within-time velocity on the platform). On the mattress, group B cats completed the task faster at Treatment ($p < 0.001$) and Recov-1 ($p = 0.003$) compared to Baseline.

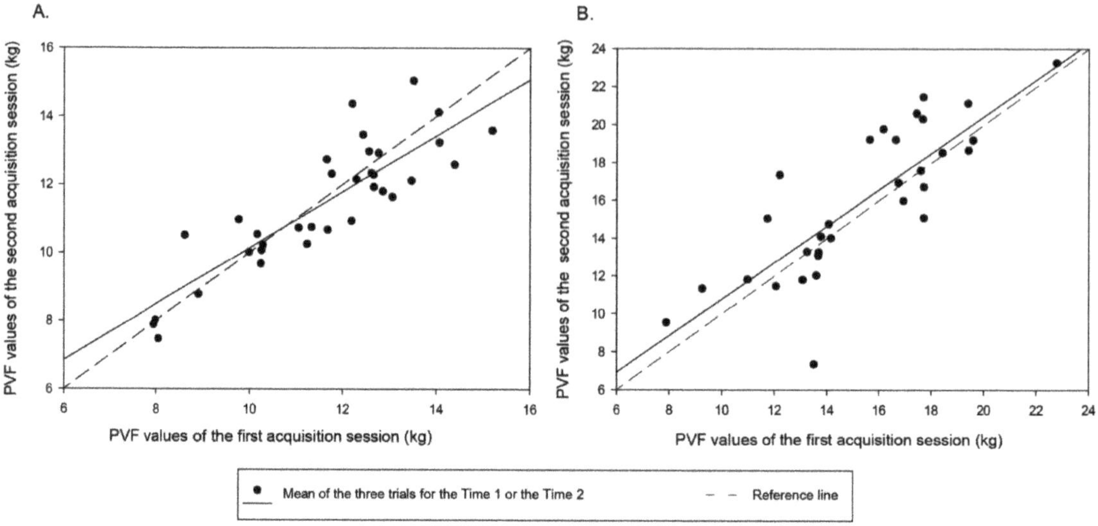

Figure 1. Concordance plot for the PVF values obtained during the first (x axis) and second (y axis) baseline acquisition sessions for (**A**) the thoracic limbs and (**B**) the pelvic limbs. Each point corresponds to the mean of the three valid trials for one cat. A perfect concordance is reflected by a 45° slope (dotted line).

Table 2. Best normalization process for Effort Path values.

	Peak Vertical Force (kg)		Vertical Impulse (kg*s)	
	Thoracic Limbs	**Pelvic Limbs**	**Thoracic Limbs**	**Pelvic Limbs**
Raw Data				
Mean values (Min–Max)	11.7 (7.5–15.2)	15.5 (7.3–23.2)	1.0 (0.7–1.7)	1.5 (0.9–8.1)
Coefficient of dispersion Inter-individual	11.9%	21.2%	17.2%	26.0%
Normalization Process				
Best normalization	Ground to Shoulders	Body Weight	Body Weight	Body Weight
Coefficient of dispersion Inter-individual	**9.9%**	**14.6%**	**10.1%**	**21.6%**

Raw data of the thoracic or pelvic peak vertical force and vertical impulse are presented for the baseline period. The variable resulting in the best normalization, basing on the data dispersion, is presented. The coefficient of dispersion is indicated for raw data and after normalization process.

The thoracic PVF decreased in the pooled treatment group, from Baseline to Recov-1 ($p = 0.004$), and the decrease was close to statistical significance ($p = 0.051$) from Treatment to the same Recov-1. The pooled treatment group thoracic PVF was higher than for the placebo group during Treatment ($p = 0.043$) and Recov-2 ($p = 0.034$). Comparing the different dose-groups, group A cats, receiving the highest dose of firocoxib, had a decreased PVF at Recov-1 ($p = 0.026$) compared to Baseline.

The pooled treatment group of pelvic PVF increased from the Baseline to Recov-1 timepoint ($p = 0.025$) and tended to be higher at Treatment ($p = 0.066$) and Recov-2 ($p = 0.076$).

The thoracic VI, in the pooled treatment group, decreased from Baseline to Treatment ($p = 0.021$) and to Recov-1 ($p = 0.001$). Compared to Baseline, a significant decrease was reported at Recov-1 ($p = 0.004$) for group B. No difference was observed within-time or between groups for pelvic VI. The descriptive data of PVF and VI are reported in Table 3.

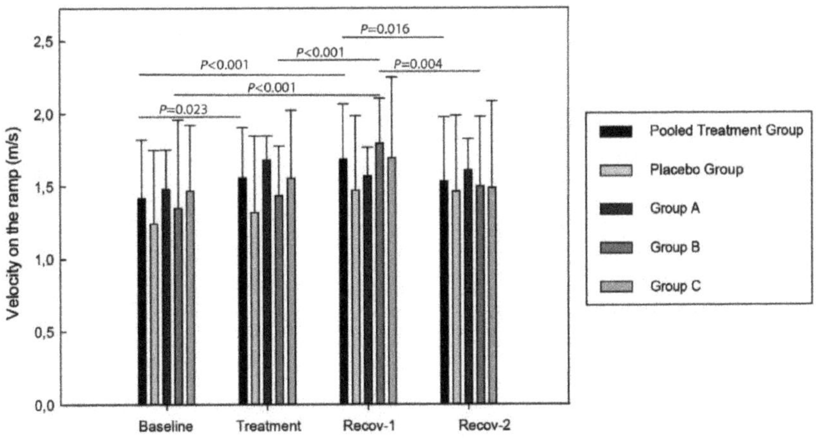

Figure 2. Cat velocity on the platform before jumping down. *p*-values are adjusted using Bonferroni correction. Group A = 0.40 mg/kg, Group B = 0.25 mg/kg, Group C = 0.15 mg/kg of Firocoxib. Recov-1 and Recov-2 = first and second recovery periods.

Table 3. Descriptive analysis of peak vertical force and vertical impulse raw data according to treatment phases.

Group	Baseline	Treatment	Recov-1	Recov-2
		Peak vertical force—Thoracic limbs (kg)		
Pooled Treatment	11.9 (8.6–15.2)	**11.7 (9.2–14.3)** [2]	**11.2 (8.7–15.1)** [1]	**11.4 (8.3–14.5)** [2]
Placebo	11.1 (7.5–14.1)	10.8 (8.2–12.5)	10.9 (8.4–12.3)	10.4 (5.8–12.7)
A	11.4 (8.8–14.1)	11.1 (9.2–13.9)	10.5 (8.7–13.1) [1]	11.1 (8.5–13.7)
B	11.7 (9.7–15.0)	12.1 (9.9–14.3)	11.6 (8.9–15.1)	11.7 (10.3–14.5)
C	12.5 [10.7–15.2]	12.1 (9.9–14.2)	11.7 (10.0–14.0)	11.6 (8.3–13.9)
		Peak vertical force—Pelvic limbs (kg)		
Pooled Treatment	16.1 (9.3–23.2)	16.5 (9.9–21.7)	**16.7 (9.7–23.2)** [1]	16.4 (7.4–22.3)
Placebo	13.8 (7.3–21.1)	14.8 (6.9–21.9)	14.7 (11.2–19.2)	14.8 (8.5–21.8)
A	14.2]9.3–19.2)	14.6 (10.9–17.3)	14.8 (10.5–18.9)	14.9 (10.7–18.2)
B	16.8 (9.7–23.2)	17.1 (13.4–21.7)	17.6 (14.0–23.2)	16.9 (11.6–22.3)
C	17.4 (13.1–21.4)	17.8 (9.9–21.1)	17.9 (9.7–22.3)	17.3 (7.4–20.3)
		Vertical impulse—Thoracic limbs (kg*s)		
Pooled Treatment	1.0 (0.7–1.7)	**0.9 (0.6–1.3)** [1]	**0.9 (0.7–1.3)** [1]	0.9 (0.2–1.3)
Placebo	1.0 (0.8–1.4)	0.9 (0.7–1.1)	0.9 (0.7–1.2)	0.9 (0.7–1.1)
A	0.9 (0.8–1.3)	0.9 (0.6–1.2)	0.8 (0.7–1.1)	0.8 (0.7–1.2)
B	1.0 (0.7–1.5)	1.0 (0.7–1.3)	0.9 (0.7–1.3) [1]	1.0 (0.8–1.3)
C	1.1 (0.8–1.7)	0.9 (0.7–1.2)	0.9 (0.8–1.2)	0.9 (0.2–1.1)
		Vertical impulse—Pelvic limbs (kg*s)		
Pooled Treatment	1.5 (0.9–5.4)	1.3 (0.9–2.0)	1.3 (0.8–1.9)	1.3 (0.3–2.1)
Placebo	1.3 (1.0–1.8)	1.3 (1.0–1.6)	1.3 (1.0–1.6)	1.3 (1.0–1.7)
A	1.4 (1.1–1.8)	1.2 (0.9–1.5)	1.2 (0.9–1.7)	1.2 (0.9–1.6)
B	1.7 (0.9–5.4)	1.4 (1.0–2.0)	1.3 (0.9–1.9)	1.4 (1.0–2.1)
C	1.5 (1.1–2.5)	1.4 (1.1–1.8)	1.4 (0.8–1.8)	1.3 (0.3–1.6)
	Mean (Min–Max)			

[1] $p < 0.05$ compared to Baseline; [2] $p < 0.05$ compared to placebo group. Bonferroni adjustment was used.

2.2. Stairs Assay Compliance

Three cats were excluded from the analysis (one was not able to complete the evaluations and two presented too much variability) during Baseline. For the remaining cats, the stairs assay compliance (Stairs) values of the first and second Baseline acquisition sessions are summarized in Table 4. In general, the twenty-nine cats climbed down fewer steps than they climbed up. The time taken to go up and down the 16-steps was similar, but the dispersion of the data was higher for the time required to go upstairs. On both Baseline acquisition sessions, the inter-individual coefficient of dispersion was elevated (18.1–25.2%) for the number of steps and (35.5–75.4%) for the time necessary to climb up or down the stairs.

Table 4. Stairs assay compliance values for the first and second baseline acquisition sessions.

	Number of Steps		Time (s)	
	Going up	**Going down**	**Going up**	**Going down**
First session				
Mean values (Min–Max)	95 (41–144)	84 (32–112)	5 (2–22)	4 (1–9)
Coefficient of dispersion Inter-individual	25.2%	23.5%	75.4%	35.5%
Second session				
Mean values (Min–Max)	103 (32–160)	97 (32–160)	4 (2–9)	4 (2–17)
Coefficient of dispersion Inter-individual	18.1%	24.7%	49.7%	39.4%

The number of steps and the time to complete one passage of the Stairs at both baselines are summarized. The coefficient of dispersion reflects the dispersion of the data.

ICC values for the between sessions were as follows: 0.74 (CI_{95} 0.49–0.87) and 0.68 (CI_{95} 0.31–0.86) for the number of steps up and down, respectively. For the time required to climb up and down, ICC values were 0.24 (CI_{95} −0.15–0.56) and 0.41 (CI_{95} 0.06–0.67), respectively. Normalization according to morphometric data (i.e., height, length, and body weight of the cat) were used as an attempt to limit the dispersion of inter-individual values (Table 5). A decrease of the inter-individual dispersion was found for the number of steps up, the time required to climbed up and down, with a normalization by, respectively, the length (chest to croup), the bodyweight, and the ground to elbow height measurements. No normalization improved the uniformity of the data for the number of steps down.

Table 5. Best normalization process for the stairs assay compliance values.

	Number of Steps		Time (s)	
	Going up	**Going down**	**Going up**	**Going down**
Raw data				
Mean values (Min–Max)	98 (32–160)	90 (32–160)	4.5 (1.5–22.0)	3.9 (1.3–17.0)
Coefficient of dispersion Inter-individual	22.6%	22.4%	60.0%	38.5%
Normalization process				
Best normalization	Chest to Croup	/	Bodyweight	Ground to Elbow
Coefficient of dispersion Inter-individual	**21.6%**	/	**55.0%**	**35.5%**

The number of steps and the time to complete one passage are summarized for the raw data and after the normalization process. The variable resulting in the best normalization, according to the coefficient of dispersion, is indicated.

The finish line analysis was used as a new potent strategy to limit the data dispersion. This analysis allowed the inclusion of the two cats with the highest variability. Taking all cats performing Stairs ($n = 31$) in consideration, 32% were able to complete the finish line up and 23% the finish line down. The data dispersion associated with this distribution is summarized in Table 6. The coefficient of dispersion was improved by 3- and 17-fold, compared to the previous normalization, for the number of steps and time, respectively.

Table 6. The Finish Line Completed descriptive analysis.

	Number of Steps		Time (s)	
	Going up	**Going down**	**Going up**	**Going down**
Raw Data				
Mean values (Min–Max)	123.6 (108.0–144.0)	120.0 (112.0–136.0)	2.7 (2.0–6.0)	2.3 (2.0–3.0)
Coefficient of dispersion Inter-individual	**3%**	**7%**	**22%**	**2%**

The number of steps and the time to complete one passage are summarized for cats completing the finish line. The finish line up was used to determine the going up and the finish line down allows to distinguish cats for the going down.

By distinguishing cats into pooled treatment and placebo groups, the percentage of cats crossing the finish line was similar between groups ($p = 0.610$) and for both Baselines ($p = 0.097$). Both Baseline-values were averaged for the following analyses. The percentage of cats reaching the finish line within-time is presented in Figure 3. The placebo group was stable within-time ($p > 0.567$). The percentage of cats crossing the finish line increased hugely in the pooled treatment group, compared to Baseline, during both Treatment (up: $p = 0.008$; down: $p = 0.036$) and Recov-2 periods (up: $p = 0.018$; down: $p = 0.017$). The number of cats completing the finish line was higher than those in the placebo group during the Treatment period ($p = 0.032$). The statistical model used was not sensitive enough to detect a dose-dependent effect (Type II error).

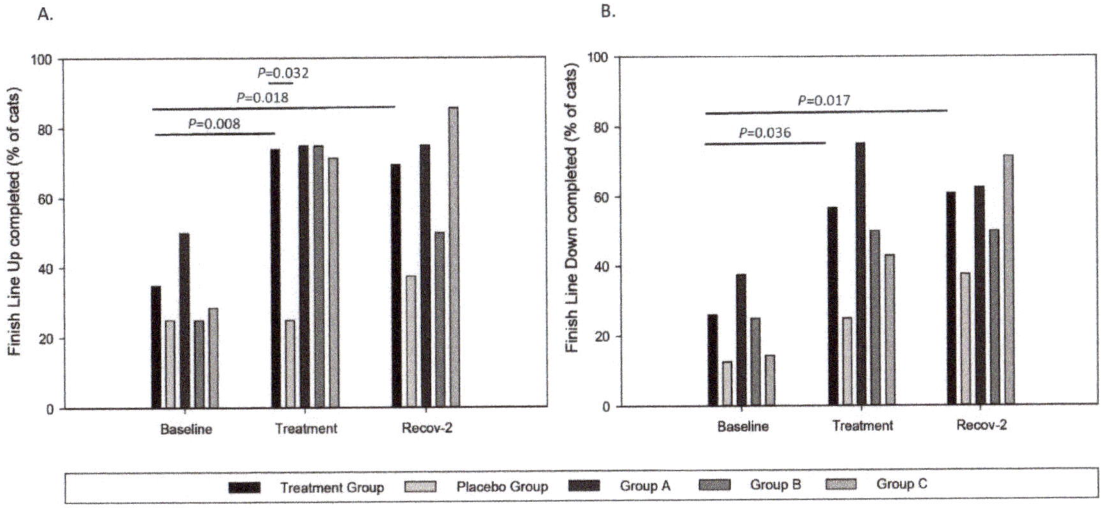

Figure 3. The Finish Line completed for up (**A**) or down (**B**) passages. Group A = 0.40 mg/kg, Group B = 0.25 mg/kg, Group C = 0.15 mg/kg of Firocoxib. Recov-2 = second recovery period.

3. Discussion

About 80% of the feline geriatric population is affected by OA [15]. Despite the wide occurrence of this disease, it remains largely underdiagnosed and consequently undermanaged [16–18]. At the present time, there is no gold standard to objectively evaluate an OA cat's functional (dis)abilities. Despite some feline OA questionnaires taking into consideration mobility-impaired activities, such as climbing stairs [19,20], the subjectivity in owner assessment always leads to a significant caregiver placebo effect [21].

As a comparison, humans affected by knee or hip OA can be assessed for their physical capacity according to specific objective exercises, such as the 6-min walk test, the stairs climbing test, the time up and go, and gait analysis [22–24]. Therefore, there is a need of performance-based objective outcome measures to better diagnose OA in cats.

Podobarometric gait analysis using a pressure-sensitive mattress has been evaluated in healthy dogs and cats [9,25] and for cats afflicted by OA [18,26]. Submitting cats to exercise before recording PVF and VI was previously reported to improve sensitivity and decrease inter-individual data variability of OA detection [27]. We kept this in mind while designing the innovative Path. Podobarometric analysis has been studied in the situation of jump reception but only in healthy cats [4]. Regarding the evaluation of cats with OA, to the best of authors' knowledge, this is the first report of forelimbs reception and hindlimbs propulsion when jumping down and up, respectively, in movement.

Focusing on Path, to test our first hypothesis, the data dispersion and reliability between both Baseline acquisition sessions were assessed with the coefficient of dispersion and ICC. At the last phase of the jump down, we observed that the cats landed on the right or left thoracic limb first, followed by landing on the pelvic limbs. This delay, however small, led to a higher value of the first limb touching on the ground, and it often changed from one trial to another. In consequence, each thoracic limb PVF presents greater variability between trials or between animals. To limit the data dispersion, the sum of both limbs was used. In both baseline acquisition sessions, the data uniformity was greater for the thoracic or pelvic PVF (sum) values (see the coefficients of dispersion values in Table 1). Additionally, PVF values were more repeatable than VI values. This could be due to the VI calculation; it is composed of two factors, i.e., the force and the time the limb is in contact with the ground. Adding a second variable could expose the data to a greater dispersion. Despite a larger inter-individual dispersion, we noted a decrease of the coefficient of dispersion for the pelvic VI values at the second Baseline acquisition session. This could be explained by a better understanding of the Path and so a decrease in variability in the duration of the limb support. This point is in concordance with the performance-based measure definition. It evaluates how an individual performs on a specific task, here the jump, and how the task is approached. It is therefore not aberrant to think that with the habituation, the jump was apprehended with a slight difference between both Baseline sessions.

A concordance plot was used to represent the agreement of both Baseline acquisition sessions for PVF data spread. Values of thoracic PVF (Figure 1A) were moderately different from the reference line (shift about 5 degrees) and the agreement between both sessions was good with a Spearman's ϱ of 0.80 and a $R^2 = 0.72$. Despite a larger spread of the pelvic PVF data ($R^2 = 0.67$), the regression curve (Figure 1B) was closest to the reference line and the correlation was as good as for the thoracic PVF data, with a Spearman's ϱ of 0.79.

Whether for PVF or VI, ICC were good to very good, except for a moderate ICC for the pelvic PVF values. The latter had more inter-trial and inter-individual variability than thoracic limbs values. It could be linked to the characteristics of our cat colony; they all are affected by the OA of at least one pelvic limb joint (most often, hip) or in the lumbo-sacral vertebral axis. Therefore, the biomechanical alterations of the OA degenerative process could lead to more influence on the pelvic than thoracic limbs. Further, thoracic limbs are passive and undergo the jump, unlike the pelvic limbs which generate a force necessary for the propulsion phase. This could explain why values from pelvic limbs were higher than thoracic limbs. Nevertheless, a recent study [28] revealed that elbow and hip joints are major contributors to energy absorption during landing in healthy cats. How the impact forces are dissipated during landing for OA cats remains to be determined.

As detailed in the literature many years ago [29] and even more recently [30,31], data normalization is relevant for dog podobarometric gait analysis. The effectiveness of the normalization process for OA cats was tested in the present study. Morphometric values (i.e., length, height), bodyweight, velocity, and time to completion were variables used in the normalization process. A slight but substantial decrease in the data dispersion of thoracic PVF was obtained by a normalizing with a ground to shoulders height. Globally, the cats with the longest shoulder height had higher PVF values. As expected [29], normalizing the pelvic PVF or VI values by bodyweight led to a decrease in the coefficient of dispersion. Normalizing simply by bodyweight does not account for the possible differences in muscular mass, bony structures, or body fat. The cat's flexibility, joint temporal, and spatial coordination, as well as the swing arm from the thoracic limbs, are also involved in the countermovement the cat executes for vertical jumping. All these factors would need to be further explored.

Therefore, the Path presented very good results for data dispersion and reliability, while normalization improved the inter-individual data variability. For the responsiveness to treatment, it is important to first highlight that the placebo group was remarkably stable within-time for all outcomes, and this helped to detect a treatment effect for the pooled treatment group. In the context of randomized controlled clinical trials, placebo responses are improvements documented in a negative control group (e.g., a group with no active intervention). The improvements can be real for the patient, such as those associated with regression-to-the-mean or a placebo by proxy ('better care") effect, or merely as perceived by the caregiver, such as those associated with a caregiver placebo effect, where the intense follow-up associated with a study can led to improved caregiver ratings on subjective measures or increased exchanges with the cat. In either case, real or perceived improvements in the negative control group can have a profound impact. Indeed, as previously reported on many occasions, using a subjective scale in naturally occurring OA-associated pain presented about 54 to 74% of success in cats receiving a placebo [19]. Significant within-time changes occurred in the pooled treatment group, regarding the velocity on the platform, the time to task completion, the PVF of both thoracic and pelvic limbs and the VI of thoracic limbs.

Treated cats moved faster on the platform, and they completed the task on the mattress, at the Treatment timepoint more rapidly than at Baseline. Importantly, thoracic PVF in the pooled treatment group was higher than in the placebo group at the same timepoint (after 15 days of treatment). This represents a real treatment effect. During the same timepoint, thoracic VI decreased compared to Baseline. This suggests that the OA cats were able to put more vertical force in the landing phase, while controlling it better over a shorter period of time. Finally, pelvic PVF increased compared to Baseline (close to statistical significance), suggesting the treated cats were able to put more force into propulsion.

The pooled treatment group presented a sustained beneficial effect at Recov-1, i.e., 4 days after stopping the treatment, for the velocity on the platform and the time to task completion (both were faster, compared to Baseline). The difference was no longer present at Recov-2, i.e., 3 weeks after stopping the treatment. At Recov-1, thoracic PVF was the most sensitive evaluation to detect the treatment withdrawal, as it was lower than Baseline, and apparent primarily in group A (highest dose of firocoxib). However, pelvic PVF remained higher than Baseline at Recov-1, and the effect persisted up to Recov-2.

Some dose-dependent effects were also detectable; the group A (highest dose) was the most sensitive to the treatment withdrawal (rebound effect?) and most beneficial changes observed in the pooled treatment group were attributable to group B (intermediate dose), whereas group C (lowest dose) had limited influence. Globally, the firocoxib-induced analgesia was reflected in each Path component, namely velocity on the platform and during the task on the mattress, as well as both jumping phases. Cats were able to increase their comfortable speed before jumping down, to jump with less joint impact but with more force, and to shorten their time to completion and to jump up with more propulsion force, all which reflect a better adaptability of the musculoskeletal system. Although studies have demonstrated that firocoxib improved the PVF of OA dogs [12], to our knowledge, this is the first publication supporting its efficacy in a feline OA pain complex task completion.

Although the number of stair steps climbed is impacted by chronic OA pain, no one to date has developed an objective count of stair compliance. We developed the Stairs task with the goal to monitor distance activity (number of steps up and down) and the velocity to realize the task (time up and down). The four minutes of assessment allowed us to distinguish different cat biomechanical alterations, and this delay was established after different trials to better engage the cats. Finally, to reflect about the possible fatigue felt by the OA cat completing the task, we proposed the finish line outcome.

In conjunction with positive enrichment, the Stairs task was successfully completed by 31 cats. Time up was the less reliable outcome measure, whereas, interestingly, steps up was more reliable. Cats were constant in the number of steps they climbed up but the time they spent to ascend changed. Overall, the inter-individual variability was higher for steps and time up than for steps and time down, possibly reflecting a higher panel of difficulty in climbing up than down in cat preferentially affected by hindlimb OA. The Stairs task is complex as many factors could affect the cat's willingness to climb the stairs up and down. Therefore, the inter-individual variability was expected to be high, and also for the same cat in different sessions. The normalization process led to a better inter-individual homogeneity. Morphometric measurements (i.e., height, length) and the bodyweight influenced the spread of the Stairs values. The length impacted the number of steps to climb up; body weight had influence on the time to go up (while it influenced the pelvic values in Path), and height influenced the time to go down (as it influenced the thoracic values in Path). However, the impact of these normalizations was limited.

The finish line was used to reduce the data dispersion by distinguishing cats as responders or not. A statistically significant and huge within-time treatment effect was detectable for the pooled treatment effect (both for up and down finish line), whereas the placebo group remained remarkably stable. The finish line up outcome revealed a real treatment effect at the Treatment period, when comparing pooled treatment and placebo groups. Moreover, the within-time improvement persisted over the recovery period. The model of analysis was not sensitive enough to detect a dose-dependent effect (type II error), but a clear trend was observable under Treatment for cats completing the finish line downwards. Cats receiving the high and intermediate doses were the cats completing more stairs passages. Regarding the effectiveness of this new "Stairs Finish Line" strategy, it will be particularly interesting to determine the median number of passages for healthy cats as a potent diagnosis tool for OA cats.

For the performance-based outcomes presented herein, the remaining inter-individual variability mostly involves the pelvic limbs. Focusing on the biomechanical aspect, the kinematic analysis of the pelvic limbs of healthy dogs during ascending and descending stairs revealed the range of motion for coxofemoral, femorotibial, and tibiotarsal joints [32,33]. Pelvic limb joints were more stressed during the climbing of stairs rather than during the descent. In contrast, the thoracic limb joints of healthy dogs seem more implicated during the descent than pelvic limb joints [34]. Interestingly, this is in concordance with the best Stairs data normalization process, meaning bodyweight influences the time taken to climb stairs and the height of thoracic limbs influences the time taken to descend. Furthermore, healthy old dogs have a decreased range of motion in all joints [35]. If we extrapolate the kinetic analysis obtained with dogs to the cats, we could say that cats solicit their pelvic limbs more to ascend stairs, and OA cats have diminished their range of motion in relation probably to their joint lesions (and age?). This could lead to an increase in variability concerning the time taken for cats to ascend stairs and the number of steps up. This is true in humans, in patients affected by OA, as they display a limited range of hip joint movement, particularly when they ascend stairs [36].

Even if we validated our hypothesis for both performance-based objective outcomes, further investigations are needed to obtain valid interpretation of the related results. The validation is based on a low degree of measurement error, either systematic (corresponding to the validity) or random (corresponding to the reliability) [37]. In other words, there are three levels for an instrument measure validation: construct precision, quantification precision, and translation precision [38]. Since OA influences the gait and the cat activity, PVF will be lowest for the most affected pelvic limb(s) and the number of steps climbed will decrease while the time taken to climb increases. Moreover, bodyweight will negatively affect pelvic activities (jumping up, Stairs time up), height will influence thoracic activities (jumping down, and Stairs time down), and length of the cat will affect the number of Stairs for steps up. This information leads to the construct precision. The quantification precision is based on the reliability, which was moderate to excellent for the Path and fair to good for Stairs. It still remains to determine the translation precision by assessing healthy cats in our innovative Path and Stairs to clearly determine the difference of activity compared to cats with OA. Our study has some limitations, described as follows: due to the sample size and the multi-joint conditions of each cat, we focused on a global assessment instead of clustering them according to their affected joints. We presented two novel functional assessments, and we are aware that analyses could be refined with a distinction in groups of activity according to the joint(s) affected by OA, the magnitude of the impairment or the body condition score. Additionally, considering the importance of central sensitization during the OA chronic pain progression, the degree of nociceptive sensitization affecting OA cats could be taken into consideration in order to favor individual mechanistic-based treatment care.

Both complex behavioral Path and Stairs tasks would need to be optimized in the future. For example, the jumping up was defined at a height of 44 cm, which was easily performed by OA cats. In contrast, a jump of 100 cm was achieved by healthy cats, as reported [4,16]. The healthy cats used the flexibility of their backs to absorb kinetic energy with higher height, but the ground reaction forces increased with the jump height [39,40]. It could be interesting to see the impact of different jump heights on OA cats.

In a world of possibilities, combining the Path and Stairs tasks could be of great interest. With a fixed number of stairs passages, the velocity, time to completion, and PVF would be recorded for each passage of the staircase. This could highlight a possible correlation between the fatigue (i.e., the number of steps climbed), the mechanical forces produced at each passage and the cat's motivation.

These new outcomes, Path and Stairs, are promising performance-based outcome measures to discriminate the dose effect of OA therapy in cats. Furthermore, the Stairs assessment requires little equipment, presents an apparent huge amplitude in analgesic responsiveness (which is a major advantage in testing new analgesic efficacy), could be optimized in the future, and even implemented in a clinic or in the cat owner's home.

4. Materials and Methods

4.1. Animal and Housing

The study was approved by the Institutional Animal Care and Use Committee (#A176-BIA19F and #CEUA-Rech-1832). All cat care and handling adhered to the Canadian Council on Animal Care's guidelines. Adult neutered geriatric (5.5–12.5 y) cats ($n = 32$; $n = 16$ females and $n = 16$ males) were selected based on radiographic evidence of naturally occurring OA. Hence, a radiographic screening was performed under sedation for thoracic (carpus, elbow, shoulder) and pelvic (tarsus, stifle, hip) limbs, including lumbo-sacral vertebral axis, with all requested views to confirm the diagnosis of radiographic OA. All X-rays were reviewed and scored, independently and blindly, by a Diplomate of the American College of Veterinary Surgeons (B.L.). The radiographic score corresponds to the summation of the scores (0–5) of the twelve joints evaluated. To be selected, a cat had to present some radiographic alterations (i.e., presence of osteophytes and/or subchondral sclerosis or cysts) in at least one appendicular joint to be designated as having OA. Lesions, such as meniscal mineralization or enthesiophytes, had to be associated with osteophytes and/or subchondral alteration to be radiographically significant.

Included cats were healthy (excepted the OA diagnosis) according to a physical exam and the absence of clinical and pathological findings. They were also selected based on their behavioral compliance. The cat's characteristics (name, sex, age, number of joints affected, radiographic and body condition scores) are presented in Appendix A. Cats were part of a colony, they were group-housed in lighting-, temperature-, and humidity-controlled rooms which contained environmental enrichment (perches, covered and uncovered beds, scratching posts, and toys). Cats were fed twice daily with commercial foods according to the manufacturer's recommendations. Fresh water was available ad libitum. Four weeks before the beginning of the experiment, cats were free of any treatment, including natural health products or veterinary diets purported to relief or ease the clinical signs of OA.

The following morphometric measurements (centimeters) were recorded for each cat: heights (ground to shoulders, ground to elbow, and ground to half of the forearm); and length (chest to croup). Cats were also weighed (kg) before each data acquisition session.

4.2. Treatment and Study Design

Cats were randomly distributed into four groups according to the firocoxib dose (Group A: 0.40, B: 0.25, C: 0.15 and D: 0.00 mg/kg bodyweight SID). The pooled treatment group refers to groups A, B, and C, whereas the placebo group corresponds to group D alone.

After acclimation over five weeks, cats were evaluated for three consecutive 3-week periods, i.e., twice during the baseline period for Path and Stairs, once for Path and Stairs during the treatment period with daily oral administration, and twice for Path and once for Stairs during the recovery (Recov-1 and Recov-2) period. Cats were continuously assessed by two registered veterinary technicians under the supervision of one registered doctor in veterinary medicine.

4.3. Effort Path

As depicted in Figure 4, the Path consisted of a custom-made initial walking ramp (427 cm long; 50 cm wide; and 100 cm high), a jump down of 56 cm, a walk over a pressure-sensitive mattress (176 cm long; 37 cm wide (Tekscan Inc, Boston, MA, USA)) and finally, a jump up of 44 cm on a second ramp. The Path was enclosed by transparent plexiglass screens to make sure the cat moved naturally and undisturbed. When the cat contacted on the pressure-sensitive mattress, a podobarometric gait analysis was performed at a resolution of 1.4 sensels/cm^2. The calibration of the pressure-sensitive mattress was carried out at the beginning of the study according to the manufacturer's recommendations.

Twice a week for five weeks, cats were conditioned to move freely at a comfortable velocity (average of 1.5 meters (m)/second (s)) across the Path using positive reinforcement (treats, petting, toys) during or at completion of the path.

Three to five trials were obtained for each cat. The first three valid trials (assessed after the experiment) were selected, and then averaged to characterize the gait profile for that session. A trial was considered as valid when a cat moved with regular and sufficient speed and in a straight direction with a good recording of ground reaction forces. We estimated a total per assessment test of 10 to 12 passages before collecting these three trials, and the maximum number of passages allowed for each session was 16. The timepoints of assessment for Path were Day −20 and Day −6 for Baseline, Day 15 for Treatment, Day 24 for Recov-1, and Day 36 for Recov-2.

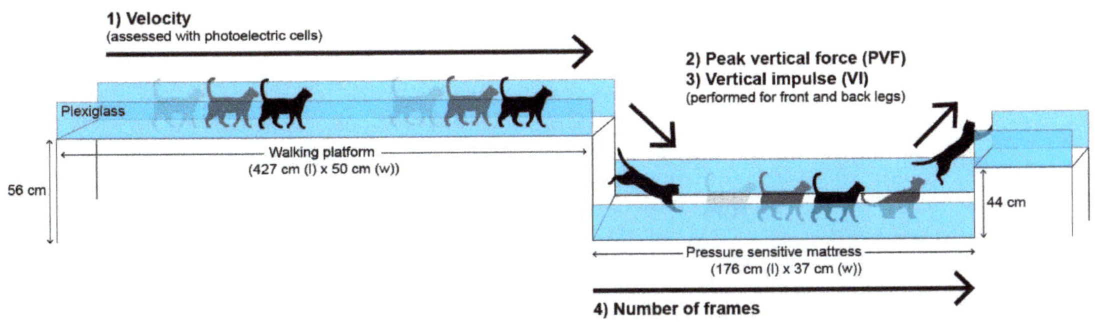

Figure 4. Illustration of the Effort Path. The cats walked/trotted across the walking ramp, jumped down onto a pressure-sensitive mattress and jumped up onto a raised ramp. Measurements were: (1) velocity (speed of movement across the walking platform), (2) peak vertical force (PVF), (3) vertical impulse (VI) as cats jumped down and up from the pressure sensitive mattress, and (4) the number of frames (reflecting the time to passing the pressure sensitive mattress). The entire path was enclosed by transparent plexiglass to allow cats to move naturally and undisturbed. The cats were positively motivated by rewards provided at the end of the Effort Path.

Performance-Based Outcome Measures for the Effort Path

The cat's velocity on the platform was monitored using a set of three photoelectric cells (LACIME; École de Technologie Supérieure, Montréal, QC, Canada). The velocity was expressed in meters per second (m/s).

Peak vertical force and vertical impulse were recorded for both thoracic limbs when the cats hit the pressure-sensitive mattress and for both pelvic limbs when jumping up on the second ramp. The thoracic or pelvic PVF and VI were expressed in kg and kg*s, respectively.

The number of frames between the first hit of the thoracic limb on the pressure-sensitive mattress until the last pelvic limb leaves the mattress was recorded. It corresponds to the time passing over the pressure sensitive mattress, i.e., the time of the task completion. Each frame was equal to 0.02 s.

4.4. Stairs Assay Compliance

The Stairs was performed using a staircase of 16 steps (step height of 20 cm). Once a week for five weeks, cats were conditioned (clicker) to climb up and down the stair using positive reinforcement (treats, petting, toys) at the top and at the bottom of the staircase. During a four-minute period, cats were encouraged to do the maximum number of up and down steps they were able to do. The timepoints of assessment for Stairs were Day −18 and Day −4 for Baseline, Day 17 for Treatment, and Day 38 for Recov-2.

Performance-Based Outcome Measures for the SAC

The number of steps reached up and down, and the time (seconds) to ascend and descend the staircase were recorded for each assay during the four-minute period. During both baseline assessments, the median value of completed up and down passages for the population sample ($n = 31$) was calculated to be 7. The number of cats (percentage) in each group crossing this "finish-line" of 7 was assessed at each subsequent timepoint.

4.5. Statistical Analysis

For each outcome measures, the mean (Min–Max) was presented as a measure of central tendency and the interval was representative of the dispersion of the data. In addition, the coefficient of dispersion was used to evaluate the dispersion of the data [10] using the formula (1):

$$\frac{\sum|xi - Median| / Sample\ size}{Median} \tag{1}$$

For the Path inter-trials coefficient of dispersion, xi was the value recorded for each trial. For the inter-individual coefficient of dispersion, xi was the mean of the three valid trials recorded. The coefficient of dispersion was expressed in percentage (%).

A process of normalization was undertaken as a potent strategy to reduce the dispersion of the data for both performance-based outcome measures using the following variables: body weight; cats' height and length; and velocity and number of frames (only for the Path). The normalization resulted in the original data divided by the selected variable. The potential of the normalized outcomes to reduce the data dispersion was evaluated with the coefficient of dispersion. Both Baseline acquisition sessions were combined, resulting in n = 64 cats for Path and n = 58 cats for Stairs.

The agreement between both Baseline acquisition sessions was determined according to a concordance plot and the Spearman's ϱ coefficient of correlation. The degree of reliability between measurements obtained at each session was determined using the intraclass coefficient correlation (ICC) index. The ICC index was interpreted as follows, >0.81 very good, >0.61 good, >0.41 moderate, >0.21 fair, and <0.20 poor reliability [41].

The treatment effect assessed was analyzed using a linear mixed model with time (i.e., timepoints), treatment groups, and their interaction as fixed factors. Trials were included as repeated factors. Univariate analysis was presented followed by post-hoc analysis when a statistically significant difference was observed between fixed factors. For Stairs, the finish line was analyzed using inferential analysis, Fisher test, or χ^2 test, depending on the sample size.

5. Conclusions

Our study described for the first time two innovative performance-based objective outcome measures with only few acclimations in OA cats. The Path and Stairs are reliable and sensitive measurements of biomechanical alterations in OA cats. Firocoxib induced an improvement in all phases of jumping, from the velocity to the propulsion for the second ramp. The stable within-time evolution of the placebo group favored the detection of studied firocoxib therapeutic effect. The response to treatment for Group B (intermediate dose) was most apparent during the treatment and recovery periods, while for group A (high dose) the response to treatment was detected after treatment withdrawal (on Path at Recov-1). Refinement in linking OA severity to analgesic responsiveness is necessary to systematically determine a dose-dependent effect. The Path and Stairs are promising outcomes to better diagnose feline OA pain and precisely detect analgesic efficacy.

Author Contributions: Conceptualization, M.M., M.D., J.-P.P., J.M.-P., B.L., and E.T.; Methodology: M.M., C.O., B.L., J.d.C., and E.T.; Validation, C.O., M.M., B.L., and E.T.; Formal analysis, A.D., M.M., C.O., M.D., J.d.C., and E.T.; Investigation, A.D., M.F., and M.M.; Resources, J.-P.P., J.M.-P., B.L., and E.T.; Data curation, A.D., C.O., M.F., and E.T.; Writing—original draft preparation, A.D., M.M., and E.T.; Writing—review and editing, A.D., M.M., C.O., M.F., M.D., J.-P.P., J.M.-P., B.L., J.d.C., and E.T.; Visualization, A.D.; Supervision, C.O., J.-P.P., J.M.-P., B.L., J.d.C., and E.T.; Project administration, M.M., J.-P.P., and E.T.; Funding acquisition, J.-P.P., J.M.-P., and E.T. All authors have read and agreed to the published version of the manuscript.

Funding: This research was funded by an operational grant of Boehringer Ingelheim Animal Health, Inc. The GREPAQ is supported by discovery grants (RGPIN #441651-2013 and #05512-2020; E.T.) for salaries, and a Collaborative Research and Development grant (RDCPJ #491953–2016; E.T.) supporting operations and salaries, from the Natural Sciences and Engineering Research Council (NSERC) of Canada, as well as by an ongoing New Opportunities Fund grant (#9483; E.T.), a Leader Opportunity Fund grant (#24601; E.T.), supporting pain/function equipment from the Canada Foundation for Innovation, and the Chair in Osteoarthritis of the Université de Montréal (J.-P.P. and J.M.-P.). C.O. was the recipient of a MITACS Canada Postdoctoral Fellowship Elevation (IT #11643).

Institutional Review Board Statement: The study was conducted in accordance with the Declaration of Helsinki and approved by two institutional committees: the Animal Care and Use Committee of the Université de Montréal (protocol no CEUA-Rech-1832, date of approval 15 November 2019) and the ArthroLab Inc. (Montréal, QC H2L 1S6, Canada) Ethical Committee (protocol no A176-BIA19F, date of approval 03 November 2019). Cats were housed in ArthroLab Inc., their cares and handling adhered to the Canadian Council on Animal Care's guidelines.

Informed Consent Statement: Not applicable.

Acknowledgments: The authors thank all the cats of the study and the personnel of ArthroLab Inc. for their technical assistance and tender loving care to the cat colony. A special thanks to Vivian S.Y. Leung for the graphism support.

Conflicts of Interest: The authors declare no conflict of interest. M.D. is a regular employee of Boehringer Ingelheim Animal health, Inc.; M.M. is regular employee of ArthroLab Inc.

Appendix A

Table A1. Characteristics of the 32 cats included in the study.

Cat ID	Sex	Age	Radiographic Score	Number of Joint Affected	Body Condition Score
F-001	F	7.5	8	2	5
F-002	M	6.5	1	1	5
F-003	M	9.5	6	4	4
F-004	F	9	2	2	5
F-006	M	10.5	5	5	5
F-008	M	6.5	2	1	6
F-025	F	9.5	6	2	6
F-010	F	10	3	2	5
F-027	F	8.5	6	6	5
F-028	M	12.5	6	2	5
F-029	M	9.5	2	2	5
F-030	M	7.5	13	6	6
F-011	M	5.5	2	2	5
F-012	M	8.5	7	3	5
F-035	M	10.5	8	2	6
F-013	F	8.5	8	2	6
F-014	F	7.5	8	2	5
F-036	F	11.5	7	7	6
F-037	F	9.5	15	6	6
F-015	F	11.5	9	5	5
F-016	F	8.5	3	3	6
F-017	M	10.5	6	2	5
F-020	F	6.5	8	2	8
F-039	M	8.5	3	3	5
F-041	F	8.5	4	3	5
F-042	M	7	3	3	4
F-043	M	7	2	2	5
F-044	M	8.5	6	2	7
F-045	F	6.5	7	3	7
F-046	F	9.5	6	4	5
F-047	F	10.5	4	4	5
F-024	M	9.5	8	3	6

The radiographic score corresponds to the sum of each joint score, for a total of twelve joints evaluated (from 0 to 5). The body condition score was assessed using a 1 to 9 scale. F = Female, M = Male.

References

1. Nielsen, L.M.; Kirkegaard, H.; Østergaard, L.G.; Bovbjerg, K.; Breinholt, K.; Maribo, T. Comparison of self-reported and performance-based measures of functional ability in elderly patients in an emergency department: Implications for selection of clinical outcome measures. *BMC Geriatr.* **2016**, *16*, 199. [CrossRef] [PubMed]
2. Dobson, F.; Hinman, R.S.; Roos, E.M.; Abbott, J.H.; Stratford, P.; Davis, A.M.; Buchbinder, R.; Snyder-Mackler, L.; Henrotin, Y.; Thumboo, J.; et al. OARSI recommended performance-based tests to assess physical function in people diagnosed with hip or knee osteoarthritis. *Osteoarthr. Cartil.* **2013**, *21*, 1042–1052. [CrossRef] [PubMed]
3. Guedes, A.G.P.; Meadows, J.M.; Pypendop, B.H.; Johnson, E.G.; Zaffarano, B. Assessment of the effects of gabapentin on activity levels and owner-perceived mobility impairment and quality of life in osteoarthritic geriatric cats. *J. Am. Vet. Med. Assoc.* **2018**, *253*, 579–585. [CrossRef] [PubMed]
4. Stadig, S.M.; Bergh, A.K. Gait and jump analysis in healthy cats using a pressure mat system. *J. Feline Med. Surg.* **2015**, *17*, 523–529. [CrossRef]
5. Shipley, H.; Flynn, K.; Tucker, L.; Wendt-Hornickle, E.; Baldo, C.; Almeida, D.; Allweiler, S.; Guedes, A. Owner evaluation of quality of life and mobility in osteoarthritic cats treated with amantadine or placebo. *J. Feline Med. Surg.* **2021**, *23*, 568–574. [CrossRef]
6. Sharon, K.P.; Thompson, C.M.; Lascelles, B.D.X.; Parrish, R.S. Novel use of an activity monitor to model jumping behaviors in cats. *Am. J. Vet. Res.* **2020**, *81*, 334–343. [CrossRef]
7. Yamazaki, A.; Edamura, K.; Tanegashima, K.; Tomo, Y.; Yamamoto, M.; Hirao, H.; Seki, M.; Asano, K. Utility of a novel activity monitor assessing physical activities and sleep quality in cats. *PLoS ONE* **2020**, *15*, e0236795. [CrossRef]
8. Moreau, M.; Lussier, B.; Ballaz, L.; Troncy, E. Kinetic measurements of gait for osteoarthritis research in dogs and cats. *Can. Vet. J.* **2014**, *55*, 1057–1065.
9. Schnabl, E.; Bockstahler, B. Systematic review of ground reaction force measurements in cats. *Vet. J.* **2015**, *206*, 83–90. [CrossRef]
10. Monteiro, B.P.; Otis, C.; del Castillo, J.R.E.; Nitulescu, R.; Brown, K.; Arendt-Nielsen, L.; Troncy, E. Quantitative sensory testing in feline osteoarthritic pain—A systematic review and meta-analysis. *Osteoarthr. Cartil.* **2020**, *28*, 885–896. [CrossRef]
11. Pollmeier, M.; Toulemonde, C.; Fleishman, C.; Hanson, P.D. Clinical evaluation of firocoxib and carprofen for the treatment of dogs with osteoarthritis. *Vet. Rec.* **2006**, *159*, 547–551. [CrossRef] [PubMed]
12. Vijarnsorn, M.; Kwananocha, I.; Kashemsant, N.; Jarudecha, T.; Lekcharoensuk, C.; Beale, B.; Peirone, B.; Lascelles, B.D.X. The effectiveness of marine based fatty acid compound (PCSO-524) and firocoxib in the treatment of canine osteoarthritis. *BMC Vet. Res.* **2019**, *15*, 349. [CrossRef] [PubMed]
13. Adrian, D.; King, J.N.; Parrish, R.S.; King, S.B.; Budsberg, S.C.; Gruen, M.E.; Lascelles, B.D.X. Robenacoxib shows efficacy for the treatment of chronic degenerative joint disease-associated pain in cats: A randomized and blinded pilot clinical trial. *Sci. Rep.* **2021**, *11*, 7721. [CrossRef] [PubMed]
14. McCann, M.E.; Rickes, E.L.; Hora, D.F.; Cunningham, P.K.; Zhang, D.; Brideau, C.; Black, W.C.; Hickey, G.J. In vitro effects and in vivo efficacy of a novel cyclooxygenase-2 inhibitor in cats with lipopolysaccharide-induced pyrexia. *Am. J. Vet. Res.* **2005**, *66*, 1278–1284. [CrossRef]
15. Slingerland, L.I.; Hazewinkel, H.A.; Meij, B.P.; Picavet, P.; Voorhout, G. Cross-sectional study of the prevalence and clinical features of osteoarthritis in 100 cats. *Vet. J.* **2011**, *187*, 304–309. [CrossRef]
16. Lascelles, B.D.; Henry, J.B., 3rd; Brown, J.; Robertson, I.; Sumrell, A.T.; Simpson, W.; Wheeler, S.; Hansen, B.D.; Zamprogno, H.; Freire, M.; et al. Cross-sectional study of the prevalence of radiographic degenerative joint disease in domesticated cats. *Vet. Surg.* **2010**, *39*, 535–544. [CrossRef]
17. Bennett, D.; Zainal Ariffin, S.M.; Johnston, P. Osteoarthritis in the cat: 1. how common is it and how easy to recognise? *J. Feline Med. Surg.* **2012**, *14*, 65–75. [CrossRef]
18. Guillot, M.; Moreau, M.; d'Anjou, M.A.; Martel-Pelletier, J.; Pelletier, J.P.; Troncy, E. Evaluation of osteoarthritis in cats: Novel information from a pilot study. *Vet. Surg.* **2012**, *41*, 328–335. [CrossRef]
19. Zamprogno, H.; Hansen, B.D.; Bondell, H.D.; Sumrell, A.T.; Simpson, W.; Robertson, I.D.; Brown, J.; Pease, A.P.; Roe, S.C.; Hardie, E.M.; et al. Item generation and design testing of a questionnaire to assess degenerative joint disease-associated pain in cats. *Am. J. Vet. Res.* **2010**, *71*, 1417–1424. [CrossRef]
20. Enomoto, M.; Lascelles, B.D.X.; Gruen, M.E. Development of a checklist for the detection of degenerative joint disease-associated pain in cats. *J. Feline Med. Surg.* **2020**, *22*, 1137–1147. [CrossRef]
21. Gruen, M.E.; Dorman, D.C.; Lascelles, B.D.X. Caregiver placebo effect in analgesic clinical trials for cats with naturally occurring degenerative joint disease-associated pain. *Vet. Rec.* **2017**, *180*, 473. [CrossRef] [PubMed]
22. Zeni, J., Jr.; Abujaber, S.; Pozzi, F.; Raisis, L. Relationship between strength, pain, and different measures of functional ability in patients with end-stage hip osteoarthritis. *Arthritis Care Res.* **2014**, *66*, 1506–1512. [CrossRef] [PubMed]
23. Nur, H.; Sertkaya, B.S.; Tuncer, T. Determinants of physical functioning in women with knee osteoarthritis. *Aging Clin. Exp. Res.* **2018**, *30*, 299–306. [CrossRef] [PubMed]
24. Kim, W.B.; Kim, B.R.; Kim, S.R.; Han, E.Y.; Nam, K.W.; Lee, S.Y.; Ji, S.M.; Kim, J.H. Comorbidities in Patients With End-Stage Knee OA: Prevalence and Effect on Physical Function. *Arch. Phys. Med. Rehabil.* **2019**, *100*, 2063–2070. [CrossRef] [PubMed]
25. Kano, W.T.; Rahal, S.C.; Agostinho, F.S.; Mesquita, L.R.; Santos, R.R.; Monteiro, F.O.; Castilho, M.S.; Melchert, A. Kinetic and temporospatial gait parameters in a heterogeneous group of dogs. *BMC Vet. Res.* **2016**, *12*, 2. [CrossRef] [PubMed]

26. Guillot, M.; Moreau, M.; Heit, M.; Martel-Pelletier, J.; Pelletier, J.P.; Troncy, E. Characterization of osteoarthritis in cats and meloxicam efficacy using objective chronic pain evaluation tools. *Vet. J.* **2013**, *196*, 360–367. [CrossRef] [PubMed]
27. Moreau, M.; Guillot, M.; Pelletier, J.P.; Martel-Pelletier, J.; Troncy, E. Kinetic peak vertical force measurement in cats afflicted by coxarthritis: Data management and acquisition protocols. *Res. Vet. Sci.* **2013**, *95*, 219–224. [CrossRef]
28. Wu, X.; Pei, B.; Pei, Y.; Wu, N.; Zhou, K.; Hao, Y.; Wang, W. Contributions of Limb Joints to Energy Absorption during Landing in Cats. *Appl. Bionics Biomech.* **2019**, *2019*, 3815612. [CrossRef]
29. Budsberg, S.C.; Verstraete, M.C.; Soutas-Little, R.W. Force plate analysis of the walking gait in healthy dogs. *Am. J. Vet. Res.* **1987**, *48*, 915–918.
30. Della Valle, G.; Caterino, C.; Aragosa, F.; Balestriere, C.; Piscitelli, A.; Di Palma, C.; Pasolini, M.P.; Fatone, G. Relationship between Ground Reaction Forces and Morpho- Metric Measures in Two Different Canine Phenotypes Using Regression Analysis. *Vet. Sci.* **2022**, *9*, 325. [CrossRef]
31. Conzemius, M.G.; Torres, B.T.; Muir, P.; Evans, R.; Krotscheck, U.; Budsberg, S. Best practices for measuring and reporting ground reaction forces in dogs. *Vet. Surg.* **2022**, *51*, 385–396. [CrossRef] [PubMed]
32. Durant, A.M.; Millis, D.L.; Headrick, J.F. Kinematics of stair ascent in healthy dogs. *Vet. Comp. Orthop. Traumatol.* **2011**, *24*, 99–105. [CrossRef] [PubMed]
33. Millard, R.P.; Headrick, J.F.; Millis, D.L. Kinematic analysis of the pelvic limbs of healthy dogs during stair and decline slope walking. *J. Small Anim. Pract.* **2010**, *51*, 419–422. [CrossRef] [PubMed]
34. Kopec, N.L.; Williams, J.M.; Tabor, G.F. Kinematic analysis of the thoracic limb of healthy dogs during descending stair and ramp exercises. *Am. J. Vet. Res.* **2018**, *79*, 33–41. [CrossRef] [PubMed]
35. Lorke, M.; Willen, M.; Lucas, K.; Beyerbach, M.; Wefstaedt, P.; Murua Escobar, H.; Nolte, I. Comparative kinematic gait analysis in young and old Beagle dogs. *J. Vet. Sci.* **2017**, *18*, 521–530. [CrossRef]
36. Hall, M.; Wrigley, T.V.; Kean, C.O.; Metcalf, B.R.; Bennell, K.L. Hip biomechanics during stair ascent and descent in people with and without hip osteoarthritis. *J. Orthop. Res.* **2017**, *35*, 1505–1514. [CrossRef]
37. Higgins, P.A.; Straub, A.J. Understanding the error of our ways: Mapping the concepts of validity and reliability. *Nurs. Outlook* **2006**, *54*, 23–29. [CrossRef]
38. Kelly, P.A.; O'Malley, K.J.; Kallen, M.A.; Ford, M.E. Integrating validity theory with use of measurement instruments in clinical settings. *Health Serv. Res.* **2005**, *40*, 1605–1619. [CrossRef]
39. Zhang, Z.; Yang, J.; Yu, H. Effect of Flexible Back on Energy Absorption during Landing in Cats: A Biomechanical Investigation. *J. Bionic Eng.* **2014**, *11*, 506–516. [CrossRef]
40. Wang, M.; Song, Y.; Valentin, S.; Baker, J.S.; Gu, Y. Kinetic analysis of felines landing from different heights. *PeerJ* **2019**, *7*, e8007. [CrossRef]
41. Oliver, V.; De Rantere, D.; Ritchie, R.; Chisholm, J.; Hecker, K.G.; Pang, D.S. Psychometric assessment of the Rat Grimace Scale and development of an analgesic intervention score. *PLoS ONE* **2014**, *9*, e97882. [CrossRef] [PubMed]

International Journal of
Molecular Sciences

MDPI

Article

Inhibition of TREM-2 Markedly Suppresses Joint Inflammation and Damage in Experimental Arthritis

Alexander B. Sigalov

SignaBlok, Inc., P.O. Box 4064, Shrewsbury, MA 01545, USA; sigalov@signablok.com; Tel.: +1-203-505-3807

Abstract: The triggering receptors expressed on myeloid cells (TREMs) are a family of activating immune receptors that regulate the inflammatory response. TREM-1, which is expressed on monocytes and/or macrophages and neutrophils, functions as an inflammation amplifier and plays a role in the pathogenesis of rheumatoid arthritis (RA). Unlike TREM-1, the role in RA of TREM-2, which is expressed on macrophages, immature monocyte-derived dendritic cells, osteoclasts, and microglia, remains unclear and controversial. TREM-2 ligands are still unknown, adding further uncertainty to our understanding of TREM-2 function. Previously, we demonstrated that TREM-1 blockade, using a ligand-independent TREM-1 inhibitory peptide sequence GF9 rationally designed by our signaling chain homooligomerization (SCHOOL) model of cell signaling, ameliorates collagen-induced arthritis (CIA) severity in mice. Here, we designed a TREM-2 inhibitory peptide sequence IA9 and tested it in the therapeutic CIA model, either as a free 9-mer peptide IA9, or as a part of a 31-mer peptide IA31 incorporated into lipopeptide complexes (IA31-LPC), for targeted delivery. We demonstrated that administration of IA9, but not a control peptide, after induction of arthritis diminished release of proinflammatory cytokines and dramatically suppressed joint inflammation and damage, suggesting that targeting TREM-2 may be a promising approach for the treatment of RA.

Keywords: triggering receptors expressed on myeloid cells; TREM-1; TREM-2; inflammation; innate immunity; signal transduction; macrophages; cytokines; nanomedicine; drug delivery systems; rheumatoid arthritis

Citation: Sigalov, A.B. Inhibition of TREM-2 Markedly Suppresses Joint Inflammation and Damage in Experimental Arthritis. *Int. J. Mol. Sci.* **2022**, *23*, 8857. https://doi.org/10.3390/ijms23168857

Academic Editor: Chih-Hsin Tang

Received: 25 July 2022
Accepted: 7 August 2022
Published: 9 August 2022

1. Introduction

Rheumatoid arthritis (RA) is an autoimmune and inflammatory disease that affects 0.24–1% of the world population [1,2]. Uncontrolled joint inflammation in RA results in cartilage damage and bone destruction and, eventually, in disability [3]. Life expectancy of patients with RA is reduced by 3–18 years [4] and 80% of RA patients are disabled after 20 years [5]. Despite recent advances [1,6,7], there is no cure for RA yet and 30–50% of RA patients do not respond, or respond poorly, to the first-line standard treatments [8,9], and, among those who respond, 50% relapse shortly after treatment cessation [9], showing an urgent need for new therapies.

Myeloid cells, including macrophages, play a central role in the pathogenesis of RA [10,11]. The abundance and activation of macrophages in the inflamed synovial membrane have been demonstrated to significantly correlate with the severity of RA [10,12,13]. Only those therapies that reduce the number of synovial sublining macrophages are likely to be clinically meaningful [14]. Proinflammatory cytokines, such as tumor necrosis factor-α (TNFα), interleukin-1 (IL-1), and IL-6, as well as macrophage colony-stimulating factor (M-CSF, also known as CSF-1) are involved in macrophage development, activation, growth, and differentiation, representing promising targets in RA [15]. Blocking IL-6 is known to decrease the number of osteoclasts [16] and inhibit joint damage in collagen-induced arthritis (CIA) [17], as well as in human RA [18]. Several biologics that block specific cytokines were approved to treat RA, including blockers of TNFα (e.g., Humira®) and Remicade®) and IL-1 receptor (Kineret®). Due to excessive immunosuppression, the use of these and similar agents can cause fatal infections, malignancies and septic arthritis [19–21]. In RA patients with a high baseline TNF, a higher dose of Remicade® is necessary, whereas lower doses are sufficient for those with a low baseline TNF [22,23], leading to the critical need for personalization [24]. This further outlines an immediate need for efficient, safe and well-tolerable RA therapy. Importantly, targeted delivery, such as therapy to myeloid cells of interest (e.g., macrophages) would not only strike the cells that mediate or amplify most of the permanent tissue destruction but also spare other cells that do not affect joint damage [13,25].

Triggering receptors expressed by myeloid cells 1 and 2 (TREM-1 and TREM-2, respectively) are involved in inflammation and activate myeloid cells through their signaling partner, DAP-12 [26]. TREM-1, which is expressed on monocytes, macrophages and neutrophils, mediates release of TNFα, IL-1β, IL-6, and CSF-1 [27,28], and is highly upregulated in the synovium of RA patients [27]. In experimental arthritis, therapeutic inhibition of TREM-1 ameliorates disease [29,30] and, importantly, can blunt excessive inflammation without affecting pathogen clearance [31]. Certain macrophages and neutrophils express both TREM-1 and TREM-2, whereas dendritic cells, osteoclasts, and microglia exhibit predominant expression of TREM-2 [26]. While the detrimental role of TREM-1 in inflammatory diseases, including RA, has been well established in most studies [32], that of TREM-2 has been largely controversial. Contrarily to TREM-1, that acts as an inflammation amplifier, TREM-2 has been shown to act either as a negative [33–38] or positive [39–42] regulator of inflammation in various inflammatory diseases.

High upregulation of TREM-2 in active RA synovium and its subsequent downregulation in inactive RA suggest a role of TREM-2 in RA-induced inflammation [43]. TREM-2 has been shown to be upregulated in the synovial tissue of rats with CIA [44]. However, to the author's knowledge, no studies have yet investigated the effect of inhibition of TREM-2 in experimental arthritis.

Similarly to TREM-1, numerous molecules were proposed as potential ligand(s) for TREM-2, ranging from various anionic molecules, such as phospholipids and proteoglycans, to apolipoproteins (apos) and heat shock proteins [45]. This suggests that the actual nature of the TREM-2 ligand(s) and mechanisms of TREM-2 signaling are still not yet well understood, impeding the development of clinically relevant inhibitors of TREM-2.

In the present study, we used the basic molecular principles of the signaling chain homooligomerization (SCHOOL) model of multichain immune recognition receptor (MIRR)-mediated cell signaling [46–48] to rationally design the peptide sequence IA9 for inhibition of TREM-2, a member of the MIRR family (Figure 1A). This nonapeptide employs a novel, ligand-independent mechanism of inhibition and can reach its site of action in the cell membrane from both outside and inside the cell (Figure 1B). As for other ligand-independent peptide inhibitors of various cell receptors (SCHOOL peptides) [48], this mechanism of action not only overcomes the uncertainty of TREM-2 ligand(s), but also allows the use of IA9, either in the form of free peptide, to target TREM-2 on virtually all TREM-2-expressing cells (Figure 1A, Route 1), or formulated into self-assembling lipopeptide complexes (LPC) that mimic human high density lipoproteins (HDL) for targeted intracellular delivery of IA9 to macrophages (Figure 1A, Route 2). To formulate IA9 sequence-containing LPC, we applied a strategy similar to that previously used to design targeted TREM-1 peptide therapy for arthritis [30] and combined the TREM-2 inhibitory peptide sequence IA9 with the 22 amino acid residues long peptide sequence of the apo A-I helix 6 (PA22) (Figure 1C). The resulting peptide IA31 interacts with lipids forming nanosized LPC (IA31-LPC). Due to a sulfoxidized methionine residue in the PA22 domain, these LPC provide targeted delivery of IA31 to cells (e.g., macrophages) via interaction with scavenger receptors (e.g., type A scavenger receptor, SR-A, most abundantly expressed on macrophages [49]) (Figure 1C). Interestingly, SR-A plays a role in excessive synovial osteoclastogenesis, a hallmark of RA [50]. SR-A is mainly involved in an early phase of this process and its level of expression declines during osteoclast differentiation [51].

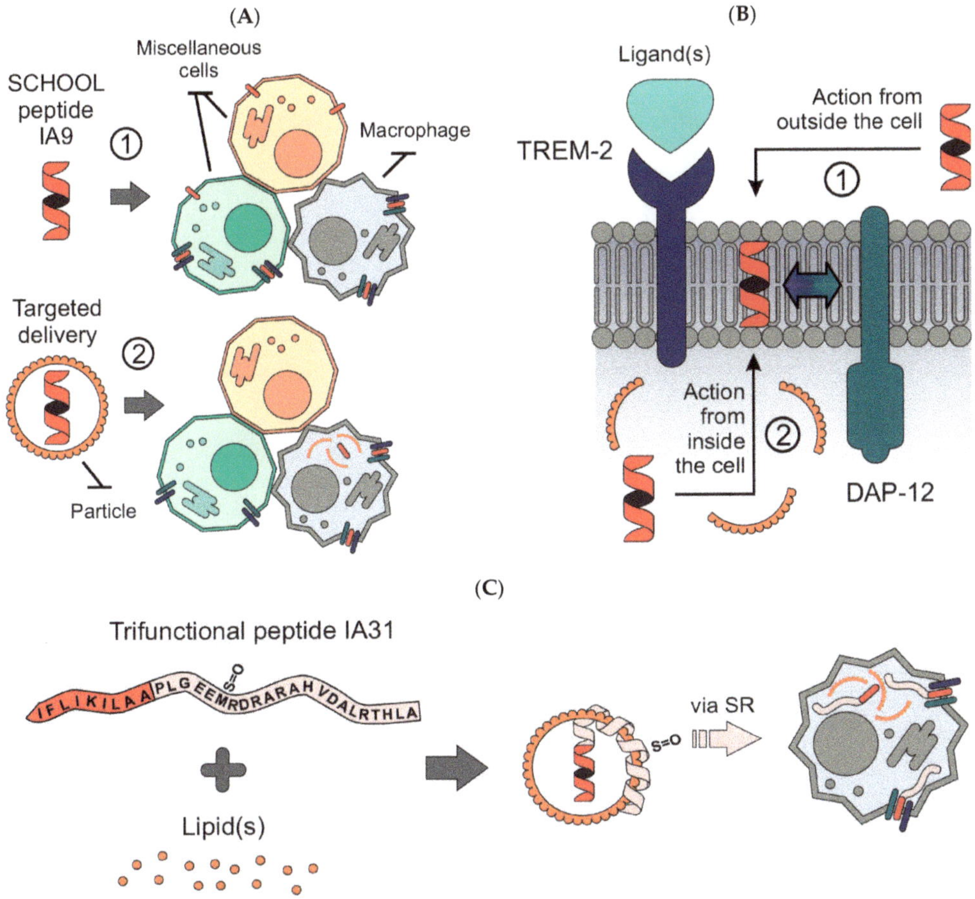

Figure 1. Schematic depiction for the proposed concepts of ligand-independent TREM-2 inhibition and macrophage-targeted drug delivery. (**A**) Peptide IA9 self-inserts into the cell membrane from outside and inhibits TREM-2 on any TREM-2-expressing cell (1). IA9 delivered into macrophages self-inserts into the cell membrane from inside and inhibits TREM-2 expressed on these cells (2). (**B**) Similar to SCHOOL peptide inhibitors of other cell receptors [48], IA9 employs ligand-independent mechanisms of action and blocks interactions between TREM-2 and its signaling partner DAP-12 in the cell membrane. (**C**) Schematic representation of a trifunctional peptide IA31 capable of formation of lipopeptide complexes (IA31-LPC) upon interaction with lipids. Due to sulfoxidized methionine in the PA22 domain, IA31-LPC deliver IA31 to cells (e.g., macrophages) via interaction with scavenger receptor (e.g., type A scavenger receptor, SR-A), where the released IA31 inhibits TREM-2.

We demonstrated, for the first time, that in the CIA mouse model, IA9 and IA31-LPC systemically administered after induction of arthritis both markedly suppress the rate of disease progression and joint inflammation, diminish release of plasma and joint proinflammatory cytokines and CSF-1, and significantly decrease synovial tissue sublining CD68, F4/80, TREM-1 and TREM-2 expression. We also comparatively studied TREM-1 inhibitory SCHOOL peptide sequence GF9 in the form of free peptide GF9, and formulated into macrophage-targeted LPC, as part of a trifunctional peptide GA31 (GA31-LPC) [30]. We showed that IA9 and IA31-LPC tend to have higher efficacy in the therapeutic CIA model used in this study compared to that of GF9 and GA31-LPC. Collectively, our data suggest that TREM-2 inhibition, using ligand-independent inhibitory SCHOOL peptides, can be a safe, effective and well-tolerable alternative therapy for the treatment of RA.

2. Results

2.1. Reduction of Inflammation and Suppression of Arthritis in a Therapeutic CIA Model

Previously [30], we used our proposed molecular mechanisms of transmembrane signaling [46,47] and targeted drug and imaging agent delivery [52,53] to design TREM-1 inhibitory peptide sequence GF9, and demonstrated that prophylactic administration of GF9 as a free peptide GF9 or delivered in the HDL-mimicking macrophage-targeted LPC formulations, efficiently reduces arthritis progression and protects against bone and cartilage damage in mice with CIA, the most widely studied autoimmune model of RA [54].

In this study, we used the same concepts to design free and LPC-bound TREM-2 inhibitory IA9 sequences (Figure 1), evaluated their anti-inflammatory and anti-arthritic effects in the therapeutic CIA mouse model and compared them with those of free and LPC-bound GF9 sequence-based inhibitors of TREM-1.

When systemically (intraperitoneally, i.p.) administered at 25 mg/kg, IA9, but not a control peptide IA9-G, ameliorated arthritis severity compared to vehicle-treated mice (Figure 2A). The difference between the IA9- and vehicle-treated groups started on day 29 and continued until day 42 (Figure 2A). Therapeutic treatment with IA9, but not vehicle or IA9-G, significantly reduced the arthritic score by day 42 showing the anti-arthritic effect not significantly different from that of 10 mg/kg oral prednisolone used as a positive control (Figure 2A). No therapeutic activity was observed for 2.5 mg/kg IA9 suggesting its effect is dose dependent. Therapeutic effect has also been observed for GF9 at a dose of 25 but not 2.5 mg/kg administered daily, starting day 28 for 14 consecutive days (Figure 2A). In contrast to the previously demonstrated prophylactic effect of 25 mg/kg of GF9 in CIA that was not significantly different from that of 0.1 mg/kg dexamethasone used as positive control [30], the therapeutic effect of 25 mg/kg GF9 observed here was significantly lower compared to that of the positive control (Figure 2A).

To test whether incorporation of TREM-2 inhibitory peptide sequence IA9 as a part of trifunctional peptide IA31 (Figure 1C) into macrophage-targeted LPC (IA31-LPC) affects its therapeutic efficacy in CIA, we used IA31 and POPC to prepare IA31-LPC1 with a mean particle diameter of 94 nm and polydispersity index (PDI) < 0.2 indicating monodispersity of these particles. GA31-LPC1 particles of similar size and size distribution (a mean particle diameter of 96 nm and PDI < 0.2) were also prepared and studied comparatively.

Earlier studies of liposomes loaded with superoxide dismutase in arthritic rats [55,56] demonstrated that small-sized liposomal formulations have significant advantages over large-sized formulations in terms of localization at arthritic sites and anti-arthritic activity. Recent studies of dexamethasone-loaded liposomes showed that the smallest liposomes (75 nm mean diameter with PDI < 0.2) were the ones that resulted in the higher anti-arthritic efficacy in arthritic rats in terms of suppression of paw thickness, and reduction of arthritic scores, proinflammatory cytokines and transaminase levels compared to two other liposomal formulations with similar dexamethasone content but larger sizes (150 and 300 nm mean diameters; both with PDI < 0.2) [57]. To test a possible particle size effect on the therapeutic activity of the LPC-based formulations used in this study, GA31-LPC3 with a mean particle diameter of 140 nm and PDI < 0.2 were prepared using GA31, POPC, cholesterol, and cholesteryl oleate, and studied comparatively.

IA31-LPC1, GA31-LPC1 and GA31-LPC3 were i.p. administered (all at the same dose of 13 mg peptide/kg) daily starting day 28 for 14 consecutive days. Despite a 2-fold decrease in the administered dose of peptide inhibitor, therapeutic treatment with IA31-LPC1 resulted in the observed anti-arthritic efficacy (Figure 2B), comparable to that observed for 25 mg/kg free IA9 (Figure 2A) and the positive control (Figure 2B). The therapeutic effect of 13 mg of GA31/kg GA31-LPC1, while significant compared to vehicle-treated mice, was significantly lower compared to that of the positive control (Figure 2B). In contrast, a significant decrease in the rate of disease progression was observed in the first several days of treatment with GA31-LPC3, which later disappeared (Figure 2B). Interestingly, in our previous studies in the prophylactic CIA mouse model [30], LPC of similar size (140 nm and PDI < 0.2), prepared using POPC, cholesterol, cholesteryl oleate, and an equimolar mixture of two trifunctional TREM-1 inhibitory peptides GA31 and GE31 (GA/E31-LPC), delayed and reduced arthritis progression exerting persistent prophylactic anti-arthritic effects that was comparable to that of the positive control. In line with the findings reported for dexamethasone-loaded liposomes of different sizes [57], our data likely indicate that the larger size of GA31-LPC3, compared to that of GA31-LPC1 and IA31-LPC1, may prevent their efficient accumulation at the local (joint) inflammatory sites. Systemic and local events in inflammatory arthritis are thought to be discrete processes, driven by multiple mediators with distinct temporospatial profiles [58,59]. Thus, when given before arthritis begins, the 140 nm-sized TREM-1 inhibitory LPC formulations may effectively prevent CIA, most likely by means of inhibiting systemic inflammatory response [30]. However, when injected after onset of joint inflammation, while initially highly effective, these formulations rapidly lose their anti-arthritic efficacy (Figure 2B), probably due to their inability to access the joint and suppress local inflammation.

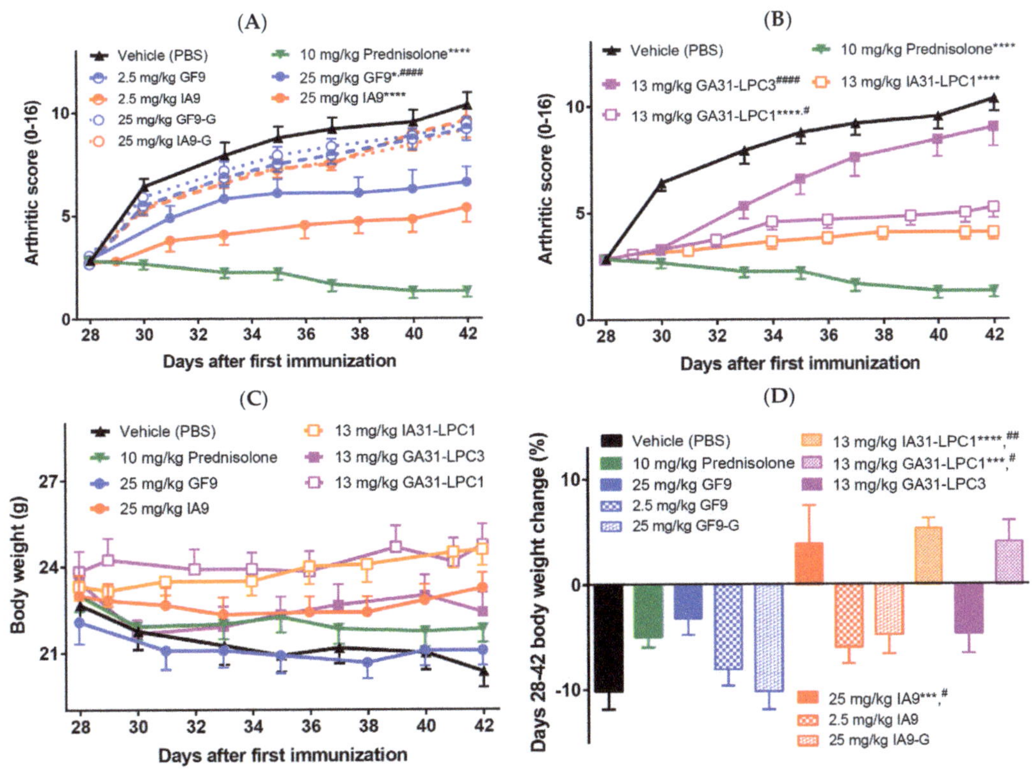

Figure 2. Effect of therapeutic treatment with free (**A**) and LPC-bound (**B**) IA9 and GF9 sequences on the severity of collagen-induced arthritis (**A**,**B**) and body weight (**C**,**D**). Data are shown as mean ± SEM ($n = 12$ mice per group). *, $p < 0.05$; ***, $p < 0.001$; and ****, $p < 0.0001$ versus vehicle. #, $p < 0.05$; ##, $p < 0.01$; and ####, $p < 0.0001$ versus prednisolone.

In terms of body weight, administration of IA9 and IA31-LPC1 resulted in an increase in body weight in contrast to the decrease observed in vehicle- or prednisolone-treated mice with CIA (Figure 2C,D), suggesting a good tolerability of TREM-2 inhibitory formulations.

In summary, these findings collectively indicate that, in the current study, IA9 and IA31-LPC1 exerted anti-inflammatory and anti-arthritic therapeutic effects comparable to those of prednisolone used as a positive control, thereby providing further experimental in vivo evidence of the usability of the SCHOOL model to design clinically relevant ligand-independent peptide inhibitors of MIRRs [48,60]. Incorporation of IA9 sequence into macrophage-specific LPC substantially increased their therapeutic efficacy, probably because of its targeted delivery to the inflammatory sites and/or the prolonged circulatory half-life of the peptide afforded by this strategy.

2.2. Reduction of Joint Damage and Bone Erosion in CIA

To gain insight into in situ pathological processes and determine whether therapeutic treatment of CIA mice with free and LPC-bound TREM-2 inhibitory IA9 sequences reduces chronic inflammation of synovial tissue, pannus formation, cartilage destruction, and bone erosion, we next examined the histopathology of six joints from each animal including fore paws, hind paws, and knees (Figure 3).

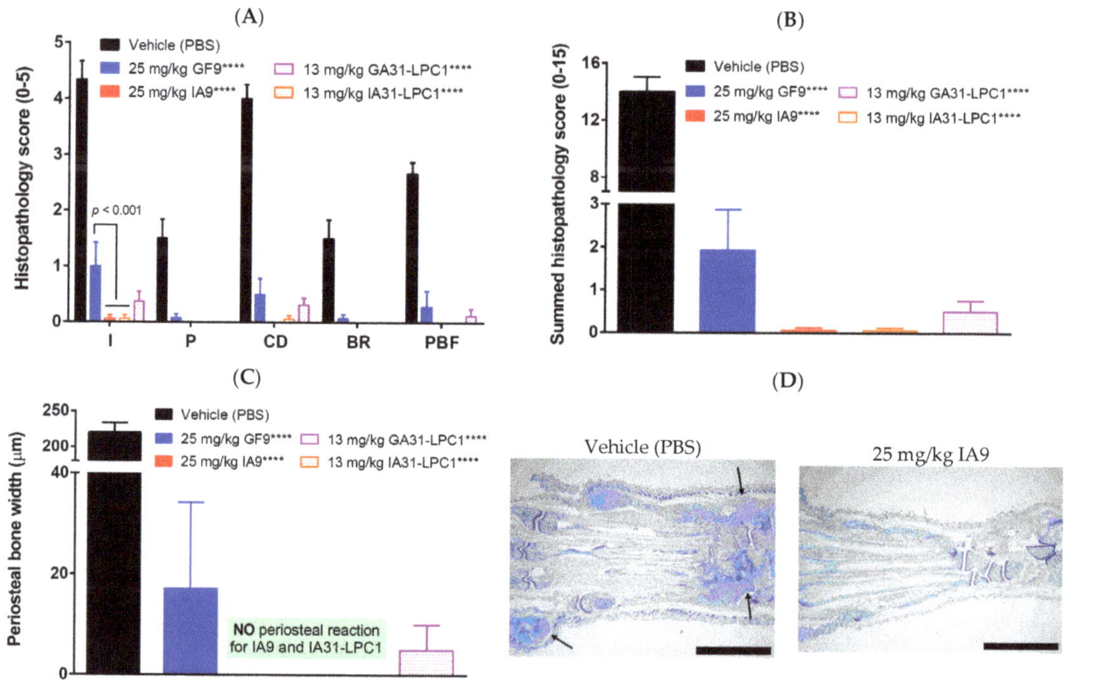

Figure 3. Effect of therapeutic treatment with free and LPC-bound IA9 and GF9 sequences on histopathological scores of inflammation (I), pannus (P), cartilage damage (CD), bone resorption (BR), and periosteal new bone formation (PBF) (**A**), summed histopathological score (**B**) and periosteal bone width (**C**). No periosteal reaction was observed in IA9- and IA31-LPC1-treated mice (**C**). Photomicrographs of hind paws of vehicle- and IA9-treated arthritic mice stained with toluidine blue (animals with the approximate mean summed paw score for the group were selected) (**D**). Arrows identify representative affected joints. The scale bars at the bottom right of the images indicate 5 mm. Data are shown as mean ± SEM ($n = 8$). ****, $p < 0.0001$ versus vehicle.

Vehicle-treated arthritic mice had histopathology changes, consistent with those seen in type II CIA, including infiltration of synovium and periarticular tissue with neutrophils and mononuclear inflammatory cells (inflammation), marginal zone pannus and bone resorption and cartilage damage (proteoglycan loss, chondrocyte death and collagen matrix destruction). Histopathological parameters in arthritic mice treated with 2.5 mg/kg IA9 or GF9, as well as with 25 mg/kg IA9-G or GF9-G, starting day 28 for 14 consecutive days did not differ significantly from those observed in vehicle-treated mice (data not shown). In contrast, therapeutic treatment of CIA mice with higher doses of IA9 or GF9 (25 mg/kg), as well as with 13 mg/kg IA31-LPC1 or 13 mg/kg GA31-LPC1, overall significantly reduced all six-joint mean histopathological parameters compared to vehicle-treated mice (Figure 3).

When compared to vehicle-treated mice, mice therapeutically treated with 25 mg/kg IA9 or 13 mg/kg IA31-LPC1 had significantly reduced inflammation (99 and 96% reduction, respectively), pannus formation (100% for both agents), cartilage damage (100 and 98%, respectively), bone resorption (100% for both agents), and periosteal bone formation (100% for both agents) (Figure 3A). A similar tendency was observed in mice treated with either 25 mg/kg GF9 or 13 mg/kg GA31-LPC1 (Figure 3A). Interestingly, IA9 and IA31-LPC1 were significantly more efficient than GF9 in suppressing inflammation in terms of neutrophils and mononuclear inflammatory cells infiltrated into the synovium and periarticular tissue (Figure 3A).

In line with our clinical data (Figure 2A,B), we observed a 99–100% reduction of summed histopathological scores in arthritic mice therapeutically treated with either 25 mg/kg IA9 or 13 mg/kg IA31-LPC1 compared to vehicle-treated mice (Figure 3B). While not statistically significant, there was a trend toward higher efficacy with IA9 or IA31-LPC1 than with GF9 or GA31-LPC1 at the same doses in one study. No histopathological changes were observed in arthritic mice treated with either a lower dose of IA9 (2.5 mg/kg) or control peptide (25 mg/kg IA9-G) compared to vehicle-treated mice (data not shown).

No or little periosteal reaction was observed in arthritic mice therapeutically treated with IA9, IA31-LPC1, GF9, and GA31-LPC1 (Figure 3C). The lack of bone resorption and periosteal reaction in IA9- and IA31-LPC1-treated mice (Figure 3A,C) suggests that, along with inhibiting local inflammatory cells, these agents may directly inhibit TREM-2 expressed on osteoclasts, the cells that are of central importance in the structural damage of chronic inflammatory joint disease [61]. The hind paw joints of vehicle-treated arthritic mice showed inflammation and destruction of articular structures, whereas the joints of IA9-treated CIA mice showed retained structure with no lesions (Figure 3D).

Thus, in line with clinical findings, the histopathology data demonstrated that therapeutic treatment with TREM-2 and TREM-1 inhibitory peptides (IA9 and GF9, respectively) as well as with targeted LPC-bound formulations of IA9 and GF9 sequences (IA31-LPC1 and GA31-LPC1, respectively) significantly reduced joint damage and bone erosion in CIA in a specific and dose-dependent manner.

2.3. Reduction of Plasma and Joint Proinflammatory Cytokine Levels in CIA

In experimental and clinical arthritis, TREM-1 is well known to mediate the release of proinflammatory cytokines and chemokines, including CSF-1 [27,30,62–64], that are all implicated in RA disease pathogenesis [65]. In contrast, the role of TREM-2 in RA is not yet well elucidated. TREM-2 is widely thought to function as an immunomodulatory receptor, which negatively regulates inflammation [34,66,67]. Contrary to this understanding, TREM-2 is upregulated in active RA synovium and subsequently downregulated in inactive RA, suggesting a role of TREM-2 as a positive regulator of RA-induced inflammation [43].

To further elucidate the molecular mechanisms underlying the significant reduction in CIA severity observed in mice treated with IA9 and IA31-LPC1 rationally designed to inhibit TREM-2, we next analyzed the plasma and joint (knee) proinflammatory cytokine levels on day 42 at the end of the study (Figure 4). Plasma and knee tissue of mice treated with the TREM-1 inhibitory formulations used in this study (GF9, GA31-LPC1 and GA31-LPC3) were assayed comparatively.

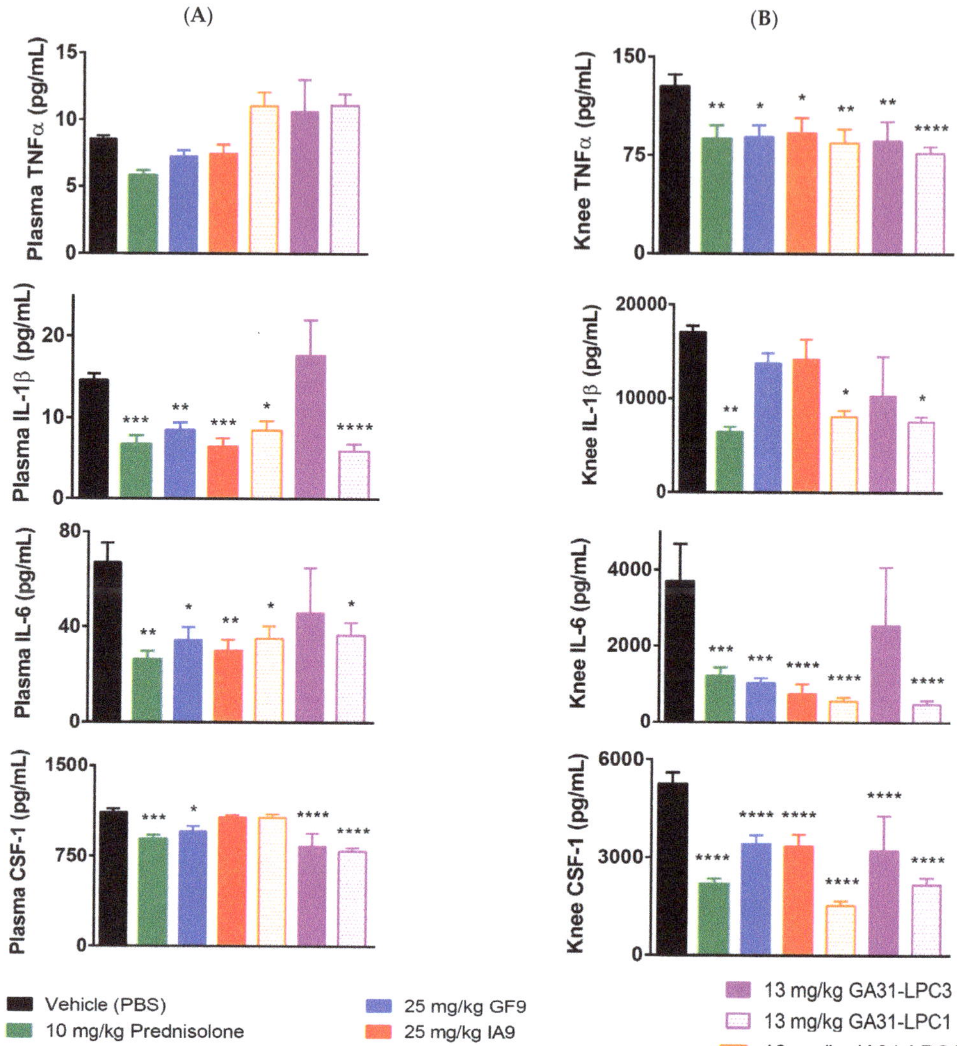

Figure 4. Effect of therapeutic treatment with free and LPC-bound IA9 and GF9 sequences on plasma (**A**) and joint (knee) (**B**) levels of proinflammatory cytokines. Data are shown as mean ± SEM ($n = 12$). *, $p < 0.05$; **, $p < 0.01$; ***, $p < 0.001$; and ****, $p < 0.0001$ versus vehicle.

No differences in plasma levels of TNFα were observed on day 42 in all treatment groups, including prednisolone-treated mice, as compared to vehicle-treated controls (Figure 4A). In contrast, treatment either with oral prednisolone or i.p. administered IA9, GF9, IA31-LPC1, GA31-LPC1 or GA31-LPC3 resulted in significantly reduced knee levels of TNFα. (Figure 4B). Interestingly, plasma and knee levels of IL-1β and IL-6 in mice treated with GA31-LPC3 did not differ from those in vehicle-treated controls (Figure 4A,B). Plasma levels of IL-1β and IL-6 in mice treated with prednisolone, IA9, IA31-LPC1, GF9 and GA31-LPC1, but not in mice treated with GA31-LPC3, were significantly reduced compared to those in vehicle-treated controls (Figure 4A). In contrast, no differences in knee levels of IL-1β were observed between mice treated with vehicle, IA9 or GF9 (Figure 4B).

Therapeutic treatment with prednisolone, GF9, GA31-LPC1 or GA31-LPC3, but not IA9 or IA31-LPC1, decreased plasma levels of CSF-1 compared to vehicle-treated mice (Figure 4A). However, marked reduction of knee levels of CSF-1 was observed in all treatment groups, with groups treated with IA31-LPC1 and GA31-LPC1 presenting the greatest decrease (Figure 4B). No significant differences were observed in plasma and knee cytokine levels in CIA mice treated with 2.5 mg IA9 or GF9 as well as with 25 mg/kg IA9-G or GF9-G, compared to those in vehicle-treated mice (data not shown).

Thus, cytokine data indicated that in the therapeutic CIA model, TREM-2 and TREM-1 inhibitory peptides (IA9 and GF9, respectively), as well as targeted LPC-bound formulations of these peptide sequences, reduced plasma and/or joint proinflammatory cytokine levels in a specific and dose-dependent manner.

2.4. Immunohistochemical Analysis for F4/80, CD68, Collagen IV, TREM-1 and TREM-2

To further characterize the anti-inflammatory and anti-arthritic effects exhibited in this study by the peptide sequence IA9 and its LPC-bound formulation IA31-LPC1, we next performed immunohistochemical (IHC) staining of joint tissues for F4/80, CD68, collagen IV, TREM-1 and TREM-2. Joint tissues of CIA mice treated with GF9 and GA31-LPC1 were analyzed comparatively.

In the synovial lining of arthritic joints of vehicle-treated mice, the mean CD68-, F4/80+, TREM-2, and TREM-1-immunopositive cell count varied from 15 to 30, depending on the marker (Figure 5A). In line with clinical and histopathological findings, all treatment groups exhibited significant reduction of CD68- and F4/80-immunopositive cell counts, compared to those of the vehicle-treated control group, with the effect being most pronounced for IA9 and IA31-LPC1 (Figure 5A). No CD68-immunopositive cells were observed in joints of mice treated either with IA9 or IA31-LPC1 (Figure 5A). TREM-1-stained sections had distinctive and fairly easy to quantify immuno-positive macrophages in, and around, the inflamed joints, and TREM-2-stained sections had distinctive, and fairly easy to quantify, immuno-positive osteoclasts and macrophages lining the endosteal and periosteal surfaces of bone. Therapeutic treatment with IA9, GF9, IA31-LPC1 or GA31-LPC1 resulted in significant reduction of TREM-1- and TREM-2-immunopositive cell counts compared to those of vehicle-treated mice (Figure 5A).

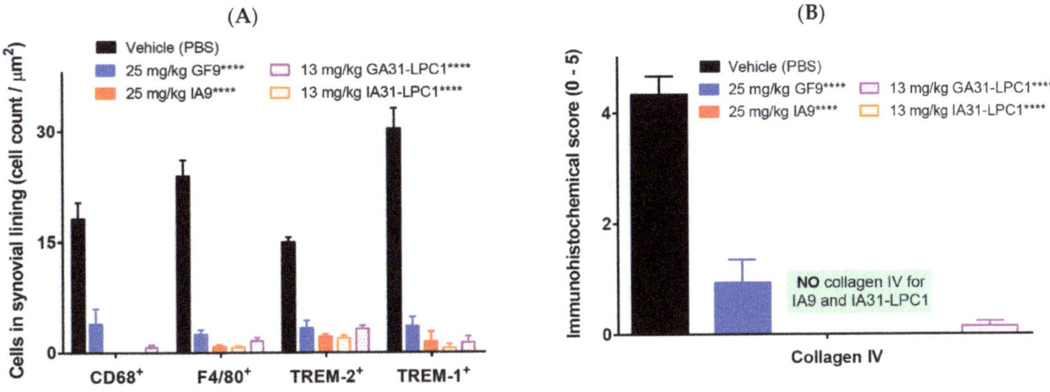

Figure 5. Immunohistochemical analysis of collagen-induced arthritic joints and effect of therapeutic treatment with free and LPC-bound IA9 and GF9 sequences on the number of CD68-, F4/80-, TREM-2- and TREM-1-positive cells (**A**) and collagen IV immunostaining score (**B**). Data are shown as mean ± SEM ($n = 8$). ****, $p < 0.0001$ versus vehicle.

A similar tendency was observed for collagen IV with significant increase in collagen IV immunostaining in vehicle-treated mice with CIA. Therapeutic treatment with GF9 and GA31-LPC1 resulted in significant reduction of collagen IV immunostaining score, compared to that of vehicle-treated mice (Figure 5B). No collagen IV was detected in joints of mice treated with IA9 and IA31-LPC1.

Thus, IHC findings suggest that in the therapeutic CIA model, TREM-2 and TREM-1 inhibitory peptides (IA9 and GF9, respectively), as well as targeted LPC-bound formulations of these peptide sequences, significantly reduced the number of inflammatory cells in the synovial membrane of the joints, with IA9 peptide sequences being most effective.

3. Discussion

Both autoimmune and systemic inflammatory responses play a role in development and progression of RA [68]. Proinflammatory cytokines are key drivers of inflammation in RA, and multiple cytokine-blocking agents, including orally active inhibitors, neutralizing antibodies, soluble receptors, or receptor antagonists, have been tested in patients with RA [69,70]. However, inadequate response and safety concerns, especially the potential for serious infections and malignancy, remain for TNFα and other cytokine blockers [20,71–73]. This makes a search for new therapeutic approaches to RA an area of great clinical importance. Among these approaches, targeting myeloid cells, that play a central role in the pathogenesis of RA [10,11], represents a promising perspective in this disease [74].

Despite the central role of TREM-2 in Alzheimer's disease, metabolic syndrome, cancer, and other diverse pathologies causing it to attract considerable recent attention [36], its role in RA is not well understood. Some studies have reported upregulation of TREM-2 in active RA synovium [43] and overexpression of TREM-2 in the synovial tissue of rats with CIA [44], suggesting blockade of TREM-2 signaling or depletion of TREM-2-expressing myeloid cells from synovium as potential anti-arthritic approaches. In contrast, other studies have indicated a protective function for TREM-2-expressing synovial tissue macrophages in RA [75], which questions the hypothetical advantage of TREM-2 blocking strategy.

To our best knowledge, the present study is the first to demonstrate that TREM-2 inhibition is therapeutically effective against CIA in mice, suggesting TREM-2 as a promising target for treating RA. We showed that treatment with rationally designed ligand-independent TREM-2 inhibitory peptide sequence IA9, either in the form of free peptide or as a part of trifunctional peptide IA31 formulated into macrophage-targeted LPC (IA31-LPC1), remarkably reduced the clinical arthritic score to an extent comparable to that of prednisolone used as positive control in this study. Importantly, therapeutic treatment with IA9 or IA31-LPC1 did not lead to disease-associated weight loss in CIA mice, in contrast to that observed in vehicle- or prednisolone-treated groups. Using cytokine, histopathological and IHC analyses, we further demonstrated that therapeutic treatment with IA9 and IA31-LPC significantly reduced systemic inflammatory response and inflammatory macrophage joint infiltration, as well as joint inflammation, pannus, cartilage damage, bone resorption, and periosteal bone formation, compared to vehicle-treated controls. As predicted by the SCHOOL mechanisms of TREM-2 signaling [46,47], no therapeutic effect was observed for control peptide IA9-G with lysine replaced by glycine, suggesting specificity of this effect. Overall, our study lays the premise that ligand-independent peptide therapies targeting TREM-2 signaling may provide a novel therapeutic strategy in treating RA.

There is one major challenge that complicates our understanding of the molecular mechanisms of TREM-2 signaling and its acting as pro- [39–42] or anti-inflammatory [33–38] regulator in inflammatory diseases. Despite TREM-2 binding to a set of potential ligands that are distinct from those recognized by TREM-1, an established inflammation amplifier [32], TREM2 and TREM-1 both signal through the same signaling partner DAP-12 (Figure 1B). In addition, certain macrophages and neutrophils express both TREM-1 and TREM-2 [26], further complicating this picture. Possibly, depending on the cell type involved, TREM-1 and/or TREM-2 ligation might activate different cytoplasmic adaptors, producing different outcomes, as suggested for osteoclasts, monocyte/macrophages and dendritic cells [42]. In this study, we showed that in experimental arthritis, inhibiting TREM-2 ameliorated arthritis and significantly reduced cartilage and joint damage, similarly to what happens when inhibiting TREM-1. Further studies are needed to differentiate the precise mechanisms of the anti-inflammatory and anti-arthritic effects of TREM-2 and TREM-1, as well as to investigate whether concurrent inhibition of TREM-2 and TREM-1 signaling would be more effective than inhibition of either pathway alone.

Previously, we demonstrated that ligand-independent TREM-1 inhibitory functionality can be combined in one sequence with seemingly unrelated functionalities of other peptides resulting in multifunctional peptides GA31 and GE31 capable of self-assembling into targeted LPC upon interaction with lipids. We further demonstrated that these LPC can therapeutically inhibit TREM-1 in various inflammatory diseases, including CIA [30], pancreatic cancer [76], retinopathy of prematurity [77], and alcoholic liver disease [78]. In the present study, we extended this concept to design a multifunctional peptide IA31 with the predicted capability to inhibit TREM-2 and showed that nanosized IA31-LPC1 particles formed upon interaction of IA31 with lipid exhibited significant anti-inflammatory and anti-arthritic activities in the therapeutic CIA mouse model. This further supports the combinatorial "molecular Lego" approach to designing multifunctional peptide therapies by combining the functionality of ligand-independent peptide inhibitors of cell receptors [48] with functionalities of other peptides, such as the native, or rationally modified, amphipathic peptide sequences of apo A-I used in this study and in our previous studies [30,52,76,77,79].

Here, we showed that, as revealed by histological and proinflammatory cytokine analyses, TREM-2 inhibitory peptide sequence IA9 in the form of free peptide or formulated into targeted IA31-LPC1 formulations exhibited a high efficacy in suppressing local (joint) inflammation and that, histologically, the observed anti-inflammatory effect of IA9 and IA31-LPC1 was significantly higher than that observed for TREM-1 inhibitors GF9 and GA31-LPC1. This is in line not only with findings in RA showing that TREM-2 is highly upregulated in active but not inactive RA synovium [43], but also with studies in IBD [42,80] that reported high levels of TREM-2 in the inflamed mucosa of patients with IBD and the virtual absence of TREM-2 in colon samples of healthy donors. Further, TREM-2 is expressed by tumor-associated macrophages (TAMs) in various tumor types [81] and plays an important role in tumor immunity [82]. In experimental cancer, inhibition of TREM-2 with anti-TREM-2 blocking monoclonal antibody (mAb) not only exhibits a robust antitumor effect when used as single-agent therapy, but also significantly improves the efficacy of immune checkpoint blockade (ICB) therapy when used in combination with anti-programmed cell death protein-1 (PD-1) treatment [81,83]. Collectively, this suggests that a rationally designed ligand-independent TREM-2 inhibitory peptide sequence IA9 can be a promising alternative to ligand-dependent anti-TREM-2 mAbs to modulate local inflammation in the management of RA, IBD, cancer and, probably, other inflammatory diseases. Considering the therapeutic efficacy of both TREM-2- and TREM-1-targeting approaches in various inflammation-associated diseases, one may suggest that concurrent targeting of TREM-2 and TREM-2 would exhibit a synergistic effect in treating these diseases. Further studies are in progress to confirm this hypothesis.

In summary, we showed the effectiveness of the TREM-2-inhibiting approach in the treatment of CIA, as demonstrated by the significant decrease in clinical signs of arthritis, joint inflammation and destruction, inflammatory cell infiltration of joint tissues, and proinflammatory cytokine levels in the plasma and joints. We also demonstrated that TREM-2 inhibitory peptide sequence IA9 is therapeutically effective, not only in the form of free peptide, but also as a part of a multifunctional peptide IA31 incorporated into LPC formulations for its targeted delivery to the inflammation sites.

4. Materials and Methods

4.1. Chemicals, Lipids and Peptides

Sodium cholate, prednisolone 21-hemisuccinate sodium salt and other chemicals were purchased from Sigma Aldrich Company (St. Louis, MO, USA). Bovine type II collagen was ordered from Chondrex, Inc. (Woodinville, WA, USA). 1-palmitoyl-2-oleoyl-sn-glycero-3-phosphocholine (POPC) and cholesterol were purchased from Avanti Polar Lipids

(Alabaster, AL, USA). Cholesteryl oleate was purchased from Nu-Chek Prep, Inc. (Elysian, MN, USA). The following two synthetic 9-mer peptides were ordered from Bachem Americas, Inc. (Torrance, CA, USA): GFLSKSLVF (human TREM-$1_{213-221}$, GF9) and GFLSGSLVF (GF9-G). Two 9-mer peptides. IFLIKILAA (human TREM-$2_{182-190}$, IA9) and IFLIGILAA (IA9-G), and two 31-mer peptides with sulfoxidized methionine residues, GFLSKSLVF-PLGEEM(O)RDRARAHVDALRTHLA (GA31) and IFLIKILAAPLGEEM(O)RDRARAHVD ALRTHLA (IA31), were synthesized by Ambiopharm Inc. (Beech Island, SC, USA). All peptides were purified by reversed-phase high-performance liquid chromatography (RP-HPLC), and their purity and net peptide content were confirmed by analytical RP-HPLC, mass spectrometry and amino acid analysis.

4.2. Lipopeptide Complexes

Lipopeptide complexes (LPC) of oxidized peptides GA31 and IA31 (GA31-LPC and IA31-LPC, respectively, both of spherical shape) were synthesized by substantially using the sodium cholate dialysis procedure, as previously described [30]. The initial molar ratio for complexes of oxidized GA31 with 3 lipids (GA31-LPC3) was 125:6:2:1:210, corresponding to POPC:cholesterol:cholesteryl oleate:GA31:sodium cholate. The initial molar ratio for complexes of oxidized GA31 and IA31 with 1 lipid (GA31-LPC1 and IA31-LPC1, respectively) was 125:1:210 corresponding to POPC:peptide:sodium cholate. All obtained LPC formulations of GA31 and IA31 were purified and characterized as described previously [30]. Mean LPC size was determined by dynamic light scattering (DLS) with a DynaPro-99-E-50 instrument. The polydispersity index (PDI) that can vary from 0 (monodisperse) to 1.0 (polydisperse) was used to evaluate LPC size distribution.

4.3. Therapeutic Collagen-Induced Arthritis (CIA) Model

All animal experiments were performed by Washington Biotechnology, Inc. (WBI; Baltimore, MD, USA). Male DBA/1J mice (7–9 weeks old) were purchased from Jackson Laboratory (Bar Harbor, MA, USA) and maintained under specific pathogen-free (SPF) conditions with food and water ad libitum. CIA was induced by immunization with bovine type II collagen as previously described [30,79]. Briefly, mice were weighed and injected subcutaneously at the base of the tail with 50 μL of Freund's complete adjuvant containing 100 μg of bovine type II collagen (2 mg/mL final concentration) on day 0. Mice were boosted on day 21 with the same dose of bovine type II collagen, but incomplete Freund's adjuvant was used to make the emulsion. Mice were weighed weekly and scored for signs of arthritis daily. Each paw was scored as follows: 0: no visible effects of arthritis; 1: edema and/or erythema of one digit; 2: edema and/or erythema of 2 joints; 3: edema and/or erythema of more than 2 joints; 4: severe arthritis of the entire paw and digits including limb deformation and ankylosis of the joint. The sum of all four scores was recorded as the arthritic score with the maximum possible value of 16. Starting day 28, the mice were i.p. injected daily for 14 consecutive days with GF9 (2.5 or 25 mg/kg), GF9-G (25 mg/kg), IA9 (2.5 or 25 mg/kg) or IA9-G (25 mg/kg) as well as with IA31-LPC1, GA31-LPC3 or GA31-LPC1 (all at a dose of 13 mg of peptide/kg) or with vehicle (phosphate-buffered saline, pH 7.4; PBS). The positive treatment control for these experiments was oral prednisolone administered at a dose of 10 mg/kg daily for 14 consecutive days starting day 28. Once the dosing regimen was initiated, the mice were weighed and scored for signs of disease three times a week and prior necropsy (day 42). On day 42, mice were euthanized for necropsy.

4.4. Histological Assessment

At the end of study, fore paws, hind paws, and knees were harvested, fixed in 10% neutral buffered formalin (NBF) for 1–2 days, and then decalcified in 5% formic acid for 4–5 days before standard processing for paraffin embedding. Sections (8 μm) were cut and stained with toluidine blue (T blue) essentially as described [84]. Hind paws, fore paws, and knees were embedded and sectioned in the frontal plane. Six joints from each animal were processed for histopathological evaluation. The joints were then evaluated by a board-certified veterinary pathologist using light microscopy using 0–5 scale for inflammation, pannus formation, cartilage damage, bone resorption, and periosteal new bone formation as previously reported [30]. A summed histopathology score (sum of five parameters, 0–25 scale) was also determined.

4.5. Plasma and Joint Cytokine Analysis

Plasma and joint tissues were collected by the end of day 42. The knees were minced and flash frozen in liquid nitrogen and stored at −80 °C. Then, the collected knees were thawed to 4–8 °C and homogenized in 1 mL 2X cell lysis buffer (Cell Signaling Technology, Inc.; Danvers, MA, USA) followed by sonication. The homogenates were centrifuged for 15 min and the supernatants were stored at −80 °C until analyzed. Cytokines were analyzed in the collected plasma and knee homogenates using ELISA kits (R&D Systems, Minneapolis, MN, USA) according to the manufacturer's instructions.

4.6. Immunohistochemical Analysis

Immunohistochemical (IHC) staining in formalin-fixed, paraffin-embedded (FFPE) mouse limb sections was conducted using the Bond RXm platform (Leica Biosystems, Deer Park, IL, USA) and antibodies to F4/80 (Absolute Antibody, [CI:A3-1], Ab00106-23.0), CD68 (Abcam, ab125212), collagen IV (Abcam, ab6586), TREM-1 (LS-Bio, LS-C312743) and TREM-2 (LS-Bio, LS-C489619). Antibody binding was detected using an horseradish peroxidase (HRP)-conjugated secondary polymer, followed by chromogenic visualization with diaminobenzidine (DAB). A hematoxylin counterstain was used to visualize nuclei. IHC staining of collagen IV was scored on a scale of 0 to 5 based on increases in the percent area of disease-associated staining: 0: normal; 0.5: very minimal, <1% of area at risk affected; 1: minimal, approximately 1–10% of area at risk affected; 2: mild, approximately 11–25% of area at risk affected; 3: moderate, approximately 26–50% of area at risk affected; 4: marked, approximately 51–75% of area at risk affected; and 5: severe, approximately 76–100% of area at risk affected. Areas of normal background staining (distal digit nail beds, skin, periosteum, endosteum, and osteocyte lacunae) were not included in the % area affected/scores. CD68, F4/80, TREM-1, and TREM-2 immuno-positive cells were counted at 400x magnification in a defined square micron area in synovium/exudate (10×100 units = 25×250 μm = 6250 μm^2), and the percentage of positive cells was calculated.

4.7. Statistical Analysis

All statistical analyses were performed using GraphPad Prism 6.0 software (GraphPad, La Jolla, CA, USA). Results are expressed as the mean ± SEM. Statistical differences were analyzed using analysis of variance with Bonferroni adjustment. p values less than 0.05 were considered significant.

4.8. Sequence Accession Numbers

Accession numbers (UniProtKB/Swiss-Prot knowledgebase, http://www.uniprot.org/, accessed on 22 July 2022) for the protein sequences discussed in this article are as the follows: human TREM-2, Q9NZC2; human TREM-1, Q9NP99.

5. Conclusions

In this study, we demonstrated that TREM-2 can be a promising target in therapy of RA. We further provided compelling in vivo evidence of the therapeutic potential of targeting TREM-2 in RA using the TREM-2 inhibitory peptide sequence IA9 rationally designed using the SCHOOL model of cell signaling. This further expands the applicability of our SCHOOL concept of ligand-independent inhibition of various cell receptors in multiple diseases and disorders, where blockade of these receptors is of clinical value.

Funding: This work was partly supported by a grant R44AR077456 (ABS; Alexander B. Sigalov, Principal investigator) from National Institute of Arthritis and Musculoskeletal and Skin Diseases of the National Institutes of Health. The additional funding has come from SignaBlok, Inc. The funding sources have no role in the design of the study, conduction of the experiments, interpretation of the data, and writing of the manuscript.

Institutional Review Board Statement: All animal experiments were performed by Washington Biotechnology, Inc. (WBI; Baltimore, MD, USA), a contract research organization, on a fee-for-service basis in strict accordance with the recommendations in the Guide for the Care and Use of Laboratory Animals of the National Institutes of Health (NIH) and in the United States Department of Agriculture (USDA) Animal Welfare Act (9 CFR, Parts 1, 2, and 3). All experimental procedures were approved by the Institutional Animal Care and Use Committee of WBI for compliance with regulations prior to study initiation (Animal Welfare Assurance number A7649-16) and all experiments were performed in accordance with the approved protocol No. CIA-SBI-1.

Informed Consent Statement: Not applicable.

Data Availability Statement: The data obtained in this study are available in the article.

Acknowledgments: We are grateful to Washington Biotechnology, Inc. for animal experiments. We also owe a debt of gratitude to Sean O'Neill, Yongping Chen, Valerie Lowe and Anna Freeman, who did an excellent job conducting mouse studies, for their important expertise, experience, and skills and for numerous valuable discussions.

Conflicts of Interest: Sigalov is an employee of SignaBlok, Inc. No non-financial conflicts of interest exist for the author with respect to this study.

Abbreviations

RA	Rheumatoid arthritis
IL	Interleukin
TNF	Tumor necrosis factor
M-CSF	Macrophage-colony stimulating factor
CIA	Collagen-induced arthritis
SEM	Standard error of the mean
TREM-1	Triggering receptors expressed by myeloid cells 1
TREM-2	Triggering receptors expressed by myeloid cells 2
DAP-12	DNAX-activating protein of 12 kDa
SCHOOL	Signaling chain homo-oligomerization
MIRR	Multichain immune recognition receptor
LPC	Lipopeptide complex
HDL	High density lipoproteins
Apo	Apolipoprotein
SR-A	Type A scavenger receptor
IP	Intraperitoneally
I	Inflammation
P	Pannus
CD	Cartilage damage
PBF	Periosteal bone formation
POPC	1-Palmitoyl-2-oleoyl-sn-glycero-3-phosphocholine
IBD	Inflammatory bowel disease
mAb	Monoclonal antibody
ICB	Immune checkpoint blockade
PD-1	Programmed cell death protein 1
RP-HPLC	Reversed-phase high-performance liquid chromatography
DLS	Dynamic light scattering
PDI	Polydispersity index
SPF	Specific pathogen-free
PBS	Phosphate-buffered saline
NBF	Neutral buffered formalin
T blue	Toluidine blue

DAB	Diaminobenzidine
IHC	Immunohistochemistry
HRP	Horseradish peroxidase
ELISA	Enzyme-linked immunosorbent assay
FFPE	Formalin-fixed, paraffin-embedded

References

1. Prasad, P.; Verma, S.; Surbhi; Ganguly, N.K.; Chaturvedi, V.; Mittal, S.A. Rheumatoid arthritis: Advances in treatment strategies. *Mol. Cell. Biochem.* **2022**. [CrossRef] [PubMed]
2. Gibofsky, A. Overview of epidemiology, pathophysiology, and diagnosis of rheumatoid arthritis. *Am. J. Manag. Care* **2012**, *18*, S295–S302. [PubMed]
3. Smolen, J.S.; Aletaha, D.; Barton, A.; Burmester, G.R.; Emery, P.; Firestein, G.S.; Kavanaugh, A.; McInnes, I.B.; Solomon, D.H.; Strand, V.; et al. Rheumatoid arthritis. *Nat. Rev. Dis. Primers* **2018**, *4*, 18001. [CrossRef] [PubMed]
4. Pincus, T.; Callahan, L.F. Taking mortality in rheumatoid arthritis seriously–predictive markers, socioeconomic status and comorbidity. *J. Rheumatol.* **1986**, *13*, 841–845. [PubMed]
5. Scott, D.L.; Symmons, D.P.; Coulton, B.L.; Popert, A.J. Long-term outcome of treating rheumatoid arthritis: Results after 20 years. *Lancet* **1987**, *1*, 1108–1111. [CrossRef]
6. McInnes, I.B.; O'Dell, J.R. State-of-the-art: Rheumatoid arthritis. *Ann. Rheum. Dis.* **2010**, *69*, 1898–1906. [CrossRef]
7. Siegel, J. Comparative effectiveness of treatments for rheumatoid arthritis. *Ann. Intern. Med.* **2008**, *148*, 162–163. [CrossRef]
8. Bansard, C.; Lequerre, T.; Daveau, M.; Boyer, O.; Tron, F.; Salier, J.P.; Vittecoq, O.; Le-Loet, X. Can rheumatoid arthritis responsiveness to methotrexate and biologics be predicted? *Rheumatology* **2009**, *48*, 1021–1028. [CrossRef]
9. Smolen, J.S.; Aletaha, D.; McInnes, I.B. Rheumatoid arthritis. *Lancet* **2016**, *388*, 2023–2038. [CrossRef]
10. Kinne, R.W.; Brauer, R.; Stuhlmuller, B.; Palombo-Kinne, E.; Burmester, G.R. Macrophages in rheumatoid arthritis. *Arthritis Res.* **2000**, *2*, 189–202. [CrossRef]
11. Alivernini, S.; Tolusso, B.; Ferraccioli, G.; Gremese, E.; Kurowska-Stolarska, M.; McInnes, I.B. Driving chronicity in rheumatoid arthritis: Perpetuating role of myeloid cells. *Clin. Exp. Immunol.* **2018**, *193*, 13–23. [CrossRef] [PubMed]
12. Mulherin, D.; Fitzgerald, O.; Bresnihan, B. Synovial tissue macrophage populations and articular damage in rheumatoid arthritis. *Arthritis Rheum.* **1996**, *39*, 115–124. [CrossRef] [PubMed]
13. Kinne, R.W.; Stuhlmuller, B.; Burmester, G.R. Cells of the synovium in rheumatoid arthritis. Macrophages. *Arthritis Res. Ther.* **2007**, *9*, 224. [CrossRef]
14. Bresnihan, B.; Gerlag, D.M.; Rooney, T.; Smeets, T.J.; Wijbrandts, C.A.; Boyle, D.; Fitzgerald, O.; Kirkham, B.W.; McInnes, I.B.; Smith, M.; et al. Synovial macrophages as a biomarker of response to therapeutic intervention in rheumatoid arthritis: Standardization and consistency across centers. *J. Rheumatol.* **2007**, *34*, 620–622. [PubMed]
15. Li, J.; Hsu, H.C.; Mountz, J.D. Managing macrophages in rheumatoid arthritis by reform or removal. *Curr. Rheumatol. Rep.* **2012**, *14*, 445–454. [CrossRef] [PubMed]
16. Axmann, R.; Bohm, C.; Kronke, G.; Zwerina, J.; Smolen, J.; Schett, G. Inhibition of interleukin-6 receptor directly blocks osteoclast formation in vitro and in vivo. *Arthritis Rheum.* **2009**, *60*, 2747–2756. [CrossRef] [PubMed]
17. Takagi, N.; Mihara, M.; Moriya, Y.; Nishimoto, N.; Yoshizaki, K.; Kishimoto, T.; Takeda, Y.; Ohsugi, Y. Blockage of interleukin-6 receptor ameliorates joint disease in murine collagen-induced arthritis. *Arthritis Rheum.* **1998**, *41*, 2117–2121. [CrossRef]
18. Smolen, J.S.; Avila, J.C.; Aletaha, D. Tocilizumab inhibits progression of joint damage in rheumatoid arthritis irrespective of its anti-inflammatory effects: Disassociation of the link between inflammation and destruction. *Ann. Rheum. Dis.* **2012**, *71*, 687–693. [CrossRef]
19. Benucci, M.; Saviola, G.; Baiardi, P.; Manfredi, M.; Sarzi Puttini, P.; Atzeni, F. Determinants of Risk Infection During Therapy with Anti TNF-Alpha Blocking Agents in Rheumatoid Arthritis. *Open Rheumatol. J.* **2012**, *6*, 33–37. [CrossRef]
20. Choy, E.H.; Kavanaugh, A.F.; Jones, S.A. The problem of choice: Current biologic agents and future prospects in RA. *Nat. Rev. Rheumatol.* **2013**, *9*, 154–163. [CrossRef]
21. Bongartz, T.; Sutton, A.J.; Sweeting, M.J.; Buchan, I.; Matteson, E.L.; Montori, V. Anti-TNF antibody therapy in rheumatoid arthritis and the risk of serious infections and malignancies: Systematic review and meta-analysis of rare harmful effects in randomized controlled trials. *JAMA* **2006**, *295*, 2275–2285. [CrossRef] [PubMed]
22. Edrees, A.F.; Misra, S.N.; Abdou, N.I. Anti-tumor necrosis factor (TNF) therapy in rheumatoid arthritis: Correlation of TNF-alpha serum level with clinical response and benefit from changing dose or frequency of infliximab infusions. *Clin. Exp. Rheumatol.* **2005**, *23*, 469–474. [PubMed]
23. Takeuchi, T.; Miyasaka, N.; Tatsuki, Y.; Yano, T.; Yoshinari, T.; Abe, T.; Koike, T. Baseline tumour necrosis factor alpha levels predict the necessity for dose escalation of infliximab therapy in patients with rheumatoid arthritis. *Ann. Rheum. Dis.* **2011**, *70*, 1208–1215. [CrossRef] [PubMed]
24. American College of Rheumatology Ad Hoc Committee on Clinical Guidelines. Guidelines for monitoring drug therapy in rheumatoid arthritis. *Arthritis Rheum.* **1996**, *39*, 723–731.
25. Garrood, T.; Pitzalis, C. Targeting the inflamed synovium: The quest for specificity. *Arthritis Rheum.* **2006**, *54*, 1055–1060. [CrossRef]

26. Colonna, M. TREMs in the immune system and beyond. *Nat. Rev. Immunol.* **2003**, *3*, 445–453. [CrossRef]
27. Kuai, J.; Gregory, B.; Hill, A.; Pittman, D.D.; Feldman, J.L.; Brown, T.; Carito, B.; O'Toole, M.; Ramsey, R.; Adolfsson, O.; et al. TREM-1 expression is increased in the synovium of rheumatoid arthritis patients and induces the expression of pro-inflammatory cytokines. *Rheumatology* **2009**, *48*, 1352–1358. [CrossRef]
28. Dower, K.; Ellis, D.K.; Saraf, K.; Jelinsky, S.A.; Lin, L.L. Innate immune responses to TREM-1 activation: Overlap, divergence, and positive and negative cross-talk with bacterial lipopolysaccharide. *J. Immunol.* **2008**, *180*, 3520–3534. [CrossRef]
29. Murakami, Y.; Akahoshi, T.; Aoki, N.; Toyomoto, M.; Miyasaka, N.; Kohsaka, H. Intervention of an inflammation amplifier, triggering receptor expressed on myeloid cells 1, for treatment of autoimmune arthritis. *Arthritis Rheum.* **2009**, *60*, 1615–1623. [CrossRef]
30. Shen, Z.T.; Sigalov, A.B. Rationally designed ligand-independent peptide inhibitors of TREM-1 ameliorate collagen-induced arthritis. *J. Cell. Mol. Med.* **2017**, *21*, 2524–2534. [CrossRef]
31. Weber, B.; Schuster, S.; Zysset, D.; Rihs, S.; Dickgreber, N.; Schurch, C.; Riether, C.; Siegrist, M.; Schneider, C.; Pawelski, H.; et al. TREM-1 Deficiency Can Attenuate Disease Severity without Affecting Pathogen Clearance. *PLoS Pathog.* **2014**, *10*, e1003900. [CrossRef] [PubMed]
32. Tammaro, A.; Derive, M.; Gibot, S.; Leemans, J.C.; Florquin, S.; Dessing, M.C. TREM-1 and its potential ligands in non-infectious diseases: From biology to clinical perspectives. *Pharmacol. Ther.* **2017**, *177*, 81–95. [CrossRef]
33. Gao, X.; Dong, Y.; Liu, Z.; Niu, B. Silencing of triggering receptor expressed on myeloid cells-2 enhances the inflammatory responses of alveolar macrophages to lipopolysaccharide. *Mol. Med. Rep.* **2013**, *7*, 921–926. [CrossRef] [PubMed]
34. Turnbull, I.R.; Gilfillan, S.; Cella, M.; Aoshi, T.; Miller, M.; Piccio, L.; Hernandez, M.; Colonna, M. Cutting edge: TREM-2 attenuates macrophage activation. *J. Immunol.* **2006**, *177*, 3520–3524. [CrossRef] [PubMed]
35. Li, T.; Lu, L.; Pember, E.; Li, X.; Zhang, B.; Zhu, Z. New Insights into Neuroinflammation Involved in Pathogenic Mechanism of Alzheimer's Disease and Its Potential for Therapeutic Intervention. *Cells* **2022**, *11*, 1925. [CrossRef] [PubMed]
36. Deczkowska, A.; Weiner, A.; Amit, I. The Physiology, Pathology, and Potential Therapeutic Applications of the TREM2 Signaling Pathway. *Cell* **2020**, *181*, 1207–1217. [CrossRef] [PubMed]
37. Sun, H.; Feng, J.; Tang, L. Function of TREM1 and TREM2 in Liver-Related Diseases. *Cells* **2020**, *9*, 2626. [CrossRef]
38. Rai, V.; Dietz, N.E.; Dilisio, M.F.; Radwan, M.M.; Agrawal, D.K. Vitamin D attenuates inflammation, fatty infiltration, and cartilage loss in the knee of hyperlipidemic microswine. *Arthritis Res. Ther.* **2016**, *18*, 203. [CrossRef]
39. Wang, M.; Gao, X.; Zhao, K.; Chen, H.; Xu, M.; Wang, K. Effect of TREM2 on Release of Inflammatory Factor from LPS-stimulated Microglia and Its Possible Mechanism. *Ann. Clin. Lab. Sci.* **2019**, *49*, 249–256.
40. Suchankova, M.; Bucova, M.; Tibenska, E.; Tedlova, E.; Demian, J.; Majer, I.; Novosadova, H.; Tedla, M.; Paulovicova, E.; Kantarova, D. Triggering receptor expressed on myeloid cells-1 and 2 in bronchoalveolar lavage fluid in pulmonary sarcoidosis. *Respirology* **2013**, *18*, 455–462. [CrossRef]
41. Sharif, O.; Gawish, R.; Warszawska, J.M.; Martins, R.; Lakovits, K.; Hladik, A.; Doninger, B.; Brunner, J.; Korosec, A.; Schwarzenbacher, R.E.; et al. The triggering receptor expressed on myeloid cells 2 inhibits complement component 1q effector mechanisms and exerts detrimental effects during pneumococcal pneumonia. *PLoS Pathog.* **2014**, *10*, e1004167. [CrossRef] [PubMed]
42. Genua, M.; Rutella, S.; Correale, C.; Danese, S. The triggering receptor expressed on myeloid cells (TREM) in inflammatory bowel disease pathogenesis. *J. Transl. Med.* **2014**, *12*, 293. [CrossRef] [PubMed]
43. Crotti, T.N.; Dharmapatni, A.A.; Alias, E.; Zannettino, A.C.; Smith, M.D.; Haynes, D.R. The immunoreceptor tyrosine-based activation motif (ITAM)-related factors are increased in synovial tissue and vasculature of rheumatoid arthritic joints. *Arthritis Res. Ther.* **2012**, *14*, R245. [CrossRef] [PubMed]
44. Ye, P.; Li, J.H.; Xu, J.H.; Huang, S.H.; Liu, G.W.; Zhang, W.Q.; Zheng, P.Z.; Huang, J.R. Triggering receptor expressed on myeloid cells 2 in synovial tissue of rheumatoid arthritis rats. *Chin. J. Tissue Eng. Res.* **2015**, *19*, 2807–2813. [CrossRef]
45. Kober, D.L.; Brett, T.J. TREM2-Ligand Interactions in Health and Disease. *J. Mol. Biol.* **2017**, *429*, 1607–1629. [CrossRef]
46. Sigalov, A.B. Multichain immune recognition receptor signaling: Different players, same game? *Trends Immunol.* **2004**, *25*, 583–589. [CrossRef]
47. Sigalov, A.B. Immune cell signaling: A novel mechanistic model reveals new therapeutic targets. *Trends Pharmacol. Sci.* **2006**, *27*, 518–524. [CrossRef]
48. Sigalov, A.B. SCHOOL of nature: Ligand-independent immunomodulatory peptides. *Drug Discov. Today* **2020**, *25*, 1298–1306. [CrossRef]
49. Greaves, D.R.; Gordon, S. Thematic review series: The immune system and atherogenesis. Recent insights into the biology of macrophage scavenger receptors. *J. Lipid Res.* **2005**, *46*, 11–20. [CrossRef]
50. Lin, Y.L.; de Villiers, W.J.S.; Garvy, B.; Post, S.R.; Nagy, T.R.; Safadi, F.F.; Faugere, M.C.; Wang, G.; Malluche, H.H.; Williams, J.P. The effect of class a scavenger receptor deficiency in bone. *J. Biol. Chem.* **2007**, *282*, 4653–4660. [CrossRef]
51. Takemura, K.; Sakashita, N.; Fujiwara, Y.; Komohara, Y.; Lei, X.; Ohnishi, K.; Suzuki, H.; Kodama, T.; Mizuta, H.; Takeya, M. Class A scavenger receptor promotes osteoclast differentiation via the enhanced expression of receptor activator of NF-kappaB (RANK). *Biochem. Biophys. Res. Commun.* **2010**, *391*, 1675–1680. [CrossRef] [PubMed]
52. Sigalov, A.B. Nature-inspired nanoformulations for contrast-enhanced in vivo MR imaging of macrophages. *Contrast Media Mol. Imaging* **2014**, *9*, 372–382. [CrossRef] [PubMed]

53. Sigalov, A.B. A novel ligand-independent peptide inhibitor of TREM-1 suppresses tumor growth in human lung cancer xenografts and prolongs survival of mice with lipopolysaccharide-induced septic shock. *Int. Immunopharmacol.* **2014**, *21*, 208–219. [CrossRef] [PubMed]
54. Brand, D.D.; Latham, K.A.; Rosloniec, E.F. Collagen-induced arthritis. *Nat. Protoc.* **2007**, *2*, 1269–1275. [CrossRef] [PubMed]
55. Corvo, M.L.; Boerman, O.C.; Oyen, W.J.; Van Bloois, L.; Cruz, M.E.; Crommelin, D.J.; Storm, G. Intravenous administration of superoxide dismutase entrapped in long circulating liposomes. II. In vivo fate in a rat model of adjuvant arthritis. *Biochim. Biophys. Acta (BBA)-Biomembr.* **1999**, *1419*, 325–334. [CrossRef]
56. Corvo, M.L.; Boerman, O.C.; Oyen, W.J.; Jorge, J.C.; Cruz, M.E.; Crommelin, D.J.; Storm, G. Subcutaneous administration of superoxide dismutase entrapped in long circulating liposomes: In vivo fate and therapeutic activity in an inflammation model. *Pharm. Res.* **2000**, *17*, 600–606. [CrossRef]
57. Wang, S.; Yang, S.; Lai, X.; Song, Y.; Hu, L.; Li, C.; Shi, T.; Liu, X.; Deng, Y.; Chen, G. Sialic Acid Conjugate-Modified Liposomal Dexamethasone Palmitate Targeting Neutrophils for Rheumatoid Arthritis Therapy: Influence of Particle Size. *AAPS PharmSciTech* **2021**, *22*, 16. [CrossRef]
58. Stolina, M.; Bolon, B.; Dwyer, D.; Middleton, S.; Duryea, D.; Kostenuik, P.J.; Feige, U.; Zack, D.J. The evolving systemic and local biomarker milieu at different stages of disease progression in rat collagen-induced arthritis. *Biomarkers* **2008**, *13*, 692–712. [CrossRef]
59. Stolina, M.; Bolon, B.; Middleton, S.; Dwyer, D.; Brown, H.; Duryea, D.; Zhu, L.; Rohner, A.; Pretorius, J.; Kostenuik, P.; et al. The evolving systemic and local biomarker milieu at different stages of disease progression in rat adjuvant-induced arthritis. *J. Clin. Immunol.* **2009**, *29*, 158–174. [CrossRef]
60. Sigalov, A.B. The SCHOOL of nature: III. From mechanistic understanding to novel therapies. *Self Nonself* **2010**, *1*, 192–224. [CrossRef]
61. Schett, G. Cells of the synovium in rheumatoid arthritis. Osteoclasts. *Arthritis Res. Ther.* **2007**, *9*, 203. [CrossRef] [PubMed]
62. Joosten, L.A.; Helsen, M.M.; Saxne, T.; van De Loo, F.A.; Heinegard, D.; van Den Berg, W.B. IL-1 alpha beta blockade prevents cartilage and bone destruction in murine type II collagen-induced arthritis, whereas TNF-alpha blockade only ameliorates joint inflammation. *J. Immunol.* **1999**, *163*, 5049–5055. [PubMed]
63. Ohno, H.; Uemura, Y.; Murooka, H.; Takanashi, H.; Tokieda, T.; Ohzeki, Y.; Kubo, K.; Serizawa, I. The orally-active and selective c-Fms tyrosine kinase inhibitor Ki20227 inhibits disease progression in a collagen-induced arthritis mouse model. *Eur. J. Immunol.* **2008**, *38*, 283–291. [CrossRef] [PubMed]
64. Fan, D.; He, X.; Bian, Y.; Guo, Q.; Zheng, K.; Zhao, Y.; Lu, C.; Liu, B.; Xu, X.; Zhang, G.; et al. Triptolide Modulates TREM-1 Signal Pathway to Inhibit the Inflammatory Response in Rheumatoid Arthritis. *Int. J. Mol. Sci.* **2016**, *17*, 498. [CrossRef]
65. Burmester, G.R.; Stuhlmuller, B.; Keyszer, G.; Kinne, R.W. Mononuclear phagocytes and rheumatoid synovitis. Mastermind or workhorse in arthritis? *Arthritis Rheum.* **1997**, *40*, 5–18. [CrossRef]
66. Pandupuspitasari, N.S.; Khan, F.A.; Huang, C.J.; Chen, X.; Zhang, S. Novel Attributions of TREMs in Immunity. *Curr. Issues Mol. Biol.* **2016**, *20*, 47–54. [CrossRef]
67. Jay, T.R.; Miller, C.M.; Cheng, P.J.; Graham, L.C.; Bemiller, S.; Broihier, M.L.; Xu, G.; Margevicius, D.; Karlo, J.C.; Sousa, G.L.; et al. TREM2 deficiency eliminates TREM2+ inflammatory macrophages and ameliorates pathology in Alzheimer's disease mouse models. *J. Exp. Med.* **2015**, *212*, 287–295. [CrossRef]
68. Rommel, C.; Camps, M.; Ji, H. PI3K delta and PI3K gamma: Partners in crime in inflammation in rheumatoid arthritis and beyond? *Nat. Rev. Immunol.* **2007**, *7*, 191–201. [CrossRef]
69. Dinarello, C.A. Inflammation in human disease: Anticytokine therapy. *Biol. Blood Marrow Transplant.* **2009**, *15*, 134–136. [CrossRef]
70. Curtis, J.R.; Singh, J.A. Use of biologics in rheumatoid arthritis: Current and emerging paradigms of care. *Clin. Ther.* **2011**, *33*, 679–707. [CrossRef]
71. Mewar, D.; Wilson, A.G. Treatment of rheumatoid arthritis with tumour necrosis factor inhibitors. *Br. J. Pharmacol.* **2011**, *162*, 785–791. [CrossRef] [PubMed]
72. Atzeni, F.; Sarzi-Puttini, P.; Botsios, C.; Carletto, A.; Cipriani, P.; Favalli, E.G.; Frati, E.; Foschi, V.; Gasparini, S.; Giardina, A.; et al. Long-term anti-TNF therapy and the risk of serious infections in a cohort of patients with rheumatoid arthritis: Comparison of adalimumab, etanercept and infliximab in the GISEA registry. *Autoimmun. Rev.* **2012**, *12*, 225–229. [CrossRef] [PubMed]
73. Galloway, J.B.; Hyrich, K.L.; Mercer, L.K.; Dixon, W.G.; Ustianowski, A.P.; Helbert, M.; Watson, K.D.; Lunt, M.; Symmons, D.P. Risk of septic arthritis in patients with rheumatoid arthritis and the effect of anti-TNF therapy: Results from the British Society for Rheumatology Biologics Register. *Ann. Rheum. Dis.* **2011**, *70*, 1810–1814. [CrossRef]
74. Sica, A.; Massarotti, M. Myeloid suppressor cells in cancer and autoimmunity. *J. Autoimmun.* **2017**, *85*, 117–125. [CrossRef] [PubMed]
75. Alivernini, S.; MacDonald, L.; Elmesmari, A.; Finlay, S.; Tolusso, B.; Gigante, M.R.; Petricca, L.; Di Mario, C.; Bui, L.; Perniola, S.; et al. Distinct synovial tissue macrophage subsets regulate inflammation and remission in rheumatoid arthritis. *Nat. Med.* **2020**, *26*, 1295–1306. [CrossRef] [PubMed]
76. Shen, Z.T.; Sigalov, A.B. Novel TREM-1 Inhibitors Attenuate Tumor Growth and Prolong Survival in Experimental Pancreatic Cancer. *Mol. Pharm.* **2017**, *14*, 4572–4582. [CrossRef]
77. Rojas, M.A.; Shen, Z.T.; Caldwell, R.B.; Sigalov, A.B. Blockade of TREM-1 prevents vitreoretinal neovascularization in mice with oxygen-induced retinopathy. *Biophys. Acta (BBA)-Mol. Basis Dis.* **2018**, *1864*, 2761–2768. [CrossRef]

78. Tornai, D.; Furi, I.; Shen, Z.T.; Sigalov, A.B.; Coban, S.; Szabo, G. Inhibition of Triggering Receptor Expressed on Myeloid Cells 1 Ameliorates Inflammation and Macrophage and Neutrophil Activation in Alcoholic Liver Disease in Mice. *Hepatol. Commun.* **2019**, *3*, 99–115. [CrossRef]
79. Shen, Z.T.; Sigalov, A.B. SARS Coronavirus Fusion Peptide-Derived Sequence Suppresses Collagen-Induced Arthritis in DBA/1J Mice. *Sci. Rep.* **2016**, *6*, 28672. [CrossRef]
80. Correale, C.; Genua, M.; Vetrano, S.; Mazzini, E.; Martinoli, C.; Spinelli, A.; Arena, V.; Peyrin-Biroulet, L.; Caprioli, F.; Passini, N.; et al. Bacterial sensor triggering receptor expressed on myeloid cells-2 regulates the mucosal inflammatory response. *Gastroenterology* **2013**, *144*, 346–356 e343. [CrossRef]
81. Molgora, M.; Esaulova, E.; Vermi, W.; Hou, J.; Chen, Y.; Luo, J.; Brioschi, S.; Bugatti, M.; Omodei, A.S.; Ricci, B.; et al. TREM2 Modulation Remodels the Tumor Myeloid Landscape Enhancing Anti-PD-1 Immunotherapy. *Cell* **2020**, *182*, 886–900.e817. [CrossRef] [PubMed]
82. Cheng, X.; Wang, X.; Nie, K.; Cheng, L.; Zhang, Z.; Hu, Y.; Peng, W. Systematic Pan-Cancer Analysis Identifies TREM2 as an Immunological and Prognostic Biomarker. *Front. Immunol.* **2021**, *12*, 646523. [CrossRef] [PubMed]
83. Binnewies, M.; Pollack, J.L.; Rudolph, J.; Dash, S.; Abushawish, M.; Lee, T.; Jahchan, N.S.; Canaday, P.; Lu, E.; Norng, M.; et al. Targeting TREM2 on tumor-associated macrophages enhances immunotherapy. *Cell Rep.* **2021**, *37*, 109844. [CrossRef] [PubMed]
84. Schmitz, N.; Laverty, S.; Kraus, V.B.; Aigner, T. Basic methods in histopathology of joint tissues. *Osteoarthr. Cartil.* **2010**, *18* (Suppl. 3), S113–S116. [CrossRef] [PubMed]

International Journal of
Molecular Sciences

MDPI

Article

IL-17 Facilitates VCAM-1 Production and Monocyte Adhesion in Osteoarthritis Synovial Fibroblasts by Suppressing miR-5701 Synthesis

Tsung-Ju Wu [1,†], Sunny Li-Yun Chang [2,†], Chih-Yang Lin [3], Chao-Yang Lai [4], Xiu-Yuan He [2], Chun-Hao Tsai [5,6], Chih-Yuan Ko [6], Yi-Chin Fong [5,6,7], Chen-Ming Su [5,*] and Chih-Hsin Tang [2,4,8,9,*]

1 Department of Physical Medicine and Rehabilitation, Changhua Christian Hospital, Changhua 500209, Taiwan; 134330@cch.org.tw
2 Graduate Institute of Biomedical Sciences, China Medical University, Taichung 404333, Taiwan; sunnylyc@gmail.com (S.L.-Y.C.); hchp99812@gmail.com (X.-Y.H.)
3 Translational Medicine Center, Shin-Kong Wu Ho-Su Memorial Hospital, Taipei 111045, Taiwan; T016406@ms.skh.org.tw
4 Department of Medical Laboratory Science and Biotechnology, Asia University, Taichung 413305, Taiwan; chaoyang@asia.edu.tw
5 Department of Sports Medicine, College of Health Care, China Medical University, Taichung 406040, Taiwan; ritsai8615@gmail.com (C.-H.T.); yichin.fong@gmail.com (Y.-C.F.)
6 Department of Orthopedic Surgery, China Medical University Hospital, Taichung 404327, Taiwan; d14333@mail.cmuh.org.tw
7 Department of Orthopaedic Surgery, China Medical University Beigang Hospital, Yunlin 651012, Taiwan
8 Department of Pharmacology, School of Medicine, China Medical University, Taichung 406040, Taiwan
9 Chinese Medicine Research Center, China Medical University, Taichung 406040, Taiwan
* Correspondence: cmsu@mail.cmu.edu.tw (C.-M.S.); chtang@mail.cmu.edu.tw (C.-H.T.); Tel.: +886-2205-3366 (ext. 7616) (C.-M.S.); +886-2205-2121 (ext. 7726) (C.-H.T.)
† These authors contributed equally to this work.

Citation: Wu, T.-J.; Chang, S.L.-Y.; Lin, C.-Y.; Lai, C.-Y.; He, X.-Y.; Tsai, C.-H.; Ko, C.-Y.; Fong, Y.-C.; Su, C.-M.; Tang, C.-H. IL-17 Facilitates VCAM-1 Production and Monocyte Adhesion in Osteoarthritis Synovial Fibroblasts by Suppressing miR-5701 Synthesis. *Int. J. Mol. Sci.* **2022**, *23*, 6804. https://doi.org/10.3390/ijms23126804

Academic Editor: Francesca Oliviero

Received: 28 April 2022
Accepted: 15 June 2022
Published: 18 June 2022

Abstract: Osteoarthritis (OA) is characterized by the infiltration and adhesion of monocytes into the inflamed joint synovium. Interleukin (IL)-17 is a critical inflammatory mediator that participates in the progression of OA, although the mechanisms linking IL-17 and monocyte infiltration are not well understood. Our analysis of synovial tissue samples retrieved from the Gene Expression Omnibus (GEO) dataset exhibited higher monocyte marker (CD11b) and vascular cell adhesion molecule 1 (VCAM-1) levels in OA samples than in normal, healthy samples. The stimulation of human OA synovial fibroblasts (OASFs) with IL-17 increased VCAM-1 production and subsequently enhanced monocyte adhesion. IL-17 affected VCAM-1-dependent monocyte adhesion by reducing miR-5701 expression through the protein kinase C (PKC)-α and c-Jun N-terminal kinase (JNK) signaling cascades. Our findings improve our understanding about the effect of IL-17 on OA progression and, in particular, VCAM-1 production and monocyte adhesion, which may help with the design of more effective OA treatments.

Keywords: IL-17; osteoarthritis; monocytes; VCAM-1; adhesion

1. Introduction

Osteoarthritis (OA) is a joint disorder that is accompanied by the migration and invasion of monocytes into the synovial membrane, leading to synovial inflammation, cartilage degradation, and bone breakdown [1,2], evoking pain and adversely affecting the patient's quality of life. As the disease progresses, critical steps in the joint microenvironment regarding the synthesis of proinflammatory factors and chondrolytic mediators enhance the breakdown of cartilage and loss of bone [3,4]. Numerous OA synovial fibroblasts (OASFs) in the joint microenvironment control the development of OA by synthesizing proinflammatory factors and catabolic mediators [3,5,6], indicating that remedying the state of the synovium is appropriate for OA treatment [7,8].

Macrophage and monocyte infiltration into the joint microenvironment and their adhesion to the synovial membrane is an important mediator of OA development [9]. Several adhesion molecules regulate the infiltration and migration of macrophages and monocytes during OA development, including vascular cell adhesion molecule 1 (VCAM-1) [9,10]. Higher VCAM-1 expression is documented in human OA synovium than in normal synovium [10]. The inhibition of VCAM-1 levels in OA synovium reportedly lowers the inflammatory response during OA progression [11,12].

Accumulating evidence indicates that the interleukin (IL)-17 family of cytokines regulates the pathogenesis of OA [13]. A higher expression of IL-17 in OA serum and synovial fluid is reflected by radiographic OA severity scores [13,14]. *IL-17* gene polymorphisms have been linked to the development of OA in several populations [15,16], while injections of IL-17 into the rabbit knee joint induces OA [17]. Moreover, IL-17 enhances osteoclastogenesis, and bone erosion plays an important role in arthritic diseases [18]. Thus, it is worth targeting IL-17 as a novel therapeutic for managing OA disease.

MicroRNAs (miRNAs, single-stranded noncoding RNAs) regulate the production of target genes at the post-transcriptional stage [19,20]. Several miRNAs mediate the development of OA by negatively or positively regulating synovial cell inflammation, differentiation, angiogenesis, and survival [21,22]. However, it is not clear as to whether IL-17 regulates miRNA-mediated VCAM-1 synthesis and the adhesion of monocytes during OA progression. Here, we found higher levels of the monocyte marker CD11b and VCAM-1 expression in OA synovial tissue than in normal, healthy tissue. Our results also indicate that IL-17 facilitates VCAM-1 production and promotes monocyte adhesion in human OASFs by decreasing miR-5701 expression in the protein kinase C (PKC)-α and c-Jun N-terminal kinase (JNK) signaling cascades, indicating that IL-17 may be worth targeting when treating OA.

2. Results

2.1. IL-17 Promotes Monocyte Adhesion in Human OASFs by Enhancing VCAM-1 Production

The infiltration of macrophages and monocytes and their adhesion to synovial membrane, where they promote a proinflammatory response, is a critical step in OA development [23]. Since CD11b is a major monocyte marker for OA disease, we examined the expression of CD11b in raw data from OA (n = 22) and healthy synovial tissue samples (n = 28) downloaded from the Gene Expression Omnibus (GEO) dataset (accession code: GSE89408). The analyses revealed significantly higher levels of the monocyte marker CD11b in OA synovial samples than in normal controls (Figure 1A), which was also the case in our histopathologic analysis of CD11b expression in our samples of human OA synovial tissue (n = 4) and healthy control samples (n = 4) (Figure 1B,C, Supplementary Figure S1A). OASFs were stimulated with IL-17 for 2 h, and then the culture was changed to a serum-free medium for the next 24 h (to exclude the direct effect of IL-17 on monocytes), and monocytes (THP-1 cells) were added to a monolayer of OASFs for 1 h. Monocyte adhesion analysis revealed that IL-17 treatment dose-dependently enhanced monocyte adhesion in OASFs (Figure 1D,E, Supplementary Figure S1B). Treatment of monocytes with IL-17 for 1 h did not increase their adherence to OASFs (Supplementary Figure S2). Stimulation of OASFs with TNF-α also promoted monocyte adherence (Supplementary Figure S3). Thus, IL-17 promotes monocyte adhesion in human OASFs; the other pathways, such as TNF-α, also have similar effects.

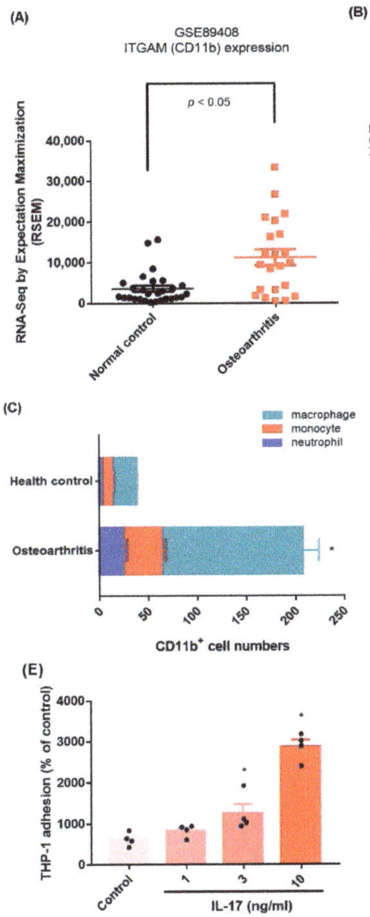

Figure 1. IL-17 promotes monocyte adhesion in OASFs. (**A**) Levels of CD11b were investigated in OA and healthy control synovial tissue collected from the GEO database. (**B**,**C**) IHC staining for CD11b$^+$ (neutrophil, monocyte, and macrophage) in synovium samples from OA patients and healthy individuals. (**D**,**E**) OASFs were stimulated with vehicle or IL-17 (1–10 ng/mL) for 24 h. Monocytes (THP-1 cells) were then applied to the OASFs. Adherent THP-1 cells were photographed and quantified under fluorescence microscopy. Size bar = 320 μm. * $p < 0.05$ compared with the control group.

VCAM-1-regulated adhesion of macrophages and monocytes to the synovial membrane is crucial for OA [24]. Data from the GEO database and our clinical samples displayed higher expression of VCAM-1 in OA synovial tissue than in healthy tissue (Figure 2A–D, Supplementary Figure S4A), and we observed a significant positive correlation between CD11b and VCAM-1 levels (Figure 2E,F). Treatment of OASFs with IL-17 promoted the transcription of VCAM-1 mRNA and the translation of VCAM-1 protein (Figure 2G,H). Transfection of OASFs with VCAM-1 siRNA without IL-17 treatment inhibited VCAM-1 expression (Figure 2I). In addition, transfection of OASFs with VCAM-1 siRNA and IL-17 treatment abolished IL-17-induced promotion of VCAM-1 expression and monocyte adhesion (Figure 2J–M, Supplementary Figure S4B). VCAM-1 siRNA completely inhibited IL-17-induced promotion of VCAM-1 expression. Thus, IL-17 facilitates the adhesion of monocytes to human OASFs by facilitating VCAM-1 synthesis.

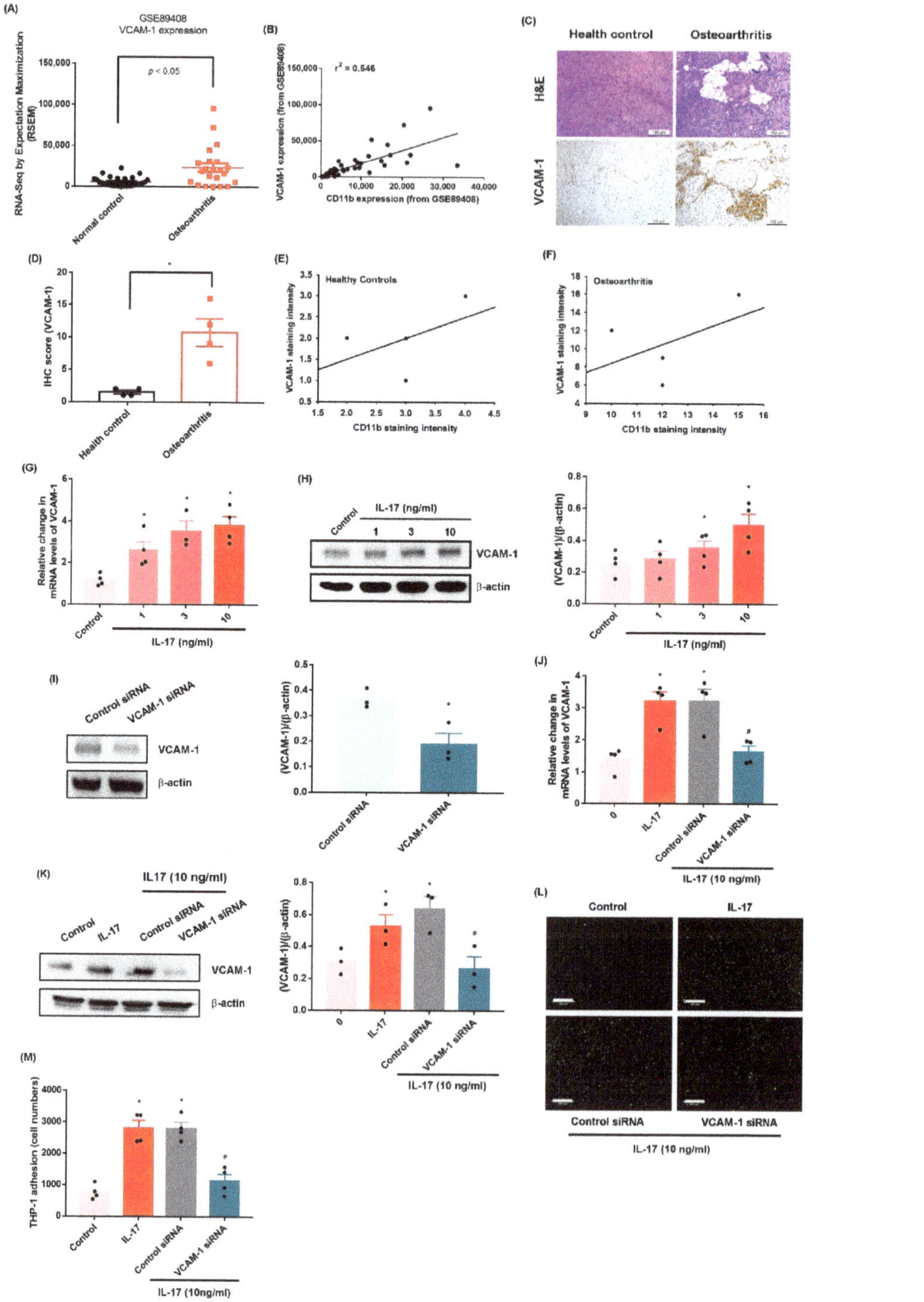

Figure 2. IL-17 promotes monocyte adhesion in OASFs through upregulating VCAM-1 production.

(**A**) Levels of VCAM-1 were investigated in synovial tissue collected from the GEO database containing OA patients and healthy controls. (**B**) Spearman's rank correlation coefficient testing identified significant, positive correlations between VCAM-1 and CD11b. (**C–F**) IHC staining for VCAM-1 in synovium samples from OA patients and healthy individuals. (**G**,**H**) OASFs were stimulated with IL-17 for 24 h, and VCAM-1 synthesis was performed by qPCR and Western blot. (**I–M**) OASFs were transfected with a VCAM-1 siRNA for 24 h and then treated with or without IL-17 (10 ng/mL). VCAM-1 expression was examined by Western blot and qPCR. Adherent THP-1 cells were photographed and quantified under fluorescence microscopy. Size bar = 320 μm. * $p < 0.05$ compared with the control group; # $p < 0.05$ compared with the IL-17-stimulated group.

2.2. IL-17 Promotes VCAM-1-Dependent Monocyte Adhesion in OASFs via the PKC-α and JNK Signaling Pathways

PKC activation is an important event in OA development [12,25]. Treatment of OASFs with the pan PKC inhibitor (GF109203X) and PKC-α/β inhibitor (Gö6976) or PKC-α siRNA antagonized IL-17-induced increases in VCAM-1 synthesis and monocyte adhesion (Figure 3A–F, Supplementary Figure S5A,B). The PKC inhibitors (GF109203X and Gö6976) did not affect the basal levels of VCAM-1 mRNA expression (Figure 3A). Transfection of OASFs with PKC-α siRNA inhibited PKC-α expression (Figure 3G); the knockdown of PKC-α produced similar effects (Figure 3H). In addition, Western blot analysis found that IL-17 facilitated PKC-α phosphorylation (Figure 3I).

JNK is a downstream molecule of PKC in VCAM-1-mediated cell adhesion [12]. Both the JNK inhibitor (SP600125) and JNK siRNA reversed IL-17-induced promotion of VCAM-1 synthesis and monocyte adhesion (Figure 4A–F, Supplementary Figure S6A,B). Transfection of OASFs with JNK siRNA inhibited JNK expression (Figure 4G). IL-17 also enhanced the phosphorylation of JNK (Figure 4H), which was diminished by pretreatment with the PKC inhibitors (Figure 4I). In contrast, the JNK inhibitor inhibited IL-17-promoted JNK but not PKC-α phosphorylation (Figure 4J), suggesting that PKC-α-dependent JNK activation mediates IL-17-induced enhancement of VCAM-1 synthesis and monocyte adhesion in OASFs.

2.3. IL-17 Enhances VCAM-1 Synthesis and Monocyte Adhesion by Suppressing miR-5701 Expression

Numerous miRNAs are found at different levels of expression in normal and OA synovial tissue and regulate OA progression [26,27]. Analyses of six open-source software programs predicted that 21 miRNAs interfere with VCAM-1 mRNA transcription (Figure 5A). Our analysis of the GEO database found that among these miRNAs, eighteen (including miR-5701) exhibited lower levels of expression in OA patients than in normal, healthy individuals (Figure 5B). When OASFs were treated with IL-17, the expression of miR-5701 was suppressed by a markedly greater extent compared with the other miRNAs (Figure 5C). In addition, IL-17 concentration-dependently abolished miR-5701 synthesis (Figure 5D,E). Transfecting OASFs with miR-5701 mimic lowered VCAM-1 synthesis and monocyte adhesion (Figure 5F–I, Supplementary Figure S7). Treating OASFs with inhibitors and siRNAs of PKC-α and JNK antagonized IL-17-induced inhibition of miR-5701 synthesis (Figure 5J,K), indicating that IL-17 suppresses miR-5701 synthesis through the PKC-α and JNK signaling pathways.

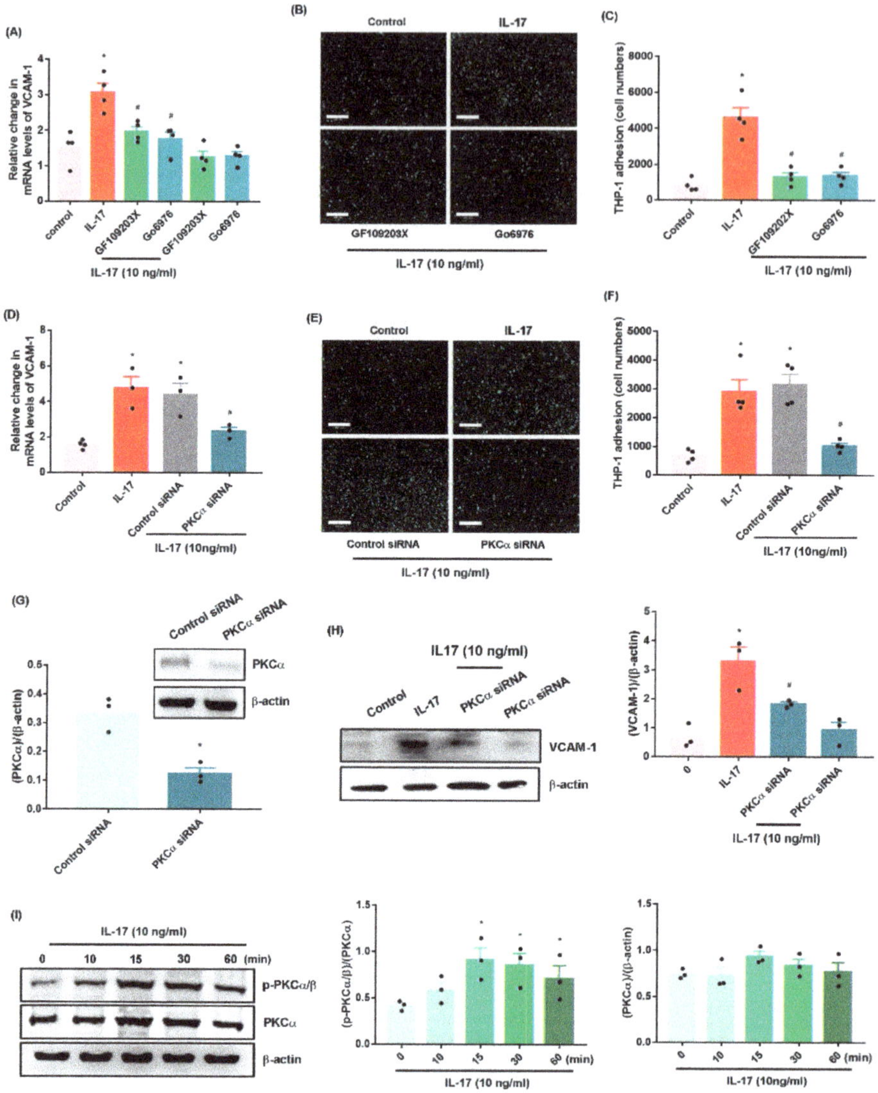

Figure 3. The PKC-α pathway mediates IL-17-induced promotion of VCAM-1 synthesis and monocyte adhesion in OASFs. (**A**,**D**,**H**) OASFs were stimulated with PKC inhibitors (GF109203X, 10 nM and Gö6976, 10 nM) for 30 min or transfected with a PKC-α siRNA for 24 h and then treated with or without IL-17 (10 ng/mL) for 24 h. Quantification of VCAM-1 expression was performed by qPCR and Western blot. (**B**,**C**,**E**,**F**) Adherent THP-1 cells were photographed and quantified under fluorescence microscopy. (**G**) PKC-α protein levels were measured by Western blot. (**I**) OASFs were stimulated with IL-17 for the indicated time intervals. PKC-α phosphorylation was performed by Western blot. Size bar = 320 μm. * $p < 0.05$ compared with the control group; # $p < 0.05$ compared with the IL-17-stimulated group.

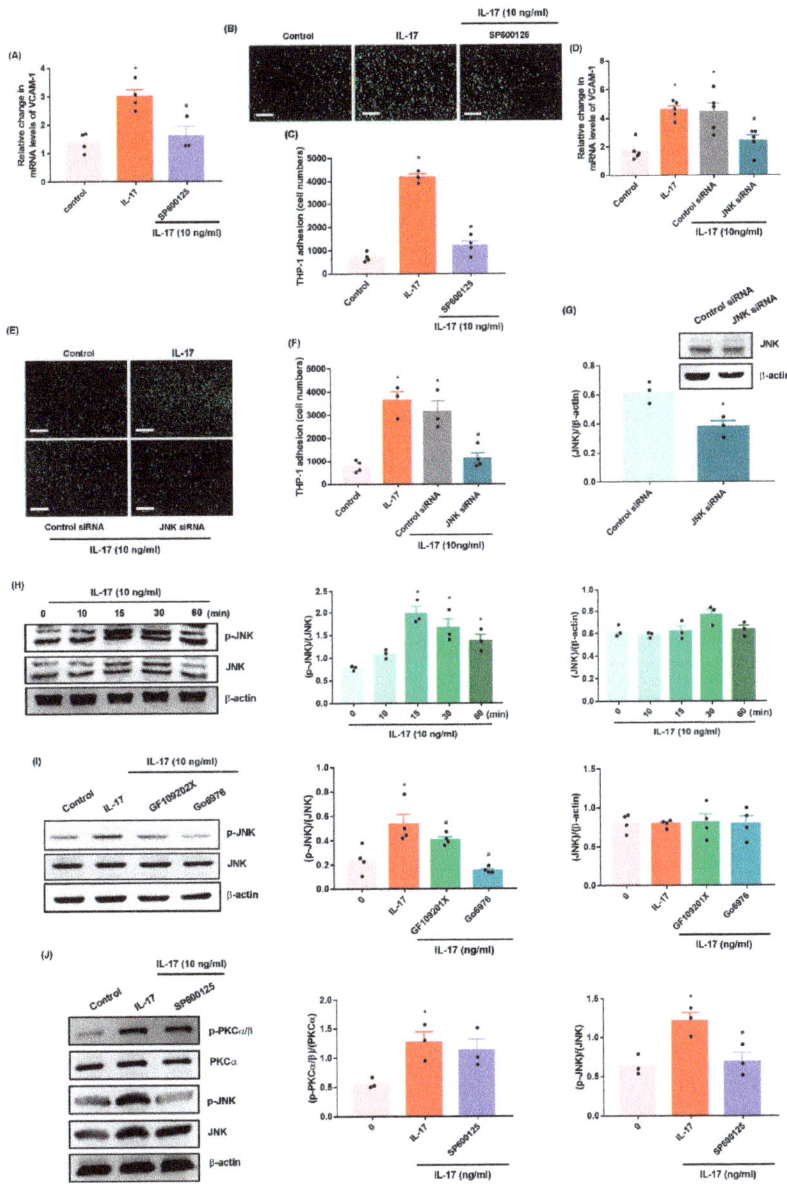

Figure 4. The JNK pathway mediates IL-17-induced promotion of VCAM-1 synthesis and monocyte adhesion in OASFs. (**A**,**D**) OASFs were stimulated with a JNK inhibitor (SP600125, 10 nM) for 30 min or transfected with a JNK siRNA for 24 h and then treated with IL-17 (10 ng/mL) for 24 h. VCAM-1 levels were quantified by qPCR. (**B**,**C**,**E**,**F**) Adherent THP-1 cells were photographed and quantified under fluorescence microscopy. (**G**) JNK protein levels were measured by Western blot. (**H–J**) OASFs were stimulated with IL-17 for the indicated time intervals or pretreated with PKC or JNK inhibitors and then incubated with IL-17 (10 ng/mL). JNK or PKC phosphorylation was performed by Western blot. Size bar = 320 μm. * $p < 0.05$ compared with the control group; # $p < 0.05$ compared with the IL-17-stimulated group.

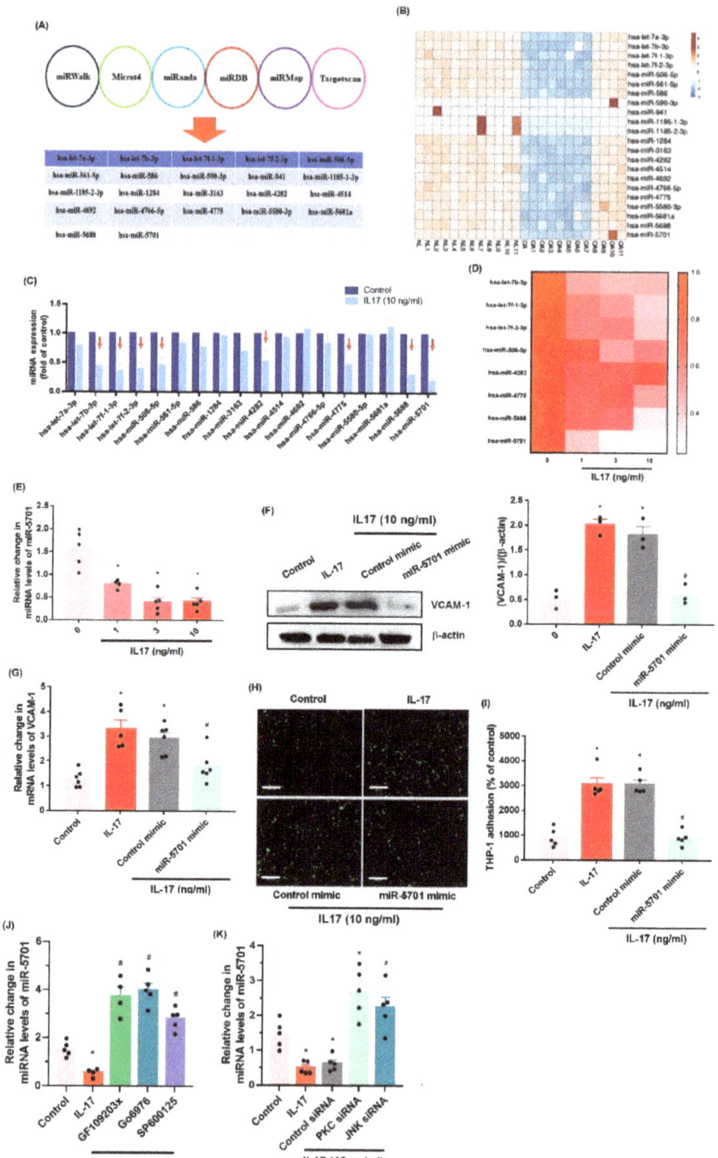

Figure 5. IL-17 enhances VCAM-1 production by inhibiting miR-5701 expression. (**A**) Six software databases were examined to predict which miRNAs interfere with VCAM-1 transcription. (**B**) Levels of miRNAs were investigated in OA and normal, healthy synovial tissue collected from the GEO database. (**C–E**) OASFs were treated with IL-17 (10 ng/mL). miRNA expression was examined by qPCR. (**F,G**) OASFs were transfected with miR-5701 mimic and then treated with IL-17 (10 ng/mL). VCAM-1 expression was examined by Western blot and qPCR. (**H,I**) Adherent THP-1 cells were photographed and quantified under fluorescence microscopy. (**J,K**) OASFs were stimulated with PKC and JNK inhibitors for 30 min or the respective siRNAs for 24 h and then incubated with IL-17 (10 ng/mL). miR-5701 expression was examined by qPCR. Size bar = 320 μm. * $p < 0.05$ compared with the control group; # $p < 0.05$ compared with the IL-17-stimulated group.

3. Discussion

OA causes much physical disability [1]. Much remains unknown about the pathogenesis of OA; however, synovial inflammation is well-recognized [28], so treatment targeting the synovium may inhibit disease progression [7,29]. Elevated levels of macrophage and monocyte expression are found in the OA joint [30]. In this study, an analysis of the GEO database and our clinical results found higher levels of the monocyte marker CD11b in synovial tissue from OA patients than in tissue from normal, healthy individuals. IL-17 appears to aggravate the symptoms of OA [13]. Higher IL-17 levels have been reported in the serum and synovial fluid of OA patients than in healthy controls [13,14]. In this study, we demonstrated that IL-17 enhanced monocyte adhesion in human OASFs by upregulating VCAM-1 production. Moreover, the suppression of miR-5701 expression via PKC-α and JNK signaling regulated the effects of IL-17. The anti-IL17 monoclonal antibody secukinumab is approved for the treatment of psoriasis [31]. Whether anti-IL-17 agents are appropriate in OA treatment needs to be clarified.

VCAM-1-dependent mononuclear cell infiltration and adhesion in synovial tissue influences arthritic progression [24,32]. In this study, the GEO database records and our clinical samples displayed higher VCAM-1 expression in synovial tissue from OA patients compared with that from normal, healthy controls. A positive correlation between CD11b and VCAM-1 levels indicates that these cytokines contribute to OA disease progression. Here, we found that VCAM-1 is a response mediator in IL-17 stimulation, promoting monocyte adhesion. This effect was antagonized when OASFs were transfected with VCAM-1 siRNA, which suggests that IL-17 facilitates VCAM-1-induced monocyte adhesion in human OASFs.

PKC activation is crucial for regulating different cellular events [33], such as the promotion of cell motility and adhesion [12,34]. Our data found that IL-17 enhances PKC-α phosphorylation, while the PKC inhibitor or siRNA diminished IL-17-facilitated promotion of VCAM-1 synthesis and monocyte adhesion in OASFs. JNK is essential for regulating the inflammatory process during OA disease [35,36]. Our data showed that a JNK inhibitor or siRNA antagonized IL-17-facilitated VCAM-1-dependent monocyte adhesion. Our findings also reveal that IL-17 enhances JNK phosphorylation, which was reversed by the PKC inhibitor, indicating that PKC-α-dependent JNK activation regulates IL-17-induced synthesis of VCAM-1 and monocyte adhesion in human OASFs.

miRNAs are critical post-transcriptional mediators of gene production and are found in several diseases, including OA [37,38]. It has been proposed that pharmacotherapy capable of controlling miRNA levels would inhibit OA inflammatory progression and thus be an appropriate therapeutic approach for this disease [37,39]. Here, our analysis of six miRNA software databases predicted that miR-5701 interferes with VCAM-1 transcription. This was supported by the study data showing lower miR-5701 expression in OA synovial tissue than in normal, healthy tissue. We found that IL-17 treatment inhibits miR-5701 expression, and treatment of OASFs with miR-5701 mimic antagonizes IL-17-induced promotion of VCAM-1 synthesis and monocyte adhesion. PKC-α and JNK inhibitors, as well as their respective siRNAs, antagonized IL-17-enhanced inhibition of miR-5701 synthesis, suggesting that IL-17 promotes VCAM-1 synthesis and monocyte adhesion in human OASFs by reducing miR-5701 production through the PKC-α and JNK pathways. Our results also suggest that the development of IL-17, PKC, JNK, and VCAM-1 antagonists inhibit OA progression.

4. Materials and Methods

Antibodies against PKC-α, JNK, VCAM-1, CD11b, and β-actin were purchased from GeneTex (Hsinchu, Taiwan). Antibodies against p-PKCα and p-JNK were purchased from Cell Signaling Technology (Danvers, MA, USA). 2′,7′-Bis(2-carboxyethyl)-5(6)-carboxyfluorescein tetrakis(acetoxymethyl) ester (BCECF-AM) and GF109203X, Gö6976 and SP600125 inhibitors were obtained from Sigma-Aldrich (St. Louis, MO, USA).

4.1. Cell Culture

Synovial tissues freshly obtained from OA patients were washed with phosphate-buffered saline (PBS), minced thoroughly using a scalpel, and then subjected to 4 h of enzymatic digestion in serum-free DMEM medium with 2 mg/mL type I collagenase in an incubator at 37 °C, before removal of collagenase by centrifugation. OASFs were cultured in DMEM containing 10% fetal bovine serum (FBS), penicillin, and streptomycin (Invitrogen; Carlsbad, CA, USA) [25]. A total of 2 passages were performed of culture when the adherent cells approached 70% confluence, and experiments were performed using cells grown in vitro for 3–6 passages.

THP-1 cells (human monocytes) were purchased from the Bioresource Collection and Research Center (Hsinchu, Taiwan) and maintained in RPMI-1640 medium supplemented with 10% FBS, 2 mM L-glutamine, 0.05 mM β-mercaptoethanol, 10 mM HEPES, 100 U/mL penicillin, and 100 μg/mL streptomycin at 37 °C in a humidified 5% CO_2 atmosphere. THP-1 cells were kept at a minimum density of 3×10^5 cells and were passaged when the density reached 8×10^5 cells.

4.2. Monocyte Adhesion Analysis

Human OASFs (1×10^5 cells) were cultured in 24-well culture plates and treated with IL-17 for 2 h, before changing the culture medium to serum-free conditions for 24 h. THP-1 cells were treated with BCECF-AM (10 μM; a pH-sensitive fluorescent dye used for determining living cells) at 37 °C for 1 h and subsequently washed twice with PBS by centrifugation. BCECF-AM-labeled THP-1 cells (2.5×10^5 cells/mL) were added to a monolayer of OASFs at 37 °C for 1 h. Nonadherent THP-1 cells were cleaned off using PBS. Adherent THP-1 cells were quantified under fluorescence microscopy. We counted the number of cells in three random fields under each condition.

4.3. Human Clinical Samples

The collection of synovial samples from patients with OA and those with trauma/joint injuries (serving as normal, healthy controls) was approved by the Institutional Review Board of China Medical University Hospital. Informed written consent was obtained from all patients.

4.4. Real-Time Quantitative PCR Analysis of mRNA and miRNA

Total RNA was isolated from OASFs using TRIzol reagent (MDBio; Taipei, Taiwan). RNA (1 μg) was reverse-transcribed into cDNA with oligo-DT primer, according to the manufacturer's procedure (Invitrogen; Carlsbad, CA, USA). qPCR was performed using SYBR Green with sequence-specific primers (Invitrogen; Carlsbad, CA, USA) (Supplementary Table S1). Levels of GAPDH or U6 snRNA expression served as the endogenous controls for normalization purposes. qPCR assays were performed with StepOnePlus (Applied Biosystems; Foster City, CA, USA) [11,40].

4.5. Western Blot

OASFs were treated with RIPA buffer. Isolated proteins were subjected to SDS-PAGE and transferred to polyvinylidene difluoride membranes (Merck; Darmstadt, Germany) [41,42]. The membranes were blocked with 5% nonfat milk and then treated with primary antibodies. The membranes were then washed and treated with secondary antibodies and then visualized using the ImageQuant™ LAS 4000 biomolecular imager [43–45].

4.6. Measurement of Data from the Gene Expression Omnibus (GEO) Database

Data on CD11b and VCAM-1 expression from normal, healthy control samples and OA samples were obtained from the GEO database, as according to our previous studies [46,47].

4.7. *Immunohistochemistry (IHC)*

Human synovial tissues were stained with anti-CD11b or VCAM-1 antibody and quantified according to the protocol described in our previous work [48,49]. The sum of the intensity and percentage scores was used as the final staining score [47].

4.8. *Small Interfering RNA (siRNA) Transfection*

ON-TARGETplus siRNAs of PKC (L-003523-00), JNK (L00351400), VCAM-1 (L-013351-00), and control (D0018101005) were purchased from Dharmacon Research (Lafayette, CO, USA). Transient transfection of siRNAs was carried out using DharmaFECT1 transfection reagent (T-2001-01). All siRNAs (100 nM) were formulated with DharmaFECT1 transfection reagent, according to the manufacturer's instructions.

4.9. *Statistical Analysis*

All values are given as the mean ± standard deviation (S.D.). The Student's *t*-test assessed between-group differences. A p value of < 0.05 was considered to be statistically significant.

5. Conclusions

Our study indicates that IL-17 promotes VCAM-1 production in OASFs and facilitates monocyte adhesion by suppressing miR-5701 production via the PKC-α and JNK signaling cascades (Figure 6). We now have a better understanding about how IL-17-induced monocyte adhesion contributes to OA pathogenesis, which may help scientists design more effective therapy for OA.

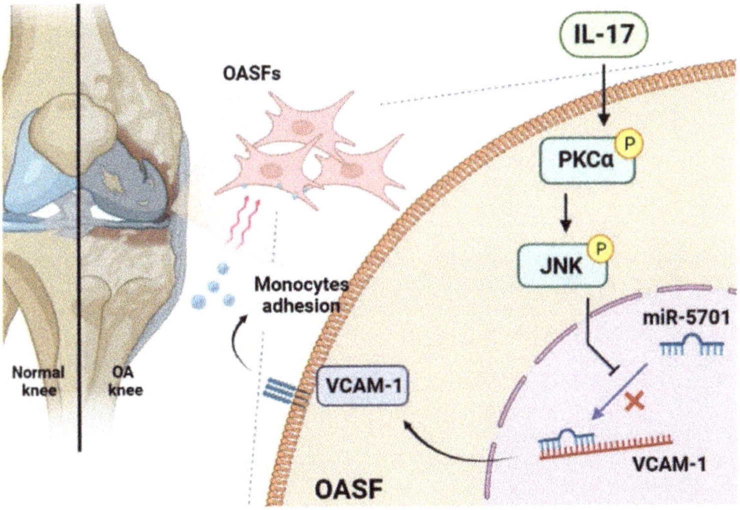

Figure 6. Schematic diagram summarizes the mechanisms by which IL-17 facilitates VCAM-1 production and monocyte adhesion in human OASFs. IL-17 promotes VCAM-1 synthesis and enhances monocyte adhesion in human OASFs by suppressing miR-5701 production in the PKC-α and JNK signaling cascades.

Supplementary Materials: The following supporting information can be downloaded at: https://www.mdpi.com/article/10.3390/ijms23126804/s1.

Author Contributions: Conceptualization, T.-J.W. and S.L.-Y.C.; methodology, C.-Y.L. (Chih-Yang Lin); validation, C.-Y.L. (Chih-Yang Lin) and C.-Y.L. (Chao-Yang Lai); formal analysis, X.-Y.H.; investigation, C.-H.T. (Chun-Hao Tsai) and Y.-C.F.; resources, C.-H.T. (Chih-Hsin Tang); data curation,

C.-H.T. (Chun-Hao Tsai); writing—original draft preparation, C.-Y.K.; writing—review and editing, C.-M.S.; visualization, T.-J.W. and S.L.-Y.C.; funding acquisition, C.-H.T. (Chih-Hsin Tang) All authors have read and agreed to the published version of the manuscript.

Funding: This work was supported by a grant from the Ministry of Science and Technology of Taiwan (MOST 110-2314-B-195-003-; MOST 110-2314-B-039-008-), China Medical University (CMU110-ASIA-08), and China Medical University Hospital (DMR-110-176; DMR-111-108; DMR-111-229; DMR-111-165).

Institutional Review Board Statement: The study protocol was approved by the Institutional Review Board (IRB) of China Medical University Hospital (CMUH108-REC3-039).

Informed Consent Statement: None of the authors of this paper has any financial or personal relationships with other people or organizations that could inappropriately influence this work.

Data Availability Statement: The original data to this present study are available from the corresponding authors.

Acknowledgments: We would like to thank Iona J. MacDonald from China Medical University for her English language revision of this manuscript.

Conflicts of Interest: None of the authors of this paper has any financial or personal relationships with other people or organizations that could inappropriately influence this work.

References

1. Yuan, X.; Meng, H.; Wang, Y.; Peng, J.; Guo, Q.; Wang, A.; Lu, S. Bone–cartilage interface crosstalk in osteoarthritis: Potential pathways and future therapeutic strategies. *Osteoarthr. Cartil.* **2014**, *22*, 1077–1089. [CrossRef] [PubMed]
2. MacDonald, I.J.; Liu, S.C.; Su, C.M.; Wang, Y.H.; Tsai, C.H.; Tang, C.H. Implications of angiogenesis involvement in arthritis. *Int. J. Mol. Sci.* **2018**, *19*, 2012. [CrossRef] [PubMed]
3. Kuo, S.J.; Yang, W.H.; Liu, S.C.; Tsai, C.H.; Hsu, H.C.; Tang, C.H. Transforming growth factor beta1 enhances heme oxygenase 1 expression in human synovial fibroblasts by inhibiting microrna 519b synthesis. *PLoS ONE* **2017**, *12*, e0176052. [CrossRef] [PubMed]
4. Chen, S.S.; Tang, C.H.; Chie, M.J.; Tsai, C.H.; Fong, Y.C.; Lu, Y.C.; Chen, W.C.; Lai, C.T.; Wei, C.Y.; Tai, H.C.; et al. Resistin facilitates vegf-a-dependent angiogenesis by inhibiting mir-16-5p in human chondrosarcoma cells. *Cell Death Dis.* **2019**, *10*, 31. [CrossRef] [PubMed]
5. Benito, M.J.; Veale, D.J.; FitzGerald, O.; van den Berg, W.B.; Bresnihan, B. Synovial tissue inflammation in early and late osteoarthritis. *Ann. Rheum. Dis.* **2005**, *64*, 1263–1267. [CrossRef] [PubMed]
6. Dehghan, M.; Asgharian, S.; Khalesi, E.; Ahmadi, A.; Lorigooini, Z. Comparative study of the effect of thymus daenensis gel 5% and diclofenac in patients with knee osteoarthritis. *Biomedicine* **2019**, *9*, 9. [CrossRef]
7. Sellam, J.; Berenbaum, F. The role of synovitis in pathophysiology and clinical symptoms of osteoarthritis. *Nat. Rev. Rheumatol.* **2010**, *6*, 625–635. [CrossRef]
8. Xu, Z.Y.; Liu, Y.L.; Lin, J.B.; Cheng, K.L.; Wang, Y.G.; Yao, H.L.; Wei, P.; Wu, H.Y.; Su, W.W.; Shaw, P.C.; et al. Preparative expression and purification of a nacreous protein n16 and testing its effect on osteoporosis rat model. *Int. J. Biol. Macromol.* **2018**, *111*, 440–445. [CrossRef]
9. Zhang, H.; Cai, D.; Bai, X. Macrophages regulate the progression of osteoarthritis. *Osteoarthr. Cartil.* **2020**, *28*, 555–561. [CrossRef]
10. Schett, G.; Kiechl, S.; Bonora, E.; Zwerina, J.; Mayr, A.; Axmann, R.; Weger, S.; Oberhollenzer, F.; Lorenzini, R.; Willeit, J. Vascular cell adhesion molecule 1 as a predictor of severe osteoarthritis of the hip and knee joints. *Arthritis Rheum.* **2009**, *60*, 2381–2389. [CrossRef]
11. Lee, H.-P.; Liu, S.-C.; Wang, Y.-H.; Chen, B.-C.; Chen, H.-T.; Li, T.-M.; Huang, W.-C.; Hsu, C.-J.; Wu, Y.-C.; Tang, C.-H. Cordycerebroside a suppresses vcam-dependent monocyte adhesion in osteoarthritis synovial fibroblasts by inhibiting mek/erk/ap-1 signaling. *J. Funct. Foods* **2021**, *86*, 104712. [CrossRef]
12. Chen, W.C.; Lin, C.Y.; Kuo, S.J.; Liu, S.C.; Lu, Y.C.; Chen, Y.L.; Wang, S.W.; Tang, C.H. Resistin enhances vcam-1 expression and monocyte adhesion in human osteoarthritis synovial fibroblasts by inhibiting mir-381 expression through the pkc, p38, and jnk signaling pathways. *Cells* **2020**, *9*, 1369. [CrossRef] [PubMed]
13. Liu, Y.; Peng, H.; Meng, Z.; Wei, M. Correlation of il-17 level in synovia and severity of knee osteoarthritis. *Med. Sci. Monit. Int. Med. J. Exp. Clin. Res.* **2015**, *21*, 1732–1736.
14. Jin, Y.; Chen, X.; Gao, Z.; Liu, K.; Hou, Y.; Zheng, J. Expression levels of il-15 and il-17 in synovial fluid of rheumatoid arthritis animal model. *Exp. Ther. Med.* **2018**, *16*, 3377–3382. [CrossRef]
15. Bai, Y.; Gao, S.; Liu, Y.; Jin, S.; Zhang, H.; Su, K. Correlation between interleukin-17 gene polymorphism and osteoarthritis susceptibility in han chinese population. *BMC Med. Genet.* **2019**, *20*, 20. [CrossRef]

16. Eftedal, R.; Vrgoc, G.; Jotanovic, Z.; Dembic, Z. Alternative interleukin 17a/f locus haplotypes are associated with increased risk to hip and knee osteoarthritis. *J. Orthop. Res. Off. Publ. Orthop. Res. Soc.* **2019**, *37*, 1972–1978. [CrossRef]
17. Wang, Z.; Zheng, C.; Zhong, Y.; He, J.; Cao, X.; Xia, H.; Ba, H.; Li, P.; Wu, S.; Peng, C. Interleukin-17 can induce osteoarthritis in rabbit knee joints similar to hulth's method. *BioMed Res. Int.* **2017**, *2017*, 2091325. [CrossRef]
18. Moon, Y.M.; Yoon, B.Y.; Her, Y.M.; Oh, H.J.; Lee, J.S.; Kim, K.W.; Lee, S.Y.; Woo, Y.J.; Park, K.S.; Park, S.H.; et al. Il-32 and il-17 interact and have the potential to aggravate osteoclastogenesis in rheumatoid arthritis. *Arthritis Res. Ther.* **2012**, *14*, R246. [CrossRef]
19. Lee, R.C.; Feinbaum, R.L.; Ambros, V. The c. Elegans heterochronic gene lin-4 encodes small rnas with antisense complementarity to lin-14. *Cell* **1993**, *75*, 843–854. [CrossRef]
20. Tehrani, S.S.; Zaboli, E.; Sadeghi, F.; Khafri, S.; Karimian, A.; Rafie, M.; Parsian, H. Microrna-26a-5p as a potential predictive factor for determining the effectiveness of trastuzumab therapy in her-2 positive breast cancer patients. *BioMedicine* **2021**, *11*, 30–39.
21. Asahara, H. Current status and strategy of microrna research for cartilage development and osteoarthritis pathogenesis. *J. Bone Metab.* **2016**, *23*, 121–127. [CrossRef] [PubMed]
22. Lin, Y.Y.; Ko, C.Y.; Liu, S.C.; Wang, Y.H.; Hsu, C.J.; Tsai, C.H.; Wu, T.J.; Tang, C.H. Mir-144-3p ameliorates the progression of osteoarthritis by targeting il-1beta: Potential therapeutic implications. *J. Cell. Physiol.* **2021**, *236*, 6988–7000. [CrossRef] [PubMed]
23. Zhang, H.; Lin, C.; Zeng, C.; Wang, Z.; Wang, H.; Lu, J.; Liu, X.; Shao, Y.; Zhao, C.; Pan, J.; et al. Synovial macrophage m1 polarisation exacerbates experimental osteoarthritis partially through r-spondin-2. *Ann. Rheum. Dis.* **2018**, *77*, 1524–1534. [CrossRef] [PubMed]
24. Liu, J.F.; Hou, S.M.; Tsai, C.H.; Huang, C.Y.; Hsu, C.J.; Tang, C.H. Ccn4 induces vascular cell adhesion molecule-1 expression in human synovial fibroblasts and promotes monocyte adhesion. *Biochim. Biophys. Acta* **2013**, *1833*, 966–975. [CrossRef] [PubMed]
25. Kuo, S.J.; Liu, S.C.; Huang, Y.L.; Tsai, C.H.; Fong, Y.C.; Hsu, H.C.; Tang, C.H. Tgf-beta1 enhances foxo3 expression in human synovial fibroblasts by inhibiting mir-92a through ampk and p38 pathways. *Aging* **2019**, *11*, 4075–4089. [CrossRef] [PubMed]
26. Wu, T.J.; Lin, C.Y.; Tsai, C.H.; Huang, Y.L.; Tang, C.H. Glucose suppresses il-1beta-induced mmp-1 expression through the fak, mek, erk, and ap-1 signaling pathways. *Environ. Toxicol.* **2018**, *33*, 1061–1068. [CrossRef]
27. Taipaleenmaki, H. Regulation of bone metabolism by micrornas. *Curr. Osteoporos. Rep.* **2018**, *16*, 1–12. [CrossRef]
28. Gao, B.; Gao, W.; Wu, Z.; Zhou, T.; Qiu, X.; Wang, X.; Lian, C.; Peng, Y.; Liang, A.; Qiu, J.; et al. Melatonin rescued interleukin 1beta-impaired chondrogenesis of human mesenchymal stem cells. *Stem Cell Res. Ther.* **2018**, *9*, 162. [CrossRef]
29. Mathiessen, A.; Conaghan, P.G. Synovitis in osteoarthritis: Current understanding with therapeutic implications. *Arthritis Res. Ther.* **2017**, *19*, 18. [CrossRef]
30. Zhu, X.; Lee, C.W.; Xu, H.; Wang, Y.F.; Yung, P.S.H.; Jiang, Y.; Lee, O.K. Phenotypic alteration of macrophages during osteoarthritis: A systematic review. *Arthritis Res. Ther.* **2021**, *23*, 110. [CrossRef]
31. Wasilewska, A.; Winiarska, M.; Olszewska, M.; Rudnicka, L. Interleukin-17 inhibitors. A new era in treatment of psoriasis and other skin diseases. *Postepy Dermatol. Alergol.* **2016**, *33*, 247–252. [CrossRef] [PubMed]
32. Lin, Y.M.; Hsu, C.J.; Liao, Y.Y.; Chou, M.C.; Tang, C.H. The ccl2/ccr2 axis enhances vascular cell adhesion molecule-1 expression in human synovial fibroblasts. *PLoS ONE* **2012**, *7*, e49999. [CrossRef] [PubMed]
33. Chen, C.Y.; Su, C.M.; Hsu, C.J.; Huang, C.C.; Wang, S.W.; Liu, S.C.; Chen, W.C.; Fuh, L.J.; Tang, C.H. Ccn1 promotes vegf production in osteoblasts and induces endothelial progenitor cell angiogenesis by inhibiting mir-126 expression in rheumatoid arthritis. *J. Bone Miner. Res. Off. J. Am. Soc. Bone Miner. Res.* **2017**, *32*, 34–45. [CrossRef] [PubMed]
34. Horng, C.T.; Shieh, P.C.; Tan, T.W.; Yang, W.H.; Tang, C.H. Paeonol suppresses chondrosarcoma metastasis through up-regulation of mir-141 by modulating pkcdelta and c-src signaling pathway. *Int. J. Mol. Sci.* **2014**, *15*, 11760–11772. [CrossRef]
35. Liu, J.F.; Chi, M.C.; Lin, C.Y.; Lee, C.W.; Chang, T.M.; Han, C.K.; Huang, Y.L.; Fong, Y.C.; Chen, H.T.; Tang, C.H. PM2.5 facilitates il-6 production in human osteoarthritis synovial fibroblasts via ask1 activation. *J. Cell. Physiol.* **2021**, *236*, 2205–2213. [CrossRef]
36. Wu, M.H.; Tsai, C.H.; Huang, Y.L.; Fong, Y.C.; Tang, C.H. Visfatin promotes il-6 and tnf-alpha production in human synovial fibroblasts by repressing mir-199a-5p through erk, p38 and jnk signaling pathways. *Int. J. Mol. Sci.* **2018**, *19*, 190. [CrossRef]
37. Nugent, M. Micrornas: Exploring new horizons in osteoarthritis. *Osteoarthr. Cartil.* **2016**, *24*, 573–580. [CrossRef]
38. Law, Y.Y.; Lin, Y.M.; Liu, S.C.; Wu, M.H.; Chung, W.H.; Tsai, C.H.; Fong, Y.C.; Tang, C.H.; Wang, C.K. Visfatin increases icam-1 expression and monocyte adhesion in human osteoarthritis synovial fibroblasts by reducing mir-320a expression. *Aging* **2020**, *12*, 18635–18648. [CrossRef]
39. Al-Modawi, R.N.; Brinchmann, J.E.; Karlsen, T.A. Multi-pathway protective effects of micrornas on human chondrocytes in an in vitro model of osteoarthritis. *Mol. Ther.-Nucleic Acids* **2019**, *17*, 776–790. [CrossRef]
40. Lee, H.-P.; Wu, Y.-C.; Chen, B.-C.; Liu, S.-C.; Li, T.-M.; Huang, W.-C.; Hsu, C.-J.; Tang, C.-H. Soya-cerebroside reduces interleukin production in human rheumatoid arthritis synovial fibroblasts by inhibiting the erk, nf-κb and ap-1 signalling pathways. *Food Agric. Immunol.* **2020**, *31*, 740–750. [CrossRef]
41. Lee, H.P.; Wang, S.W.; Wu, Y.C.; Lin, L.W.; Tsai, F.J.; Yang, J.S.; Li, T.M.; Tang, C.H. Soya-cerebroside inhibits vegf-facilitated angiogenesis in endothelial progenitor cells. *Food Agric. Immunol.* **2020**, *31*, 193–204. [CrossRef]
42. Cheng, F.J.; Huynh, T.K.; Yang, C.S.; Hu, D.W.; Shen, Y.C.; Tu, C.Y.; Wu, Y.C.; Tang, C.H.; Huang, W.C.; Chen, Y.; et al. Hesperidin is a potential inhibitor against sars-cov-2 infection. *Nutrients* **2021**, *13*, 2800. [CrossRef] [PubMed]
43. Lee, H.P.; Wang, S.W.; Wu, Y.C.; Tsai, C.H.; Tsai, F.J.; Chung, J.G.; Huang, C.Y.; Yang, J.S.; Hsu, Y.M.; Yin, M.C.; et al. Glucocerebroside reduces endothelial progenitor cell-induced angiogenesis. *Food Agric. Immunol.* **2019**, *30*, 1033–1045. [CrossRef]

44. Su, C.M.; Tang, C.H.; Chi, M.J.; Lin, C.Y.; Fong, Y.C.; Liu, Y.C.; Chen, W.C.; Wang, S.W. Resistin facilitates vegf-c-associated lymphangiogenesis by inhibiting mir-186 in human chondrosarcoma cells. *Biochem. Pharmacol.* **2018**, *154*, 234–242. [CrossRef] [PubMed]
45. Wu, K.M.; Hsu, Y.M.; Ying, M.C.; Tsai, F.J.; Tsai, C.H.; Chung, J.G.; Yang, J.S.; Tang, C.H.; Cheng, L.Y.; Su, P.H.; et al. High-density lipoprotein ameliorates palmitic acid-induced lipotoxicity and oxidative dysfunction in h9c2 cardiomyoblast cells via ros suppression. *Nutr. Metab.* **2019**, *16*, 36. [CrossRef]
46. Liu, S.C.; Tsai, C.H.; Wu, T.Y.; Tsai, C.H.; Tsai, F.J.; Chung, J.G.; Huang, C.Y.; Yang, J.S.; Hsu, Y.M.; Yin, M.C.; et al. Soya-cerebroside reduces il-1 beta-induced mmp-1 production in chondrocytes and inhibits cartilage degradation: Implications for the treatment of osteoarthritis. *Food Agric. Immunol.* **2019**, *30*, 620–632. [CrossRef]
47. Achudhan, D.; Liu, S.C.; Lin, Y.Y.; Lee, H.P.; Wang, S.W.; Huang, W.C.; Wu, Y.C.; Kuo, Y.H.; Tang, C.H. Antcin k inhibits vegf-dependent angiogenesis in human rheumatoid arthritis synovial fibroblasts. *J. Food Biochem.* **2022**, *46*, e14022. [CrossRef]
48. Su, C.-H.; Lin, C.-Y.; Tsai, C.-H.; Lee, H.-P.; Lo, L.-C.; Huang, W.-C.; Wu, Y.-C.; Hsieh, C.-L.; Tang, C.-H. Betulin suppresses tnf-α and il-1β production in osteoarthritis synovial fibroblasts by inhibiting the mek/erk/nf-κb pathway. *J. Funct. Foods* **2021**, *86*, 104729. [CrossRef]
49. Lee, K.T.; Su, C.H.; Liu, S.C.; Chen, B.C.; Chang, J.W.; Tsai, C.H.; Huang, W.C.; Hsu, C.J.; Chen, W.C.; Wu, Y.C.; et al. Cordycerebroside a inhibits icam-1-dependent m1 monocyte adhesion to osteoarthritis synovial fibroblasts. *J. Food Biochem.* **2022**, e14108. [CrossRef]

International Journal of
Molecular Sciences

MDPI

Article

Anti-Inflammatory Effects of Endogenously Released Adenosine in Synovial Cells of Osteoarthritis and Rheumatoid Arthritis Patients

Rebecca Sohn [1,†], Marius Junker [1,†], Andrea Meurer [1], Frank Zaucke [1], Rainer H. Straub [2,‡] and Zsuzsa Jenei-Lanzl [1,*,‡]

1 Dr. Rolf M. Schwiete Research Unit for Osteoarthritis, Department of Orthopedics (Friedrichsheim), University Hospital Frankfurt, Goethe University, 60528 Frankfurt/Main, Germany; rebecca.sohn@kgu.de (R.S.); marius.junker@kgu.de (M.J.); andrea.meurer@kgu.de (A.M.); frank.zaucke@kgu.de (F.Z.)

2 Laboratory of Experimental Rheumatology and Neuroendocrine Immunology, Department of Internal Medicine, University Hospital Regensburg, 93053 Regensburg, Germany; rainer.straub@ukr.de

* Correspondence: zsuzsa.jenei-lanzl@kgu.de; Tel.: +49-69-6301-94-408

† Contributed equally as first author.

‡ Contributed equally as senior author.

Abstract: Exogenous adenosine and its metabolite inosine exert anti-inflammatory effects in synoviocytes of osteoarthritis (OA) and rheumatoid arthritis (RA) patients. We analyzed whether these cells are able to synthesize adenosine/inosine and which adenosine receptors (ARs) contribute to anti-inflammatory effects. The functionality of synthesizing enzymes and ARs was tested using agonists/antagonists. Both OA and RA cells expressed CD39 (converts ATP to AMP), CD73 (converts AMP to adenosine), ADA (converts adenosine to inosine), ENT1/2 (adenosine transporters), all AR subtypes (A_1, A_{2A}, A_{2B} and A_3) and synthesized predominantly adenosine. The CD73 inhibitor AMPCP significantly increased IL-6 and decreased IL-10 in both cell types, while TNF only increased in RA cells. The ADA inhibitor DAA significantly reduced IL-6 and induced IL-10 in both OA and RA cells. The A_{2A}AR agonist CGS 21680 significantly inhibited IL-6 and induced TNF and IL-10 only in RA, while the A_{2B}AR agonist BAY 60-6583 had the same effect in both OA and RA. Taken together, OA and RA synoviocytes express the complete enzymatic machinery to synthesize adenosine/inosine; however, mainly adenosine is responsible for the anti- (IL-6 and IL-10) or pro-inflammatory (TNF) effects mediated by A_{2A}- and A_{2B}AR. Stimulating CD39/CD73 with simultaneous ADA blockage in addition to TNF inhibition might represent a promising therapeutic strategy.

Keywords: adenosine; inosine; rheumatoid arthritis; osteoarthritis; synoviocytes; inflammation

Citation: Sohn, R.; Junker, M.; Meurer, A.; Zaucke, F.; Straub, R.H.; Jenei-Lanzl, Z. Anti-Inflammatory Effects of Endogenously Released Adenosine in Synovial Cells of Osteoarthritis and Rheumatoid Arthritis Patients. *Int. J. Mol. Sci.* **2021**, 22, 8956. https://doi.org/10.3390/ijms22168956

Academic Editors: Chih-Hsin Tang and David A. Hart

Received: 27 July 2021
Accepted: 18 August 2021
Published: 19 August 2021

Publisher's Note: MDPI stays neutral with regard to jurisdictional claims in published maps and institutional affiliations.

1. Introduction

Rheumatoid arthritis (RA) is a systemic, chronic inflammatory autoimmune disorder affecting around 1% of the population worldwide [1]. RA results in symmetric primary inflammatory polyarthritis characterized by painful swelling in multiple joints [2]. Uncontrolled active synovial inflammation in RA results in joint damage and causes chronic pain, disabilities, decreased quality of life, as well as different comorbidities such as cardiovascular, gastrointestinal, renal and pulmonary diseases or fatigue [3]. To date, RA remains an incurable disease; mainly symptomatic treatment exists [4], although significant progress in knowledge about its pathogenesis has been achieved in recent years.

After RA induction by an initiating factor such as infection or environmental exposure (e.g., smoking or chronic stress) [5], synovial lining cells become activated and start to release matrix-degrading enzymes, pro-inflammatory cytokines and chemokines, which in turn recruit immune cells [6]. A vicious cycle arises, resulting in synoviocyte- and osteoclast-mediated cartilage and bone destruction [7]. Synovial cells in inflamed synovium contain fibroblasts, macrophages, B- and T lymphocytes and dendritic cells, which release different cytokines [8,9]. Key cytokines driving inflammatory processes in RA synovium are IL-6 and TNF. The major IL-6 producers are synovial fibroblasts and pro-inflammatory M1 macrophages. The more anti-inflammatory IL-10 is synthesized mainly by B cells and anti-inflammatory M2 macrophages, while highly pro-inflammatory cytokine TNF is released by T cells, monocytes, and M1 macrophages [10,11].

Recent symptomatic RA therapies are primarily based on disease-modifying antirheumatic drugs (DMARDs), which are often combined with biologicals such as TNF inhibitors that target synovitis and systemic inflammation [12]. However, in many cases, the clinically active disease persists in spite of RA-modifying medications [3,13]. Therefore, alternative therapy options have to be developed. In contrast to RA, osteoarthritis (OA) is mainly a chronic degenerative and not primary inflammatory disorder of the joints even though a low-grade inflammation of the synovium was described [14]. Therefore, OA synoviocytes are often used as a control in studies analyzing inflammatory processes in RA cell cultures.

Previous studies demonstrated that the nucleoside adenosine and its metabolite inosine exert anti-inflammatory effects in different tissues in the human body, such as the lung, liver or kidney after binding to specific G protein-coupled adenosine receptors (Ars) [15,16]. In general, four AR subtypes do exist (A_1, A_{2A}, A_{2B} and A_3) [17–19]. All four subtypes have been detected in the synovial tissue of RA patients in earlier studies [20], and indeed, exogenously applied adenosine and inosine exhibited anti-inflammatory effects in synovial cells from rheumatoid arthritis (RA) patients in vitro [21]. Similar anti-inflammatory effects were reported in murine models of experimental RA by mainly reducing TNF, but also inhibiting IL-1β, and IL-8 release. The majority of these effects were shown to be mediated by the AR subtypes A_{2A}, A_{2B} or A_3 [22–25].

However, most cell culture studies were performed under 20% O_2 concentration, which represents neither a physiological nor a pathophysiological microenvironment. In a healthy synovial tissue, O_2 concentrations of 2–4% predominate, while an inflamed synovium contains only 1–3% O_2 [26]. The anti-inflammatory effect of applied adenosine or inosine, as well as of specific receptor subtype agonists targeting A_{2A}AR and A_3AR during RA manifestation, was also confirmed in a few animal studies [23,27]. Thus, in these earlier studies, the anti-inflammatory acting adenosine, inosine, or AR agonists/antagonists were applied as a drug externally. However, the human body itself is capable of producing adenosine and inosine [28], and one might use the internal source for experiments.

Different cell types such as cardiomyocytes, circulating lymphocytes, or cancer-associated fibroblasts in the lung are able to convert ATP to AMP by CD39 followed by AMP conversion to adenosine by CD73 both intra- and extracellularly [29]. Regarding RA, only a few studies exist that describe the fact that regulatory T cells in the synovial fluid express CD73 [30], or M2 macrophages in the blood co-express CD39/CD73 [31]. OA synovial tissue and fluid have not yet been investigated in this regard. Moreover, the transmembrane Equilibrative Nucleoside Transporters ENT1 and ENT2 are responsible for adenosine transport between intra- and extracellular space, thereby influencing the extracellularly acting levels of adenosine [32]. Additionally, last but not least, the enzyme adenosine deaminase (ADA), which catalyzes the conversion of adenosine to inosine, belongs to the machinery regulating nucleoside homeostasis [33].

ADA was detected in the synovial fluid of OA and RA patients as well as in RA synovial fibroblasts [34]. However, the existence of these enzymes and transporters has not yet been investigated in mixed synovial cell cultures containing fibroblasts, macrophages, lymphocytes, and dendritic cells [8].

Thus, at present, no study is available demonstrating that OA and RA mixed synoviocytes do express all enzymes of adenosine and inosine synthesis. It is also unclear how, and via which ARs, endogenously released nucleosides could contribute to possible anti-inflammatory events in the synovium. Therefore, we analyzed the entire adenosine synthesizing and transporting machinery in OA and RA mixed synovial cell culture.

2. Results

2.1. CD39/CD73 and ADA Expression as well as Adenosine/Inosine Release

In order to analyze whether synoviocytes are capable of synthesizing adenosine and inosine, cells were examined for the presence of CD39 and CD73. Double immunostaining revealed that mixed synoviocytes from both OA and RA patients co-expressed CD39 and CD73 (Figure 1A). In order to investigate whether the cells are able to convert adenosine to its metabolite inosine, ADA was stained immunohistochemically. Both OA and RA synovial cells expressed ADA without any differences between the groups (Figure 1B). In addition, after cultivation for 24 h under hypoxia, synovial cells spontaneously released physiologically relevant amounts of adenosine and inosine; however, OA synoviocytes synthesized significantly higher nucleoside concentrations compared to RA cells (mean ± SEM: adenosine: OA 23.8 ± 8.7 ng/mL, RA 4.6 ± 2.7 ng/mL, $p = 0.008$; inosine: OA 73.4 ± 37.5 ng/mL, RA 10.4 ± 8.3 ng/mL, $p = 0.002$) (Figure 1C). No age- or gender-dependent differences were detected.

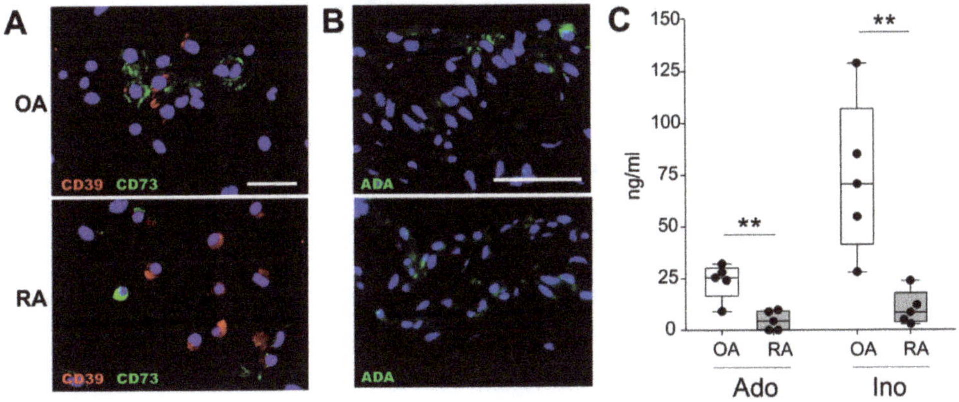

Figure 1. CD39/CD73 expression, ADA expression, and adenosine/inosine release. (**A**) Representative fluorescent micrographs of OA and RA mixed synoviocytes immunostained for CD39 (red) and CD73 (green) and counterstained nuclei with DAPI (blue) (bar: 25 µm). (**B**) Representative fluorescent micrographs of OA and RA mixed synoviocytes immunostained for ADA (green) and counterstained nuclei with DAPI (blue) (bar: 50 µm). (**C**) Quantification of spontaneous adenosine and inosine release in OA and RA mixed synoviocytes. Data are represented as box plots, where the boxes represent the 25th to 75th percentiles, the lines within the boxes represent the median, and the lines outside the boxes represent the 10th and 90th percentiles. Each black circle represents the synovial cells of an individual patient (n = 5). Significant *p*-values are presented as ** $p \leq 0.01$. Abbreviations: ADA—adenosine deaminase; Ado—adenosine; DAPI—4′,6-diamidino-2-phenylindole; Ino—inosine; OA—osteoarthritis; RA—rheumatoid arthritis.

2.2. ENT1/2 Expression

To investigate the ability of synovial tissue to transport endogenous adenosine across the cell membrane, immunohistochemical staining of the respective transporters was performed. Both OA and RA synovial cells possess these transporters (ENT1 and ENT2) without any obvious differences between the groups (Figure 2).

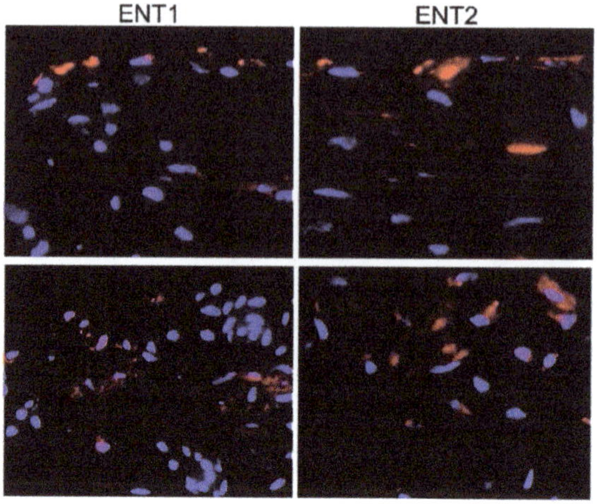

Figure 2. ENT1/2 expression in the synovium. Representative fluorescent micrographs of OA and RA synovial tissues immunostained for ENT1 and ENT2 (red) and counterstained for nuclei with DAPI (blue) (bar: 50 µm). Abbreviations: DAPI—4′,6-diamidino-2-phenylindole; ENT—equilibrative nucleoside transporter; OA—osteoarthritis; RA—rheumatoid arthritis.

2.3. Expression of AR Subtypes

In order to determine the possible ability to respond to adenosine, synovial tissue was screened immunohistochemically for all different AR subtypes. In general, all AR subtypes were detectable in OA and RA synovium (Figure 3). A_1- and A_{3A}R expression levels were similar in OA and RA, while the expression of A_{2A}- and A_{2B}AR seemed to be more pronounced in RA tissue (Figure 3). No further AR quantification was performed, because earlier studies reported and quantified the same phenomenon, namely a dominant A_{2B}AR expression in the synovium of RA patients [20].

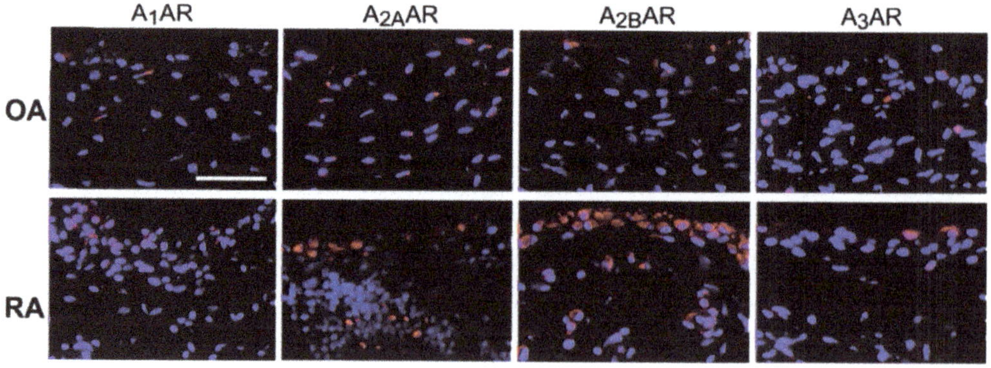

Figure 3. Expression of adenosine receptors (ARs) in the synovium. Representative fluorescent micrographs of OA and RA synovial tissues immunostained for A_1-, A_{2A}-, A_{2B}-, and A_3AR (red) and counterstained for nuclei with DAPI (blue) (bar: 50 µm). Abbreviations: see legends to Figure 1.

2.4. Effects of CD73 and ADA Inhibition

To better understand the role of endogenously synthesized adenosine within the synovium, its last synthesis step, as well as its conversion to inosine, were blocked by treating mixed synovial cells with the CD37 inhibitor AMPCP or the ADA inhibitor DAA, respectively. The absolute levels of released cytokine concentrations in untreated control groups were as follows: OA IL-6 205.5 ± 72.9 μg/mL, TNF 348.7 ± 135.3 pg/mL, IL-10 254.0 ± 179.2 pg/mL; RA IL-6 364.5 ± 174.4 μg/mL, TNF 580.2 ± 387.9 pg/mL, IL-10 455.7 ± 235.2 pg/mL. Although RA cells seem to release higher cytokine concentrations, the differences between OA and RA cells were not significant. No age- or gender-dependent differences were detected.

The treatment of both OA and RA cells with the CD37-blocker AMPCP resulted in significantly increased IL-6 concentrations compared to untreated control cells (OA: 10^{-6} M $p = 0.036$, 10^{-5} M $p = 0.013$, 10^{-4} M $p < 0.001$; RA: 10^{-6} M $p < 0.001$, 10^{-5} M $p < 0.001$, 10^{-4} M $p < 0.001$) (Figure 4A). The same treatment conditions also significantly increased TNF release in OA and RA cells compared to the control (OA: 10^{-6} M $p = 0.024$, 10^{-5} M $p = 0.001$, 10^{-4} M $p = 0.002$; RA: 10^{-6} M $p = 0.008$, 10^{-5} M $p < 0.001$, 10^{-4} M $p < 0.001$) (Figure 4A). In contrast, IL-10 concentrations decreased after applying 10^{-4} M AMPCP in RA ($p = 0.043$), but not in OA mixed synoviocytes (Figure 4A).

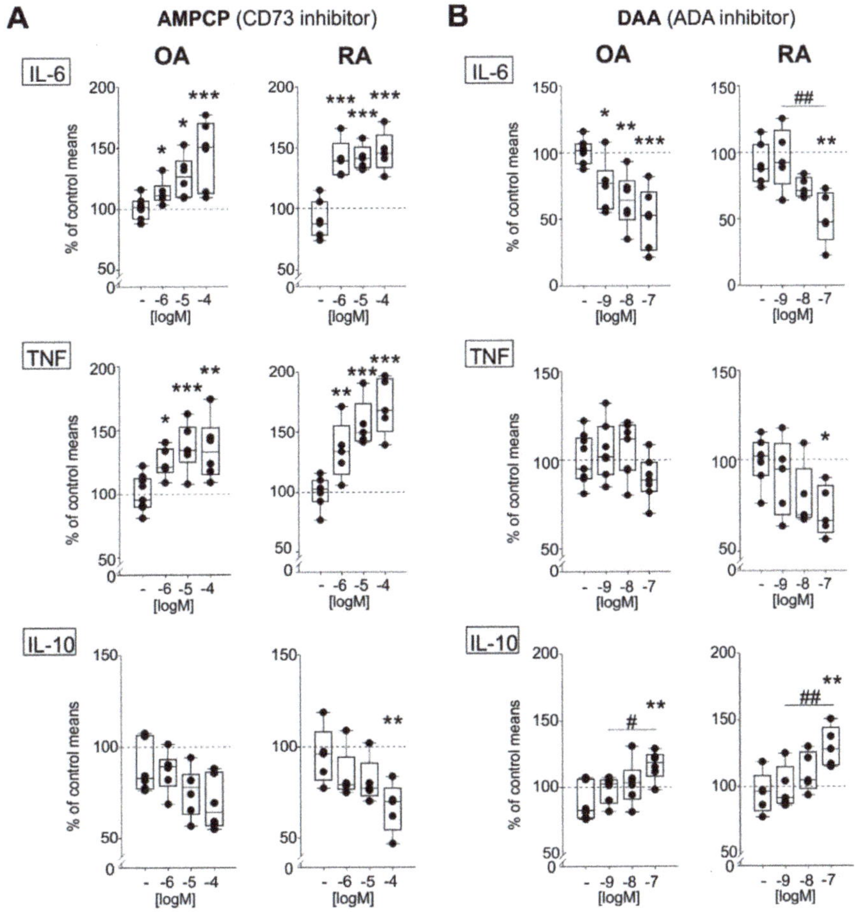

Figure 4. Effects of CD73 and ADA inhibition. (**A**) IL-6, TNF, and IL-10 release in OA and RA mixed synoviocyte cultures after CD37 inhibition using AMPCP (10^{-6} M to 10^{-4} M). (**B**) IL-6, TNF, and IL-10 release in OA and RA mixed synoviocyte cultures after ADA inhibition using DAA (10^{-9} M to 10^{-7} M). Data are represented as box plots (as explained in the legend of Figure 1). Values are expressed as percent of untreated control (untreated control is represented as "-"; the mean of untreated controls is represented as dashed line = 100%). Significant *p*-values are presented as * $p \leq 0.05$ ** $p \leq 0.01$ *** $p \leq 0.001$ when compared to untreated controls or as # $p \leq 0.05$ ## $p \leq 0.01$ when two treatment groups were compared. Abbreviations: see legends to Figures 1 and 2.

Treatment with the adenosine deaminase blocker DAA significantly reduced IL-6 release in OA synovial cells, while in RA cells, only the highest DAA concentration, 10^{-7} M, caused a significant IL-6 reduction (OA: 10^{-9} M $p = 0.022$, 10^{-8} M $p = 0.004$, 10^{-7} M $p < 0.001$; RA: 10^{-7} M $p = 0.003$, 10^{-9} M compared to 10^{-7} M $p = 0.003$) (Figure 4B). Compared to untreated controls, TNF levels in OA and RA mixed synoviocytes were only slightly affected; the only significant reduction was observed in RA cells at 10^{-7} M ($p = 0.043$) (Figure 4B). Moreover, 10^{-7} M DAA significantly increased IL-10 concentration in OA and RA synoviocytes (OA: 10^{-7} M $p = 0.02$, 10^{-9} M compared to 10^{-7} M $p = 0.29$; RA: 10^{-7} M $p = 0.004$, 10^{-9} M compared to 10^{-7} M $p = 0.005$) (Figure 4B).

2.5. Effect of ENT1/2 Inhibiton

Since the transport of adenosine between intra- and extracellular space might influence its inflammatory effects, the impact of blocking adenosine transfer across the cell membrane was analyzed using the ENT1/ENT2 inhibitor DIP. This treatment did not modulate cytokine release in both OA and RA cells, and neither IL-6, TNF, nor IL-10 concentrations changed significantly compared to controls (Supplementary Materials Figure S1).

2.6. Effects of AR Agonists on IL-6 Release

In order to study effects at specific ARs in mixed synoviocytes in vitro, we used agonists. IL-6 release in OA synoviocyte cultures was reduced only by the A_{2B}AR agonist BAY 60-6583, but at all concentrations (10^{-10} M $p = 0.014$, 10^{-9} M $p = 0.031$, 10^{-8} M $p = 0.002$, Figure 5). In contrast, in RA synoviocytes, the treatment with the A_{2A}AR agonist CGS 21680 also resulted in a significant IL-6 reduction; however, only at the higher concentration of 10^{-8} M (CGS 21680 $p = 0.002$, BAY 60-6583 $p < 0.001$) (Figure 5). The A_1AR agonist ccpA and the A_3AR agonist HEMADO showed no effect on either OA or RA synovial cell cultures regarding IL-6 release (Figure 5).

2.7. Effects of AR Agonists on TNF Release

Similar to the effects on IL-6, the A_{2A}AR agonist CGS 21680 significantly increased TNF release in RA but not in OA synoviocytes (10^{-9} M $p = 0.039$, 10^{-8} M $p = 0.003$, 10^{-7} M $p = 0.002$) (Figure 6). However, the A_{2B}AR agonist BAY 60-6583 significantly enhanced the TNF levels in both OA ad RA synovial cell cultures (OA: 10^{-9} M $p = 0.007$, 10^{-8} M $p < 0.001$, 10^{-10} M compared to 10^{-9} M $p = 0.023$, 10^{-10} M compared to 10^{-8} M $p < 0.001$; RA: 10^{-10} M $p = 0.021$, 10^{-9} M $p = 0.003$, 10^{-8} M $p < 0.001$) (Figure 6). Furthermore, the A_1AR agonist ccpA and the A_3AR agonist HEMADO did not affect TNF release, neither in OA nor in RA synoviocyte cultures (Figure 6).

2.8. Effects of AR Agonists on IL-10 Release

In contrast to the effects on IL-6 and TNF, the treatment with CGS 21680 in high concentrations significantly elevated IL-10 release in both OA and RA synovial cells (OA: 10^{-7} M $p = 0.005$; RA: 10^{-8} M $p = 0.022$, 10^{-7} M $p = 0.03$) (Figure 7). In contrast, the A_{2B}AR agonist BAY 60-6583 increased IL-10 synthesis only in RA but not in OA cells (10^{-9} M $p = 0.036$, 10^{-8} M $p = 0.012$, 10^{-10} M compared to 10^{-8} M $p = 0.036$) (Figure 7). Again, the A_1AR agonist ccpA and the A_3AR agonist HEMADO did not affect IL-10 release, neither in OA nor in RA synoviocyte cultures (Figure 7).

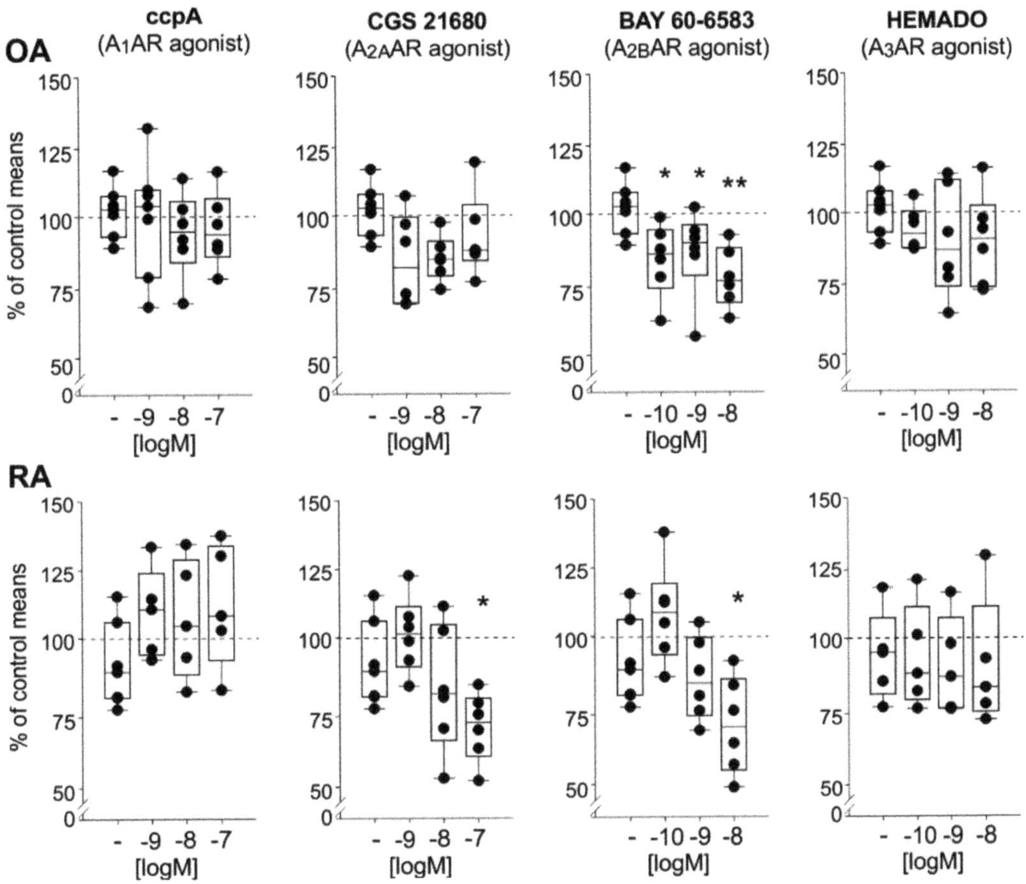

Figure 5. IL-6 release in OA and RA mixed synoviocyte cultures after activation of individual adenosine receptor subtypes by applying different AR agonists. Data are represented as box plots (as explained in the legend of Figure 1) (n = 5–6). Values are expressed as percent of untreated control (untreated control is represented as "-"; the mean of untreated controls is represented as dashed line = 100%). Significant p-values compared to untreated control are presented as * $p \leq 0.05$ ** $p \leq 0.01$ when compared to untreated controls. Abbreviations: see legend to Figure 1.

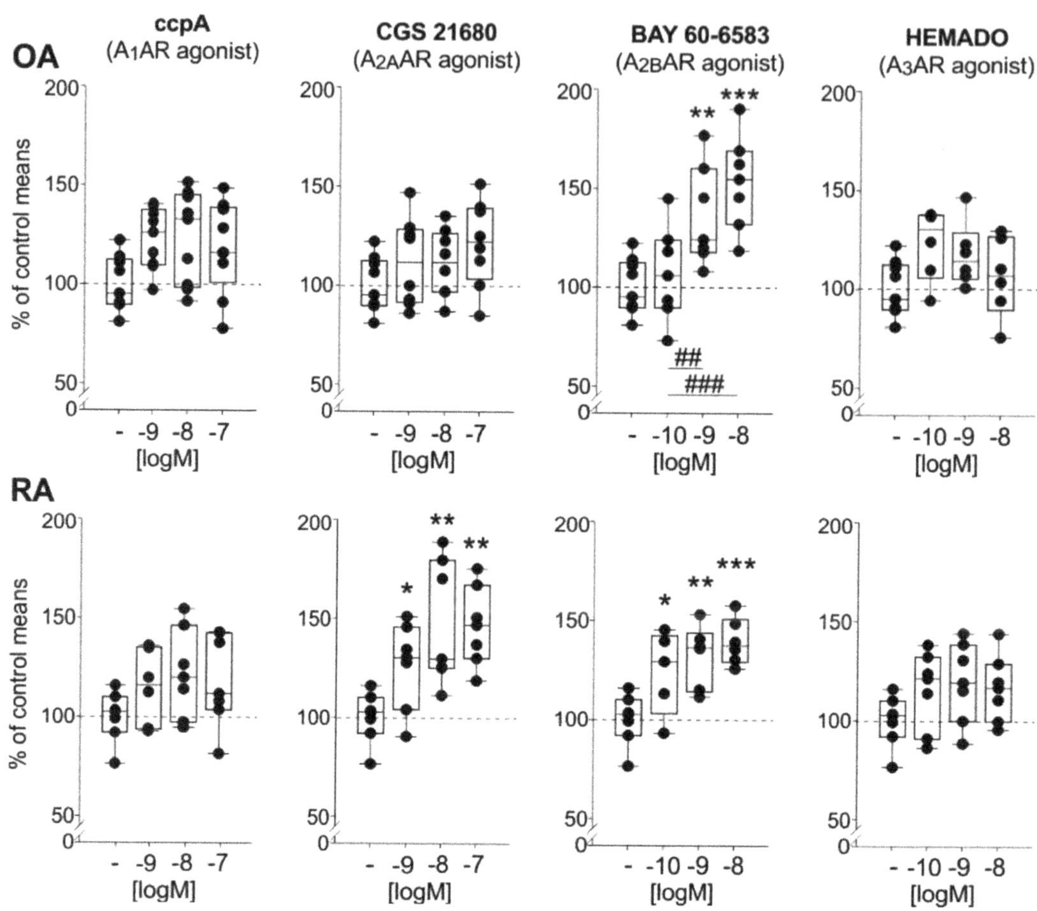

Figure 6. TNF release in OA and RA mixed synoviocyte cultures after activation of individual adenosine receptor subtypes by applying different AR agonists. Data are represented as box plots (as explained in the legend of Figure 1) (n = 5–6). Values are expressed as percent of untreated control (untreated control is represented as "-"; the mean of untreated controls is represented as dashed line = 100%). Significant p-values compared to untreated control are presented as p * ≤ 0.05. ** $p \leq 0.01$. *** $p \leq 0.001$ when compared to untreated controls or as ## $p \leq 0.05$ ### $p \leq 0.001$ when two treatment groups were compared. Abbreviations: see legend to Figure 1.

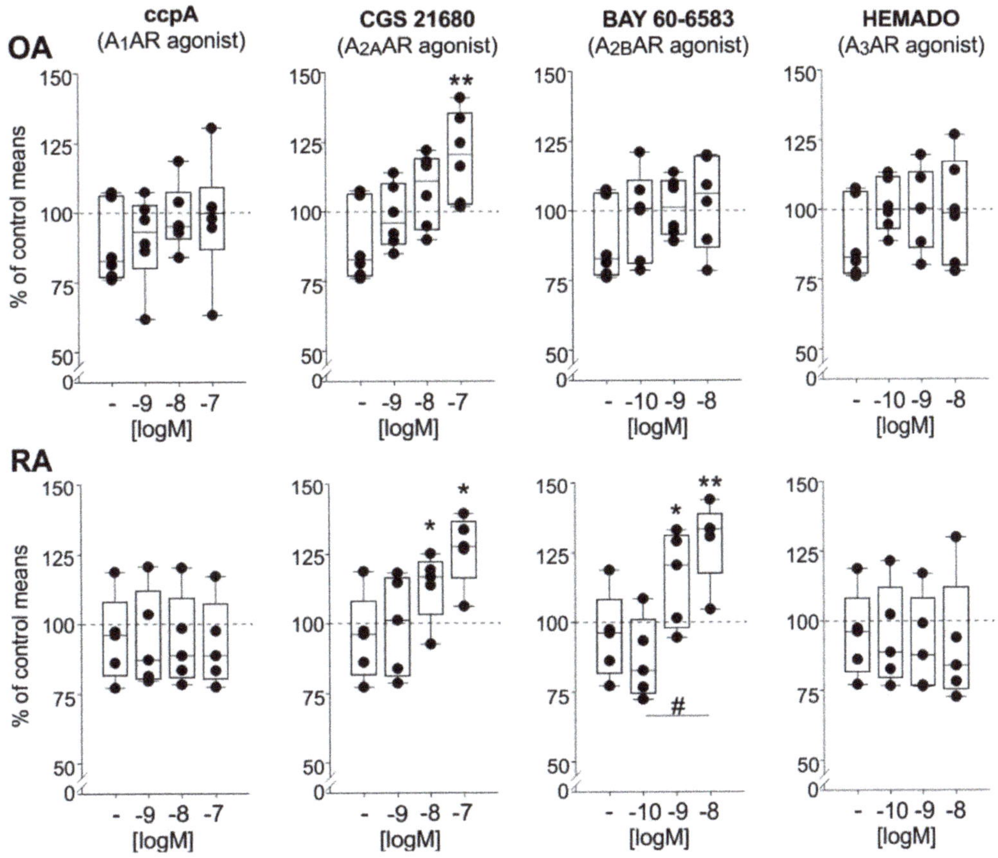

Figure 7. IL-10 release in OA and RA mixed synoviocyte cultures after activation of individual adenosine receptor subtypes by applying different AR agonists. Data are represented as box plots (as explained in the legend of Figure 1) (n = 5–6). Values are expressed as percent of untreated control (untreated control is represented as "-"; the mean of untreated controls is represented as dashed line = 100%). Significant p-values compared to untreated control are presented as * $p \leq 0.05$ ** $p \leq 0.01$ when compared to untreated controls or as # $p \leq 0.05$ when two treatment groups were compared. Abbreviations: see legend to Figure 1.

3. Discussion

A number of previous studies in humans and mice described that exogenously applied adenosine and inosine exert anti-inflammatory effects during RA pathogenesis [21], but it was never investigated whether synovial cells themselves are capable of producing these nucleosides, and if so, by which ARs autocrine effects might be exhibited. The present study demonstrates that both OA and RA synoviocytes express the complete enzymatic machinery to synthesize adenosine and inosine endogenously, which then mediate dual, predominantly anti-inflammatory but for the smaller part also pro-inflammatory, autocrine effects, mainly by activating the A_{2A}- and A_{2B}AR subtypes.

The initial step in this study was to analyze whether mixed synoviocytes from OA and RA patients express CD39 and CD73, the two cell surface enzymes that are known to convert ATP to adenosine, as well as ADA, being responsible for the conversion of adenosine to inosine [35]. We demonstrated that synovial cells from both patient groups expressed CD39 and CD73 to a comparable extent. This fits with the earlier studies mentioned above, demonstrating that regulatory T cells in RA synovial fluid express

CD73 [30], and M2 macrophages in the blood of RA patients co-express CD39/CD73 [31]. Thus, the prerequisite for adenosine synthesis is given in mixed synovial cells. In order to convert adenosine to inosine, cells should express the enzyme ADA. We demonstrated that both OA and RA mixed synovial cells are ADA-positive. This is in line with previous studies that show that ADA was expressed by RA synovial fibroblasts [34], while similar data do not exist for OA fibroblasts or OA and RA synovial immune cells.

In addition, we demonstrated that the detected enzymes CD39, CD73 and ADA are active because synovial cells spontaneously release physiologically relevant amounts of adenosine and inosine. Nucleoside synthesis in synovial cells was never investigated before now. Until now, only endogenous catecholamine synthesis in mixed synovial cells from OA and RA patients has been described in our earlier studies [8,9]. However, OA synoviocytes produced significantly higher nucleoside concentrations compared to RA cells. The reason for this difference might be a decreased functionality of CD39 and CD73, or an elevated expression of adenosine- and inosine-degrading enzymes in RA due to the highly inflammatory situation [36]. In a chronic inflammatory microenvironment, which is accompanied by hypoxia, mitochondrial dysfunction and in turn decreased ATP synthesis occurs. This might lead to reduced adenosine levels as described by other studies [21]. Additionally, it has been reported that ADA activity is higher in RA synovial fluid compared to healthy or OA synovial fluids [37,38]. This could lead to the reduction in adenosine concentrations in RA tissue.

One prerequisite for a possible adenosine effect, besides the presence of adenosine itself, is the existence of ARs on target cells [21]. In general, all AR subtypes were detectable in both OA and RA synovium. This confirmed some results of our earlier study that demonstrated that isolated mixed synovial cells expressed all AR subtypes [9]. However, the expression levels of the different AR subtypes in synovial sections were different between OA and RA. In particular, the expression of A_{2A}AR and A_{2B}AR seemed to be more pronounced in RA synovial tissue. Until now, no study compared the expression of the different AR subtypes in the synovial tissue from OA and RA patients at the protein level. One possible reason for the elevated AR expression levels in RA might be the highly inflammatory microenvironment. Indeed, TNF, IL-β and LPS have been shown to upregulate A_{2A}AR expression in human and equine monocytes [39,40]. This might be a compensatory mechanism for a higher ADA expression and function [37,38].

As the first evidence for the possible autocrine effects of endogenously synthesized adenosine, the release of the most prominent RA-related cytokines, namely IL-6, TNF and IL-10, were quantified after blocking CD73 activity, which is the rate-limiting step of adenosine production [35]. In general, we observed that RA synoviocytes release higher cytokine concentrations than OA cells, but the differences were not significant due to naturally occurring variation in human primary cultures [41,42]. A further reason for these differences might be the fact that the source of RA synoviocytes is a highly inflamed synovium containing more immune cells, while only a low-grade inflammation is present in OA synovium [43]. The fact that CD73 inhibition, causing an adenosine deficit, led to an increased pro-inflammatory (IL-6 and TNF) and decreased anti-inflammatory (IL-10) cytokine release, but ADA inhibition, leading to adenosine accumulation, resulted in the opposite, suggests that mainly endogenously released adenosine, and not inosine, is responsible for the anti-inflammatory effects in the synovium. This confirms the findings of earlier studies that show that adenosine treatment of RA synovial cells results in the inhibition of pro-inflammatory cytokines [22–25]. Moreover, it is astonishing that RA synoviocytes responded to CD73 or ADA inhibition in a similar manner as OA cells even though the concentration of endogenously produced adenosine or inosine was much lower in RA culture. This could be explained by a potentially higher nucleoside sensitivity of RA cells due to stronger A_{2A}- and A_{2B}AR expression or signal transduction.

Apparently, ENT1 and ENT2 do not influence the intra- and extracellular adenosine concentrations. The most likely explanation for this could be that ENT1/2 activity was balanced regarding adenosine transport between extra-and intracellular space without any significant gradient between these compartments. This result suggests that no ENT1/2 dysregulation takes place in OA or RA synovial cells during inflammation, although the opposite has been reported in studies investigating inflammatory bowel disease in mice, where ENT1/2 inhibition dampened intestinal inflammation [44]. In addition, this result also indicates that no intracellular adenosine, and accordingly its transport to extracellular space, is required to achieve anti-inflammatory effects.

The AR agonist treatments resulted in clear anti-inflammatory effects because the release of IL-6 was significantly reduced but IL-10 synthesis was induced. On the other hand, the same treatments also induced TNF, thus, ARs also mediate pro-inflammatory effects at the same time. We demonstrated that mainly the A_{2A}- and A_{2B}AR subtypes were responsible for these effects. The latter is in line with previous studies that showed that the majority of anti-inflammatory effects caused by exogenously applied adenosine was mediated by exactly these AR subtypes [22–25]. However, A_3AR has also been described to exert anti-inflammatory effects in the RA synovium [45], which could not be confirmed in our study. One possible reason for this discrepancy might be that the concentration of endogenously synthesized adenosine in our study is lower and A_3ARs possess lower affinity to adenosine compared to A_{2A}Rs [17]. Therefore, mainly the A_{2A}ARs have been targeted by the released adenosine.

The fact that the pro-inflammatory cytokine IL-6 was inhibited but the anti-inflammatory IL-10 was induced by A_{2A}AR agonists is in agreement with the existing literature that shows similar effects in synoviocytes and peripheral lymphocytes of RA patients after adenosine or AR agonist application [9,22–24]. However, opposite to most previous studies, TNF release increased after the activation of A_{2A}ARs. Two reasons might be responsible for this phenomenon. Firstly, the majority of former studies performed their experiments under hyperoxic conditions and not under hypoxia [23,46]. Secondly, AR desensitization due to continuous stimulation can lead to uncoupling of the receptors from the stimulatory Gαs protein, being the dominant signaling partners of the A_{2A}ARs, and following coupling to other G proteins, such as the inhibitory Gαi [47]. Thus, TNF increase is likely the consequence of a pro-inflammatory AR switch, as described by us earlier for G protein coupled receptors in the synovium [9].

Interestingly, a similar TNF inhibition did not occur after ADA treatment. This might be due to the specificity of the AR agonists used (https://www.tocris.com/pharmacology/adenosine-receptors, accessed on 16 August 2021). Endogenously synthesized adenosine can in principle act via all AR subtypes expressed and the sum of the effects is anti-inflammatory because TNF was also reduced. In contrast, targeting exactly one AR subtype by applying a specific agonist does not represent the same situation. Therefore, we believe that rather, the natural ligand adenosine or a subtype specific synthetic agonist should be considered for therapy options.

The fact that most effects of inhibitors and agonists were stronger in RA than in OA synoviocytes can be explained by the differences in the inflammatory pattern. It is well known that RA is a primary inflammatory systemic disorder and in contrast to OA, much higher pro-inflammatory cytokine concentrations are present in the synovial tissue or fluid [14]. Thus, it is not surprising that that the effects of adenosine are not as pronounced as in RA. However, adenosine was also able to exert beneficial effects in OA synovial cells and should therefore be investigated in more detail in order to also develop a potent therapeutic strategy for OA.

One limitation of the present study might be that we did not further analyze the different cell types in mixed synoviocyte cultures specifically; however, this could also be seen as a strength of our investigations, because all cell types interact in the synovial tissue [48]. Therefore, we believe that analyzing the net effect of all cell types together provides a more holistic picture relevant to the clinical situation. Furthermore, in an in vitro synoviocyte model, it is not possible to investigate all factors playing a role in vivo at the same time. Besides adenosine, further factors play a role in synovial inflammation during RA and OA pathogenesis, such as the cytokines TNF or IL-1β, but also the major matrix-degrading enzymes MMP-1, -2, -3, -9, and -13 [49]. So far, only one study showed that anti-TNF therapy had no effect on the serum ADA level of RA patients compared to those who received DMARD therapy [50]. Another study reported a significant positive correlation between MMP-9 concentration and ADA activity in the synovial fluid of RA patients [51]. However, the causality between other factors and clinical phenotype has not yet been investigated in greater detail. Thus, the interaction between all these inflammatory microenvironment-related factors and endogenous adenosine/inosine has to be examined in future studies. Moreover, in most studies on synovial cell cultures, investigators take a maximum of eight to ten patients (10-20 years earlier, only three to five patients). Necessarily, all questions as to the influence of age of patients, medication, biological sex, menopausal status, or duration of the disease do not represent the conditions in normal synovium or in RA/OA patients with very early disease, because synovium will be most often taken during joint replacement surgery in a chronic phase. This represents a limitation to our studies.

4. Materials and Methods

4.1. Patients

Synovial tissue from patients with OA and RA was obtained during knee joint replacement surgery (patient characteristics are given in Table 1). Patients between 56 and 84 years were included in this study (age range of patients approved by the ethics committee: 18-85 years, inclusion criteria). The diagnosis of RA was based on the established criteria according to the American College of Rheumatology (formerly, the American Rheumatism Association) [52]. We excluded patients with joint infections. Patients were informed about the purpose of the study and gave their written consent. The Ethics Committee of the University of Regensburg approved the project (number 13-101-0135). All experiments were performed in accordance with relevant guidelines and regulations.

Table 1. Characteristics of patients under study.

Patient Characteristics	Osteoarthritis	Rheumatoid Arthritis
Number	18	12
Mean age (range) (yr)	67.5 (56–84)	62.4 (56–79)
Number of women/men, n (%)	8/10 (44/56)	10/2 (83/17)
C-reactive protein (mg/l)	2.08 ± 1.88	11.44 ± 10.99
Medication		
Daily Prednisolone (mg)	n.a.	5.9
Prednisolone, n (%)	n.a.	9 (75)
Methotrexate, n (%)	n.a.	8 (67)
Leflunomide, n (%)	n.a.	1 (8)
Sulfasalazine, n (%)	n.a.	2 (17)
Hydroxychloroquinel, n (%)	n.a.	2 (17)
NSAID, n (%)	17 (94)	12 (100)
Steroids (other than Prednisolone), n (%)	n.a.	n.a
Opiod analgesics, n (%)	1 (6)	2 (17)
Biologicals, n (%)	n.a.	3 (25)

Abbreviations: yr—years, n—number, n.a.—not applicable, NSAID—non-steroidal anti-inflammatory drug.

4.2. Synovial Tissue

Synovial tissue from RA and OA patients was obtained immediately after opening the knee joint capsule. Pieces of synovial tissue of up to 9 cm^2 were excised. One part of the synovial tissue specimen was fixed for immunohistochemical analyses using 3.7% paraformaldehyde (PFA; Merck, Darmstadt, Germany), then infiltrated with increasing concentrations of sucrose (10–30%; Merck, Darmstadt, Germany), embedded in Tissue-Tek (Sakura Sakura Finetek, Zoeterwoude, The Netherlands), and cryosectioned at 6–8 μm.

4.3. Mixed Synovial Cells

For functional in vitro studies, the remaining tissue pieces were minced and placed in Dispase I (Roche Diagnostics, Penzberg, Germany). Digestion was carried out for at least 1 h at 37 °C on a shaking platform. The resulting suspension was filtered (70 μm) and spun at 300× g for 10 min. The pellet was then treated with erythrocyte lysis buffer (Merck, Darmstadt, Germany) for 5 min and recentrifuged for 10 min at 300× g. The pellet was resuspended in.RPMI 1640 (Sigma-Aldrich, Taufkirchen, Germany) with 10% fetal calf serum (FCS; Thermo Fisher Scientific, Darmstadt, Germany). The obtained mixed synovial cells contain fibroblasts, macrophages, lymphocytes, and dendritic cells, as demonstrated in an earlier study [8]. For stimulation, 50.000 mixed synovial cells per well were transferred into 96-well culture plates and cultivated physioxic conditions (1% O_2). After overnight incubation, cells were treated with different compounds, as described above. For immunocytochemical studies, untreated cells cytospinned and fixed with 3.7% PFA. Slides were then stored at −20 °C until analysis.

4.4. Immunostainings

In order to detect CD39 and CD73 co-expression by immunocytochemistry, fixed synovial cells were stained for these cell surface ectonucleotidases using the primary antibodies rabbit anti-CD39 (ab178572, Abcam, Cambridge, UK) and mouse anti-CD73 (ab133582, Abcam, Cambridge, UK). The expression of ADA, ENT1, ENT2, and ARs was investigated by immunohistochemical staining of synovial tissue samples using the primary antibodies rabbit anti-ADA (NBP1-90361, Novus Biologicals, Cambridge, UK), rabbit anti-ENT1 (NBP1-84838, Novus Biologicals, Cambridge, UK), rabbit anti-ENT2 (ab48595, Abcam, Cambridge, UK), rabbit anti-A_1AR (ab124780, Abcam, Cambridge, UK), rabbit anti-A_{2A}AR (ab260032, Abcam, Cambridge, UK), rabbit anti-A_{2B}AR (LS-C20310, LSBio, via Biozol, Eching, Germany), and rabbit anti-A_3AR (LS-A686, LSBio, via Biozol, Eching, Germany). After blocking (10% bovine serum albumine, 10% chicken serum, and 10% goat serum), cytospin or tissue slides were incubated with primary antibodies overnight at 4 °C. Primary staining was visualized using Alexa Fluor-labeled secondary antibodies (goat anti-rabbit Alexa Fluor 594 or goat anti-mouse or anti-rabbit Alexa Fluor 488; Thermo Fisher/Life technologies, Schwerte, Germany). Cell nuclei were counterstained with DAPI (Merck, Darmstadt, Germany). Slides without primary antibody served as negative controls (Supplementary Materials Figure S2).

4.5. Adenosine and Inosine Quantification

Spontaneous adenosine as well as inosine release was determined 24 h after cell seeding by HPLC as described earlier [53,54].

4.6. Synovial Cell Stimulation

After overnight incubation with standard medium, synoviocytes were treated with the CD73 inhibitor A,B-Methylenadenosine 5'diphosphate (AMPCP), the ADA inhibitor 1-Deazaadenosine (DAA) and the ENT1/2 inhibitor Dipyridamole (DIP). While AMPCP suppresses adenosine synthesis, DAA keeps the adenosine level high by preventing the conversion of adenosine to inosine. ENT1/2 are responsible for the transport of adenosine between the intra- and extracellular space.

To identify the AR subtypes responsible for possible adenosine-dependent effects, different selective AR subtype agonists (A_1AR agonist 6-chloro-N6-cyclopentyladenosine (ccpA), A_{2A}AR agonist CGS 21680 hydrochloride (CGS 21680), A_{2B}AR agonist BAY 60–6583, A_3AR agonist 2-(1-Hexynyl)-N-methyladenosine (HEMADO), all from Tocris Bioscience Wiesbaden-Nordenstadt, Germany, were used. After treatments for 24 h under physioxia, cell culture supernatants were collected and released. IL-6, TNF, and IL-10 concentrations were quantified by ELISA and Luminex assays.

4.7. Data Analysis

All experiments were carried out with synovial cells of at least five patients. Data are presented as box plots, as % of non-treated controls due to naturally occurring variation in primary culture. To test for normality, the Kolmogorov–Smirnov test was used. Differences between groups were calculated using the non-parametric ANOVA (when data were normally distributed) or ANOVA on ranks (when normality was not given) followed by the Bonferroni or Student–Newman–Keuls correction method (pairwise comparison of all groups), as suggested for the respective analysis by the statistics software (SigmaPlot V.11, Systat Software, Erkrath, Germany). p values less than 0.05 were considered significant.

5. Conclusions

Taken together, the present study clearly demonstrates that OA and RA synoviocytes express the full functional enzymatic machinery necessary for adenosine synthesis, namely CD39 and CD73.

Since the inhibition of CD73 resulted in clear pro-inflammatory effects, we speculate that CD73 might be a novel therapeutic target and promoting its activity might represent a novel treatment option. It has been shown for an in vitro microvascular endothelial model that the transcriptional activation of functional CD73 was induced by its product adenosine [55]. In the synovium, a similar positive feedback loop might result in the perpetuation of anti-inflammatory adenosine effects. We believe that the inhibition of ADA and the subsequent adenosine accumulation could lead to an increased CD73 activity.

Besides adenosine feedback regulation, hypoxia has been shown to impair CD73 function mediated by hypoxia-inducible factor-1 (HIF-1) in epithelial cells [21,56]. Since HIF-1 expression is increased in an inflamed synovium [57], we hypothesize that inhibiting HIF-1 would result in a functional rehabilitation of CD73 and in turn in elevated adenosine synthesis. Methotrexate, a standard and frequently used disease-modifying drug in RA therapy, has been described to increase adenosine levels besides numerous further possible mechanisms of action [58]. However, quite obviously, the adenosine induction by methotrexate is not sufficient to create or maintain the anti-inflammatory state. Therefore, further research is required to investigate whether CD73 induction can be induced in RA synovial cells using ADA and/or HIF-1 blocking drugs in addition to standard strategies.

In addition, we demonstrated that endogenously released adenosine exerted its anti-inflammatory effects mainly via A_{2A}- and A_{2B}ARs. Therefore, an alternative activation of these receptors using specific synthetic agonists also represents an attractive approach for the treatment of synovial inflammation in both OA and RA.

All things considered, we conclude that stimulating the CD39/CD73 enzymatic machinery and, at the same time, inhibiting ADA activity in the synovial tissue could be a useful addition to existing standard medications. This concept might not only represent a promising anti-inflammatory therapeutic strategy for RA patients but could also be beneficial for OA patients.

Supplementary Materials: The following are available online at https://www.mdpi.com/article/10.3390/ijms22168956/s1.

Author Contributions: Conceptualization, R.H.S. and Z.J.-L.; methodology, R.S., M.J., and Z.J.-L.; validation, R.H.S., F.Z. and Z.J.-L.; formal analysis, R.S., M.J., R.H.S. and Z.J.-L.; investigation, R.S., M.J., and Z.J.-L.; resources, R.H.S., A.M. and F.Z.; writing—original draft preparation, R.S., M.J., R.H.S. and C writing—review and editing, A.M., F.Z., R.H.S. and Z.J.-L.; visualization, R.S., M.J., R.H.S. and Z.J.-L.; supervision, A.M., F.Z., R.H.S. and Z.J.-L.; project administration, R.H.S. and Z.J.-L.; funding acquisition, F.Z., R.H.S. and Z.J.-L. All authors have read and agreed to the published version of the manuscript.

Funding: This research was funded by the Deutsche Forschungsgemeinschaft FOR2407 (JE 642/4-2 to Z.J.-L. (project number 277277765)), STR 511/32-1 to R.H.S. (project number 243785207), and FOR2722 (FZ 561/3-1 to F.Z. (project number 407168728).

Institutional Review Board Statement: The study was conducted according to the guidelines of the Declaration of Helsinki, and approved by the Institutional Ethics Committee of the University of Regensburg (protocol code 13-101-0135, date of approval 18 July 2013).

Informed Consent Statement: Informed consent was obtained from all subjects involved in the study. Written informed consent has been obtained from the patient(s) to publish this paper.

Data Availability Statement: The data presented in this study are available on request from the corresponding author.

Acknowledgments: The authors thank Elena Underberg, Madlen Melzer and Angelika Gräber for their excellent technical assistance.

Conflicts of Interest: The authors declare no conflict of interest. The funders had no role in the design of the study; in the collection, analyses, or interpretation of data; in the writing of the manuscript, or in the decision to publish the results.

Abbreviations

ADA	Adenosine deaminase
Ado	Adenosine
AMP	Adenosine monophosphate
AMPCP	A: B-Methylenadenosine 5′ diphosphate
AR	Adenosine receptor
ATP	Adenosine triphosphate
BAY	BAY 60-6583
ccPA	2-chloro-N6-cyclopentyladenosine
CD39	Ectonucleoside triphosphate diphosphohydrolase 1
CD73	Ecto 5′ nucleotidase
CGS	CGS 21680
DAA	1-Deazaadenosine
DAPI	4′,6-diamidino-2-phenylindole
DIP	Dipyridamole
DMARDs	Disease-modifying antirheumatic drugs
ENT1	Equilibrative Nucleoside Transporter 1
ENT2	Equilibrative Nucleoside Transporter 2
FCS	Fetal calf serum
HEMADO	2-(1-Hexynyl)-N-methyladenosine
HIF-1	Hypoxia-inducible factor-1
HPLC	High pressure liquid chromatography
IL-6	Interleukin 6
IL-10	Interleukin 10
Ino	Inosine
MMP	Matrix metalloproteinase
N	Number
n.a.	Not applicable
NSAID	Non-steroidal anti-inflammatory drug
OA	Osteoarthritis
PFA	Paraformaldehyde
RA	Rheumatoid arthritis
TNF	Tumor necrosis factor
yr	Years

References

1. Aletaha, D.; Smolen, J.S. Diagnosis and Management of Rheumatoid Arthritis: A Review. *JAMA* **2018**, *320*, 1360–1372. [CrossRef] [PubMed]
2. Sweeney, S.E.; Firestein, G.S. Rheumatoid arthritis: Regulation of synovial inflammation. *Int. J. Biochem. Cell Biol.* **2004**, *36*, 372–378. [CrossRef]
3. Scott, D.L.; Wolfe, F.; Huizinga, T.W. Rheumatoid arthritis. *Lancet* **2010**, *376*, 1094–1108. [CrossRef]

4. Yu, M.B.; Firek, A.; Langridge, W.H.R. Predicting methotrexate resistance in rheumatoid arthritis patients. *Inflammopharmacology* **2018**, *26*, 699–708. [CrossRef] [PubMed]
5. Deane, K.D.; Demoruelle, M.K.; Kelmenson, L.B.; Kuhn, K.A.; Norris, J.M.; Holers, V.M. Genetic and environmental risk factors for rheumatoid arthritis. *Best Pract. Res. Clin. Rheumatol.* **2017**, *31*, 3–18. [CrossRef]
6. Schönfeld, C.; Pap, T.; Neumann, E.; Müller-Ladner, U. Fibroblasts as pathogenic cells in rheumatic inflammation. *Z. Fur Rheumatol.* **2015**, *74*, 33–38. [CrossRef]
7. McInnes, I.B.; Schett, G. Pathogenetic insights from the treatment of rheumatoid arthritis. *Lancet* **2017**, *389*, 2328–2337. [CrossRef]
8. Capellino, S.; Cosentino, M.; Wolff, C.; Schmidt, M.; Grifka, J.; Straub, R.H. Catecholamine-producing cells in the synovial tissue during arthritis: Modulation of sympathetic neurotransmitters as new therapeutic target. *Ann. Rheum. Dis.* **2010**, *69*, 1853–1860. [CrossRef] [PubMed]
9. Jenei-Lanzl, Z.; Zwingenberg, J.; Lowin, T.; Anders, S.; Straub, R.H. Proinflammatory receptor switch from Gαs to Gαi signaling by β-arrestin-mediated PDE4 recruitment in mixed RA synovial cells. *Brain Behav. Immun.* **2015**, *50*, 266–274. [CrossRef] [PubMed]
10. McInnes, I.B.; Buckley, C.D.; Isaacs, J.D. Cytokines in rheumatoid arthritis—Shaping the immunological landscape. *Nat. Rev. Rheumatol.* **2016**, *12*, 63–68. [CrossRef]
11. McInnes, I.B.; Schett, G. Cytokines in the pathogenesis of rheumatoid arthritis. *Nat. Rev. Immunol.* **2007**, *7*, 429–442. [CrossRef] [PubMed]
12. Schett, G.; Emery, P.; Tanaka, Y.; Burmester, G.; Pisetsky, D.S.; Naredo, E.; Fautrel, B.; van Vollenhoven, R. Tapering biologic and conventional DMARD therapy in rheumatoid arthritis: Current evidence and future directions. *Ann. Rheum. Dis.* **2016**, *75*, 1428–1437. [CrossRef]
13. Vlachogiannis, N.I.; Gatsiou, A.; Silvestris, D.A.; Stamatelopoulos, K.; Tektonidou, M.G.; Gallo, A.; Sfikakis, P.P.; Stellos, K. Increased adenosine-to-inosine RNA editing in rheumatoid arthritis. *J. Autoimmun.* **2020**, *106*, 102329. [CrossRef] [PubMed]
14. Scanzello, C.R. Role of low-grade inflammation in osteoarthritis. *Curr. Opin. Rheumatol.* **2017**, *29*, 79–85. [CrossRef]
15. Milne, G.R.; Palmer, T.M. Anti-inflammatory and immunosuppressive effects of the A2A adenosine receptor. *Sci. World J.* **2011**, *11*, 320–339. [CrossRef]
16. Odashima, M.; Bamias, G.; Rivera-Nieves, J.; Linden, J.; Nast, C.C.; Moskaluk, C.A.; Marini, M.; Sugawara, K.; Kozaiwa, K.; Otaka, M.; et al. Activation of A2A adenosine receptor attenuates intestinal inflammation in animal models of inflammatory bowel disease. *Gastroenterology* **2005**, *129*, 26–33. [CrossRef] [PubMed]
17. Fredholm, B.B.; AP, I.J.; Jacobson, K.A.; Linden, J.; Müller, C.E. International Union of Basic and Clinical Pharmacology. LXXXI. Nomenclature and classification of adenosine receptors—An update. *Pharmacol. Rev.* **2011**, *63*, 1–34. [CrossRef] [PubMed]
18. Sattin, A.; Rall, T.W. The effect of adenosine and adenine nucleotides on the cyclic adenosine 3′, 5′-phosphate content of guinea pig cerebral cortex slices. *Mol. Pharmacol.* **1970**, *6*, 13–23.
19. Vecchio, E.A.; White, P.J.; May, L.T. Targeting Adenosine Receptors for the Treatment of Cardiac Fibrosis. *Front. Pharmacol.* **2017**, *8*, 243. [CrossRef]
20. Stamp, L.K.; Hazlett, J.; Roberts, R.L.; Frampton, C.; Highton, J.; Hessian, P.A. Adenosine receptor expression in rheumatoid synovium: A basis for methotrexate action. *Arthritis Res. Ther.* **2012**, *14*, R138. [CrossRef]
21. Cronstein, B.N.; Sitkovsky, M. Adenosine and adenosine receptors in the pathogenesis and treatment of rheumatic diseases. *Nat. Rev. Rheumatol.* **2017**, *13*, 41–51. [CrossRef] [PubMed]
22. Campo, G.M.; Avenoso, A.; D'Ascola, A.; Nastasi, G.; Micali, A.; Puzzolo, D.; Pisani, A.; Prestipino, V.; Scuruchi, M.; Calatroni, A.; et al. Combined treatment with hyaluronan inhibitor Pep-1 and a selective adenosine A2 receptor agonist reduces inflammation in experimental arthritis. *Innate Immun.* **2013**, *19*, 462–478. [CrossRef] [PubMed]
23. Flögel, U.; Burghoff, S.; van Lent, P.L.; Temme, S.; Galbarz, L.; Ding, Z.; El-Tayeb, A.; Huels, S.; Bönner, F.; Borg, N.; et al. Selective activation of adenosine A2A receptors on immune cells by a CD73-dependent prodrug suppresses joint inflammation in experimental rheumatoid arthritis. *Sci. Transl. Med.* **2012**, *4*, 146ra108. [CrossRef]
24. Li, Q.H.; Xie, W.X.; Li, X.P.; Huang, K.T.; Du, Z.H.; Cong, W.J.; Zhou, L.H.; Ye, T.S.; Chen, J.F. Adenosine A2A Receptors Mediate Anti-Inflammatory Effects of Electroacupuncture on Synovitis in Mice with Collagen-Induced Arthritis. *Evid. Complementary Altern. Med. eCAM* **2015**, *2015*, 809560. [CrossRef]
25. Magni, G.; Ceruti, S. Adenosine Signaling in Autoimmune Disorders. *Pharmaceuticals* **2020**, *13*, 260. [CrossRef] [PubMed]
26. Muz, B.; Khan, M.N.; Kiriakidis, S.; Paleolog, E.M. Hypoxia. The role of hypoxia and HIF-dependent signalling events in rheumatoid arthritis. *Arthritis Res. Ther.* **2009**, *11*, 201. [CrossRef] [PubMed]
27. Fishman, P.; Cohen, S. The A3 adenosine receptor (A3AR): Therapeutic target and predictive biological marker in rheumatoid arthritis. *Clin. Rheumatol.* **2016**, *35*, 2359–2362. [CrossRef]
28. Novotný, J. Adenosine and its role in physiology. *Ceskoslovenska Fysiol.* **2015**, *64*, 35–44.
29. Giatromanolaki, A.; Kouroupi, M.; Pouliliou, S.; Mitrakas, A.; Hasan, F.; Pappa, A.; Koukourakis, M.I. Ectonucleotidase CD73 and CD39 expression in non-small cell lung cancer relates to hypoxia and immunosuppressive pathways. *Life Sci.* **2020**, *259*, 118389. [CrossRef]
30. Zhang, R.; Miao, J.; Zhang, K.; Zheng, Z.; Zhu, P. Increased percentage and defective inhibitory function of CD4(+)CD25(−) FOXP3(+) T cells in synovial fluid of patients with rheumatoid arthritis. *Xi Bao Yu Fen Zi Mian Yi Xue Za Zhi Chin. J. Cell. Mol. Immunol.* **2019**, *35*, 961–966.

31. Ohradanova-Repic, A.; Machacek, C.; Charvet, C.; Lager, F.; Le Roux, D.; Platzer, R.; Leksa, V.; Mitulovic, G.; Burkard, T.R.; Zlabinger, G.J.; et al. Extracellular Purine Metabolism Is the Switchboard of Immunosuppressive Macrophages and a Novel Target to Treat Diseases With Macrophage Imbalances. *Front. Immunol.* **2018**, *9*, 852. [CrossRef] [PubMed]
32. Baldwin, S.A.; Beal, P.R.; Yao, S.Y.; King, A.E.; Cass, C.E.; Young, J.D. The equilibrative nucleoside transporter family, SLC29. *Pflug. Arch. Eur. J. Physiol.* **2004**, *447*, 735–743. [CrossRef]
33. Van der Weyden, M.B.; Kelley, W.N. Human adenosine deaminase. Distribution and properties. *J. Biol. Chem.* **1976**, *251*, 5448–5456. [CrossRef]
34. Nakamachi, Y.; Koshiba, M.; Nakazawa, T.; Hatachi, S.; Saura, R.; Kurosaka, M.; Kusaka, H.; Kumagai, S. Specific increase in enzymatic activity of adenosine deaminase 1 in rheumatoid synovial fibroblasts. *Arthritis Rheum.* **2003**, *48*, 668–674. [CrossRef] [PubMed]
35. Szabo, C.; Pacher, P. The outsiders: Emerging roles of ectonucleotidases in inflammation. *Sci. Transl. Med.* **2012**, *4*, 146ps114. [CrossRef]
36. Coates, L.C.; FitzGerald, O.; Helliwell, P.S.; Paul, C. Psoriasis, psoriatic arthritis, and rheumatoid arthritis: Is all inflammation the same? *Semin. Arthritis Rheum.* **2016**, *46*, 291–304. [CrossRef]
37. Yuksel, H.; Akoğlu, T.F. Serum and synovial fluid adenosine deaminase activity in patients with rheumatoid arthritis, osteoarthritis, and reactive arthritis. *Ann. Rheum. Dis.* **1988**, *47*, 492–495. [CrossRef] [PubMed]
38. Zakeri, Z.; Izadi, S.; Niazi, A.; Bari, Z.; Zendeboodi, S.; Shakiba, M.; Mashhadi, M.; Narouie, B.; Ghasemi-Rad, M. Comparison of adenosine deaminase levels in serum and synovial fluid between patients with rheumatoid arthritis and osteoarthritis. *Int. J. Clin. Exp. Med.* **2012**, *5*, 195–200. [PubMed]
39. Khoa, N.D.; Montesinos, M.C.; Reiss, A.B.; Delano, D.; Awadallah, N.; Cronstein, B.N. Inflammatory cytokines regulate function and expression of adenosine A(2A) receptors in human monocytic THP-1 cells. *J. Immunol.* **2001**, *167*, 4026–4032. [CrossRef]
40. Sun, W.C.; Berghaus, L.J.; Moore, J.N.; Hurley, D.J.; Vandenplas, M.L.; Thompson, R.; Linden, J. Lipopolysaccharide and TNF-alpha modify adenosine A(2A) receptor expression and function in equine monocytes. *Vet. Immunol. Immunopathol.* **2010**, *135*, 289–295. [CrossRef] [PubMed]
41. Altschuler, S.J.; Wu, L.F. Cellular heterogeneity: Do differences make a difference? *Cell* **2010**, *141*, 559–563. [CrossRef]
42. Thomas, S.; Rouilly, V.; Patin, E.; Alanio, C.; Dubois, A.; Delval, C.; Marquier, L.G.; Fauchoux, N.; Sayegrih, S.; Vray, M.; et al. The Milieu Intérieur study—An integrative approach for study of human immunological variance. *Clin. Immunol.* **2015**, *157*, 277–293. [CrossRef] [PubMed]
43. Robinson, W.H.; Lepus, C.M.; Wang, Q.; Raghu, H.; Mao, R.; Lindstrom, T.M.; Sokolove, J. Low-grade inflammation as a key mediator of the pathogenesis of osteoarthritis. *Nat. Rev. Rheumatol.* **2016**, *12*, 580–592. [CrossRef]
44. Aherne, C.M.; Collins, C.B.; Rapp, C.R.; Olli, K.E.; Perrenoud, L.; Jedlicka, P.; Bowser, J.L.; Mills, T.W.; Karmouty-Quintana, H.; Blackburn, M.R.; et al. Coordination of ENT2-dependent adenosine transport and signaling dampens mucosal inflammation. *JCI Insight* **2018**, *3*, e121521. [CrossRef] [PubMed]
45. Bar-Yehuda, S.; Silverman, M.H.; Kerns, W.D.; Ochaion, A.; Cohen, S.; Fishman, P. The anti-inflammatory effect of A3 adenosine receptor agonists: A novel targeted therapy for rheumatoid arthritis. *Expert Opin. Investig. Drugs* **2007**, *16*, 1601–1613. [CrossRef]
46. Ochaion, A.; Bar-Yehuda, S.; Cohen, S.; Amital, H.; Jacobson, K.A.; Joshi, B.V.; Gao, Z.G.; Barer, F.; Patoka, R.; Del Valle, L.; et al. The A3 adenosine receptor agonist CF502 inhibits the PI3K, PKB/Akt and NF-kappaB signaling pathway in synoviocytes from rheumatoid arthritis patients and in adjuvant-induced arthritis rats. *Biochem. Pharmacol.* **2008**, *76*, 482–494. [CrossRef] [PubMed]
47. Daaka, Y.; Luttrell, L.M.; Lefkowitz, R.J. Switching of the coupling of the beta2-adrenergic receptor to different G proteins by protein kinase A. *Nature* **1997**, *390*, 88–91. [CrossRef] [PubMed]
48. Aarvak, T.; Natvig, J.B. Cell-cell interactions in synovitis: Antigen presenting cells and T cell interaction in rheumatoid arthritis. *Arthritis Res.* **2001**, *3*, 13–17. [CrossRef]
49. Burrage, P.S.; Mix, K.S.; Brinckerhoff, C.E. Matrix metalloproteinases: Role in arthritis. *Front. Biosci. A J. Virtual Libr.* **2006**, *11*, 529–543. [CrossRef] [PubMed]
50. Erer, B.; Yilmaz, G.; Yilmaz, F.M.; Koklu, S. Assessment of adenosine deaminase levels in rheumatoid arthritis patients receiving anti-TNF-alpha therapy. *Rheumatol. Int.* **2009**, *29*, 651–654. [CrossRef]
51. Iwaki-Egawa, S.; Watanabe, Y.; Matsuno, H. Correlations between matrix metalloproteinase-9 and adenosine deaminase isozymes in synovial fluid from patients with rheumatoid arthritis. *J. Rheumatol.* **2001**, *28*, 485–489. [PubMed]
52. Arnett, F.C.; Edworthy, S.M.; Bloch, D.A.; McShane, D.J.; Fries, J.F.; Cooper, N.S.; Healey, L.A.; Kaplan, S.R.; Liang, M.H.; Luthra, H.S.; et al. The American Rheumatism Association 1987 revised criteria for the classification of rheumatoid arthritis. *Arthritis Rheum.* **1988**, *31*, 315–324. [CrossRef] [PubMed]
53. Huang, L.F.; Guo, F.Q.; Liang, Y.Z.; Li, B.Y.; Cheng, B.M. Simple and rapid determination of adenosine in human synovial fluid with high performance liquid chromatography-mass spectrometry. *J. Pharm. Biomed. Anal.* **2004**, *36*, 877–882. [CrossRef] [PubMed]
54. Straub, R.H.; Pongratz, G.; Günzler, C.; Michna, A.; Baier, S.; Kees, F.; Falk, W.; Schölmerich, J. Immunoregulation of IL-6 secretion by endogenous and exogenous adenosine and by exogenous purinergic agonists in splenic tissue slices. *J. Neuroimmunol.* **2002**, *125*, 73–81. [CrossRef]
55. Narravula, S.; Lennon, P.F.; Mueller, B.U.; Colgan, S.P. Regulation of endothelial CD73 by adenosine: Paracrine pathway for enhanced endothelial barrier function. *J. Immunol.* **2000**, *165*, 5262–5268. [CrossRef]

56. Synnestvedt, K.; Furuta, G.T.; Comerford, K.M.; Louis, N.; Karhausen, J.; Eltzschig, H.K.; Hansen, K.R.; Thompson, L.F.; Colgan, S.P. Ecto-5′-nucleotidase (CD73) regulation by hypoxia-inducible factor-1 mediates permeability changes in intestinal epithelia. *J. Clin. Investig.* **2002**, *110*, 993–1002. [CrossRef] [PubMed]
57. Hu, F.; Liu, H.; Xu, L.; Li, Y.; Liu, X.; Shi, L.; Su, Y.; Qiu, X.; Zhang, X.; Yang, Y.; et al. Hypoxia-inducible factor-1α perpetuates synovial fibroblast interactions with T cells and B cells in rheumatoid arthritis. *Eur. J. Immunol.* **2016**, *46*, 742–751. [CrossRef]
58. Friedman, B.; Cronstein, B. Methotrexate mechanism in treatment of rheumatoid arthritis. *Jt. Bone Spine* **2019**, *86*, 301–307. [CrossRef] [PubMed]

International Journal of
Molecular Sciences

MDPI

Article

Hyperbilirubinemia Maintained by Chronic Supplementation of Unconjugated Bilirubin Improves the Clinical Course of Experimental Autoimmune Arthritis

Tomas Sykora [1,*], Pavel Babal [1], Kristina Mikus-Kuracinova [1], Frantisek Drafi [2], Silvester Ponist [2], Monika Dvorakova [3], Pavol Janega [1] and Katarina Bauerova [2]

1 Department of Pathology, Faculty of Medicine, Comenius University in Bratislava, Spitalska 24, 81372 Bratislava, Slovakia; pavel.babal@fmed.uniba.sk (P.B.); kristina.kuracinova@fmed.uniba.sk (K.M.-K.); pavol.janega@fmed.uniba.sk (P.J.)

2 Centre of Experimental Medicine, Institute of Experimental Pharmacology and Toxicology, Slovak Academy of Sciences, Dúbravská Cesta 9, 84104 Bratislava, Slovakia; frantisek.drafi@savba.sk (F.D.); exfasipo@savba.sk (S.P.); exfakbau@savba.sk (K.B.)

3 Department of Medical Chemistry, Biochemistry and Clinical Biochemistry, Faculty of Medicine, Comenius University in Bratislava, Spitalska 24, 81372 Bratislava, Slovakia; monika.dvorakova@fmed.uniba.sk

* Correspondence: tomas.sykora@nudch.eu

Citation: Sykora, T.; Babal, P.; Mikus-Kuracinova, K.; Drafi, F.; Ponist, S.; Dvorakova, M.; Janega, P.; Bauerova, K. Hyperbilirubinemia Maintained by Chronic Supplementation of Unconjugated Bilirubin Improves the Clinical Course of Experimental Autoimmune Arthritis. *Int. J. Mol. Sci.* **2021**, *22*, 8662. https://doi.org/10.3390/ijms22168662

Academic Editor: Chih-Hsin Tang

Received: 15 July 2021
Accepted: 6 August 2021
Published: 12 August 2021

Abstract: Rheumatoid arthritis (RA) is a chronic multisystem disease, therapy of which remains a challenge for basic research. The present work examined the effect of unconjugated bilirubin (UCB) administration in adjuvant-induced arthritis (AIA)—an experimental model, in which oxidative stress (OS), inflammation and inadequate immune response are often similar to RA. Male Lewis rats were randomized into groups: CO—control, AIA—untreated adjuvant-induced arthritis, AIA-BIL—adjuvant-induced arthritis administrated UCB, CO-BIL—control with administrated UCB. UCB was administered *intraperitoneally* 200 mg/kg of body weight daily from 14th day of the experiment, when clinical signs of the disease are fully manifested, to 28th day, the end of the experiment. AIA was induced by a single intradermal immunization at the base of the tail with suspension of *Mycobacterium butyricum* in incomplete Freund's adjuvant. Clinical, hematologic, biochemical and histologic examinations were performed. UCB administration to animals with AIA lead to a significant decrease in hind paws volume, plasma levels of C-reactive protein (CRP) and ceruloplasmin, drop of leukocytes, lymphocytes, erythrocytes, hemoglobin and an increase in platelet count. UCB administration caused significantly lowered oxidative damage to DNA in arthritic animals, whereas in healthy controls it induced considerable oxidative damage to DNA. UCB administration also induced atrophy of the spleen and thymus in AIA and CO animals comparing to untreated animals. Histological signs of joint damage assessed by neutrophils infiltration and deposition of fibrin were significantly reduced by UCB administration. The effects of exogenously administered UCB to the animals with adjuvant-induced arthritis might be identified as therapeutic, in contrast to the effects of UCB administration in healthy animals rather classified as toxic.

Keywords: adjuvant-induced arthritis; bilirubin; immunomodulation; inflammation; white blood cells

1. Introduction

Rheumatoid arthritis (RA) is a complex inflammatory disease of joints, which typically affect small joints of the hand and feet. If left untreated, it leads to a progressive joint cartilage destruction and disability. Moreover, this disease can damage a wide variety of body systems, including the skin, eyes, lungs, heart and blood vessels. The prevalence of RA in population is around 1% [1]. RA is predominantly classified on the basis of the clinical phenotype, autoantibody production, influenced by both genetic and environmental factors [2,3]. Joint synovium is normally a structure with low cellularity and a delicate intimal lining. Activation of signal pathways of cytokines and other inflammation markers lead to infiltration of the synovium by CD4$^+$ T-cells, B-cells, macrophages and neutrophils [4,5]. Increased numbers of macrophage-like and fibroblast-like synoviocytes result in synovial hyperplasia. Locally released degradation enzymes, including metalloproteinases, serine proteases and aggrecanases, digest the extracellular matrix and destroy the articular structures. T-cell activation is part of the process but the reason of systemic loss of tolerance turning to a localized onset of inflammation in the joint is still unclear [6].

According to Smolen et al. (2014) the treatment for RA can be classified into biological original and biosimilar disease-modifying anti-rheumatic drugs (boDMARDs and bsDMARDs, respectively) and the former non-biologic DMARDs into conventional synthetic and targeted synthetic DMARDs (csDMARDs and tsDMARDs, respectively) [7]. Methotrexate (MTX) belongs to the csDMARDs and is widely used as the first-line therapy in RA [8,9]. Recent advances in RA treatment include the application of approved novel agents inhibiting IL-6, IL-17 (boDMARDs) and Janus kinase (tsDMARDs) as well as biosimilars (bsDMARDs) [6,10,11]. Although there is a number of RA treatment alternatives, many of the approved agents are not available for most of the patient and side effects as well as treatment resistance are limiting the best treatment option. Despite of advances in drug development for RA, a group of patients may benefit of alternative treatments such as antioxidant intake in form of fresh fruits/vegetables as well as food supplements [12].

Nearly a century ago, jaundiced patients were observed to have surprising and spontaneous remissions from incurable immunologic diseases including rheumatoid arthritis, allergy, and asthma. The mystery of why this phenomenon occurred remains unresolved to this day [13]. Bilirubin is a secondary breakdown product of normal heme catabolism that is excreted in bile and urine, and elevated levels may indicate certain diseases [14]. For decades was bilirubin considered as a metabolism side product with no specific purpose but recent data indicate that bilirubin exhibits potent antioxidant properties with positive clinical consequence and relatively low toxicity [15–17]. Most recently, the molecule has been found to possess immunomodulatory properties that rival its redox capacity, possibly explaining its ability to suppress inflammation [13]. Higher serum levels of bilirubin are linked with an absence of inflammatory diseases such as RA [16,18]. Gilbert's syndrome may be defined as harmless unconjugated hyperbilirubinemia due to a decreased conjugation enzymatic capacity in liver [19]. It is known that this trait in people may reduce health risks in cardiovascular diseases [15,20,21].

Unconjugated bilirubin (UCB) investigation on the adjuvant-induced arthritis (AIA) model has not been performed yet. In the presented experimental study we evaluate the tissue protective and immunomodulatory effect of UCB on the course of AIA where oxidative stress, inflammation and inadequate immune response lead to development of significant pathology [22]. In our pre-clinical research, there was an interest to find out which of the markers are modified in AIA conditions and to compare this with treated healthy controls. We have described the anti-inflammatory properties of UCB for the first time, UCB has furthermore exhibited its properties on many other markers on the AIA model. Further research of UCB may introduce interest for development of its new pharmaceutical forms to improve therapeutic outcome of RA treatment.

2. Results

2.1. Bilirubin Levels

Serum levels of total and conjugated bilirubin were measured on 28th day of the experiment. Values of total bilirubin in control group (CO) and AIA, 0.20 $\pm$ 0.07 and 0.29 $\pm$ 0.11 µM/L, are naturally very low in Lewis rats and conjugated bilirubin in these two groups was undetectable [23]. UCB administration increased its levels approximately hundred times. In adjuvant-induced arthritis group with UCB administration (AIA-BIL) was the average level of conjugated bilirubin 4.95 $\pm$ 0.39 µM/L and of total bilirubin 28.67 $\pm$ 2.23 µM/L. In control group with UCB administration (CO-BIL) was the average level of conjugated bilirubin 5.93 $\pm$ 1.35 µM/L and of total bilirubin 29.73 $\pm$ 1.82 µM/L.

2.2. Changes in Hind Paw Volume and Body Weight

Swelling of the hind paws was a marker of clinical progression [24]. Induction of AIA resulted in significant swelling of the hind paw joints evaluated as the change in hind paw volume (HPV, $p < 0.001$ vs. CO on day 14, 21 and 28). In the AIA-BIL group, UCB administration lead to a decrease of HPV compared to untreated AIA group ($p < 0.01$ vs. AIA on day 21 and 28; Figure 1a), which improved mobility of the animals. In CO-BIL was HPV on day 28 significantly decreased comparing to healthy CO animals ($p < 0.01$ vs. CO on day 28; Figure 1a). There was observed a general body weight loss of the animals with AIA and in both groups of animals administered UCB since day 14 towards the end of the experiment (for CO-BIL $p < 0.001$ vs. CO on day 21 and 28, for AIA-BIL $p < 0.05$ vs. AIA on day 28; Figure 1b).

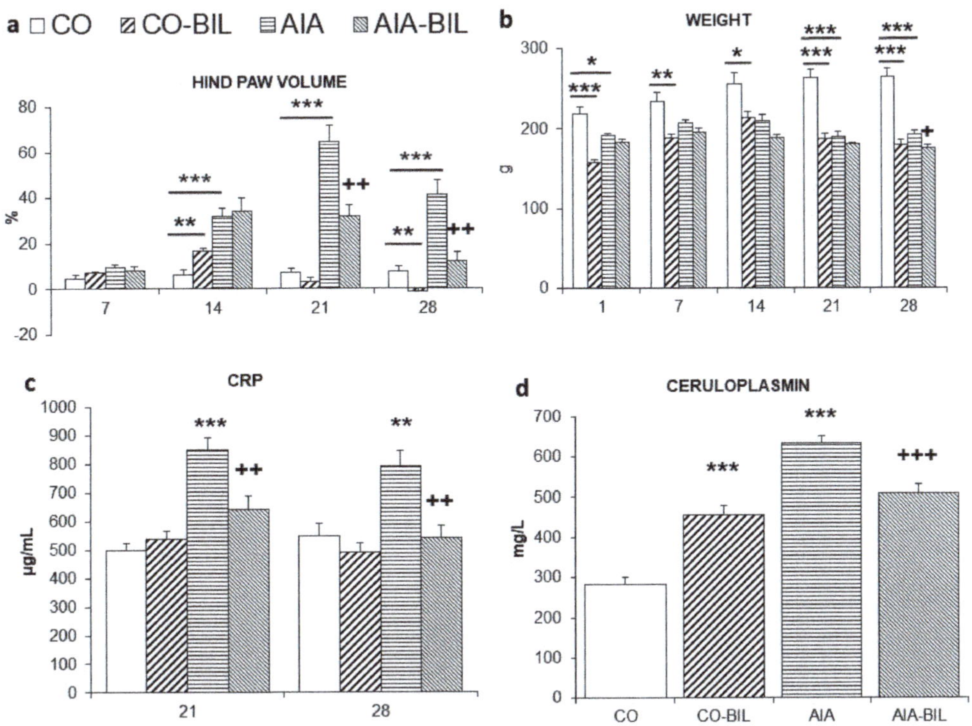

Figure 1. (**a**). Time profile of hind paw volume changes during the course of the experiment. (**b**). Body weight changes of the animals during the experiment. (**c**). CRP levels change on 21st and 28th day and (**d**). Ceruloplasmin levels at the end of the experiment. CO—control group, CO-BIL—control group administered with UCB 200 mg/kg of body weight daily i.p. from day 14, AIA—group with adjuvant induced arthritis, AIA-BIL—group with adjuvant induced arthritis administered with UCB 200 mg/kg of body weight daily i.p. from day 14. Results are expressed as mean ± SEM, n = 7–8. Significant difference between groups CO and CO-BIL, CO and AIA: *** $p < 0.001$ vs. CO, ** $p < 0.01$ vs. CO, * $p < 0.05$ vs. CO. Significant difference between groups AIA and AIA-BIL: $^{+++}$ $p < 0.001$ vs. AIA, $^{++}$ $p < 0.01$ vs. AIA, $^{+}$ $p < 0.05$ vs. AIA.

2.3. Changes in Blood Screen

Induction of AIA lead in AIA animals to an increase in leukocyte, lymphocyte and platelet counts in the peripheral blood ($p < 0.001$ vs. CO on day 14, 21 and 28; Figure 2a–c respectively). UCB administration caused a significant decrease of leukocytes ($p < 0.01$) and lymphocytes ($p < 0.01$) that continued towards the end of the experiment (Figure 2a,b). UCB administration produced significant changes in the number of red blood cells, in levels of hemoglobin and in the mean corpuscular volume (MCV) in AIA animals. In control animals administration of UCB caused significant decrease of hemoglobin level and significant decrease in MCV, thus the size of erythrocytes was smaller (Table 1). On the contrary, as demonstrated in both AIA-BIL and CO-BIL groups, UCB administration caused significant elevation of thrombocytes when compared to AIA and CO, respectively (Figure 2c).

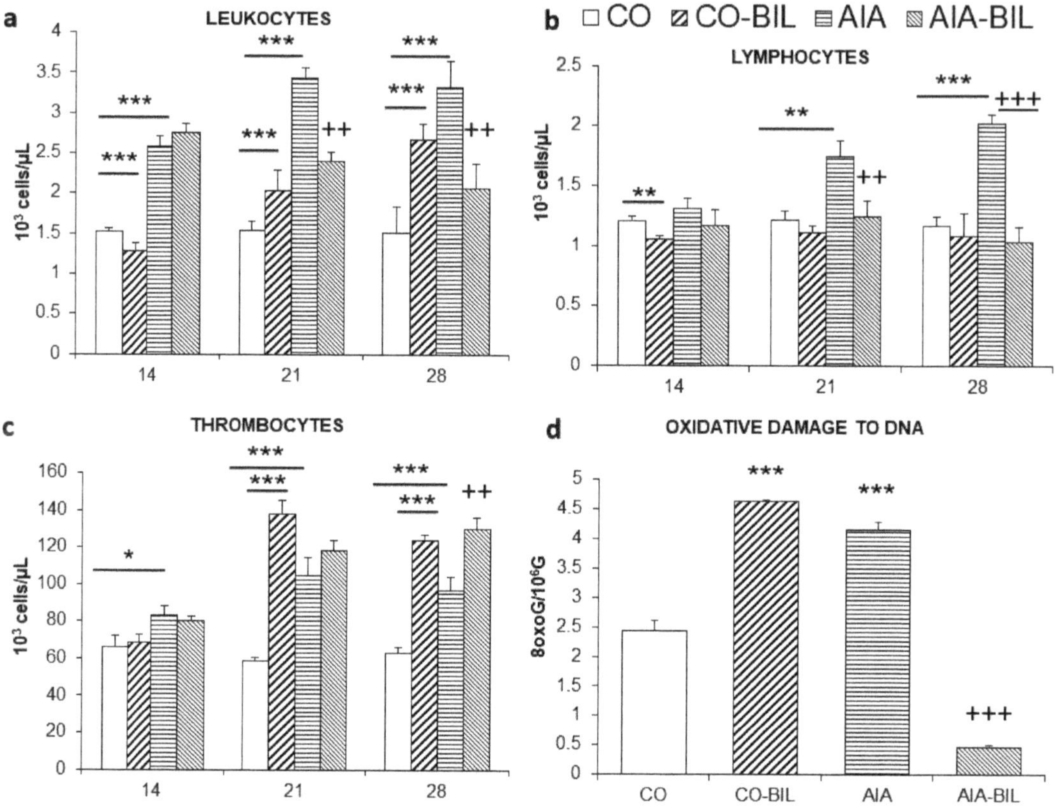

Figure 2. Time profile of changes in (**a**). leukocytes, (**b**). lymphocytes and (**c**). thrombocytes (**d**). Oxidative damage to DNA evaluated on day 28 of the experiment CO—control group, CO-BIL—control group administered with UCB 200 mg/kg of body weight daily i.p. from day 14, AIA—group with adjuvant induced arthritis, AIA-BIL—group with adjuvant induced arthritis administered with UCB 200 mg/kg of body weight daily i.p. from day 14. Results are expressed as mean ± SEM, n = 7–8. Significant difference between groups CO and CO-BIL, CO and AIA: *** $p < 0.001$ vs. CO, ** $p < 0.01$ vs. CO, * $p < 0.05$ vs. CO. Significant difference between groups AIA and AIA-BIL: +++ $p < 0.001$ vs. AIA, ++ $p < 0.01$ vs. AIA.

Table 1. Changes in erythrocytes (number of erythrocytes, hemoglobin content and corpuscular volume) parameters during the course of the experiment. MCV—mean corpuscular volume. CO—control group, CO-BIL—control group administered with UCB 200 mg/kg of body weight daily i.p. from day 14, AIA—group with adjuvant induced arthritis, AIA-BIL—group with adjuvant induced arthritis administered with UCB 200 mg/kg of body weight daily i.p. from day 14. Results are expressed as mean ± SEM, n = 7–8. Significant difference between groups CO and CO-BIL, CO and AIA: *** $p < 0.001$ vs. CO, ** $p < 0.01$ vs. CO, * $p < 0.05$ vs. CO. Significant difference between groups AIA and AIA-BIL: ++ $p < 0.01$ vs. AIA, + $p < 0.05$ vs. AIA.

		Day					
	Group	14		21		28	
Erythrocytes ($10^6/\mu L$)	CO	0.84	±0.04	0.96	±0.03	1.00	±0.03
	CO-BIL	0.94	±0.03	0.99	±0.13	0.96	±0.02
	AIA	0.86	±0.02	0.96	±0.03	1.05	±0.02
	AIA-BIL	0.84	±0.03	0.91	±0.02	0.92 ++	±0.03
Hemoglobin (g/dL)	CO	1.37	±0.05	1.63	±0.06	1.66	±0.04
	CO-BIL	1.69 **	±0.07	1.63	±0.03	1.56*	±0.02
	AIA	1.38	±0.03	1.51	±0.04	1.60	±0.04
	AIA-BIL	1.31	±0.04	1.40	±0.04	1.42 +	±0.06
MCV (μL)	CO	47.71	±0.84	46.86	±0.77	47.43	±0.72
	CO-BIL	46.63	±0.32	44.63 *	±0.26	44.71 **	±0.29
	AIA	45.00 **	±0.27	43.88 **	±0.35	42.86 ***	±0.40
	AIA-BIL	43.88 +	±0.40	42.86	±0.40	42.67	±0.33

2.4. Markers of Inflammation and Organ Weight

Administration of UCB caused in AIA-BIL significant decrease of CRP ($p < 0.01$ vs. AIA on day 21 and 28; Figure 1c) and ceruloplasmin ($p < 0.001$ vs. AIA on day 28; Figure 1d) in AIA-BIL compared to AIA, which corresponded with the clinical course of the disease in the experimental animals.

At the end of the experiment, liver, thymus and spleen were collected and weighted. Animals with UCB administration had significantly smaller spleen (CO-BIL $p < 0.05$ vs. CO, AIA-BIL $p < 0.05$ vs. AIA; Figure 3a) and thymus (CO-BIL $p < 0.001$ vs. CO; AIA-BIL $p < 0.001$ vs. AIA; Figure 1b), liver was significantly smaller in CO-BIL comparing to CO ($p < 0.01$; Figure 1b), but about the same weight in AIA and AIA-BIL (Figure 3).

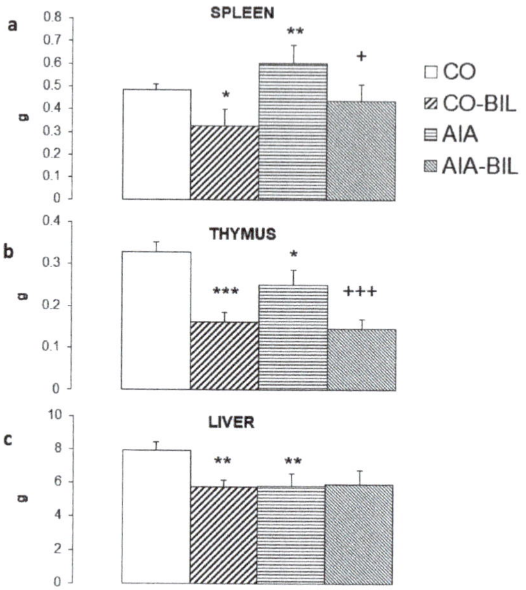

Figure 3. Weight of selected organs at the end of the experiment; (**a**). spleen, (**b**). thymus, (**c**). liver. CO—control group, CO-BIL—control group administered with UCB 200 mg/kg of body weight daily i.p. from day 14, AIA—group with adjuvant induced arthritis, AIA-BIL—group with adjuvant induced arthritis administered with UCB 200 mg/kg of body weight daily i.p. from day 14. Results are expressed as mean ± SEM, n = 7–8. Significant difference between groups CO and CO-BIL, CO and AIA: *** $p < 0.001$ vs. CO, ** $p < 0.01$ vs. CO, * $p < 0.05$ vs. CO. Significant difference between groups AIA and AIA-BIL: $^{+++}$ $p < 0.001$ vs. AIA, $^{+}$ $p < 0.05$ vs. AIA.

2.5. Oxidative Damage to DNA and Histological Examination

Oxidative damage to DNA evaluated at the end of the experiment was significantly increased in the AIA and dramatically dropped by bilirubin in the AIA-BIL group ($p < 0.001$; Figure 2d). UCB administration in CO-BIL resulted in a significantly higher oxidative DNA damage comparing to CO group ($p < 0.001$; Figure 2d).

Bilirubin treatment dramatically reduced the inflammatory cell infiltrate in AIA-BIL ($p < 0.001$ vs. AIA; Figure 4). Histological evaluation of the hind paw knee joints in animals with arthritis showed enlargement of the articular cavity and with leukocyte accumulation, interstitial edema and infiltration of the soft tissues by leukocytes. Joint inflammation was documented by dense infiltration of the periarticular tissues by neutrophilic granulocytes and their presence in the articular cavity, as demonstrated with chloroacetylesterase (CHAE) activity (Figure 5). The fibrin exudation was significantly reduced in the AIA-BIL group ($p < 0.001$ vs. AIA; Figure 6). Fibrin exudation detected by phosphotungstic acid hematoxylin (PTAH) staining, as the sign of an active inflammatory process, was in high amounts present in the joints in all AIA samples (Figure 7).

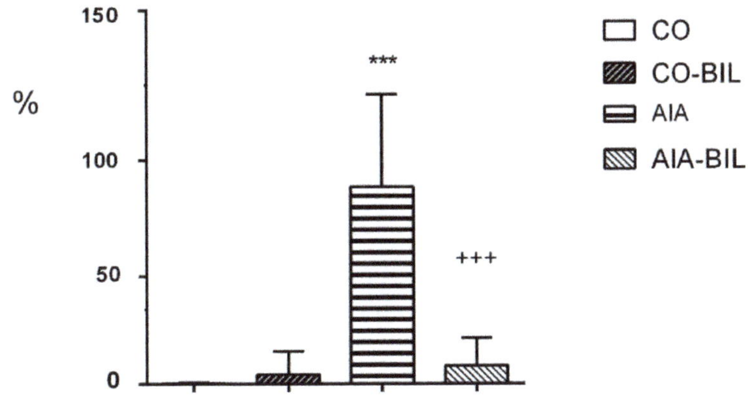

Figure 4. Infiltration of joints by granulocytes. CO—control group, CO-BIL—control group administered with UCB 200 mg/kg of body weight daily i.p. from day 14, AIA—group with adjuvant induced arthritis, AIA-BIL—group with adjuvant induced arthritis administered with UCB 200 mg/kg of body weight daily i.p. from day 14. Results are expressed as mean ± SEM, n = 7–8. Significant difference between groups CO and CO-BIL, CO and AIA: *** $p < 0.001$ vs. CO. Significant difference between groups AIA and AIA-BIL: +++ $p < 0.001$ vs. AIA.

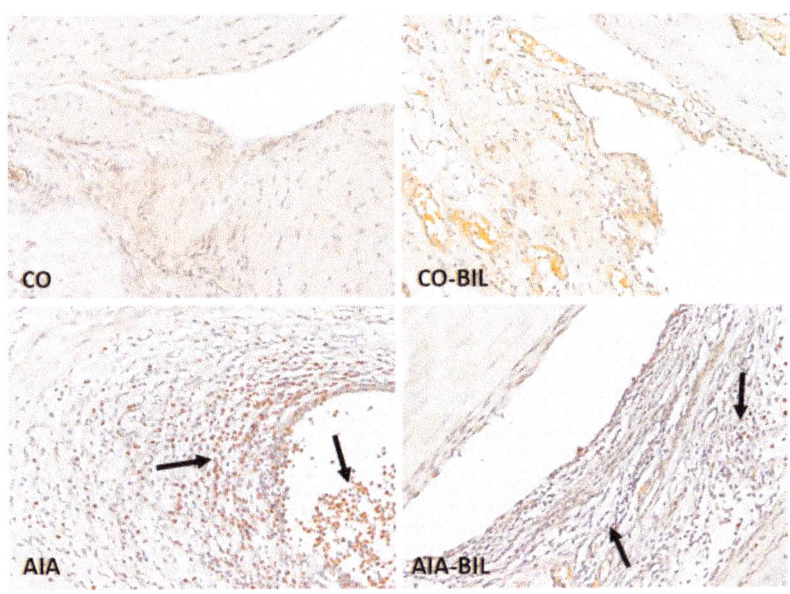

Figure 5. Infiltration of joints by granulocytes detected with naphtol-AS-D-chloroacetate esterase (CHAE) activity. Dense granulocytic infiltrate (arrow) in the inflamed joints (AIA) was reduced by UCB treatment (AIA-BIL). CO—control group, CO-BIL—control group administered with UCB 200 mg/kg of body weight daily i.p. from day 14, AIA—group with adjuvant induced arthritis, AIA-BIL—group with adjuvant induced arthritis administered with UCB 200 mg/kg of body weight daily i.p. from day 14. CHAE, 100×.

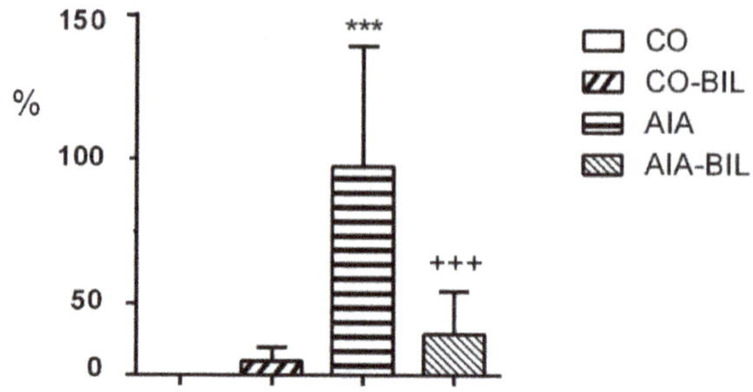

Figure 6. Fibrin exudation into joints. CO—control group, CO-BIL—control group administered with UCB 200 mg/kg of body weight daily i.p. from day 14, AIA—group with adjuvant induced arthritis, AIA-BIL—group with adjuvant induced arthritis administered with UCB 200 mg/kg of body weight daily i.p. from day 14. Results are expressed as mean ± SEM, n = 7–8. Significant difference between groups CO and CO-BIL, CO and AIA: *** $p < 0.001$ vs. CO. Significant difference between groups AIA and AIA-BIL: +++ $p < 0.001$ vs. AIA.

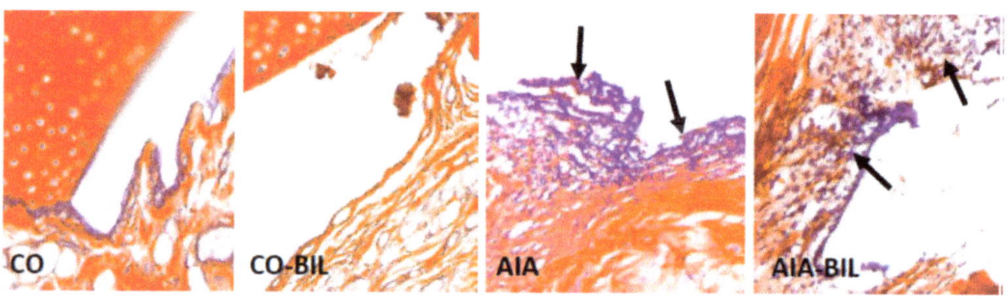

Figure 7. Detection of fibrin in joints with Mallory's phosphotungstic acid hematoxylin (PTAH) staining. Massive exudation of fibrin (arrow pointing at blue color) in the inflamed joints (AIA) was reduced by UCB treatment (AIA-BIL). CO—control group, CO-BIL—control group administered with UCB 200 mg/kg of body weight daily i.p. from day 14, AIA—group with adjuvant induced arthritis, AIA-BIL—group with adjuvant induced arthritis administered with UCB 200 mg/kg of body weight daily i.p. from day 14. PTAH, 200×.

3. Discussion

The aim of the study was to observe changes in the course of an experimentally-induced arthritis disease in the settings of unconjugated bilirubin administration. The model of AIA was chosen as a disease similar to human RA that allows to monitor progression of the disease and effects of the experimental treatment [25]. The murine models have many limitations in regard to human RA, such as the genetically-based onset of RA and the agent of disease model induction is known. However, our research team is focusing on the symptoms mitigation as well as other markers of inflammation that might be relevant for further RA pharmacotherapy, but strictly on the preclinical research level. Bilirubin presence in plasma is natural in humans, but in rats its levels are naturally low, almost undetectable in the physiological state [23], thus, the model allows to study the specific effect of UCB administration. UCB's impact on function of the immune system was described in several different experimental settings [23,26]. To our knowledge, this is the first study that documents complex changes of blood elements variables in the time course during high dose of UCB administration for the period of 14 days (Figure 2a–c, Table 1).

Adjuvant induced arthritis brought about inflammatory changes in the hind paw knee joints clinically manifested by swelling, as previously demonstrated [25]. Inflammation in hind paw joints is caused by granulocyte infiltration leading to fibrin depositions as seen in our experiments (Figures 4–7) [27,28]. Decrease of the hind paws volume, the reduction of leukocytes, granulocyte infiltration and fibrin deposition in the joints histologic evaluation proved significant effects of UCB administration on the course of the disease (Figures 1a, 2a and 4–7). Therapeutic use of UCB has not been used before in an experimental model of RA. Bonneli (2012) used UCB precursor—biliverdin as a heme oxygenase-1 end product, which successfully improved the course of murine collagen induced arthritis (CIA). Histological examination of affected joints in mice after 60 days long treatment showed lowered inflammation and bone destruction in the CIA mouse model [29]. Epidemiological study National Health and Nutrition Examination Survey by Fischman (2010) concluded that higher total bilirubin levels were linked to a reduced risk of RA and as a protective factor in humans [16]. These data, supported also by the results of our experimental findings, indicate the protective role of bilirubin administration, and also its pathological consequences.

The plausible anti-inflammatory effects of unconjugated bilirubin in our experiment were supported also by decreased levels of inflammation proteins such as CRP and ceruloplasmin (Figure 1c,d). The relationship between bilirubin and CRP and suppressing effect of bilirubin on CRP levels have already been observed in humans [30]. It has also been documented as in vitro experiment by Khan and Poduval (2011) [26], and as in vivo experiment in a mouse model of endotoxemia [31], but correlation between hyperbilirubinemia and low levels of ceruloplasmin was only part of the clinical assessment in full-term newborn infants [32].

Immunomodulative properties of UCB were part of various animal studies [13]. In general, administration of UCB showed major impact on the immune system. Experiments performed in vitro documented toxic effect of 25 μM/L concentration of UCB on unfractionated splenocytes and splenic T cells, B cells, macrophages and LPS-stimulated $CD19^+$ B cells [26]. In vivo administration of UCB to healthy animals induced atrophy of the spleen, depletion of bone marrow cells, peripheral leukopenia and decreased lymphocyte count [26]. High levels of UCB improved the outcome of experimental autoimmune encephalomyelitis. The immunomodulatory effect of UCB was attributed to possible induction of apoptosis in reactive T cells [23]. The above-mentioned findings resulted from different study designs. In our experimental setting, the spleen, the thymus and the liver were assessed by means of the change of their weight. Except for the liver, we observed atrophy of the thymus and the spleen in the AIA group caused by UCB administration (Figure 3). In addition to the evaluation of the impact of UCB on the arthritis clinical presentation changes, our data also recorded changes in the blood screen in the period of 14 days. In the experiment we showed that increased levels of UCB caused a universal decrease in the number of lymphocytes, atrophy of the spleen, thymus and the liver in both, the AIA and the CO animals (Figures 2b and 3). All these findings point at the immunomodulatory effect of high levels of UCB and with positive effect on the course of AIA.

UCB administration to AIA-BIL group deepened atrophy of the thymus in comparison with untreated AIA group (Figure 3b). Similar observation of the thymic regression as a response to the outflow of mature T lymphocytes in the context of inflammatory cells redistribution in the AIA experimental model has already been reported [25]. Analyzing the effect of UCB on the spleen, UCB administration to AIA-BIL restore the hypertrophy to the size of untreated CO group (Figure 3a). Due to high leukocytosis and the ongoing inflammation in the AIA animals, hypertrophy of the spleen may be the result. Administration of UCB in the AIA group lead to a greater thymus atrophy and a significant decrease of weight of the spleen. These results show similar course of the atrophy in the thymus and the spleen in the CO-BIL group induced by administration of UCB, which confirms the findings previously reported by others [26].

General impact of UCB on hematopoiesis is demonstrated by changes of platelets and erythrocytes parameters (Figure 2c, Table 1). The lifespan of erythrocytes in rats is approximately 60 days [33], which might explain the delayed decrease compared to the rapid changes in leukocytes. The drop of hemoglobin caused by hyperbilirubinemia has already been described by others [26]. Brito (2006), according to the observation of hyperbilirubinemic and normobilirubinemic neonates, presumed toxicity of UCB to erythrocyte's membrane [34]. In contrast to this assumption, McDonagh (2007) claimed that Gunn rats and patients with Crigler-Najjar syndrome have persistent unconjugated hyperbilirubinemia and do not suffer from extensive hemolysis [35]. Of particular interest in our experiment is the observed rise in thrombocytes after UCB administration, both in healthy and the AIA animals (Figure 2c). This is a unique observation that has not been described before. The underlying mechanism for rising numbers of platelets might be linked with the atrophy of the spleen resulting in decreased platelet removal from circulation and older platelets being allowed to circulate for a longer period of time. These suggestions will require to be confirmed by further research.

Bilirubin is known to possess powerful antioxidant properties [36,37]. Oxidative stress is an important factor of inflammation and plays an important role in the pathogenesis of autoimmune diseases such as RA and its experimental model—adjuvant induced arthritis [38]. This hypothesis was confirmed also by our results, where administration of UCB significantly decreased oxidative DNA damage in sick animals (Figure 2d). On the other hand, the results in the control group were remarkably completely the opposite. Administration of UCB caused in healthy animals a massive oxidative damage to DNA (Figure 2d). Similar results are obtained from experiments on Gunn rats that suffer naturally from unconjugated hyperbilirubinemia. The DNA fragility in leukocytes induced by radiation exposure of Gunn and Wistar rats [39] was significantly reduced when compared to the Wistar rats. On the contrary, DNA fragility was significantly higher in Gunn rats that were not irradiated. This could be accounted either to higher DNA damage itself or might indicate differences in efficiency of DNA repair [39,40].

Groups, where UCB was administered had not only smaller spleen, liver and thymus, but they had also lower body weight and smaller hind paw volumes (Figure 1a,b). This general unwanted growth retardation was present even though rats had the same access to food and better mobility due to suppressed clinical signs of AIA. As was previously observed in mice, bilirubin administration for 14 days caused reduction of the liver size and body fat, decrease of total plasma cholesterol, insulin and leptin and raise of adiponectin [41]. In human studies, hyperbilirubinemia correlated in subjects with lower BMI and was considered as a possible factor for weight loss in obese people [39,42]. In healthy mice, UCB administration, besides significant reduction of the spleen weight, resulted in decreased viability of bone marrow cells resulting in significant decrease of leukocytes, lymphocytes and hemoglobin levels [26]. These changes seem to be specific due to UCB administration.

Despite the ongoing therapy of patient with RA some clinical studies have shown increased markers of OS in these patients [43–45]. The systemic autoimmune disease RA is characterized by increased cardiovascular mortality and morbidity and is an independent cardiovascular risk factor [46]. Oxidative stress has been linked to functional and structural cardiovascular alterations in animal models of chronic arthritis and in patients with RA, suggesting a complex interplay between oxidative stress, autoimmune response and inflammation in the development of atherosclerotic cardiovascular disease in RA [47]. Reactive oxygen species and reactive nitrogen species are highly reactive chemical compounds that have the potential to damage lipids, proteins and DNA favouring expression of neoantigens and initiation of autoimmunity in predisposed individuals. Accordingly, exaggerated reactive oxygen species formation and increased levels of markers of protein and lipid oxidation have been reported in several systemic autoimmune diseases, including RA [48,49]. However, there is no standard therapeutic approach to address the OS in RA patients.

To objectify the biological impact of unconjugated bilirubin administration it is important to interpret the results depending on the clinical context. In healthy animals the effect of UCB may be perceived as unwanted side effect, but in animals with AIA, the effects employ as therapeutic.

4. Material and Methods

4.1. Animals and AIA Experimental Model

31 adult male Lewis rats weighing 160–180 g were obtained from Department of Toxicology and Laboratory Animal Breeding, Centre of Experimental Medicine, SAS, Dobrá Voda, Slovak Republic (SK CH 24016). The rats had free access to the standard pellet diet and tap water as well as dark/light regime 12 h/12 h. The experimental protocol was approved by the Ethics Committee of the Institute of Experimental Pharmacology and Toxicology, Center of Experimental Medicine SAS in Bratislava, Slovakia, (3144/16-221/3, 1.1.2011) and by the Slovak State Veterinary and Food Administration of the Slovak Republic, Bratislava in accordance with the European Convention for the Protection of Vertebrate Animals Used for Experimental and Other Scientific Purposes and with Slovak legislation.

4.2. The Design of AIA Experiment

The animals were randomized into four groups: healthy not treated animals as Control group (CO, $n = 7$), healthy animals with UCB administration (CO-BIL, $n = 8$), untreated adjuvant-induced arthritis group (AIA, $n = 8$) and adjuvant-induced arthritis group administrated with UCB (AIA-BIL, $n = 8$). AIA was induced by single intradermal shot with suspension of 0.1 mL of 12 mg/mL heat-inactivated *Mycobacterium butyricum* powder suspended in incomplete IFA (Difco Laboratories, Detroit, MI, USA) applied to the rat tail root region according to our previous experimental protocol [50–52]. Therapeutic treatment regime was as follows: UCB was administered 200 mg/kg of body weight daily i.p. from day 14, to the day 28 of the study. UCB (porcine origin, AppliChem, GmbH, Darmstadt, Germany) was stored at −20 °C until reconstitution in 0.2 M sodium hydroxide to obtain water soluble sodium salt of UCB. This solution was neutralized by 1.0 M hydrochloric acid and diluted by saline for desired concentration of 50 mg/mL. Reconstituted solution was stored at room temperature in a dark place. Handling and manipulation with UCB were under low light condition to reduce its depletion. Body weight of rats was measured regularly to calculate the precise application of doses. The body weight of the animals was measured daily. The changes in body weight are shown as weight gain (g). Weight measured on the day (*n*—day 14, 21 and 28) minus weight measured on day 1. HPV was calculated as the percentage increase of the hind paw of each animal, compared to the HPV measured at the onset of the experiment by means of an electronic water plethysmometer (UGO BASILE, Comerio-Varese, Italy). The HPV was measured at the same days as change in the weight.

4.3. Blood Tests and Oxidative Damage Evaluation

Changes in the blood count were evaluated on 14th, 21st and 28th day of the experiment using ABX Pentra 60 analyzer (Horiba Medical, Tokyo, Japan). On 28th day, when the experiment was terminated, blood and the plasma were collected and evaluated: levels of conjugated and unconjugated bilirubin using automatic analyzer Advia 2400 (Siemens AG, Munich, Germany), oxidative DNA damage was determined by the Collin's comet method, CRP by commercial ELISA kit (Immunology consultant laboratories, Inc., Portland, OR, USA) and ceruloplasmin by the method according to Pribyl [24,53,54]. All plasma samples were stored at −80 °C until biochemical analysis.

Single cell electrophoresis (comet assay) [52] was used to evaluate oxidative damage to DNA in lymphocytes isolated from the whole blood collected on 28th day. The levels of the marker for DNA oxidative damage, 8-oxoguanines, were calculated from formamidopyrimidine DNA glycosylase (Fpg) sites, represented by total damage (TD) values reduced about buffer score, where, in TD, *i* is a class of damage and N is the number of cells in each class:

$$\mathrm{TD} = \sum_{i=0}^{4} \mathrm{i.N_i}$$

using the calibration curve y = 134.97x + 7.0612, where y refers to the number of Fpg sites and x refers to breaks of DNA [55]. The concentration of 8-oxoG per 10^6 guanines was calculated as previously described [55]. The experiments were done in duplicate.

4.4. Histology and Histochemistry

At the end of the experiment, thymus, spleen, liver and hind paw knee joints were collected, weighted and processed for histological evaluation. The hind paw knee joint samples were after 24-h fixation in 4% formaldehyde decalcified in EDTA, routinely processed by embedding in paraffin, cut in 5 µm thick slices, stained with hematoxylin and eosin and evaluated by light microscopy (Leica DM2000, Wetzlar, Germany). Staining with naphtol-AS-D-chloroacetate for the detection of CHAE activity was performed to evaluate tissue infiltration by granulocytes. Conventional dyeing with PTAH was performed to evaluate the presence of fibrin in joints.

4.5. Morphometry and Statistics

Granulocyte infiltration and fibrin deposition in the knee joint samples were evaluated by morphometry using ImageJ 1.38 (National Institute of Health, San Diego, CA, USA) in 10 randomly selected microscopic fields at 40× magnification. Using digital color extraction, the proportion of selected positivity to the total area of tissue was assessed. The measured values were statistically evaluated by GraphPad Prism (GraphPad Prism, San Diego, CA, USA).

The data were expressed as arithmetic mean ± SEM, with 7–8 animals in each experimental group. AIA and CO-BIL groups were compared with CO (*) and AIA-BIL group was compared with AIA (+). For significance calculations, unpaired Student's t-test (two sample, unequal variance) was used with the following significance designations: extremely significant ($p < 0.001$), highly significant ($p < 0.01$), significant ($p < 0.05$); not significant ($p > 0.05$).

5. Conclusions

Dysregulation of the innate and adaptive immune responses occur at different stages of RA development. The inflammatory process lead to functional and structural changes of joints and internal organs. According to our findings, induced systemic unconjugated hyperbilirubinemia might have beneficial effects on the course of AIA. By administration of UCB we observed improved clinical signs, decrease of inflammation and protective role in DNA oxidative damage in studied animals. To our knowledge, this is the first study that documents complex changes of blood elements variables in the time course during high dose of UCB administration in healthy animals as well in AIA for the period of 14 days.

Our research is focused to mitigate the OS in experimental arthritis, by means of substances with known and/or unknown antioxidative properties. From our perspective we think that lowering of the OS could be a part of a more complex therapeutic approach of patients with RA, together with newer agents, which are based on blocking/modifying specific steps in the inflammatory cascade. Supplementation with substances able to reduce the OS could be a part of observational clinical studies with standard anti-rheumatic treatment.

These findings might be the basis for further research on immunomodulative properties of UCB.

Author Contributions: T.S. and P.B. are equally considered as first authors. T.S., P.B., F.D., S.P. Performed the experiment; evaluation of results and substantially participated on manuscript preparation; approved the final version of the manuscript. T.S., P.B., F.D. Contributed to the design of the article; responsible for data curation; preparation of the first draft of the manuscript; revised manuscript critically; substantially manuscript preparation; contributed to the final version of the manuscript; approved the final version of the manuscript. P.J. Provided the active substance; statistical analysis of data; revised the manuscript. M.D. Academician: Revised the manuscript. K.B. Responsible for supervision of the experiment, project administration, funding acquisition and revision of the manuscript; approved the final version of the manuscript. K.M.-K. Performed morphometric analysis and prepared figures; preparation of the first draft of the manuscript; responsible for data curation; substantially manuscript preparation. S.P., F.D. Prepared methodology and performed laboratory work; revised manuscript critically; approved the final version of the manuscript. All authors have read and agreed to the published version of the manuscript.

Funding: This research was supported by Slovak grant agency VEGA 2/0045/11, VEGA 2/0115/19 and VEGA 2/0136/20.

Institutional Review Board Statement: The study was conducted according to the guidelines of the Declaration of Helsinki and approved by the Institutional Ethics Committee the Institute of Experimental Pharmacology and Toxicology, Center of Experimental Medicine SAS in Bratislava, Slovakia (SK UCH 04018) and State Veterinary and Food Administration of the Slovak Republic, Bratislava (3144/16-221/3).

Informed Consent Statement: Not applicable.

Data Availability Statement: Data are available using this link: https://drive.google.com/file/d/1Y8DYN_CRyJ9Nka41kSFKgo0ExvTp2P88/view?usp=sharing (accessed on 12 August 2021).

Acknowledgments: We thanks to Viera Kuncirova and Danica Mihalova for technical assistance.

Conflicts of Interest: We declare no conflict of interest.

References

1. Firestein, G.S. Immunologic mechanisms in the pathogenesis of rheumatoid arthritis. *J. Clin. Rheumatol.* **2005**, *11*, S39–S44. [CrossRef]
2. Smolen, J.S.; Landewé, R.B.M.; Bijlsma, J.W.J.; Burmester, G.R.; Dougados, M.; Kerschbaumer, A.; McInnes, I.B.; Sepriano, A.; van Vollenhoven, R.F.; de Wit, M.; et al. EULAR recommendations for the management of rheumatoid arthritis with synthetic and biological disease-modifying antirheumatic drugs: 2019 update. *Ann. Rheum. Dis.* **2020**, *79*, S685–S699. [CrossRef] [PubMed]
3. McInnes, I.B.; Schett, G. The Pathogenesis of Rheumatoid Arthritis. *N. Engl. J. Med.* **2011**, *365*, 2205–2219. [CrossRef]
4. Firestein, G.S. Evolving concepts of rheumatoid arthritis. *Nature* **2003**, *423*, 356–361. [CrossRef] [PubMed]
5. Chen, L.; Deng, H.; Cui, H.; Fang, J.; Zuo, Z.; Deng, J.; Li, Y.; Wang, X.; Zhao, L. Inflammatory responses and inflammation-associated diseases in organs. *Oncotarget* **2018**, *9*, 7204–7218. [CrossRef]
6. Guo, Q.; Wang, Y.; Xu, D.; Nossent, J.; Pavlos, N.J.; Xu, J. Rheumatoid arthritis: Pathological mechanisms and modern pharmacologic therapies. *Bone Res.* **2018**, *6*, 1–14. [CrossRef] [PubMed]
7. Smolen, J.S.; Van Der Heijde, D.; Machold, K.; Aletaha, D.; Landewé, R. Proposal for a new nomenclature of disease-modifying antirheumatic drugs. *Ann. Rheum. Dis.* **2013**, *73*, 3–5. [CrossRef]
8. Cutolo, M.; Sulli, A.; Pizzorni, C.; Seriolo, B.; Straub, R.H. Anti-inflammatory mechanisms of methotrexate in rheumatoid arthritis. *Ann. Rheum. Dis.* **2001**, *60*, 729–735. [CrossRef] [PubMed]
9. Hazlewood, G.S.; Barnabe, C.; Tomlinson, G.; Marshall, D.; Devoe, D.; Bombardier, C. Methotrexate monotherapy and methotrexate combination therapy with traditional and biologic disease modifying antirheumatic drugs for rheumatoid arthritis: Abridged cochrane Systematic review and network meta-analysis. *BMJ* **2016**, *353*, i1777. [CrossRef]
10. Taams, L.S. Interleukin-17 in rheumatoid arthritis: Trials and tribulations. *J. Exp. Med.* **2020**, *217*, 48. [CrossRef] [PubMed]
11. Mahajan, T.D.; Mikuls, T.R. Recent advances in the treatment of rheumatoid arthritis. *Curr. Opin. Rheumatol.* **2018**, *30*, 231–237. [CrossRef]
12. Salehi, B.; Martorell, M.; Arbiser, J.; Sureda, A.; Martins, N.; Maurya, P.; Sharifi-Rad, M.; Kumar, P.; Sharifi-Rad, J. Antioxidants: Positive or negative actors? *Biomolecules* **2018**, *8*, 124. [CrossRef] [PubMed]
13. Jangi, S.; Otterbein, L.; Robson, S. The molecular basis for the immunomodulatory activities of unconjugated bilirubin. *Int. J. Biochem. Cell Biol.* **2013**, *45*, 2843–2851. [CrossRef]
14. Sullivan, J.I.; Rockey, D.C. Diagnosis and evaluation of hyperbilirubinemia. *Curr. Opin. Gastroenterol.* **2017**, *33*, 164–170. [CrossRef]
15. Bulmer, A.C.; Verkade, H.J.; Wagner, K.-H. Bilirubin and beyond: A review of lipid status in Gilbert's syndrome and its relevance to cardiovascular disease protection. *Prog. Lipid Res.* **2013**, *52*, 193–205. [CrossRef]
16. Fischman, D.; Valluri, A.; Gorrepati, V.S.; Murphy, M.E.; Cheriyath, I.P.P. Bilirubin as a Protective Factor for Rheumatoid Arthritis: An NHANES Study of 2003–2006 Data. *J. Clin. Med. Res.* **2010**, *2*, 256–260. [CrossRef] [PubMed]
17. Sedlak, T.W.; Snyder, S.H. Bilirubin benefits: Cellular protection by a biliverdin reductase antioxidant cycle. *Pediatrics* **2004**, *113*, 1776–1782. [CrossRef]
18. Juping, D.; Yuan, Y.; Shiyong, C.; Jun, L.; Xiuxiu, Z.; Haijian, Y.; Jianfeng, S.; Bo, S. Serum bilirubin and the risk of rheumatoid arthritis. *J. Clin. Lab. Anal.* **2017**, *31*, e22118. [CrossRef] [PubMed]
19. Fevery, J. Bilirubin in clinical practice: A review. *Liver Int.* **2008**, *28*, 592–605. [CrossRef] [PubMed]
20. Tapan, S.; Karadurmus, N.; Dogru, T.; Ercin, C.N.; Tasci, I.; Bilgi, C.; Kurt, I.; Erbil, M.K. Decreased small dense LDL levels in Gilbert's syndrome. *Clin. Biochem.* **2011**, *44*, 300–303. [CrossRef] [PubMed]

21. Vítek, L.; Jirsa, M., Jr.; Brodanová, M.; Kaláb, M.; Mareček, Z.; Danzig, V.; Novotný, L.; Kotal, P. Gilbert syndrome and ischemic heart disease: A protective effect of elevated bilirubin levels. *Atherosclerosis* **2002**, *160*, 449–456. [CrossRef]
22. Bauerova, K.; Drafi, F.; Kuncirova, V.; Ponist, S.; Mihalova, D.; Babal, P.; Sykora, T. Hyperbilirubinemia decreases physiological markers in adjuvant-induced arthritis. *Physiol. Res.* **2015**, *64*, 459–466. [CrossRef] [PubMed]
23. Liu, Y.; Li, P.; Lu, J.; Xiong, W.; Oger, J.; Tetzlaff, W.; Cynader, M. Bilirubin possesses powerful immunomodulatory activity and suppresses experimental autoimmune encephalomyelitis. *J. Immunol.* **2008**, *181*, 1887–1897. [CrossRef] [PubMed]
24. Bauerova, K.; Ponist, S.; Kuncirova, V.; Mihalova, D.; Paulovicova, E.; Volpi, N. Chondroitin sulfate effect on induced arthritis in rats. *Osteoarthr. Cartil.* **2011**, *19*, 1373–1379. [CrossRef]
25. Feketeová, L.; Jančová, P.; Moravcová, P.; Janegová, A.; Bauerová, K.; Poništ, S.; Mihalová, D.; Janega, P.; Babál, P. Effect of methotrexate on inflammatory cells redistribution in experimental adjuvant arthritis. *Rheumatol. Int.* **2011**, *32*, 3517–3523. [CrossRef] [PubMed]
26. Khan, N.M.; Poduval, T.B. Immunomodulatory and immunotoxic effects of bilirubin: Molecular mechanisms. *J. Leukoc. Biol.* **2011**, *90*, 997–1015. [CrossRef]
27. Stanescu, R.; Lider, O.; van Eden, W.; Holoshitz, J.; Cohen, I.R. Histopathology of arthritis induced in rats by active immunization to mycobacterial antigens or by systemic transfer of T lymphocyte lines. A light and electron microscopic study of the articular surface using cationized ferritin. *Arthritis Rheum.* **1987**, *30*, 779–792. [CrossRef] [PubMed]
28. Yamashita, A.; Yonemitsu, Y.; Okano, S.; Nakagawa, K.; Nakashima, Y.; Irisa, T.; Iwamoto, Y.; Nagai, Y.; Hasegawa, M.; Sueishi, K. Arthritis in Rats Adjuvant-induced severity of joint disease in fibroblast growth factor-2 determines. *J. Immunol.* **2021**, *168*, 450–457. [CrossRef]
29. Bonelli, M.; Savitskaya, A.; Steiner, C.W.; Rath, E.; Bilban, M.; Wagner, O.; Bach, F.H.; Smolen, J.S.; Scheinecker, C. Heme oxygenase-1 end-products carbon monoxide and biliverdin ameliorate murine collagen induced arthritis. *Clin. Exp. Rheumatol.* **2012**, *30*, 73–78.
30. Hwang, H.-J.; Lee, S.-W.; Kim, S.-H. Relationship between bilirubin and C-reactive protein. *Clin. Chem. Lab. Med.* **2011**, *49*, 1823–1828. [CrossRef]
31. Kadl, A.; Pontiller, J.; Exner, M.; Leitinger, N. Single bolus injection of bilirubin improves the clinical outcome in a mouse model of endotoxemia. *Shock* **2007**, *28*, 582–588. [CrossRef]
32. Corchia, C.; Balata, A.; Soletta, G.; Mastroni, P.; Meloni, G.F. Increased bilirubin production, ceruloplasmin concentrations and hyperbilirubinaemia in full-term newborn infants. *Early Hum. Dev.* **1994**, *38*, 91–96. [CrossRef]
33. Derelanko, M.J. Determination of erythrocyte life span in F-344, wistar, and sprague-dawley rats using a modification of the [H]diisopropylfluorophosphate ([H]DFP) method. *Toxicol. Sci.* **1987**, *9*, 271–276. [CrossRef]
34. Brito, M.A.; Silva, R.F.M.; Brites, D. Bilirubin toxicity to human erythrocytes: A review. *Clin. Chim. Acta* **2006**, *374*, 46–56. [CrossRef] [PubMed]
35. McDonagh, A.F. Bilirubin toxicity to human erythrocytes: A more sanguine view. *Pediatrics* **2007**, *120*, 175–178. [CrossRef]
36. Jansen, T.; Daiber, A. Direct antioxidant properties of bilirubin and biliverdin. Is there a role for biliverdin reductase? *Front. Pharmacol.* **2012**, *3*, 30. [CrossRef] [PubMed]
37. McDonagh, A.F. The biliverdin–bilirubin antioxidant cycle of cellular protection: Missing a wheel? *Free Radic. Biol. Med.* **2010**, *49*, 814–820. [CrossRef] [PubMed]
38. Bauerova, K.; Acquaviva, A.; Ponist, S.; Gardi, C.; Vecchio, D.; Drafi, F.; Arezzini, B.; Bezakova, L.; Kuncirova, V.; Mihalova, D.; et al. Markers of inflammation and oxidative stress studied in adjuvant-induced arthritis in the rat on systemic and local level affected by pinosylvin and methotrexate and their combination. *Autoimmunity* **2015**, *48*, 46–56. [CrossRef] [PubMed]
39. Wallner, M.; Antl, N.; Rittmannsberger, B.; Schreidl, S.; Najafi, K.; Müllner, E.; Moelzer, C.; Ferk, F.; Knasmüller, S.; Marculescu, R.; et al. Anti-genotoxic potential of bilirubin in vivo: Damage to DNA in hyperbilirubinemic human and animal models. *Cancer Prev. Res.* **2013**, *6*, 1056–1063. [CrossRef] [PubMed]
40. Collins, A.R.; Dobson, V.L.; Dusinská, M.; Kennedy, G.; Stětina, R. The comet assay: What can it really tell us. *Mutat. Res.* **1997**, *375*, 183–193. [CrossRef]
41. Liu, J.; Dong, H.; Zhang, Y.; Cao, M.; Song, L.; Pan, Q.; Bulmer, A.C.; Adams, D.B.; Dong, X.; Wang, H. Bilirubin increases insulin sensitivity by regulating cholesterol metabolism, adipokines and PPARγ levels. *Sci. Rep.* **2015**, *5*, 9886. [CrossRef] [PubMed]
42. Andersson, C.; Weeke, P.; Fosbøl, E.; Brendorp, B.; Køber, L.; Coutinho, W.; Sharma, A.M.; Van Gaal, L.; Finer, N.; James, W.P.T.; et al. Acute effect of weight loss on levels of total bilirubin in obese, cardiovascular high-risk patients: An analysis from the lead-in period of the Sibutramine Cardiovascular Outcome trial. *Metabolism* **2009**, *58*, 1109–1115. [CrossRef]
43. García-González, A.; Gaxiola-Robles, R.; Zenteno-Savín, T. Oxidative Stress in Patients with Rheumatoid Arthritis. *Rev. Investig. Clin.* **2015**, *67*, 46–53.
44. Altindag, O. Increased DNA damage and oxidative stress in patients with rheumatoid arthritis. *Clin. Biochem.* **2007**, *40*, 167–171. [CrossRef]
45. Veselinovic, M.; Barudzic, N.; Vuletic, M.; Zivkovic, V.; Tomic-Lucic, A.; Djuric, D.; Jakovljevic, V. Oxidative stress in rheumatoid arthritis patients: Relationship to diseases activity. *Mol. Cell. Biochem.* **2014**, *391*, 225–232. [CrossRef]
46. Bordy, R.; Totoson, P.; Prati, C.; Marie, C.; Wendling, D.; Demougeot, C. Microvascular endothelial dysfunction in rheumatoid arthritis. *Nat. Rev. Rheumatol.* **2018**, *14*, 404–420. [CrossRef] [PubMed]

47. England, B.R.; Thiele, G.M.; Anderson, D.R.; Mikuls, T.R. Increased cardiovascular risk in rheumatoid arthritis: Mechanisms and implications. *BMJ* **2018**, *23*, 361. [CrossRef] [PubMed]
48. Griffiths, H.R. ROS as signalling molecules in T cells—Evidence for abnormal redox signalling in the autoimmune disease, rheumatoid arthritis. *Redox. Rep.* **2005**, *10*, 273–280. [CrossRef] [PubMed]
49. Souliotis, V.L.; Vlachogiannis, N.I.; Pappa, M.; Argyriou, A.; Ntouros, P.A.; Sfikakis, P.P. DNA Damage Response and Oxidative Stress in Systemic Autoimmunity. *Int. J. Mol. Sci.* **2020**, *21*, 55. [CrossRef]
50. Bauerová, K.; Poništ, S.; Mihalová, D.; Dráfi, F.; Kuncírová, V. Utilization of adjuvant arthritis model for evaluation of new approaches in rheumatoid arthritis therapy focused on regulation of immune processes and oxidative stress. *Interdiscip. Toxicol.* **2011**, *4*, 33–39. [CrossRef]
51. Bendele, A.; McComb, J.; Gould, T.; McAbee, T.; Sennello, G.; Chlipala, E.; Guy, M. Animal models of arthritis: Relevance to human disease. *Toxicol. Pathol.* **1999**, *27*, 134–142. [CrossRef]
52. Chaudhary, A.; Vinay, P. Rheumatoid Arthritis: Etiology, treatment and animal models. *J. Drug Deliv. Ther.* **2020**, *10*, 290–298. [CrossRef]
53. Collins, A.R.; Dusinská, M.; Gedik, C.M.; Stětina, R. Oxidative damage to DNA: Do we have a reliable biomarker? *Environ. Health Perspect.* **1996**, *104* (Suppl. S3), 465–469. [CrossRef] [PubMed]
54. Pribyl, T. Serum polyphenol oxidase activity (ceruloplasmin) in conventional laboratory animals and man. *Folia Biol.* **1978**, *24*, 136–141.
55. Gedik, C.M.; Collins, A. Establishing the background level of base oxidation in human lymphocyte DNA: Results of an interlaboratory validation study. *FASEB J.* **2005**, *19*, 82–84. [PubMed]

International Journal of *Molecular Sciences*

MDPI

Article

Immunofluorescence Analysis of NF-kB and iNOS Expression in Different Cell Populations during Early and Advanced Knee Osteoarthritis

Marko Ostojic [1,2], Ante Zevrnja [3], Katarina Vukojevic [4,5,*] and Violeta Soljic [5]

1 Department of Orthopaedics and Traumatology, University Hospital Mostar, 88 000 Mostar, Bosnia and Herzegovina; marko.ostojic@mef.sum.ba
2 Department of Anatomy, School of Medicine, University of Mostar, 88 000 Mostar, Bosnia and Herzegovina
3 Public Health Centre, First Responders Unit, 21 000 Split, Croatia; antezevrnja17@gmail.com
4 Department of Anatomy, Histology and Embryology, School of Medicine, University of Split, Soltanska 2, 21 000 Split, Croatia
5 Department of Histology and Embryology, School of Medicine, University of Mostar, Kralja Petra Kresimira IV, 88 000 Mostar, Bosnia and Herzegovina; violeta.soljic@mef.sum.ba
* Correspondence: katarina.vukojevic@mefst.hr

Citation: Ostojic, M.; Zevrnja, A.; Vukojevic, K.; Soljic, V. Immunofluorescence Analysis of NF-kB and iNOS Expression in Different Cell Populations during Early and Advanced Knee Osteoarthritis. *Int. J. Mol. Sci.* **2021**, 22, 6461. https://doi.org/10.3390/ijms22126461

Academic Editor: Chih-Hsin Tang

Received: 3 May 2021
Accepted: 14 June 2021
Published: 16 June 2021

Abstract: Synovitis of the knee synovium is proven to be a precursor of knee osteoarthritis (OA), leading to a radiologically advanced stage of the disease. This study was conducted to elucidate the expression pattern of different inflammatory factors—NF-kB, iNOS, and MMP-9 in a subpopulation of synovial cells. Thirty synovial membrane intra-operative biopsies of patients (ten controls, ten with early OA, and ten with advanced OA, according to the Kellgren–Lawrence radiological score) were immunohistochemically stained for NF-kB, iNOS, and MMP9, and for different cell markers for macrophages, fibroblasts, leukocytes, lymphocytes, blood vessel endothelial cells, and blood vessel smooth muscle cells. The total number of CD68+/NF-kB+ cells/mm^2 in the intima of early OA patients (median = 2359) was significantly higher compared to the total number of vimentin+/Nf-kB+ cells/mm^2 (median = 1321) and LCA+/NF-kB+ cells/mm^2 (median = 64) ($p < 0.001$ and $p < 0.0001$, respectively). The total number of LCA+/NF-kB+ cells/mm^2 in the subintima of advanced OA patients (median = 2123) was significantly higher compared to the total number of vimentin+/NF-kB+ cells/mm^2 (median = 14) and CD68+/NF-kB+ cells/mm^2 (median = 29) ($p < 0.0001$). The total number of CD68+/iNOS+ cells/mm^2 in the intima of both early and advanced OA patients was significantly higher compared to the total number of vimentin+/iNOS+ cells/mm^2 and LCA+/iNOS+ cells/mm^2 ($p < 0.0001$ and $p < 0.001$, respectively). The total number of CD68+/MMP-9+ cells/mm^2 in the intima of both early and advanced OA patients was significantly higher compared to the total number of vimentin+/MMP-9+ cells/mm^2 and CD5+/MMP-9+ cells/mm^2 ($p < 0.0001$). Macrophages may have a leading role in OA progression through the NF-kB production of inflammatory factors (iNOS and MMP-9) in the intima, except in advanced OA, where leukocytes could have a dominant role through NF-kB production in subintima. The blocking of macrophageal and leukocyte NF-kB expression is a possible therapeutic target as a disease modifying drug.

Keywords: osteoarthritis; synovitis; inducible nitric oxide synthase; nuclear factor kappa B; macrophage

1. Introduction

Osteoarthritis (OA) is the most common disease of the synovial joints that mostly affects older adults. It indicates chronic degenerative changes in the articular cartilage that perpetuate pathological changes in other parts of the joint in a cascade manner [1]. Degenerative changes in the cartilage are both in biochemical composition and physical properties [2,3]. The pronounced pathological changes of knee osteoarthritis include cartilage damage, osteophyte formation, subchondral bone sclerosis, synovial inflammation, the degeneration of ligaments and the menisci, and the thickening of the joint capsule [1].

Current management largely emphasizes on alleviating symptoms and improving function, but for many patients, these measures do not provide adequate symptom relief [4]. With the detection of high levels of cytokines, complement and plasma proteins in the synovial fluid, it has been acknowledged that OA is a low-grade inflammatory disease with underlying mechanical disorders accelerating the failure of the joint [5–7]. Therefore, investigations of different cell populations within the synovial membrane and the expression patterns of inflammatory markers can elucidate the relationship between diagnosis and prognostic outcome [8]. The synovial membrane contains resident cells such as macrophage-like synoviocytes (MLS), fibroblast-like synoviocytes (FLS), endothelium and smooth muscle cells of blood vessels, and non-resident, inflammatory cells, such as lymphocytes and plasma-cells. It has two layers; the intima, the thin layer where the macrophages and fibroblasts are located, and the subintima, the supportive stroma [9]. MLS in the synovial membrane of OA joints contribute to cartilage breakdown by producing inflammatory cytokines as well as matrix metalloproteinases (MMPs) that lead to synovitis development [5,8]. Synovial inflammation, together with subchondral bone marrow edema, has more significance in the early phases of the disease as a result of initial cartilage lesions [10–12]. In early OA, the synovial membrane shows synovial lining cell thickness, vascularity and the expression of inflammatory cells and mediators, and nuclear transcription factors to be greater in advanced OA, determining a higher hyperplastic and inflammation component of the synovitis in that stage [11,13]. Additionally, clinically, synovitis grade is greatly associated with the severity of pain, joint dysfunction, and cartilage loss in OA [14,15].

After the initial cartilage damage, parts of the cartilage cells and matrixes are released into the synovial fluid [5,16]. Cells in the cartilage and in the synovial membrane produce inflammatory mediators, such as cytokines, angiogenic factors, chemokines, MMPs, COX-2, and inducible nitric oxide synthase (iNOS), that play a distinctive role in the further degradation of the cartilage [8,17]. These inflammatory factors are mostly produced through NF-kB transcription factor activity by the MLS in the synovial intima [8,18]. In OA, NF-kB is highly activated at sites of synovial membrane inflammation, inducing transcription of the aforementioned proinflammatory factors [19]. iNOS is located in the cartilage and synovial membrane and is mostly synthetized through the NF-kB pathway [20]. Nitric oxide (NO) is produced by iNOS, and it mediates the expression of inflammatory factors, inhibits the synthesis of collagen and proteoglycans, and induces chondrocyte apoptosis and pain [21]. Selective inhibition of iNOS reduces the tissue levels of catabolic factors; therefore, NO has an inflammatory role in OA [22]. On the contrary, some studies show a possible protective role of NO through the NF-kB feedback mechanism [23]. Different MMPs have been detected in the synovial fluid of patients with OA and have been directly correlated with the expression of inflammatory cells in the synovial membrane [24–26].

FLS and MLS are the most active innate immunity cells in inflamed synovial tissue in early osteoarthritis [27–33]. So far, only a few studies have tried to determine the differences between NF-kB, iNOS, and MMPs expression in the different cells of knee synovial tissues in early and advanced OA, and all of them were focused on MLS and FLS [27,31,32], while studies investigating the role of cells within the blood vessels and lymph nodules of the knee synovial membrane in OA are scarce [34].

Newer treatment aspirations aim for early diagnosis and the usage of disease modifying drugs that could halt the progression of OA [35,36]. There is a theory that one subpopulation of OA patients was "synovium driven" and that specifically aiming the synovitis can be a successful treatment modality [8]. Therefore, the aim of this study was to analyze the expression pattern of NF-kB, iNOS, and MMP-9 in different cells that constitute the synovial membrane in the early and advanced stages of OA according to the radiological stage of OA. Most other studies did not have a control group, and to the best of our knowledge, neither one differentiated between the two main layers of the synovial membrane. Understanding the immunophenotype of the different cells of the knee synovial tissues can help us in the development of a potential therapeutical target that can influence disease progression.

2. Results

Biopsies of the synovial membranes were divided into early OA, advanced OA, and control groups (Figure 1) according to the radiologically based Kellgren–Lawrence scale (Table 1).

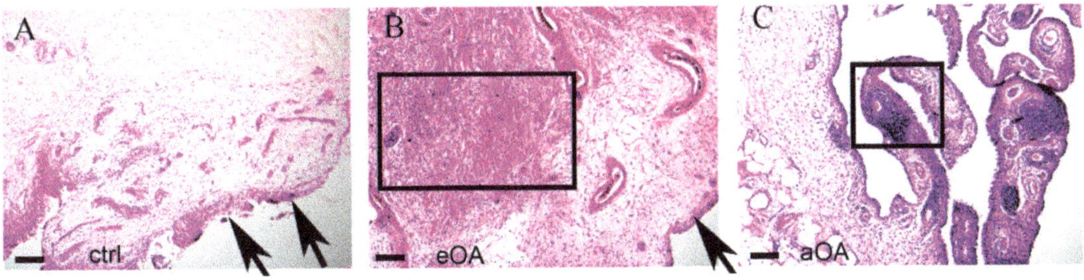

Figure 1. Hystological staining of healthy (ctrl) (**A**), early osteoarthritic synovium (eOA) (**B**), and advanced osteoarthritic synovium (aOA) (**C**). The synovial membrane of patients in the control group shows no resident cells in the subintima and the intima (arrows). In patients with early OA, the synovium contains highly visible cell infiltration (frame) in the intima (arrow). In patients with advanced OA, lymphoid nodules (frame) are shown. Haematoxylin-eosin staining. Magnification ×20, scale bar 50 µm.

Table 1. Clinical characteristics of the examined groups.

	Control	Early OA	Advanced OA	*p* Value
Age (mean ± SD, years)	20.67 ± 2.69	58 ± 6.53	70.7 ± 3.30	
BMI (mean ± SD)	-	29.05 ± 4.68	29.74 ± 4.08	0.729
ROM (mean ± SD, degrees)	-	111.50 ± 21.86	93 ± 13.98	0.037 *
Duration (mean ± SD, years)	-	3.25 ± 2.80	14.5 ± 7.62	0.000 *
WOMAC (mean ± SD)	-	43.1 ± 21.64	61.3 ± 11.18	0.030 *

chi-square test, * $p < 0.05$.

Tissue sections were analyzed with the double immunofluorescence of NF-kB, iNOS, and MMP-9, with prospective markers for different cell populations of the synovial intima and subintima (Figures 2–5). Namely, CD31 and actin were used as markers for the blood vessel wall. Vimentin was used as a marker for fibroblasts, LCA served as a marker for leukocytes while CD68 and CD5 were used as markers for macrophages and T lymphocytes, respectively.

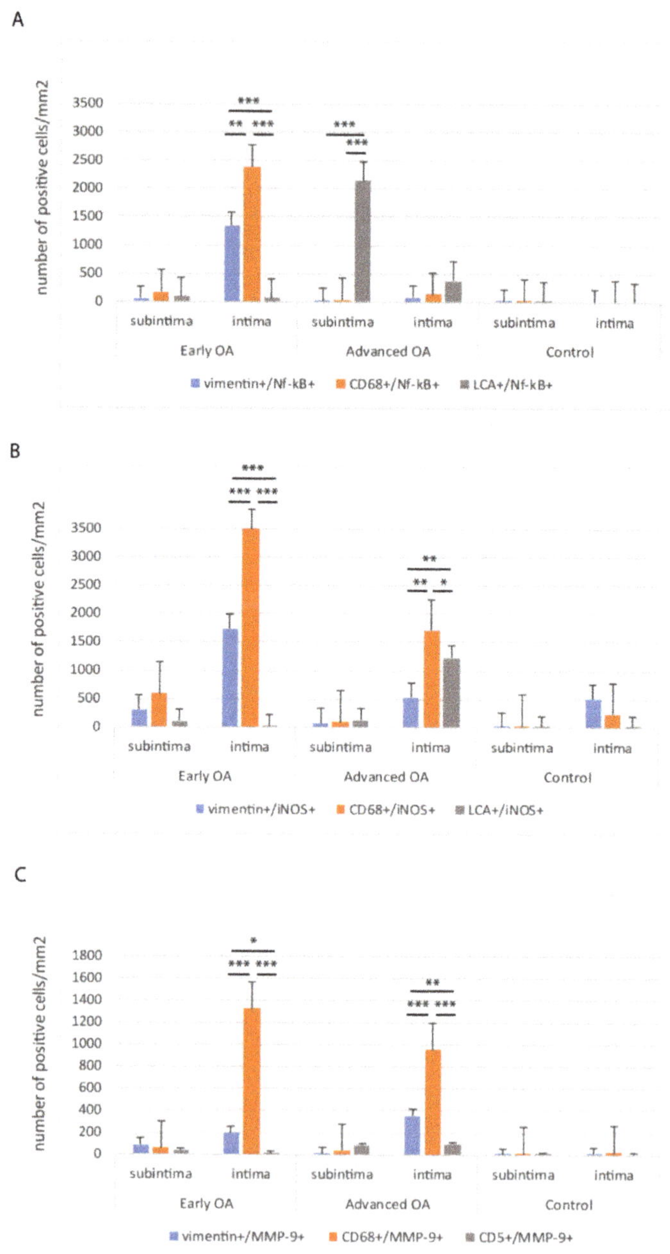

Figure 2. The distribution of vimentin+/NF-kB+, CD68+/NF-kB+, and LCA+/NF-kB+ (**A**), vimentin+/iNOS+, CD68+/iNOS+, and LCA+/iNOS+ (**B**), and vimentin+/MMP-9+, CD68+/MMP-9+, and CD5+/MMP-9 (**C**) positive cells per mm^2 in the early osteoarthritis (OA), in the advanced osteoarthritis (OA) and control groups. Data were shown as mean ± SD. Significant differences (Kruskal–Wallis) are indicated by * $p < 0.05$, ** $p < 0.001$, *** $p < 0.0001$.

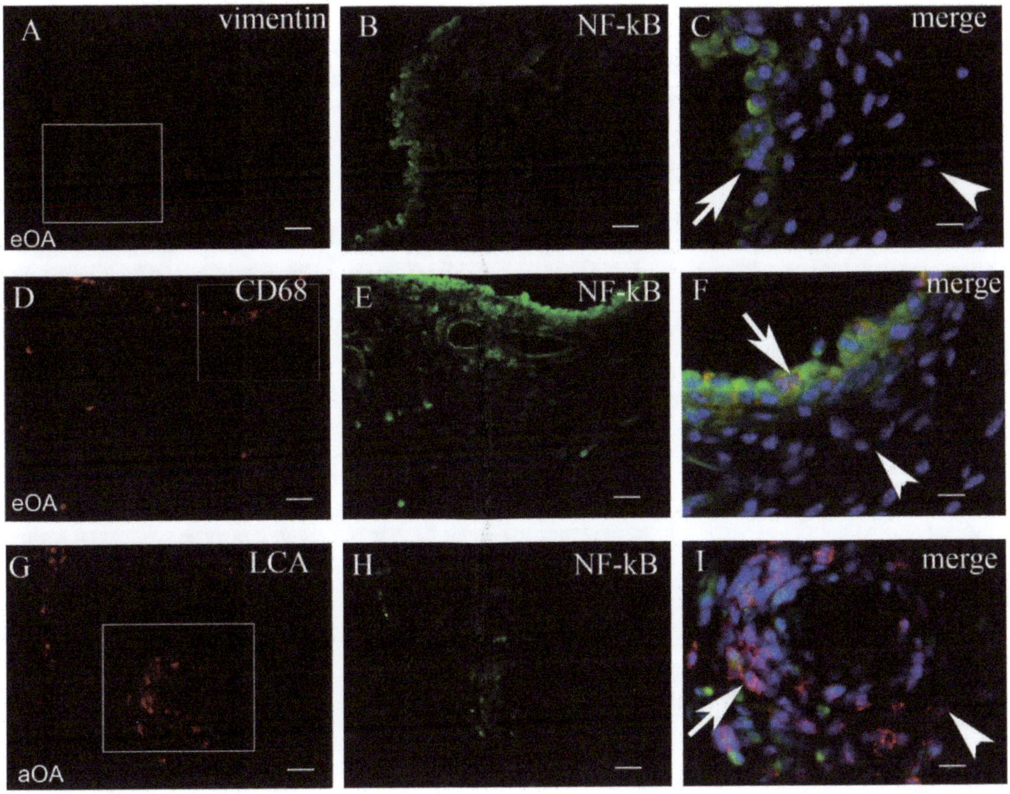

Figure 3. The synovial membrane of patients with early OA (eOA) (**A–C**). Vimentin positive (red) fibroblasts in the intima and subintima (frame), NF-kB positive cells (green) in the synovial intima and subintima (**B**). The merge of DAPI (blue) nuclear stain+vimentin+NF-kB (magnification of the frame in panel (**A**)) show numerous fibroblasts in the intima co-localized with NF-kB and vimentin (arrow), while the subintima displays vimentin positive fibroblasts (arrowhead) (**C**). The synovial membrane of patients with early OA (eOA) (**D–F**). CD68 positive (red) macrophages in the intima and subintima (frame). NF-kB positive cells (green) in the synovial intima and subintima (**E**). The merge of DAPI (blue)+CD68+NF-kB (magnification of the frame in panel (**D**)) show numerous macrophages in the intima co-localized with NF-kB and CD68 (arrow), while the subintima displayed CD68 positive macrophages(arrowhead) (**F**). The synovial membrane of patients with advanced OA (aOA) (**G–I**). LCA positive (red) lymphocytes in the intima, subintima, and lymph nodule (frame). NF-kB positive cells (green) in the synovial intima and subintima (**H**). The merge of DAPI (blue)+LCA+NF-kB (magnification of the frame in panel (**G**)) show numerous lymphocytes in the lymph nodule co-localized with NF-kB and LCA (arrow), while some lymphocytes displayed only LCA (arrowhead) (**I**). Magnification ×40 (first two columns), scale bar 25 μm and ×100 (last column), scale bar 10 μm.

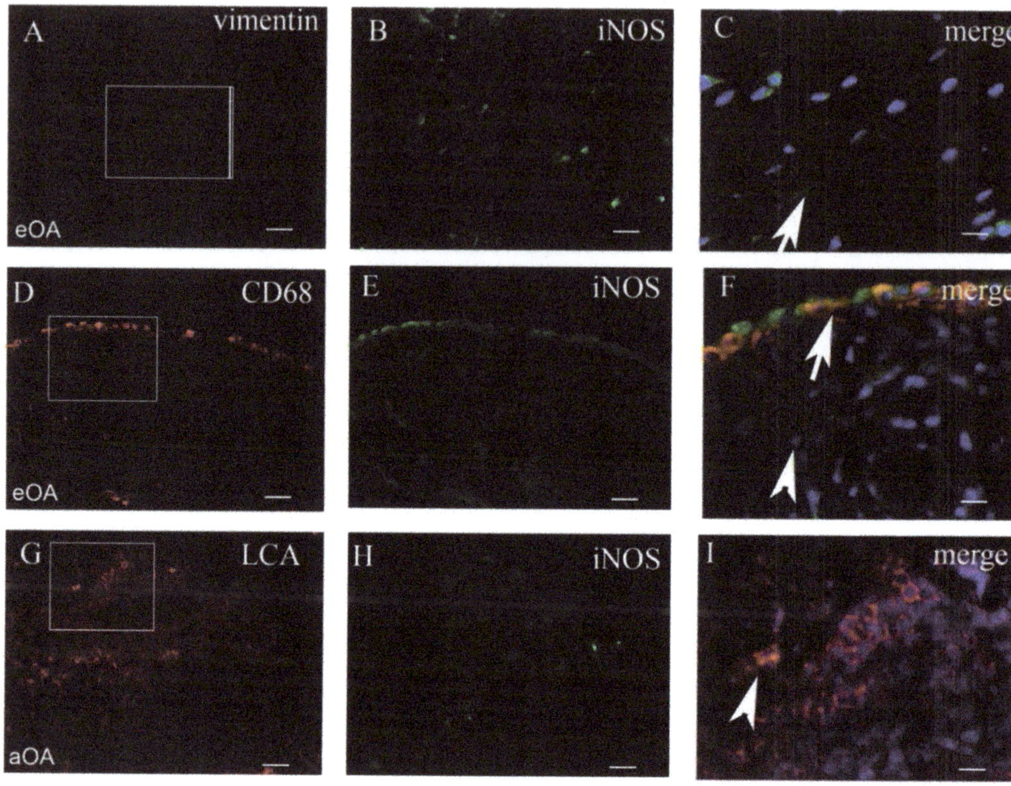

Figure 4. The synovial membrane of patients with early OA (eOA) (**A–C**). Vimentin positive (red) fibroblasts in the subintima (frame). iNOS positive cells (green) in the synovial intima and subintima (**B**). The merge of DAPI (blue) nuclear stain+vimentin+iNOS (magnification of frame in panel **A**) show occasional fibroblasts in the subintima co-localized with iNOS and vimentin (arrow) (**C**). The synovial membrane of patients with early OA (eOA) (**D–F**). CD68 positive (red) macrophages in the intima and subintima (frame). iNOS positive cells (green) in the synovial intima and subintima (**E**). The merge of DAPI (blue)+CD68+iNOS (magnification of the frame in panel (**D**)) show numerous macrophages in the intima co-localized with iNOS and CD68 (arrow), while the subintima displayed CD68 positive macrophages(arrowhead) (**F**). The synovial membrane of patients with advanced OA (aOA) (**G–I**). LCA positive (red) lymphocytes in the intima, subintima, and lymph nodule (frame). iNOS positive cells (green) in the synovial intima and subintima (**H**). The merge of DAPI (blue)+LCA+iNOS (magnification of the frame in panel (**G**)) show no co-localization of iNOS and LCA, while a numerous number of lymphocytes display only LCA (arrowhead) (**I**). Magnification ×40 (first two columns), scale bar 25 μm and ×100 (last column), scale bar 10 μm.

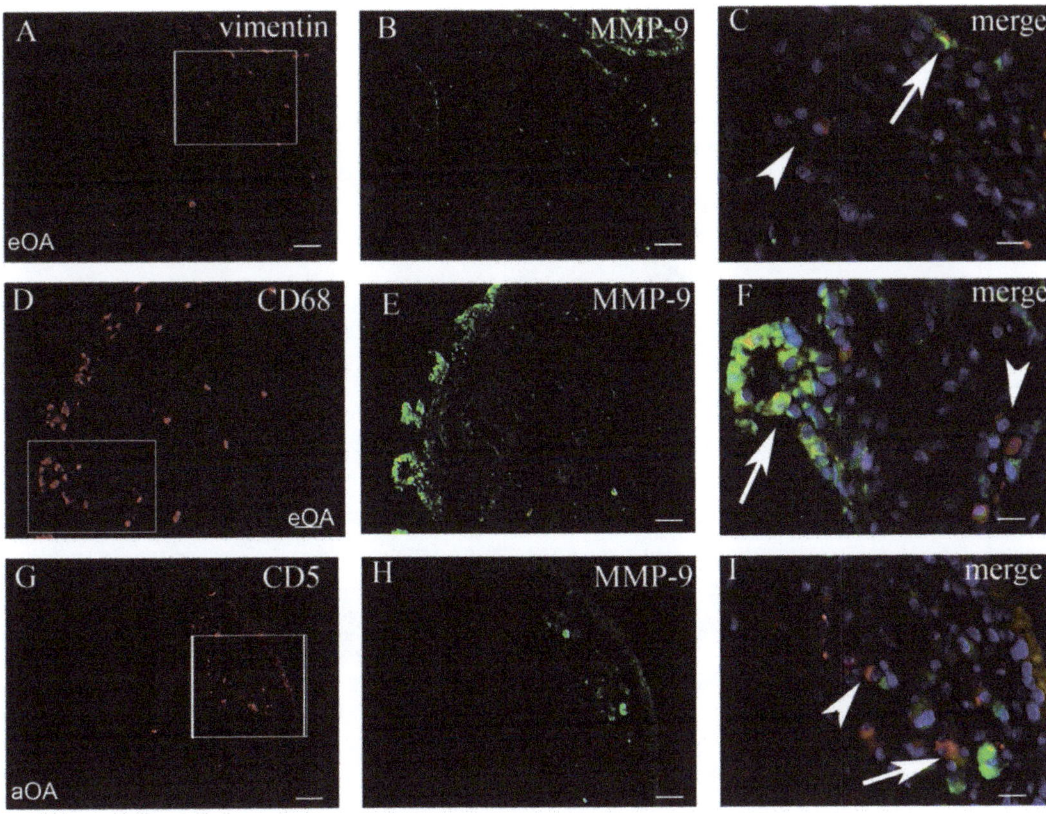

Figure 5. The synovial membrane of patients with early OA (eOA) (**A–C**). Vimentin positive (red) fibroblasts in the intima and subintima (frame). MMP-9 positive cells (green) in the synovial intima and subintima (**B**). The merge of DAPI (blue) nuclear stain+vimentin+MMP-9 (magnification of the frame in panel (**A**)) show numerous fibroblasts in the intima co-localized with MMP-9 and vimentin (arrow), while the subintima displayed vimentin positive fibroblasts (arrowhead) (**C**). The synovial membrane of patients with early OA (eOA) (**D–F**). CD68 positive (red) macrophages in the intima and subintima (frame). MMP-9 positive cells (green) in the synovial intima and subintima (**E**). The merge of DAPI. (blue)+CD68+MMP-9(magnification of the frame in panel (**D**)) show numerous macrophages in the intima co-localized with MMP-9 and CD68 (arrow), while the subintima displayed CD68 positive macrophages(arrowhead) (**F**). The synovial membrane of patients with advanced OA (aOA) (**G–I**). CD5 positive (red) lymphocytes in the subintima (frame). MMP-9 positive cells (green) in the synovial intima and subintima (**H**). The merge of DAPI (blue)+CD5+iNOS (magnification of the frame in panel (**G**)) show the co-localization of MMP-9 and CD5 (arrow), while lymphocytes occasionally display only CD5 (arrowhead) (**I**). Magnification ×40 (first two columns), scale bar 25 μm and ×100 (last column), scale bar 10 μm.

2.1. Co-Localization of iNOS+ Cells and Markers of Cell Populations in Synovial Intima and Subintima

The total number of CD68+/iNOS+ cells/mm^2 in the intima of early OA patients (median = 3492) was significantly higher compared to the total number vimentin+/iNOS+ cells/mm^2 (median = 1729) and LCA+/iNOS+ cells/mm^2 (median = 25) ($p < 0.0001$; and $p < 0.0001$, respectively). The total number of vimentin+/iNOS+ cells/mm^2 in the intima of early OA patients was significantly higher compared to the total number of LCA+/iNOS+ cells/mm^2 ($p < 0.0001$). The difference between CD68+/iNOS+ (median = 589), vimentin+/iNOS+ (median = 301), and LCA+/iNOS+ cells/mm^2 (median = 102) in the subintima of early OA patients was not statistically significant.

The total number of CD68+/iNOS+ cells/mm2 in the intima of advanced OA (median = 1701) was significantly higher compared to the total number of vimentin+/iNOS+ cells/mm^2 (median = 532) and LCA+/iNOS+ cells/mm^2 (median = 1233) ($p < 0.01$; and $p < 0.001$, respectively). The total number of LCA+/iNOS+ cells/mm^2 in the intima of advanced OA patients was significantly higher compared to the total number of vimentin+/iNOS+ cells/mm^2 ($p < 0.001$). The difference between CD68+/iNOS+ (median = 91), vimentin+/iNOS+ (median = 68), and LCA+/iNOS+ cells/mm^2 (median = 128) in the subintima of advanced OA was not statistically significant. These results were graphically summarized in Figure 2B, and positive cells were shown in Figure 4.

2.2. Co-Localization of MMP+ Cells and Markers of Cell Populations in Synovial Intima and Subintima

In order to confirm the expression of MMP-9 in different synovial membrane cells, we analyzed for the co-localization of the MMP-9 marker and prospective markers for fibroblasts, macrophages, and lymphocytes (Figure 5).

In early OA patients, macrophages strongly expressed MMP-9 (Figure 5). The total number of CD68+/MMP-9+ cells/mm^2 in the intima of early OA patients (median = 1320) was significantly higher compared to the total number of vimentin+/MMP-9+ cells/mm^2 (median = 205) and CD5+/MMP-9+ cells/mm^2 (median = 11) ($p < 0.0001$). The total number of vimentin+/MMP-9+ cells/mm^2 in the intima of early OA patients was significantly higher compared to the total number of CD5+/MMP-9+ cells/mm^2 ($p < 0.01$). Similarly, for early OA patients, the total number of CD68+/MMP-9+ cells/mm^2 in the intima of advanced OA (median = 948) was significantly higher compared to the total number of vimentin+/MMP-9+ cells/mm^2 (median = 361) and CD5+/MMP-9+ cells/mm^2 (median = 93) ($p < 0.0001$). The total number of vimentin+/MMP-9+ cells/mm2 in the intima of advanced OA patients was significantly higher compared to the total number of CD5+/MMP-9+ cells/mm^2 ($p < 0.001$). In the subintima of both early and advanced OA patients, there was not a statistically significant difference. These results were graphically summarized in Figure 2C.

The smooth muscle cells and endothelial cells the of blood vessel walls were only seen occasionally. NF-kB and iNOS were present in the endothelial and smooth muscle cells of the synovial blood vessels in early and advanced OA patients (Figure 6).

2.3. Co-Localization of NF-kB+ Cells and Markers of Cell Populations in Synovial Intima and Subintima

The total number CD68+/NF-kB+ cells/mm^2 in the intima of early OA (median = 2359) was significantly higher compared to the total number of vimentin+/NF-kB+ cells/mm^2 (median = 1321) and LCA+/NF-kB+ cells/mm^2 (median = 64) ($p < 0.001$ and $p < 0.0001$, respectively). The total number of vimentin+/NF-kB+ cells/mm^2 in the intima of early OA patients was significantly higher compared to the total number LCA+NF-kB+ cells/mm^2 ($p < 0.0001$). The difference between CD68+/NF-kB+ (median = 172), vimentin+/NF-kB+ (median = 53), and LCA+/NF-kB+ cells/mm^2 (median = 85) in the subintima of early OA was not statistically significant.

The total number of LCA+/NF-kB+ cells/mm^2 in the subintima of advanced OA patients (median = 2123) was significantly higher compared to the total number of vimentin+/NF-kB+ cells/mm^2 (median = 14) and CD68+/NF-kB+ cells/mm^2 (median = 29) ($p < 0.0001$; and $p < 0.0001$, respectively). The difference between LCA+/NF-kB+ (median = 368), vimentin+/NF-kB+ (median = 74), and CD68+/NF-kB+ cells/mm^2 (median = 131) in the intima of advanced OA patients was not statistically significant. These results were graphically summarized in Figure 2A, and positive cells were shown in Figure 3.

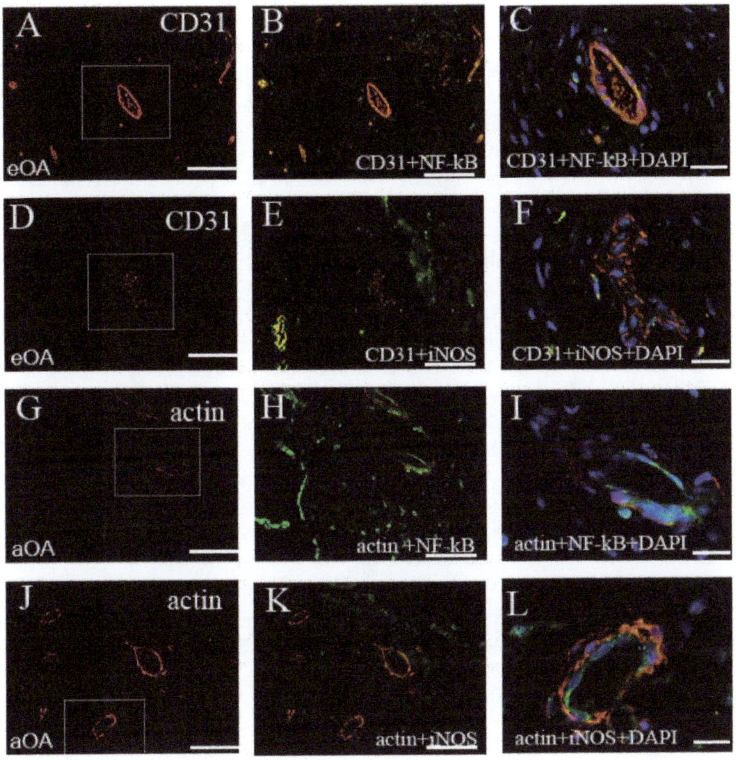

Figure 6. The synovial membrane of patients. CD31 positive cells (red) in the blood vessels (frame) (**A**). CD31+NF-kB+ (merge) in the endothelial cells (**B**). The merge of CD31+NF-kB+DAPI (blue) nuclear; stain (**C**). CD31 positive cells (red) in the blood vessels (frame) (**D**). CD31+iNOS+ (merge) in the endothelial cells (**E**). The merge of CD31+iNOS+DAPI (blue) nuclear stain (**F**). Actin positive cells (red) in the blood vessels (frame) (**G**). Actin+NF-kB+(merge) in the smooth muscle cells (**H**). The merge of Actin+NF-kB+DAPI (blue) nuclear stain (**I**). Actin positive cells (red) in the blood vessels (frame) (**J**). Actin+iNOS+(merge) in the smooth muscle cells (**K**). The merge of Actin+iNOS+DAPI (blue) nuclear stain (**L**). eOA—early OA; aOA—advanced OA. Magnification ×40 (first two columns), scale bar 50 µm and ×100 (last column), scale bar 20 µm.

3. Discussion

Synovitis has been radiologically proven to be a prognostic factor for OA development [37,38], and innate immunity plays a paramount role in early OA advancement [28]. However, the pathogenic influence of synovial tissue inflammation on early and advanced OA is not clear [39,40]. Our previous study showed the higher grade of synovitis in patients with radiologically early OA compared to advanced eOA [11]. Additionally, in the same study, NF-kB and iNOS expression was observed to be greater in early OA compared to advanced OA. Now, as a continuation of the previous study, we wanted to elucidate the exact localization of these inflammatory factors while also examining the expression of MMP-9, being aware that MMPs are the most notable degradation enzymes in cartilage deterioration [24,26]. Our main findings indicate that macrophages are the most active cells in early OA, containing most of the NF-kB, which is responsible for the production of an abundance of proinflammatory factors. In advanced OA, leukocytes contain most of the NF-kB, becoming the leading proinflammatory cells. During early OA, iNOS is mostly located in macrophages, and in advanced OA, it is expressed in leukocytes, though it still maintains presence in macrophages.

In our study, nuclear NF-kB expression in early OA was mostly pronounced in the macrophages of the intima with moderate expression in the fibroblasts. This finding is consistent with finding of others confirming that hyperplasia of the intima of the synovial membrane is due to a highly increased number of fibroblasts and macrophages, with the latter being the main source of proinflammatory cytokines [27,29]. These cytokines, especially TNFa and IL-1, are mostly produced through the NF-kB transcription factor [19], and therefore, knowing the exact location of NF-kB, we can say which cells contribute the most to the inflammation present in the synovium during early OA. We found a high expression of NF-kB in the synovial macrophages, which is direct evidence for the involvement of macrophages in the pathogenesis of knee OA. Clearly, the NF-kB pathway is not the only one through which inflammatory cytokines can be produced, but it constitutes a major ratio [18,29]. Additionally, a considerable proportion of NF-kB is expressed by the fibroblasts. Fibroblasts are the most present cells in both normal and inflamed synovium [27]. Studies have shown that by depleting macrophages, fibroblast cytokine production was also downregulated due to cytokine cross-talk [29]. Our results show this pattern regarding the NF-kB expression in these two cell types. In advanced OA, NF-kB expression in macrophages dropped ten times, lowering the expression of inflammatory cytokines, while in fibroblasts, the decrease was significant but smaller. In the synovial subintima (stroma) during advanced OA, NF-kB was mostly expressed in the leukocytes, particularly in the lymphocytes, which is a novel finding. This might implicate that subintimal leukocytes express NF-kB during the late stages of OA, keeping the inflammatory process active through this stage. In advanced osteoarthritis, the systemic pattern of disease behavior is more notable. Perivascular, nodular lymphocyte infiltration appears in response to chronic inflammation, most likely due to the autoimmune component of the disease, which also partly confirms the systemic basis of the disease [41]. The expression of NF-kB in the smooth muscle cells and the blood vessel endothelium of the synovial tissue was negligible, which was expected.

In immunohistochemical staining, iNOS is frequently used as a marker for activated macrophages, which signifies a consistent expression of this proinflammatory factor in macrophages while being active [28]. It is also secreted by fibroblasts, which constitute the dominant cellular component of the synovium [42]. iNOS expression in the intima of patients with early osteoarthritis followed a similar pattern as NF-kB, but not in in synovial the intima of advanced OA patients, where it was still expressed in the macrophages and leukocytes. This is in line with our previous study and other studies that show that the transcription of iNOS usually goes through the NF-kB pathway, but not entirely [11,19]. However, iNOS production in leukocytes in the synovial intima has grown exponentially in advanced OA. It is still unclear why, in advanced OA, most of the NF-kB presence was in the synovial subintima (stroma), whilst iNOS was mostly located in the synovial intima in the same stage of the disease.

In our study, we found MMP-9 to be predominantly produced by macrophages. Additionally, MMP production is strongly dependent on macrophage NF-kB activity, even when it is produced by fibroblasts [42,43]. Fibroblasts produce MMPs after being stimulated by cytokines, namely TNFa and IL-1 [44]. In line with these observations, in our study, we showed that in advanced OA, fibroblasts produce a higher percentage of total MMP-9 compared to early OA, but still less than the macrophages. A study by Amos et al. showed the decreased production of MMP-2, MMP-3, and MMP-9 once NF-kB had been blocked by IkB [18].

For this study, the synovium was taken from the medial and lateral gutters, parts of the knee joint with the most pronounced synovitis. The synovitis in patients with knee OA exhibits features of a T-cell immune response, with lymphocyte nodule numbers progressively growing proportionally with OA severity [41]. T-cells are mostly found in the synovial membrane and in the Hoffa fat pad of OA knees as proinflammatory cells [45]. These T-cells become dysfunctional phenotypes, thus contributing to the pathogenesis of knee OA [46]. With the achieved results, we favor the idea that both peripheral blood and tissue-infiltrating CD8 T-cells play an important role in the ongoing process of knee osteoarthritis [47]. These results suggest that B-cells and granulocytes may also be involved in the pathogenesis of knee OA, but, due to the scarce number of B-lymphocytes, their role is much smaller. Parts of the knee synovium in immediate contact with degrading cartilage are the locations of most lymphocytes [48].

Regarding the limitations of the study, the definition of the severity of knee OA was based solely on radiographs. The evidence so far does not show a strong correlation between radiographic changes and pain [49,50]. Some patients in the early OA group had bucket-handle meniscal tears with knee locking, which may not genuinely reflect synovitis due to OA. Even in the absence of OA, synovitis is also a feature of meniscal tears [51,52].

In conclusion, our study results provide information about different inflammatory cell localization in the synovial membrane of early and advanced OA patients compared to healthy individuals. The exact localization of the cells and stage of the disease when cells are active have an impact on the possible treatment of OA in its early stages. A direct association between radiological parameters and histologically proven tissue inflammation associated with different inflammatory cell immunophenotype will further elucidate OA pathophysiology.

4. Materials and Methods

4.1. Patients

The Ethics Committee of the School of Medicine, University of Mostar and the University Hospital Mostar, Bosnia and Herzegovina approved the study, and all patients gave written, informed consent. This study included 30 patients admitted to the Department of Orthopaedics and Traumatology of University Hospital Mostar. The inclusion and exclusion criteria were in accordance with the American College of Rheumatology Diagnostic and Therapeutic Criteria for knee OA [53], explained in detail in our previous study [11]. Four weeks prior to surgery, patients did not receive any anti-inflammatory drugs [54]. From the patients' histories, we collected data about gender, age, body mass index (BMI), range of motion (ROM), knee axis, symptom duration in months (pain and contracture), and clinical stage of the disease by Western Ontario and McMaster Universities Arthritis Index (WOMAC) [55].

Twenty patients (over 40 years old) had primary OA, and they were divided into two groups according to radiological, Kellgren–Lawrence (K–L), classification [56]: ten patients with early OA and 10 patients with advanced OA. Early OA was considered as stage 1 and stage 2 according to K–L classification, while advance OA was stage 3 and stage 4 according to K–L classification. In the control group, there were ten younger aged patients (16–40 years) admitted for fresh meniscal injury without arthroscopically visible hyaline cartilage damage (grade 0 or 1), by the International Cartilage Repair Society classification (ICRS) [57]. In early radiographic OA, patients mostly complained about pain and sometimes knee locking. Here, we performed arthroscopies with the debridement of the deteriorated cartilage and abundant synovial membrane. When there was knee locking, we usually found medial meniscus bucket-handle tears, and a partial meniscectomy was performed. Arthroscopy, a minimally invasive procedure relieves some of the pain and prevents future knee locking in patients. In advanced radiographic OA, total knee endoprosthesis was implanted.

4.2. Synovial Tissue Collection

A larger sample of synovial biopsies were taken during total knee arthroplasty from ten patients with advanced OA (stage 3 and stage 4 according to K–L classification). In all cases, standard medial parapatellar exposure was used. Synovial biopsies in other groups were performed arthroscopically. Samples were taken from ten patients with early OA and from the control group. All patients from the early OA group had their samples taken from the suprapatellar pouch, medial, and lateral gutters by direct visualization of the inflamed and hypertrophied tissue. Samples from control group were taken randomly from the same joint locations. Standard knee arthroscopic portals were used for the arthroscopy.

4.3. Tissue Processing and Analysis

Tissue samples of the synovial biopsies were formalin-fixed, paraffin-embedded, serially sectioned (4 μm), and mounted on glass slides. Every 10th section underwent haematoxylin and eosin staining and were analyzed using an Olympus CX41 light microscope (Olympus, Tokyo, Japan). For every patient, there were 3 biopsies that were sectioned into ten tissue sections, making a total of 30 sections per patient. Three investigators analyzed the images of the synovial tissues independently.

4.4. Immunofluorescence

The remaining sections were deparaffinized in xylol and rehydrated in ethanol and distilled water, followed by cooking in a sodium citrate buffer (pH 6.0) for 10 min at 95 °C. Before the primary antibody application, non-specific staining was prevented by using Protein Block (ab64226; Abcam, UK). The appropriate combination of primary antibodies was incubated overnight in a humidified chamber (Table 1). The next day, the sections were rinsed in PBS and incubated in appropriate combinations of the secondary antibodies (Table 2) for one hour. After a final rinse in PBS, nuclei were stained using 4,6-diamidino-2-phenylindole (DAPI), and sections were then cover-slipped (Immuno-Mount, Thermo Shandon, Pittsburgh, PA, USA) and examined by a fluorescence microscope (Olympus BX51, Tokyo, Japan) equipped with a DP71 digital camera (Olympus, Tokyo, Japan). Images were taken at ×40 magnification and assembled using Adobe Photoshop.

Table 2. Primary and secondary antibodies used.

Antibodies	Host	Dilution	Structures Identified by Antibodies	Source
SC-109 (polyclonal antibody)	Rabbit	1:200	Nf-kB p65	Santacruz Biotechnology (Santa Cruz, CA, USA)
SC-651 (monoclonal antibody)	Rabbit	1:200	iNOS	Santacruz Biotechnology (Santa Cruz, CA, USA)
A0150 (polyclonal antibody)	Rabbit	1:100	MMP-9	DAKO (Gloustrup, Denmark)
M0823 (monoclonal antibody)	Mouse	1:20	CD31 (endothelial cells of blood vessels)	DAKO (Gloustrup, Denmark)
M0851 (monoclonal antibody)	Mouse	1:40	Actin (smooth muscle cells of blood vessels)	DAKO (Gloustrup, Denmark)
M0725 (monoclonal antibody)	Mouse	1:50	Vimentin (fibroblasts)	DAKO (Gloustrup, Denmark)
M0876 (monoclonal antibody)	Mouse	1:75	CD68 (macrophages)	DAKO (Gloustrup, Denmark)
M0742 (monoclonal antibody)	Mouse	1:100	LCA (leukocytes)	DAKO (Gloustrup, Denmark)
M7194 (monoclonal antibody)	Mouse	1:50	CD5 (lymphocytes)	DAKO (Gloustrup, Denmark)
Rhodamine Goat AP124R	Mouse	1:100	Secondary antibody	MerckMillipore (Billerica, MA, USA)
Fluorescein Goat AP132F	Rabbit	1:100	Secondary antibody	MerckMillipore (Billerica, MA, USA)

Double immunofluorescence with primary antibodies to NF-kB, iNOS, and MMP9 (Santacruz Biotechnology, Santa Cruz, CA, USA, SC-109 and SC-651, respectively) was used in combination with different specific cell type markers (Table 1) to determine the number of positive cells in the surface layer of cells (intima) and the underlying tissue (subintima) of the synovial membrane. For negative control, primary antibodies were excluded from the staining procedures. As a positive control, we used the lymph node and tonsil tissue. We only counted cells that displayed both markers in the same cell (red or green signal) in the nucleus or cytoplasm. The cell count was performed using the Olympus CellB (Olympus, Tokyo, Japan) and ImageJ software [58]. The total number of vimentin+/NF-kB+, CD68+/NF-kB+, LCA+/NF-kB+, vimentin+/iNOS+, CD68+/iNOS+, LCA+/iNOS+ and vimentin/MMP-9, CD68+/MMP-9, and CD5+/MMP-9 positive cells were calculated as number of cells per mm2 in the intima and subintima of the synovial membrane. The final total number per patient was the mean of 30 sections that were counted.

4.5. Statistical Analysis

The data were analyzed using SPSS17 software (SPSS Inc., Chicago, IL, USA). Non-parametric variables were presented as frequencies and percentages. Parametric variables were shown as median and interquartile range due to deviations from the normal distribution. To test differences between groups for categorical variables, we used chi-square test and Fisher's exact test. To test differences between the parametric variables, we used the Mann–Whitney U test and Kruskal–Wallis test when the distribution of the data significantly deviated from normal. To test the correlation between the studied variables, Spearman's correlation coefficient was used. Probability level $p < 0.05$ in all tests was taken as statistically significant.

Author Contributions: Conceptualization, M.O., K.V. and V.S.; formal analysis, M.O., K.V., and V.S.; methodology, M.O., K.V., and V.S.; writing—original draft, M.O., A.Z., K.V., and V.S.; writing—review & editing, M.O., A.Z., K.V., and V.S. All authors have read and agreed to the published version of the manuscript.

Funding: This research received no external funding.

Institutional Review Board Statement: This study was conducted according to the guidelines of the Declaration of Helsinki and approved by the Institutional Review Board (or Ethics Committee) of The Ethics Committee of the University School of Medicine Class 01-669/13, issued in Mostar 29 May 2013.

Informed Consent Statement: Informed consent was obtained from all subjects involved in the study.

Data Availability Statement: The study did not report any data.

Conflicts of Interest: The authors declare no conflict of interest.

References

1. Loeser, R.F.; Goldring, S.R.; Scanzello, C.R.; Goldring, M.B. Osteoarthritis: A disease of the joint as an organ. *Arthritis Rheum.* **2012**, *64*, 1697–1707. [CrossRef]
2. Sokolove, J.; Lepus, C.M. Role of inflammation in the pathogenesis of osteoarthritis: Latest findings and interpretations. *Ther. Adv. Musculoskelet. Dis.* **2013**, *5*, 77–94. [CrossRef] [PubMed]
3. Geurts, J.; Nasi, S.; Distel, P.; Müller-Gerbl, M.; Prolla, T.A.; Kujoth, G.C.; Walker, U.A.; Hügle, T. Prematurely aging mitochondrial DNA mutator mice display subchondral osteopenia and chondrocyte hypertrophy without further osteoarthritis features. *Sci. Rep.* **2020**, *10*, 1296–1297. [CrossRef] [PubMed]
4. Walsh, D.A.; Stocks, J. New Therapeutic Targets for Osteoarthritis Pain. *SLAS Discov. Adv. Life Sci. R&D* **2017**, *22*, 931–949. [CrossRef]
5. Robinson, W.H.; Lepus, C.M.; Wang, Q.; Raghu, H.; Mao, R.; Lindstrom, T.M.; Sokolove, J. Low-grade inflammation as a key mediator of the pathogenesis of osteoarthritis. *Nat. Rev. Rheumatol.* **2016**, *12*, 580–592. [CrossRef] [PubMed]
6. Scanzello, C.R. Role of low-grade inflammation in osteoarthritis. *Curr. Opin. Rheumatol.* **2017**, *29*, 79–85. [CrossRef]
7. Koller, U.; Waldstein, W.; Krenn, V.; Windhager, R.; Boettner, F. Varus knee osteoarthritis: Elevated synovial CD15 counts correlate with inferior biomechanical properties of lateral-compartment cartilage. *J. Orthop. Res.* **2017**, *36*, 841–846. [CrossRef]
8. Siebuhr, A.S.; Bay-Jensen, A.C.; Jordan, J.M.; Kjelgaard-Petersen, C.F.; Christiansen, C.; Abramson, S.B.; Attur, M.; Berenbaum, F.; Kraus, V.; Karsdal, M.A. Inflammation (or synovitis)-driven osteoarthritis: An opportunity for personalizing prognosis and treatment? *Scand. J. Rheumatol.* **2015**, *45*, 87–98. [CrossRef] [PubMed]

9. Smith, M.D. The Normal Synovium. *Open Rheumatol. J.* **2011**, *5*, 100–106. [CrossRef]
10. Hugle, T.; Geurts, J. What drives osteoarthritis?—Synovial versus subchondral bone pathology. *Rheumatology* **2017**, *56*, 1461–1471.
11. Ostojic, M.; Soljic, V.; Vukojevic, K.; Dapic, T. Immunohistochemical characterization of early and advanced knee osteoarthritis by NF-κB and iNOS expression. *J. Orthop. Res.* **2016**, *35*, 1990–1997. [CrossRef] [PubMed]
12. Geurts, J.; Patel, A.; Hirschmann, M.T.; Pagenstert, G.I.; Müller-Gerbl, M.; Valderrabano, V.; Hügle, T. Elevated marrow inflammatory cells and osteoclasts in subchondral osteosclerosis in human knee osteoarthritis. *J. Orthop. Res.* **2015**, *34*, 262–269. [CrossRef] [PubMed]
13. Benito, M.J.; Veale, D.J.; FitzGerald, O.; Berg, W.B.V.D.; Bresnihan, B. Synovial tissue inflammation in early and late osteoarthritis. *Ann. Rheum. Dis.* **2005**, *64*, 1263–1267. [CrossRef]
14. Ostojic, M.; Ostojic, M.; Prlic, J.; Soljic, V. Correlation of anxiety and chronic pain to grade of synovitis in patients with knee osteoarthritis. *Psychiatr. Danub.* **2019**, *31* (Suppl. 1), S126–S130.
15. Sellam, J.; Berenbaum, F. The role of synovitis in pathophysiology and clinical symptoms of osteoarthritis. *Nat. Rev. Rheumatol.* **2010**, *6*, 625–635. [CrossRef]
16. Liu-Bryan, R. Synovium and the Innate Inflammatory Network in Osteoarthritis Progression. *Curr. Rheumatol. Rep.* **2013**, *15*, 1–7. [CrossRef] [PubMed]
17. Scanzello, C.R.; Goldring, S.R. The role of synovitis in osteoarthritis pathogenesis. *Bone* **2012**, *51*, 249–257. [CrossRef]
18. Amos, N.; Lauder, S.; Evans, A.; Feldmann, M.; Bondeson, J. Adenoviral gene transfer into osteoarthritis synovial cells using the endogenous inhibitor IκBα reveals that most, but not all, inflammatory and destructive mediators are NFκB dependent. *Rheumatology* **2006**, *45*, 1201–1209. [CrossRef]
19. Lepetsos, P.; Papavassiliou, K.A.; Papavassiliou, A.G. Redox and NF-κB signaling in osteoarthritis. *Free Radic. Biol. Med.* **2019**, *132*, 90–100. [CrossRef]
20. Ahmed, A.S.; Gedin, P.; Hugo, A.; Bakalkin, G.; Kanar, A.; Hart, D.A.; Druid, H.; Svensson, C.; Kosek, E. Activation of NF-κB in Synovium versus Cartilage from Patients with Advanced Knee Osteoarthritis: A Potential Contributor to Inflammatory Aspects of Disease Progression. *J. Immunol.* **2018**, *201*, 1918–1927. [CrossRef]
21. Suantawee, T.; Tantavisut, S.; Adisakwattana, S.; Tanpowpong, T.; Tanavalee, A.; Yuktanandana, P.; Anomasiri, W.; Deepaisarnsakul, B.; Honsawek, S. Upregulation of inducible nitric oxide synthase and nitrotyrosine expression in primary knee osteoarthritis. *J. Med. Assoc. Thail.* **2015**, *98*, 91–97.
22. Pelletier, J.-P.; Jovanovic, D.; Fernandes, J.C.; Manning, P.; Connor, J.R.; Currie, M.G.; Di Battista, J.A.; Martel-Pelletier, J. Reduced progression of experimental osteoarthritis in vivo by selective inhibition of inducible nitric oxide synthase. *Arthritis Rheum.* **1998**, *41*, 1275–1286. [CrossRef]
23. Rosa, S.C.; Judas, F.; Lopes, M.C.; Mendes, A.F. Nitric oxide synthase isoforms and NF-κB activity in normal and osteoarthritic human chondrocytes: Regulation by inducible nitric oxide. *Nitric Oxide* **2008**, *19*, 276–283. [CrossRef] [PubMed]
24. Požgan, U.; Caglič, D.; Rozman, B.; Nagase, H.; Turk, V.; Turk, B. Expression and activity profiling of selected cysteine cathepsins and matrix metalloproteinases in synovial fluids from patients with rheumatoid arthritis and osteoarthritis. *Biol. Chem.* **2010**, *391*, 571–579. [CrossRef] [PubMed]
25. Blom, A.B.; van Lent, P.L.; Libregts, S.; Holthuysen, A.E.; van der Kraan, P.M.; van Rooijen, N.; van den Berg, W.B. Crucial role of macrophages in matrix metalloproteinase-mediated cartilage destruction during experimental osteoarthritis: Involvement of matrix metalloproteinase 3. *Arthritis Rheum.* **2007**, *56*, 147–157. [CrossRef] [PubMed]
26. Marini, S.; Fasciglione, G.F.; Monteleone, G.; Maiotti, M.; Tarantino, U.; Coletta, M. A correlation between knee cartilage degradation observed by arthroscopy and synovial proteinases activities. *Clin. Biochem.* **2003**, *36*, 295–304. [CrossRef]
27. Manferdini, C.; Paolella, F.; Gabusi, E.; Silvestri, Y.; Gambari, L.; Cattini, L.; Filardo, G.; Fleury-Cappellesso, S.; Lisignoli, G. From osteoarthritic synovium to synovial-derived cells characterization: Synovial macrophages are key effector cells. *Arthritis Res.* **2016**, *18*, 83. [CrossRef]
28. Büyükavcı, R.; Aktürk, S.; Sağ, S. Comparison of blood platelet distribution width and neutrophil-lymphocyte ratio in patients with different grades of knee osteoarthritis. *J. Back Musculoskelet. Rehabil.* **2018**, *31*, 1035–1039. [CrossRef]
29. Bondeson, J.; Blom, A.B.; Wainwright, S.; Hughes, C.; Caterson, B.; Berg, W.B.V.D. The role of synovial macrophages and macrophage-produced mediators in driving inflammatory and destructive responses in osteoarthritis. *Arthritis Rheum.* **2010**, *62*, 647–657. [CrossRef] [PubMed]
30. Zhang, L.; Xing, R.; Huang, Z.; Zhang, N.; Li, X.; Wang, P. Inhibition of Synovial Macrophage Pyroptosis Alleviates Synovitis and Fibrosis in Knee Osteoarthritis. *Mediat. Inflamm.* **2019**, *2019*, 1–11. [CrossRef] [PubMed]
31. Xie, J.; Huang, Z.; Yu, X.; Zhou, L.; Pei, F. Clinical implications of macrophage dysfunction in the development of osteoarthritis of the knee. *Cytokine Growth Factor Rev.* **2019**, *46*, 36–44. [CrossRef] [PubMed]
32. Kragstrup, T.W.; Sohn, D.H.; Lepus, C.M.; Onuma, K.; Wang, Q.; Robinson, W.H.; Sokolove, J. Fibroblast-like synovial cell production of extra domain A fibronectin associates with inflammation in osteoarthritis. *BMC Rheumatol.* **2019**, *3*, 1–8. [CrossRef] [PubMed]
33. Ding, X.; Zhang, Y.; Huang, Y.; Liu, S.; Lu, H.; Sun, T. Cadherin-11 involves in synovitis and increases the migratory and invasive capacity of fibroblast-like synoviocytes of osteoarthritis. *Int. Immunopharmacol.* **2015**, *26*, 153–161. [CrossRef]

34. Rollín, R.; Marco, F.; Jover, J.A.; García-Asenjo, J.A.; Rodríguez, L.; López-Durán, L.; Fernandez-Gutierrez, B. Early lymphocyte activation in the synovial microenvironment in patients with osteoarthritis: Comparison with rheumatoid arthritis patients and healthy controls. *Rheumatol. Int.* **2008**, *28*, 757–764. [CrossRef]
35. Roemer, F.W.; Kwoh, C.K.; Hayashi, D.; Felson, D.T.; Guermazi, A. The role of radiography and MRI for eligibility assessment in DMOAD trials of knee OA. *Nat. Rev. Rheumatol.* **2018**, *14*, 372–380. [CrossRef]
36. Roman-Blas, J.A.; Jimenez, S.A. NF-κB as a potential therapeutic target in osteoarthritis and rheumatoid arthritis. *Osteoarthr. Cartil.* **2006**, *14*, 839–848. [CrossRef]
37. Felson, D.; Niu, J.; Neogi, T.; Goggins, J.; Nevitt, M.; Roemer, F.; Torner, J.; Lewis, C.; Guermazi, A. Synovitis and the risk of knee osteoarthritis: The MOST Study. *Osteoarthr. Cartil.* **2016**, *24*, 458–464. [CrossRef]
38. Atukorala, I.; Kwoh, C.K.; Guermazi, A.; Roemer, F.W.; Boudreau, R.M.; Hannon, M.J.; Hunter, D.J. Synovitis in knee osteoarthritis: A precursor of disease? *Ann. Rheum. Dis.* **2016**, *75*, 390–395. [CrossRef] [PubMed]
39. Caric, D.; Tomas, S.Z.; Filipovic, N.; Soljic, V.; Benzon, B.; Glumac, S.; Rakovac, I.; Vukojevic, K. Expression Pattern of iNOS, BCL-2 and MMP-9 in the Hip Synovium Tissue of Patients with Osteoarthritis. *Int. J. Mol. Sci.* **2021**, *22*, 1489. [CrossRef]
40. Kaufman, J.; Caric, D.; Vukojevic, K. Expression pattern of Syndecan-1 and HSP-70 in hip tissue of patients with osteoarthritis. *J. Orthop.* **2020**, *17*, 134–138. [CrossRef]
41. Sakkas, L.I.; Platsoucas, C.D. The role of T cells in the pathogenesis of osteoarthritis. *Arthritis Rheum.* **2007**, *56*, 409–424. [CrossRef]
42. Han, D.; Fang, Y.; Tan, X.; Jiang, H.; Gong, X.; Wang, X.; Hong, W.; Tu, J.; Wei, W. The emerging role of fibroblast-like synoviocytes-mediated synovitis in osteoarthritis: An update. *J. Cell. Mol. Med.* **2020**, *24*, 9518–9532. [CrossRef] [PubMed]
43. Bondeson, J.; Wainwright, S.D.; Lauder, S.; Amos, N.; Hughes, C.E. The role of synovial macrophages and macrophage-produced cytokines in driving aggrecanases, matrix metalloproteinases, and other destructive and inflammatory responses in osteoarthritis. *Arthritis Res.* **2006**, *8*, R187. [CrossRef]
44. Fuchs, S.; Skwara, A.; Bloch, M.; Dankbar, B. Differential induction and regulation of matrix metalloproteinases in osteoarthritic tissue and fluid synovial fibroblasts. *Osteoarthr. Cartil.* **2004**, *12*, 409–418. [CrossRef]
45. Klein-Wieringa, I.R.; de Lange-Brokaar, B.J.; Yusuf, E.; Andersen, S.N.; Kwekkeboom, J.C.; Kroon, H.M.; van Osch, G.J.; Zuurmond, A.-M.; Stojanovic-Susulic, V.; Nelissen, R.; et al. Inflammatory Cells in Patients with Endstage Knee Osteoarthritis: A Comparison between the Synovium and the Infrapatellar Fat Pad. *J. Rheumatol.* **2016**, *43*, 771–778. [CrossRef]
46. Liu, J.; Khalil, R.A. Matrix Metalloproteinase Inhibitors as Investigational and Therapeutic Tools in Unrestrained Tissue Remodeling and Pathological Disorders. *Prog. Mol. Biol. Transl. Sci.* **2017**, *148*, 355–420. [CrossRef] [PubMed]
47. Apinun, J.; Sengprasert, P.; Yuktanandana, P.; Ngarmukos, S.; Tanavalee, A.; Reantragoon, R. Immune Mediators in Osteoarthritis: Infrapatellar Fat Pad-Infiltrating CD8+ T Cells Are Increased in Osteoarthritic Patients with Higher Clinical Radiographic Grading. *Int. J. Rheumatol.* **2016**, *2016*, 1–8. [CrossRef] [PubMed]
48. Li, Y.-S.; Luo, W.; Zhu, S.-A.; Lei, G.-H. T Cells in Osteoarthritis: Alterations and Beyond. *Front. Immunol.* **2017**, *8*, 356. [CrossRef] [PubMed]
49. Kinds, M.; Welsing, P.; Vignon, E.; Bijlsma, J.; Viergever, M.; Marijnissen, A.; Lafeber, F. A systematic review of the association between radiographic and clinical osteoarthritis of hip and knee. *Osteoarthr. Cartil.* **2011**, *19*, 768–778. [CrossRef]
50. Bedson, J.; Croft, P.R. The discordance between clinical and radiographic knee osteoarthritis: A systematic search and summary of the literature. *BMC Musculoskelet. Disord.* **2008**, *9*, 116. [CrossRef]
51. Roemer, F.W.; Felson, D.T.; Yang, T.; Niu, J.; Crema, M.D.; Englund, M.; Nevitt, M.C.; Zhang, Y.; Lynch, J.A.; El Khoury, G.Y.; et al. The association between meniscal damage of the posterior horns and localized posterior synovitis detected on T1-weighted contrast-enhanced MRI—The MOST study. *Semin. Arthritis Rheum.* **2013**, *42*, 573–581. [CrossRef]
52. Scanzello, C.R.; McKeon, B.; Swaim, B.H.; Dicarlo, E.; Asomugha, E.U.; Kanda, V.; Nair, A.; Lee, D.M.; Richmond, J.C.; Katz, J.N.; et al. Synovial inflammation in patients undergoing arthroscopic meniscectomy: Molecular characterization and relationship to symptoms. *Arthritis Rheum.* **2010**, *63*, 391–400. [CrossRef]
53. Altman, R.; Asch, E.; Bloch, D.; Bole, G.; Borenstein, D.; Brandt, K.; Christy, W.; Cooke, T.D.; Greenwald, R.; Hochberg, M.; et al. Development of criteria for the classification and reporting of osteoarthritis: Classification of osteoarthritis of the knee. *Arthritis Rheum.* **1986**, *29*, 1039–1049. [CrossRef] [PubMed]
54. Brenner, S.S.; Klotz, U.; Alscher, D.M.; Mais, A.; Lauer, G.; Schweer, H.; Seyberth, H.W.; Fritz, P.; Bierbach, U. Osteoarthritis of the knee—Clinical assessments and inflammatory markers. *Osteoarthr. Cartil.* **2004**, *12*, 469–475. [CrossRef]
55. McConnell, S.; Kolopack, P.; Davis, A. The Western Ontario and McMaster Universities Osteoarthritis Index (WOMAC): A review of its utility and measurement properties. *Arthritis Rheum.* **2001**, *45*, 453–461. [CrossRef]
56. Kellgren, J.H.; Lawrence, J.S. Radiological Assessment of Osteo-Arthrosis. *Ann. Rheum. Dis.* **1957**, *16*, 494–502. [CrossRef] [PubMed]
57. Brittberg, M.; Winalski, C.S. Evaluation of Cartilage Injuries and Repair. *J. Bone Jt. Surg.* **2003**, *85*, 58–69. [CrossRef]
58. Schneider, C.A.; Rasband, W.S.; Eliceiri, K.W. NIH Image to ImageJ: 25 years of image analysis. *Nat. Methods* **2012**, *9*, 671–675. [CrossRef] [PubMed]

International Journal of *Molecular Sciences*

MDPI

Article

Kurarinone Attenuates Collagen-Induced Arthritis in Mice by Inhibiting Th1/Th17 Cell Responses and Oxidative Stress

Kuo-Tung Tang [1,2,3,†], Chi-Chien Lin [1,4,5,6,7,†], Shih-Chao Lin [8,†], Jou-Hsuan Wang [9] and Sen-Wei Tsai [9,10,*]

1 Program in Translational Medicine, National Chung Hsing University, Taichung 402, Taiwan; dirac1982@vghtc.gov.tw (K.-T.T.); lincc@email.nchu.edu.tw (C.-C.L.)
2 Faculty of Medicine, National Yang-Ming University, Taipei 112, Taiwan
3 Division of Allergy, Immunology and Rheumatology, Taichung Veterans General Hospital, Taichung 407, Taiwan
4 Institute of Biomedical Science, The iEGG and Animal Biotechnology Center, National Chung-Hsing University, Taichung 402, Taiwan
5 Department of Medical Research, China Medical University Hospital, Taichung 404, Taiwan
6 Department of Medical Research, Taichung Veterans General Hospital, Taichung 407, Taiwan
7 Department of Pharmacology, College of Medicine, Kaohsiung Medical University, Kaohsiung 807, Taiwan
8 Bachelor Degree Program in Marine Biotechnology, College of Life Sciences, National Taiwan Ocean University, Keelung 202, Taiwan; sclin@mail.ntou.edu.tw
9 Department of Physical Medicine and Rehabilitation, Taichung Tzu Chi Hospital, Buddhist Tzu Chi Medical Foundation, Taichung 427, Taiwan; doris8569@smail.nchu.edu.tw
10 School of Medicine, Tzu Chi University, Hualien 970, Taiwan
* Correspondence: swtsai@tzuchi.com.tw
† These authors contributed equally to this work.

Abstract: Kurarinone is a flavanone, extracted from *Sophora flavescens* Aiton, with multiple biological effects. Here, we determine the therapeutic potential of kurarinone and elucidate the interplay between kurarinone and the autoimmune disease rheumatoid arthritis (RA). Arthritis was recapitulated by induction of bovine collagen II (CII) in DBA/1 mice as a collagen-induced arthritis (CIA) model. After the establishment of the CIA, kurarinone was given orally from day 21 to 42 (100 mg/kg/day) followed by determination of the severity based on a symptom scoring scale and with histopathology. Levels of cytokines, anti-CII antibodies, and the proliferation and lineages of T cells from the draining lymph nodes were measured using ELISA and flow cytometry, respectively. The expressional changes, including STAT1, STAT3, Nrf2, KEAP-1, and heme oxygenase-1 (HO-1) changes in the paw tissues, were evaluated by Western blot assay. Oxidative stress featured with malondiadehyde (MDA) and hydrogen peroxide (H_2O_2) activities in paw tissues were also evaluated. Results showed that kurarinone treatment reduced arthritis severity of CIA mice, as well as their levels of proinflammatory cytokines, TNF-α, IL-6, IFN-γ, and IL-17A, in the serum and paw tissues. T cell proliferation was also reduced by kurarinone even under the stimulation of CII and anti-CD3 antibody. In addition, kurarinone reduced STAT1 and STAT3 phosphorylation and the proportions of Th1 and Th17 cells in lymph nodes. Moreover, kurarinone suppressed the production of MDA and H_2O_2. All while promoting enzymatic activities of key antioxidant enzymes, SOD and GSH-Px. In the paw tissues, upregulation of Nrf-2 and HO-1, and downregulation of KEAP-1 were observed. Overall, kurarinone showed an anti-inflammatory effect by inhibiting Th1 and Th17 cell differentiation and an antioxidant effect exerted in part through activating the Nrf-2/KEAP-1 pathway. These beneficial effects in CIA mice contributed to the amelioration of their arthritis, indicating that kurarinone might be an adjunct treatment option for rheumatoid arthritis.

Keywords: kurarinone; arthritis; Th1; Th17; STAT1; STAT3; oxidative stress

Citation: Tang, K.-T.; Lin, C.-C.; Lin, S.-C.; Wang, J.-H.; Tsai, S.-W. Kurarinone Attenuates Collagen-Induced Arthritis in Mice by Inhibiting Th1/Th17 Cell Responses and Oxidative Stress. *Int. J. Mol. Sci.* **2021**, *22*, 4002. https://doi.org/10.3390/ijms22084002

Academic Editor: Chih-Hsin Tang

Received: 18 March 2021
Accepted: 9 April 2021
Published: 13 April 2021

1. Introduction

Rheumatoid arthritis (RA) is a chronic autoimmune disease characterized by joint inflammation, cartilage damage, and joint destruction [1], that leads to negative impacts on the physical movement and life quality of patients. The pathogenesis of RA has been implied to be associated with uncontrolled autoimmunity and the resulting inflammation from antigen presenting cells, such as dendritic cells and macrophages, and lymphocytes, such as T and B cells [2–4]. The systemic inflammatory response targets the synovial membrane, leading to joint destruction through cartilage degradation and osteoclast activation [5,6]. Numerous studies have demonstrated the importance of activated T cells in RA pathogenesis. For example, experiments utilizing the collagen-induced arthritis (CIA) animal model have indicated the involvement of activated pro-inflammatory Th1 and Th17 cells and suppressed Treg cells could be involved in the RA pathogenesis [7]. Oxidative stress, a result of accumulated reactive oxygen species (ROS), also contributes to the synovitis development in RA. ROS can degrade proteoglycans and hypochlorous acid (HOCl) in the cartilage, leading to collagen fragmentations and proteoglycan synthesis suppression [8,9]. Increased oxidative stress has also been reported in RA patients [10].

At present, RA pharmacotherapy remains unsatisfactory, with various side effects [11–13]. Some RA patients are refractory to traditional disease modifying anti-rheumatic drugs (DMARDs) [14]. Some biological agents, though are good for refractory disease, cause serious infection problems [11]. There is a need for novel therapeutics with a favorable safety and efficacy profile. Kurarinone, a natural lavandulylated flavanone isolated from the medicinal herb *Sophora flavescens* Aiton, has immunosuppressive and antioxidant effects [15,16]. For example, it inhibits the differentiation of Th1/Th2/Th17 cells and promotes the differentiation of Treg cells. Its mechanism of action involves the regulation of multiple kinases signaling pathways, like JAK/STAT, T-cell receptor (TCR)-mediated Src family tyrosine kinase, PI3K/Akt, and p38 MAPK signaling. This results in suppression of psoriasis- and contact dermatitis-like inflammatory dermatitis in mice [16]. Kurarinone also inhibits the progression of murine autoimmune encephalomyelitis (EAE) by inhibiting Th1 and Th17 cell differentiation and proliferation [15]. Moreover, it activates the KEAP1/Nrf2 pathway, a major regulator of oxidative stress [17], and it overexpresses antioxidant enzymes, like heme oxygenase-1 (HO-1), thereby exerting immunosuppression on the lipopolysaccharide (LPS)-induced production of inflammatory mediators in RAW264.7 macrophages [18]. Based on these findings, we hypothesized that kurarinone has a therapeutic effect on RA through regulating Th1/Th17 cell balance and antioxidative activity. In this study, we attempted to evaluate kurarinone in the murine model of collagen-induced arthritis (CIA).

2. Results

2.1. Kurarinone Reduced the Severity of CIA

To determine the effect on arthritis in CIA, symptom scores were measured [19]. As shown in Figure 1, the administration of bovine CII emulsion in DBA/1 mice led to the development of arthritic symptoms (Figure 1A), which included swelling and erythema of the hind paws (Figure 1B,C). Symptom scores of experimental mice were lower after daily treatment with 100 mg/kg kurarinone for three weeks. Consistent with that, histopathologic findings in these animals on day 42 after primary immunization showed less joint inflammation (synovitis), pannus formation, cartilage destruction, and bone erosions compared to the control (Figure 1D,E). Moreover, treatment with kurarinone also reduced serum levels of CII-specific IgG (Figure 1F).

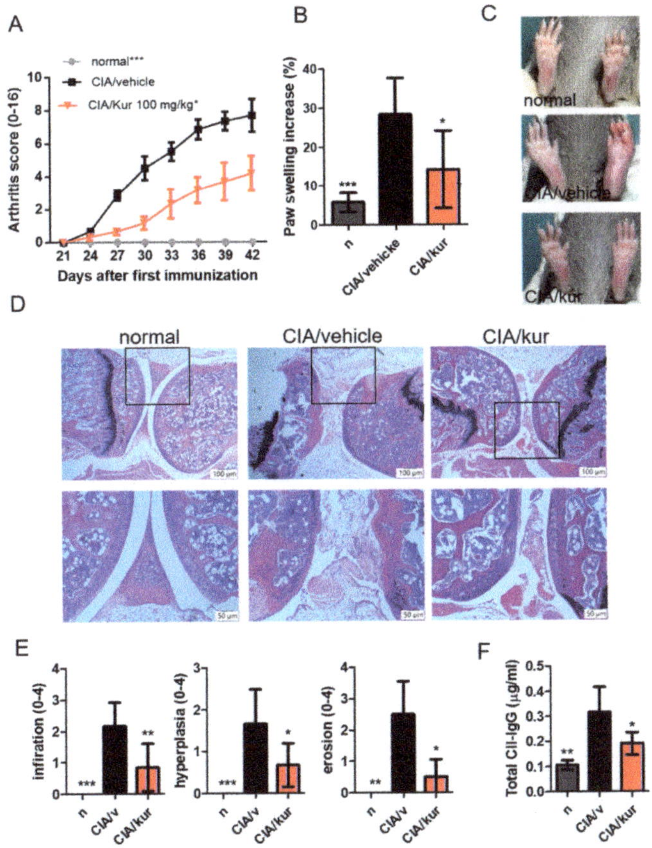

Figure 1. Effects of kurarinone on the severity of CIA. (**A**) Mice were immunized with bovine type II collagen in complete Freund's adjuvant, and (**A**) clinical scores and (**B**) paw thickness was measured on day 42. (**C**) Representative images of a hind paw at day 42. (**D**) Mouse joints stained with hematoxylin and eosin (scale bar, 100 μM, 100×; 50 μM 200×). (**E**) Semiquantitative histological analysis. (**F**) Serum anti-CII IgG was analyzed by ELISA on day 42. Data are presented as mean ± SEM of 6 mice from one of three experiments. (*) $p < 0.05$, (**) $p < 0.01$, (***) $p < 0.001$ versus vehicle-treated CIA mice group (Two Way (**A**), or One Way (**B**,**E**,**F**) ANOVA followed by Tukey's multiple comparison test).

2.2. Kurarinone Reduced Pro-Inflammatory Cytokine Levels in the Blood and Joints

Cytokine levels in serum and paw homogenates were measured using ELISA on day 42. As shown in Figure 2, kurarinone significantly reduced serum levels of TNF-α, IL-6, IFN-γ, and IL-17A when compared with those in vehicle-treated mice (Figure 2A). Similar results on pro-inflammatory cytokine levels were found in paw homogenates (Figure 2B).

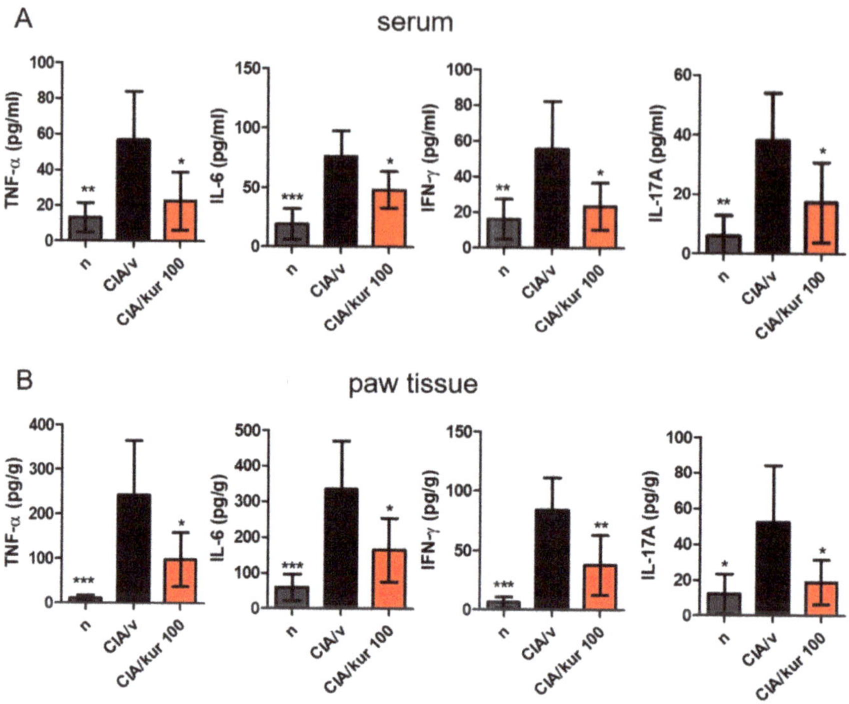

Figure 2. Effects of kurarinone on serum and paw proinflammatory cytokine productions in CIA mice. Hind paws and sera were collected on day 42 from mice. (**A**) Cytokines in serum and (**B**) paw homogenates were measured by ELISA assays. Data are presented as mean ± SEM of 6 mice from one of three experiments. (*) $p < 0.05$, (**) $p < 0.01$, (***) $p < 0.001$ versus vehicle-treated CIA mice group (One Way ANOVA followed by Tukey's multiple comparison test).

2.3. Kurarinone Treatment Attenuated CII-Specific T Cell Proliferation in CIA

Antigen-specific T-cell responses were examined on T cells isolated from the draining lymph nodes in CIA mice on day 42 after CII stimulation. While T cells obtained from vehicle-treated CIA mice showed a strong proliferative response to CII. Such a response was significantly suppressed in kurarinone-treated mice (Figure 3A). Kurarinone also significantly suppressed T cell proliferation upon stimulation with anti-CD3 antibody (Figure 3B). These results indicate that kurarinone had attenuated T cell proliferation after stimulation in CIA mice.

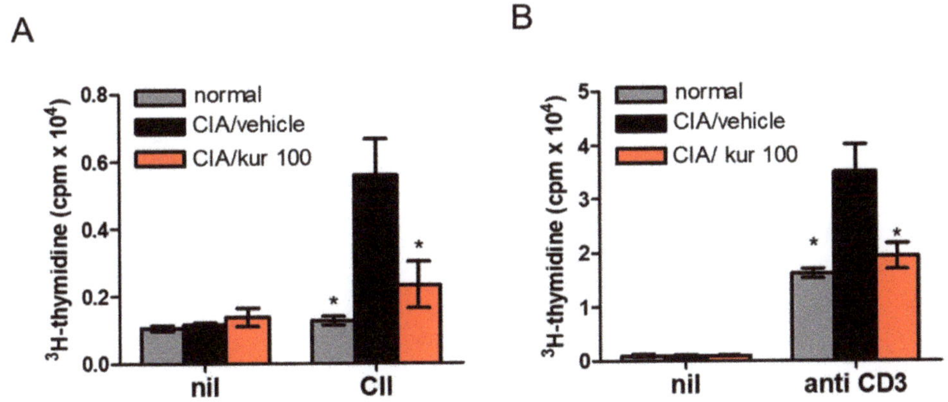

Figure 3. Effects of kurarinone on T cell proliferation in CIA. On day 42, cells from the inguinal LN were isolated for mice and were cultured for 96 hrs in the absence or presence of (**A**) 10 ug/mL CII or (**B**) anti-CD3 antibody. Proliferation was assessed after 96 h by [^{3}H] thymidine incorporation in counts per minute (cpm). Data are presented as mean ±SEM of 6 mice from one of three experiments. (*) $p < 0.05$ versus vehicle-treated CIA mice group (One Way ANOVA followed by Tukey's multiple comparison test).

2.4. Kurarinone Altered Th1/Th17 Differentiation in Lymph Nodes of CIA Mice

We further explored the possible mechanisms involved in the therapeutic effects of kurarinone on CIA mice. The abundance of Th1, Th17, and Treg in the inguinal lymph nodes was analyzed using flow cytometry. As illustrated in Figure 4A, the percentages of CD4$^+$IFN-γ^+ Th1 cells and CD4$^+$IL-17$^+$ Th17 cells isolated from the LN of kurarinone-treated CIA mice was lower than those of vehicle-treated group. However, CD4$^+$Foxp3$^+$ Treg cells appeared to have increased after kurarinone, but without reaching statistically significant levels (Figure 4A and Supplementary Figure S1). We also analyzed the lymph nodes using qPCR for the expressions of transcription factors, such as T-bet, RORγt, and Foxp3. Lower expressions of T-bet and RORγt in the lymph nodes were found in kurarinone-treated CIA mice, whereas the expression level of Foxp3 was unchanged (Figure 4B). Altogether, these findings suggest that the suppression of Th1 and Th17 differentiation is involved in the mitigation of arthritic symptoms in kurarinone-treated CIA mice.

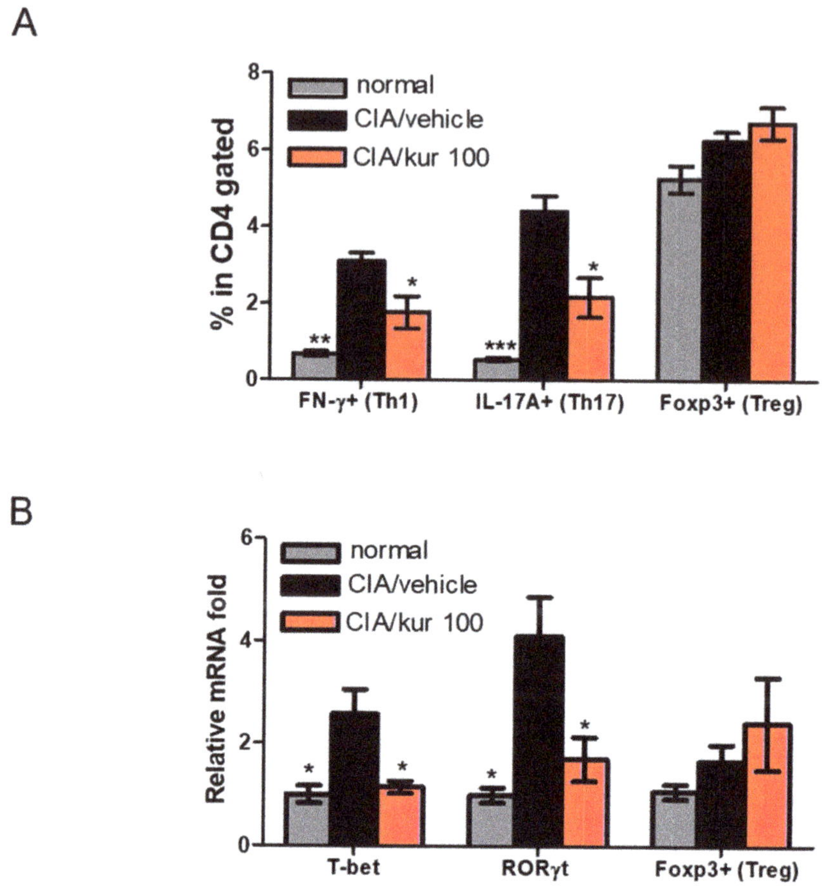

Figure 4. Effects of kurarinone on frequency of Th1 (CD4+ IFN-γ+ T cells), Th17 cells (CD4+ IL-17+ T cells) and Treg (CD4+Foxp3+ T cells) in the inguinal lymph nodes (ILNs). (**A**) Single cell suspensions were collected from ILNs on day 42, followed by stimulation with anti-CD3+ for 96 h and then stained with anti-CD4, anti-IFN-γ, anti-IL-17A, or anti-Foxp3 Abs and analyzed by flow cytometry. Statistical analysis of the percentages of Th1, Th1, and Treg in the LN. (**B**) The mRNA relative expressions of specific transcription factors for different CD4+ T cells subsets were calculated by quantitative RT-PCR using the ΔΔ CT method with the normal control group as calibrator. Data are presented as mean ± SEM of 6 mice from one of three experiments. (*) $p < 0.05$, (**) $p < 0.01$, (***) $p < 0.001$ versus vehicle-treated CIA mice group (One Way ANOVA followed by Tukey's multiple comparison test).

2.5. Kurarinone Suppressed STAT1 and STAT3 Phosphorylations in the LN of Kurarinone-Treated Mice

STAT1 and STAT3 are crucial transcription factors for Th1 and Th17 differentiation, respectively. We, therefore, measured expression levels of p-STAT1, STAT1, p-STAT3, and STAT3 in drained lymph nodes using Western blotting. Notably, significantly higher expression of phosphorylated STAT1 and STAT3 was found in the lymph nodes of CIA mice, and kurarinone treatment significantly suppressed these phosphorylation events (Figure 5A,B).

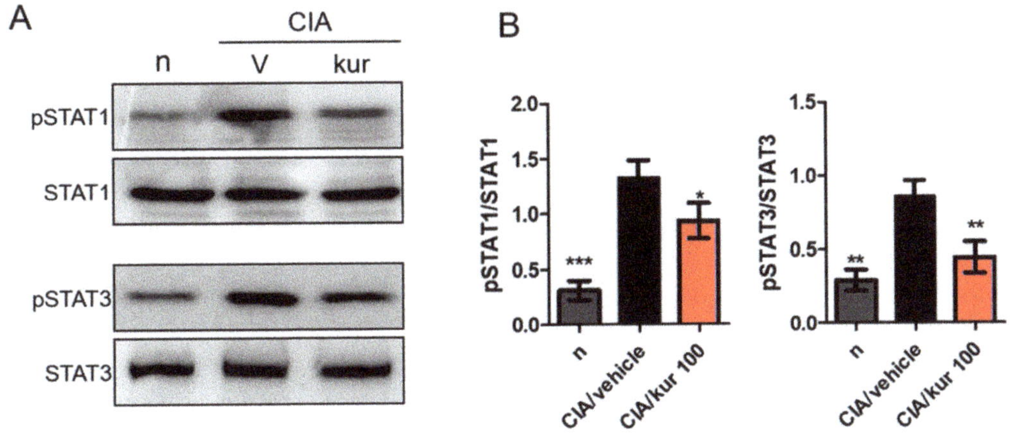

Figure 5. Effects of kurarinone on the phosphorylation of p-STAT1 and p-STAT3 in lymph nodes. Single cell suspensions were collected from ILNs on day 42, the protein expression levels of p-STAT1, STAT1, p-STAT3, and STAT3 were measured using Western blots. (**A**) Representative images of Western blot and (**B**) Densitometric analysis for protein expressions was performed using ImageJ software. Data are presented as mean ± SEM of 6 mice from one of three experiments. (*) $p < 0.05$, (**) $p < 0.01$, (***) $p < 0.001$ versus vehicle-treated CIA mice group (One Way ANOVA followed by Tukey's multiple comparison test).

2.6. Kurarinone Suppressed Joint Oxidative Stress and Increased the Activity of Antioxidant Enzymes in CIA Mice

It has been suggested that the release of free radicals and oxidizing agents, such as malondialdehyde (MDA) and hydrogen peroxide (H_2O_2), contributes to disease severity in RA. Therefore, we examined the effect of kurarinone treatment on oxidative stress in the joints of CIA mice. On day 42, MDA and H_2O_2 concentrations were drastically increased in the joints of vehicle-treated CIA mice, when compared with the control mice. This increase was significantly reversed by kurarinone treatment, as shown in Figure 6A,B. In line with this, the activity of antioxidant enzymes, like SOD and GSH-Px in paw tissues, significantly dropped in vehicle-treated CIA mice compared with control mice. Kurarinone treatment significantly increased the activity of these antioxidants when compared with vehicle-treated CIA mice (Figure 6C,D).

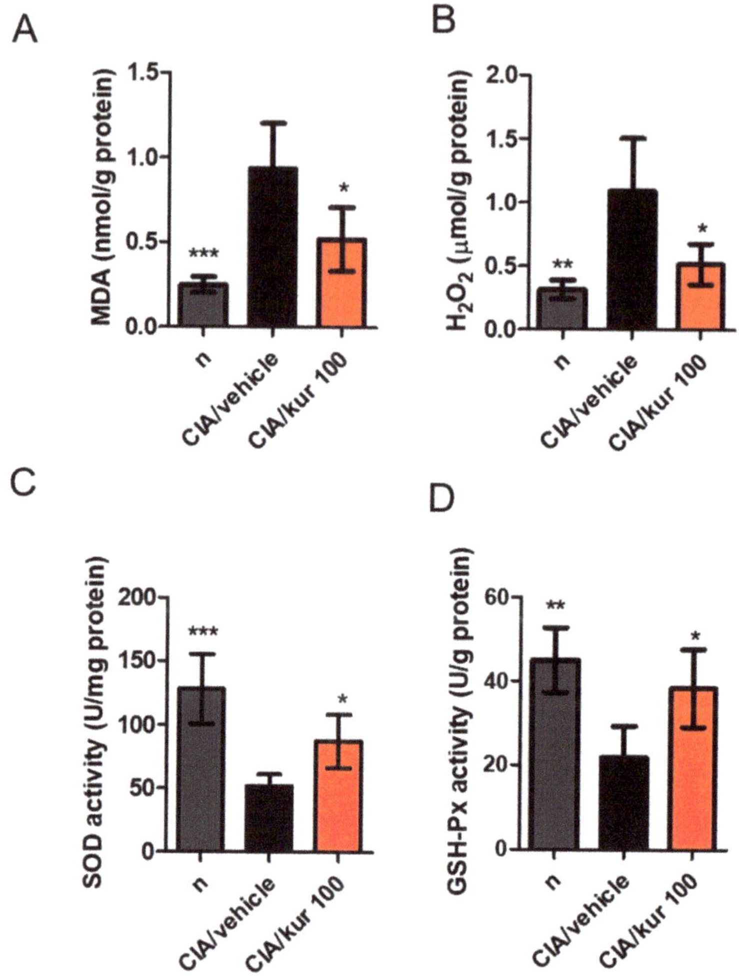

Figure 6. Effects of kurarinone on MDA, H_2O_2, SOD, and GSH-Px activities in paw tissues of CIA mice. On day 42, mice were sacrificed and the (**A**) MDA, (**B**) H_2O_2; (**C**) SOD, and (**D**) GSH-Px, expressions or activities in the paw tissues were measured as described in the methods and materials section. Data are presented as mean ± SEM of 6 mice from one of three experiments. (*) $p < 0.05$, (**) $p < 0.01$, (***) $p < 0.001$ versus vehicle-treated CIA mice group (One Way ANOVA followed by Tukey's multiple comparison test).

2.7. *Kurarinone Activated the Nrf2 Pathway in Paw Tissues of CIA Mice*

Nuclear factor, erythroid 2-like 2 (Nrf-2) is a transcription factor that plays a major role in cell protection against oxidative stress. It induces antioxidant enzymes that inactivate reactive oxygen species, like heme oxygenase-1 (HO-1), GPX, and CAT. Kurarinone is known to activate the KEAP1/Nrf2/HO-1 pathway to exert immunomodulatory effects [18]. Therefore, we further studied kurarinone's effects on expressions of Nrf2 and KEAP1 in the paw tissues of mice. We found that Nrf2 and HO-1 expressions were significantly higher in paw tissues of kuranionine-treated CIA mice (Figure 7A,B), whereas the KEAP1 expression was down-regulated. These findings suggest that Nrf2 might play an important role in the therapeutic effects of kuraninone in CIA mice.

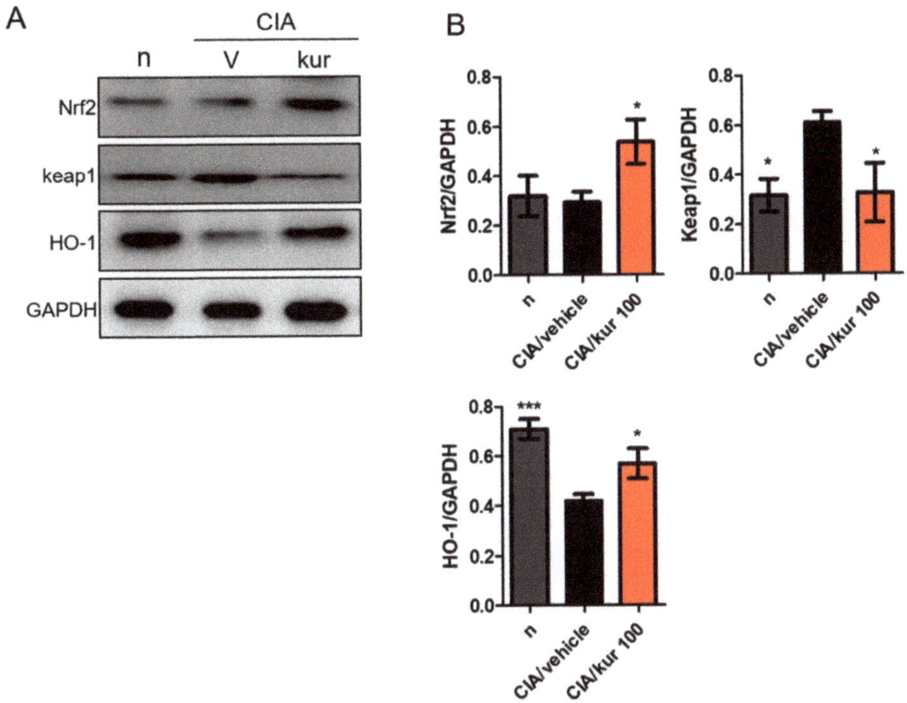

Figure 7. Effects of kurarinone on the expression of NRF2 pathway hind paw homogenates. Hind paws were collected on day 42, the protein expression levels of NRF2, Keap1, and HO-1 were measured using Western blots. (**A**) Representative images of Western blot and (**B**) Densitometric analysis for protein expressions was performed using ImageJ software. Data are presented as mean ± SEM of 6 mice from one of three experiments. (*) $p < 0.05$, (***) $p < 0.001$ versus vehicle-treated CIA mice group (One Way ANOVA followed by Tukey's multiple comparison test).

3. Discussion

Our present study is the first to demonstrate that kuraninone is therapeutically effective against CIA in a mouse animal model. The beneficial effects of kuraninone are evident by the amelioration of arthritic symptoms and histological improvements. The results are likely related to anti-inflammatory and antioxidant properties of kuraninone. The underlying mechanism includes the suppression of B and T cell responses and the elimination of oxidative stress through the up-regulation of Nrf2. Taken together, kuraninone is a potentially beneficial treatment for RA through a variety of mechanisms.

Kuraninone is a natural flavonone purified from Sophora *flavescens* Aiton, one of the traditional Chinese medicinal herbs. *Sophora flavescens* is known to have anti-inflammatory effects [20] and is used to treat inflammatory diseases such as ulcerative colitis [21], Behcet syndrome [22], arthritis [23], pulmonary fibrosis [24], asthma [25], and influenza infection [24]. Other studies have also reported anti-inflammatory effects of kuraninone through its potent inhibition of cyclooxygenase (COX)-1 [26]. Kurarinone also attenuates levels of inducible nitric oxide synthase-dependent NO, interleukin (IL)-1β. It also activates extracellular signal-regulated kinase (ERK)1/2, c-Jun N-terminal kinase (JNK), p38 MAP kinases, and nuclear factor kappa-light-chain-enhancer of activated B cells (NF-kB) in lipopolysaccharide (LPS)-stimulated RAW264.7 macrophages [18,27]. Key inflammatory cytokines (e.g., IFN-γ, IL-1α, IL-1β, IL-4, IL-6, IL-17A, IL-22, and TNF-α) and chemokines (e.g., CCL17, CCL20, CCL27, and CXCL1) are reduced by kurarinone in mice with autoimmune encephalomyelitis (EAE). Moreover, kuraninone inhibits Th1, Th2, and Th17 cell differentiation and proliferation, both in vitro and in vivo. These effects are likely related to its inhibition of EAE progression [15] and chronic inflammatory skin diseases such as psoriasis and contact dermatitis [16]. This study's results align with other reports readily available in the literature. Specifically, kuraninone exerted anti-inflammatory effects in CIA mice suppressed production of pro-inflammatory cytokines and anti-CII antibody, T cell activation, and lowered the proportions of Th1 and TH17 cells.

In addition, kuraninone is reported to have antioxidant properties in assays with 2,2′-azino-bis-3-ethylbenzothiazoline-6-sulfonic acid (ABTS), peroxynitrite ($ONOO^-$), and total ROS [28], and it inhibits oxidation of low-density lipoprotein [29]. Furthermore, treatment with kuraninone in cultured cells protects them against tert-butylhydroperoxide (t-BHP) and TNF-α/IFN-γ-induced intracellular ROS generation [16,28]. In terms of cytoprotection, KEAP1-Nrf2 pathway is the major regulatory mechanism of endogenous and exogenous oxidative stress [17]. To be noted, the treatment of prostate cancer PC3 cells with kuraninone downregulates the expression of KEAP1 and subsequently activates Nrf2, which increases the expression of heme oxygenase-1 (HO-1), an antioxidant enzyme [18]. However, this effect is not found in mouse hippocampal HT22 cells treated with kuraninone [30]. This study results in kuranionine-treated CIA mice having an upregulation of Nrf2 and HO-1, and downregulation of KEAP-1. Taken together, the antioxidative ability of kuraninone is evident. When examining the contribution of oxidative stress to the inflammatory response [31,32], these properties further enhance the anti-inflammatory effects of kuraninone.

A number of animal studies demonstrate the importance of pathogenic Th1 and Th17 cells in RA [33–35]. In addition, human studies reported similar findings early in disease progression. Higher levels of Th1 cells and IFN-γ are present in the synovial fluid and tissues in RA patients [36–38]. Other researchers also reported increased proportions of Th17 cells in the blood and bone marrow [39,40], and higher levels of IL-17 in the blood and joint fluid of RA patients [41–43]. Additionally, these levels correlate with disease progression. Based on these studies, abnormally upregulated Th1 and Th17 responses contribute to the generation of RA. Although mechanisms underlying the beneficial effects of kuraninone in CIA remain elusive, here we speculate that the therapeutic efficacy of kuraninone in CIA is partly due to the suppression of Th1 and Th17 responses. We further showed that kuraninone inhibited Th1 and Th17 responses in CIA mice via the suppression of STAT1 and STAT3 signaling, which in turn reduces T-bet and RORγt expression. Our results are compatible with reports on mouse CD4+ T cells, and human keratinocytes, and peripheral blood mononuclear cells, in which STAT1 and STAT3 activation is suppressed after kuraninone treatment [16].

In regards of T cell differentiation by kurarinone, macrophage is an antigen presenting cell that inevitably needs to be taken into consideration. While we did not provide further evidences related to macrophages, previous studies may have revealed several clues to illustrate the role of macrophages in regulating T cell functions under kurarinone treatment. It was shown that LPS activated murine macrophages, Raw 264.7 cells, to induce iNOS-dependent NO production and ROS generation as well as inflammatory cytokines, such as TNF-α, whereas kurarinone inhibited such activation via suppressing NFκB and mitogen-activated protein kinase pathways, subsequently inhibiting NO and ROS [27]. More recently, Nishikawa et al. also utilized LPS to stimulate RAW 264.7 cells and treated with kurarinone. They further confirmed that kurarione induced antioxidant enzymes, such as HO-1, to suppress iNOS and IL-1β production, rendering kurarinone being a potent antioxidant [18]. Kurarinone may also directly induce naïve T cell differentiation without the involvement of macrophages. Xie et al. purified naïve T cells and treated with kurarinone where they found that both Th1 and Th2 differentiation of T cells were dose-dependently inhibited by kurarinone [15]. Kurarinone was also shown to regulate JAK/STAT pathway to reduce the CD4 T cell differentiation [16]. Taken together, it would be reasonable to assume that kurarinone could likely inhibit T cell functions directly and indirectly through influencing macrophages.

Despite not being addressed in our study, previous studies have revealed the possible mechanisms in bone remodeling involved in RA pathogenesis. Wang et al. found that kurarinone could facilitate the differentiation of osteoblastic cells UMR 106 cells, promoting bone formation [44]. Also, a flavonoid, (2S)-2′-methoxykurarinone, which is highly similar to kurarinone in chemical structure and also abundant in *Sophora flavescent* roots, was shown by Kim et al. to downregulate the expression of receptor activator of nuclear factor-κB ligand (RANKL), subsequently inhibiting the RNAKL-induced osteoclast differentiation [45]. As a result, it is potential that kurarinone could influence the hemostasis of osteoclastogenesis and osteoblastogenesis in RA.

Kurarinone dosage used in this study showed no toxicity in mice based on body weight, behavior, and appearance [46]. Nevertheless, kuraninone has been reported to be hepatotoxic in rats [47,48]. Kurarinone could also accumulate in the liver and inhibit fatty acid β-oxidation, resulting in lipid accumulation and liver injury, a condition akin to hepatic steatosis [48]. While we have demonstrated that kurarinone can potentially ameliorate arthritic symptoms in this study, its toxicity should be thoroughly investigated before proceeding to any human studies.

4. Material and Methods

4.1. Animal Experiments

Female DBA/1J mice (20–22 g in weight) of eight-week-old were used. DBA/J strain mice were purchased from Jackson Laboratory (Bar Harbor, MA, USA) and were maintained under specific-pathogen-free (SPF) conditions with food and water ad libitum. All animals were treated in accordance with the Institutional Animal Care and Use Committee (IACUC) of National Chung Hsing University (NCHU), and the experiment was approved by the Committee on Animal Research and Care in NCHU (NO. 110030).

4.2. Establishment of CIA Animal Model and Experimental Grouping

The mouse model of collagen type II-induced arthritis (CIA) was used as described previously [49]. Briefly, chicken type II collagen (Chondrex, Inc., Woodinville, WA, USA) 2 mg/mL (dissolved in 10 mM acetic acid solution) was mixed with an equal volume of complete Freund's adjuvant (CFA) (Sigma-Aldrich, St. Louis, MO, USA) (containing *Mycobacterium tuberculosis* H37RA) and then emulsified via repeated aspiration in sterile tubes to form an emulsion of type II collagen. The mixture (100 μL/mouse) was intradermally injected on day 0 in the tail approximately 1.5 cm distal to the base. Twenty-one days later, an immunization second booster was given, using the same concentration of collagen II but this time prepared in incomplete Freund's adjuvant (IFA) (Sigma-Aldrich, MO, USA). Kurarinone was purchased from Sigma Aldrich Co. (MO, USA) and dissolved in the corn oil (Sigma-Aldrich, MO, USA)/DMSO (Santa Cruz Biotechnology Inc., Dallas, TX, USA) vehicle (v/v, 95/5). After 1-week adaptive breeding, all DBA1/J mice were randomly divided into three groups of equal numbers (n = 6) as: (1) normal/control group, in which each animal was administered a 100 μL of corn oil/DMSO from day 21 to day 41; (2) the CIA + vehicle group; and (3) the CIA + 100 mg/kg kurarinone group. We also administered 25 and 50 mg/kg kurarinone in CIA mice but no therapeutic effect was found (Supplementary Figure S2). The mice in groups 2 and 3 were then given either corn oil/DMSO or kurarinone via oral gavage (100 μL) every day from day 21 to day 41.

4.3. Mouse Arthritis Scoring System

The two investigators are specialists in these types of animal models and were blind to the experimental groupings from day 21 post-immunization. Arthritis assessment included items like erythema, edema, joint rigidity, and swelling levels of paws as measured with micro-calipers. Paw volumes were measured using a plethysmometer 37,140 (Ugo Basile SRL, Comerio, VA, Italy). The scoring of arthritis grades was based on a scale from 0 to 4, on all four paws of each animal as follows: 0: no swelling and redness; 1: the presence of redness/and or swelling of one joint or one digit; 2: the involvement of two joints; 3: more than two joints involved; 4: severe redness and swelling of the whole paw and all digits. The maximal arthritis score for each paw is 4, and therefore, the maximal total score is 16 for each animal.

4.4. Histological Analysis

Mice were sacrificed on day 42. Their knee joints were sectioned in the sagittal plane. Embedding knee joints into paraffin blocks to support the tissue structure. Blocks were cut into 5 μM thick sections, mounted onto microscope slides for analysis, and stained with hematoxylin and eosin (H&E). Histopathological changes of the joints and scoring of histopathological damages were determined under light microscopy, according to the previously defined parameters [50]. H&E sections were thus analyzed regarding the degree of cell infiltration, synovial hyperplasia, and cartilage destruction. The graded score for each feature ranged from 0 to 4 (0, no change; 1, mild change; 2, moderate change; 3, severe change; 4, total destruction of joint architecture). The maximum score for each knee was 8.

4.5. Measurement of Pro-Inflammatory Cytokine Levels

Paw tissues and serum from DBA/1 mice were collected by the end of day 42. Hind paws were homogenized in ice-cold saline using a tissue homogenizer (Mini-BeadBeater-1, BioSpec, Bartlesville, OK, USA) at 4800 rpm for 3 min. After centrifuging at 3000 rpm (4 °C, 10 min, twice), hind paw homogenates were harvested. Blood was withdrawn from the submandibular vein and centrifuged at 3000 rpm (4 °C, 10 min, twice) to collect serum. Levels of TNF-α, IL-6, IFN-γ, and IL-17A were measured in both serum and paw homogenates using murine ELISA kits (Biolegend, San Diego, CA, USA) according to the manufacturer's instructions.

4.6. Draining Lymph Node (dLN) Cells Proliferation Assay

DBA/1 mice were killed on day 42, and inguinal dLN cells (4×10^5 cells/well) were cultured with chicken CII (50 μg/mL) at 37 °C for 96 h, or with concanavalin A (ConA) (5 μg/mL) at 37 °C for 48 h. During the last 18 h of the incubation, cells were pulsed labeled with [^{3}H]-thymidine (1 μL Ci/well; NEN-DuPont, Boston, MA, USA) overnight, and radioactivity incorporation was assessed by liquid scintillation counting (Beckman Instruments, Palo Alto, CA, USA).

4.7. Fluorescence-Activated Cell Sorting (FACS)

Cell suspensions were prepared from lymph nodes obtained in sacrificed mice after 42 days. Cells (3×10^5) were seeded in a 60-mm dish and cultured with Con A (5 μg/mL) for 24 h. During the last 4 h of culture, 10 μg/mL brefeldin A was added. Afterwards, cells were trypsinized and washed in phosphate buffered saline (PBS), and cells so collected were stained with phycoerythrin- (PE-) anti-CD4 antibody for 45 min (BD Biosciences, San Diego, CA, USA), washed twice with 0.1 BSA in PBS. Cells were then permeabilized and fixed with cytofix/Cytoperm Plus solution (#51-2090KZ, BD Biosciences, San Diego, CA, USA) for 20 min. Finally, cells were stained with FITC-anti-IL-17A (#506907, Biolegend, San Diego, CA, USA), FITC-anti-IFN-γ (# RM9001, eBioscience, Waltham, MA, USA), and with anti-Foxp3 (#560407, eBioscience, Waltham, MA, USA). Cells were analyzed with the AccuriTM C5 cytometer (Accuri Cytometers, Ann Arbor, MI, USA) and data processed with the BD Accuri™ C6 Plus software.

4.8. Quantitative Real-Time (RT)-PCR Analysis

Cell suspensions were First prepared from lymph nodes of mice sacrificed after 42 days. Total RNA was extracted using Trizol reagent, and 2 μg of the RNA was RT reacted with an oligo-dT primer. Real-time PCR was carried out using the ABI 7500 Fast real-time detection system (Applied Biosystems; Thermo Fisher Scientific, Inc., Bangalore, IN, USA) with Fast SYBR™ Green Master Mix (Cat. No. 4385618, Applied Biosystems; Thermo Fisher Scientific, Woolston Warrington, UK). Cycling conditions were 95 °C for 10 min, followed by 40 cycles of 95 °C for 10 s, 60 °C for 30 s, and 72 °C for 30 s. For quantification, the target gene level was normalized to the internal standard gene, GAPDH. Primers used in the study are listed as below. RORγt forward, 5′-CCGCTGAGAGGGCTTCAC-3′, and reverse, 5′-TGCAGGAGTAGGCCA CATTACA-3′ [1]; T-bet, forward, 5′-GATCATCACCAAGCAGGGACG-3′, and reverse, 5′-TCCACACTGCACCCACTTGC-3′ [2]; Foxp3, 5′- CAAGTTCCACAACATGCGAC -3′ and reverse, 5′- ATTGAGTGTCCGCTGCTTCT-3′ [3]; Glyceraldehyde 3-phosphate dehydrogenase (GAPDH), forward, 5′–CGTGTTCCTACCCCCAATGT−3′and reverse, 5′ TGTCATCATACTTGGCAGGTTTCT−3′. All data were normalized against the expression level of GAPDH. The relative expression levels of genes in the experimental group were calculated with the ΔΔ CT method, and a water-treated control group acted as the calibrator.

4.9. Western Blot Analysis

Cells isolated from inguinal lymph nodes (ILNs) on day 42 were stimulated with Con A (5 μg/mL) (Sigma-Aldrich, St. Louis, MO, USA) for 6 h. These cells were harvested and cell pellets were lysed on ice in a RIPA buffer containing 1% protease inhibitor cocktail (Sigma-Aldrich, St. Louis, MO, USA). In addition, the hind paw tissues were homogenized in a 100 μL tissue RIPA lysis buffer for 30 min. Total protein concentration was measured with the bicinchoninic acid (BCA) assay kit (Thermo Fisher Scientific, Waltham, MA, USA). Normalized amounts of protein were separated on 10% SDS-PAGE at 100 V for 1.5 h, before transferring onto the polyvinylidene difluoride (PVDF) membrane (Millipore, Billerica, MA, USA) at 300 mA for 1 h. The membrane was blocked with BlockPRO™ Protein-Free Blocking Buffer for 1.5 h at room temperature and then incubated at 4 °C overnight with the following: anti-pSTAT1 (Cat# AF2894, R & D systems, Minneapolis, MN, USA), anti-STAT1 (Cat# 9172, Cell Signaling Technology, Danvers, MA, USA), anti-pSTAT3 (Cat# MAB1799, R & D systems, Minneapolis, MN, USA), anti-STAT3 (Cat# ab119352), anti-Nrf2 (Cat# ab89443), anti-keap1 (Cat# ab119403), anti-HO-1 (Cat# 223349) and glyceraldehyde 3-phosphate dehydrogenase (GAPDH) (Cat# ab8245, Abcam, Cambridge, MA, USA). Subsequently, the membrane was incubated with the appropriate secondary antibody, and immunoreactive bands were visualized using the LumiFlash™ Ultima Chemiluminescent substrate, HRP system (Visual protein, Taipei City, Taiwan; LF08–500). Each membrane was re-probed with the antibody against GAPDH as the internal control for an equal protein loading. The band density was analyzed with the ImageJ v1.47 program (Bethesda, Rockville, MD, USA).

4.10. Measurement of the Concentrations of Oxidative Markers

On day 42, the hind paw tissues were homogenized with 100 μL ice-cold tissue RIPA lysis buffer. The homogenate was incubated at 4 °C for 30 min and centrifuged at 12,000× *g* at 4 °C for 20 min. The supernatant was obtained as the total protein extract. Total protein concentration was measured with the bicinchoninic acid (BCA) assay kit.

The level of malondialdehyde (MDA) was determined with the Lipid Peroxidation (MDA) Assay Kit (Colorimetric/Fluorometric) (Cat# ab118970, Abcam, Cambridge, MA, USA) according to the manufacturer's instructions. Superoxide Dismutase (SOD) and glutathione peroxidase (GSH-Px) activities were determined with the Superoxide Dismutase (SOD) Colorimetric Activity Kit (Cat# EIASODC, Thermo Fisher Scientific, Waltham, MA, USA) and glutathione peroxidase ELISA Kit (Cat#11352, Cusabio Biotech Co., Ltd., Wuhan, China), all according to manufacturer's instructions. The amount of hydrogen peroxide (H_2O_2) was estimated using the Hydrogen Peroxide Assay Kit (ab102500, Abcam, Cambridge, MA, USA) according to the manufacturer's instructions.

4.11. Statistical Analysis

Numerical data were presented as mean ± SD. Comparisons among multiple treatments were Tukey's HSD (honest significant difference) test after one-way ANOVA or two-way ANOVA using GraphPad Prism (version 8 for Windows; GraphPad Software, La Jolla, CA, USA). Statistical significance was set at $p < 0.05$.

5. Conclusions

In conclusion, our results showed that kuraninone was a beneficial treatment against CIA development. Kuraninone exerted its therapeutic effects through the suppression of inflammatory cytokines and the modulation of B and T cell immune responses. Moreover, kuraninone's antioxidant properties further alleviated inflammation. Add-on kuraninone treatment could therefore be an alternative when treating RA patients. However, its use in conjunction with current RA therapies requires further studies.

Supplementary Materials: The following are available online at https://www.mdpi.com/article/10.3390/ijms22084002/s1, Figure S1: Frequencies of IFN-γ+CD4+ (Th1), IL-17A+CD4+ (Th17) and Foxp3+CD4+ (Treg) in the inguinal lymph nodes (ILNs), Figure S2: Effects of kurarinone (25 and 50 mg/kg) on the severity of CIA.

Author Contributions: C.-C.L., J.-H.W. and S.-C.L. carried out animal experimental work. C.-C.L., S.-W.T. and K.-T.T. designed the experimental work and data analysis. C.-C.L., S.-W.T. and K.-T.T. wrote the paper and data analysis. All authors have read and agreed to the published version of the manuscript.

Funding: This study was financially supported by the iEGG and Animal Biotechnology Center from the Feature Areas Research Center Program within the framework of the Higher Education Sprout Project by the Taiwan Ministry of Education (MOE-107-S-0023-E) and Buddhist Tzu Chi Medical Foundation (TTCRD-110-06).

Institutional Review Board Statement: All animals were treated in accordance with the Institutional Animal Care and Use Committee (IACUC) of National Chung Hsing University (NCHU), and the experiment was approved by the Committee on Animal Research and Care in NCHU (NO. 11030).

Informed Consent Statement: Not applicable.

Data Availability Statement: The data that support the findings of this study are available from the corresponding author upon reasonable request.

Acknowledgments: We thank Nicole Bracci from Department of Biomedical Sciences & Pathobiology, Virginia Tech, for useful comments and language editing which have greatly improved the manuscript.

Conflicts of Interest: The authors declare no conflict of interest.

References

1. Smolen, J.S.; Aletaha, D.; Barton, A.; Burmester, G.R.; Emery, P.; Firestein, G.S.; Kavanaugh, A.; McInnes, I.B.; Solomon, D.H.; Strand, V.; et al. Rheumatoid arthritis. *Nat. Rev. Dis. Primers* **2018**, *4*, 18001. [CrossRef] [PubMed]
2. Rao, D.A.; Gurish, M.F.; Marshall, J.L.; Slowikowski, K.; Fonseka, K.S.C.Y.; Liu, Y.; Donlin, L.T.; Henderson, L.A.; Wei, K.; Mizoguchi, F.; et al. Pathologically expanded peripheral T helper cell subset drives B cells in rheumatoid arthritis. *Nature* **2017**, *542*, 110–114. [CrossRef] [PubMed]
3. Du Montcel, S.T.; Michou, L.; Petit-Teixeira, E.; Osorio, J.; Lemaire, I.; Lasbleiz, S.; Pierlot, C.; Quillet, P.; Bardin, T.; Prum, B.; et al. New classification of HLA-DRB1 alleles supports the shared epitope hypothesis of rheumatoid arthritis susceptibility. *Arthritis Rheum.* **2005**, *52*, 1063–1068. [CrossRef] [PubMed]
4. Kinloch, A.; Lundberg, K.; Wait, R.; Wegner, N.; Lim, N.H.; Zendman, A.J.; Saxne, T.; Malmstrom, V.; Venables, P.J. Synovial fluid is a site of citrullination of autoantigens in inflammatory arthritis. *Arthritis Rheum.* **2008**, *58*, 2287–2295. [CrossRef]
5. Adamopoulos, I.E.; Mellins, E.D. Alternative pathways of osteoclastogenesis in inflammatory arthritis. *Nat. Rev. Rheumatol.* **2015**, *11*, 189–194. [CrossRef]
6. Goldring, S.R. Pathogenesis of bone erosions in rheumatoid arthritis. *Curr. Opin. Rheumatol.* **2002**, *14*, 406–410. [CrossRef]
7. Sarkar, S.; Cooney, L.A.; Fox, D.A. The role of T helper type 17 cells in inflammatory arthritis. *Clin. Exp. Immunol.* **2010**, *159*, 225–237. [CrossRef]
8. Hitchon, C.A.; El-Gabalawy, H.S. Oxidation in rheumatoid arthritis. *Arthritis Res. Ther.* **2004**, *6*, 265–278. [CrossRef]
9. Westman, E.; Lundberg, K.; Erlandsson Harris, H. Arthritogenicity of collagen type II is increased by chlorination. *Clin. Exp. Immunol.* **2006**, *145*, 339–345. [CrossRef]

10. da Fonseca, L.J.S.; Nunes-Souza, V.; Goulart, M.O.F.; Rabelo, L.A. Oxidative Stress in Rheumatoid Arthritis: What the Future Might Hold regarding Novel Biomarkers and Add-On Therapies. *Oxidative Med. Cell. Longev.* **2019**, *2019*, 7536805. [CrossRef]
11. Kourbeti, I.S.; Ziakas, P.D.; Mylonakis, E. Biologic therapies in rheumatoid arthritis and the risk of opportunistic infections: A meta-analysis. *Clin. Infect. Dis.* **2014**, *58*, 1649–1657. [CrossRef]
12. Caporali, R.; Caprioli, M.; Bobbio-Pallavicini, F.; Montecucco, C. DMARDS and infections in rheumatoid arthritis. *Autoimmun. Rev.* **2008**, *8*, 139–143. [CrossRef]
13. Aithal, G.P. Hepatotoxicity related to antirheumatic drugs. *Nat. Rev. Rheumatol.* **2011**, *7*, 139–150. [CrossRef]
14. Upchurch, K.S.; Kay, J. Evolution of treatment for rheumatoid arthritis. *Rheumatology* **2012**, *51*, vi28–vi36. [CrossRef]
15. Xie, L.; Gong, W.; Chen, J.; Xie, H.W.; Wang, M.; Yin, X.P.; Wu, W. The flavonoid kurarinone inhibits clinical progression of EAE through inhibiting Th1 and Th17 cell differentiation and proliferation. *Int. Immunopharmacol.* **2018**, *62*, 227–236. [CrossRef]
16. Kim, B.H.; Na, K.M.; Oh, I.; Song, I.H.; Lee, Y.S.; Shin, J.; Kim, T.Y. Kurarinone regulates immune responses through regulation of the JAK/STAT and TCR-mediated signaling pathways. *Biochem. Pharmacol.* **2013**, *85*, 1134–1144. [CrossRef]
17. Kansanen, E.; Kuosmanen, S.M.; Leinonen, H.; Levonen, A.L. The Keap1-Nrf2 pathway: Mechanisms of activation and dysregulation in cancer. *Redox Biol.* **2013**, *1*, 45–49. [CrossRef]
18. Nishikawa, S.; Inoue, Y.; Hori, Y.; Miyajima, C.; Morishita, D.; Ohoka, N.; Hida, S.; Makino, T.; Hayashi, H. Anti-Inflammatory Activity of Kurarinone Involves Induction of HO-1 via the KEAP1/Nrf2 Pathway. *Antioxidants* **2020**, *9*, 842. [CrossRef]
19. Brand, D.D.; Latham, K.A.; Rosloniec, E.F. Collagen-induced arthritis. *Nat. Protoc.* **2007**, *2*, 1269–1275. [CrossRef]
20. Zhu, N.; Hou, J. Molecular mechanism of the anti-inflammatory effects of Sophorae Flavescentis Aiton identified by network pharmacology. *Sci. Rep.* **2021**, *11*, 1005. [CrossRef]
21. Chen, M.; Ding, Y.; Tong, Z. Efficacy and Safety of Sophora flavescens (Kushen) Based Traditional Chinese Medicine in the Treatment of Ulcerative Colitis: Clinical Evidence and Potential Mechanisms. *Front. Pharmacol.* **2020**, *11*, 603476. [CrossRef]
22. Ma, Q.H.; Ren, M.Y.; Luo, J.B. San Wu Huangqin decoction regulates inflammation and immune dysfunction induced by influenza virus by regulating the NF-κB signaling pathway in H1N1-infected mice. *J. Ethnopharmacol.* **2021**, *264*, 112800. [CrossRef]
23. Jin, J.H.; Kim, J.S.; Kang, S.S.; Son, K.H.; Chang, H.W.; Kim, H.P. Anti-inflammatory and anti-arthritic activity of total flavonoids of the roots of Sophora flavescens. *J. Ethnopharmacol.* **2010**, *127*, 589–595. [CrossRef]
24. Gao, Y.; Yao, L.F.; Zhao, Y.; Wei, L.M.; Guo, P.; Yu, M.; Cao, B.; Li, T.; Chen, H.; Zou, Z.M. The Chinese Herbal Medicine Formula mKG Suppresses Pulmonary Fibrosis of Mice Induced by Bleomycin. *Int. J. Mol. Sci.* **2016**, *17*, 238. [CrossRef]
25. Yu, M.; Jia, H.M.; Cui, F.X.; Yang, Y.; Zhao, Y.; Yang, M.H.; Zou, Z.M. The Effect of Chinese Herbal Medicine Formula mKG on Allergic Asthma by Regulating Lung and Plasma Metabolic Alternations. *Int. J. Mol. Sci.* **2017**, *18*, 602. [CrossRef]
26. Chi, Y.S.; Jong, H.G.; Son, K.H.; Chang, H.W.; Kang, S.S.; Kim, H.P. Effects of naturally occurring prenylated flavonoids on enzymes metabolizing arachidonic acid: Cyclooxygenases and lipoxygenases. *Biochem. Pharmacol.* **2001**, *62*, 1185–1191. [CrossRef]
27. Han, J.M.; Jin, Y.Y.; Kim, H.Y.; Park, K.H.; Lee, W.S.; Jeong, T.S. Lavandulyl flavonoids from Sophora flavescens suppress lipopolysaccharide-induced activation of nuclear factor-κB and mitogen-activated protein kinases in RAW264.7 cells. *Biol. Pharm. Bull.* **2010**, *33*, 1019–1023. [CrossRef]
28. Jung, H.A.; Jeong, D.M.; Chung, H.Y.; Lim, H.A.; Kim, J.Y.; Yoon, N.Y.; Choi, J.S. Re-evaluation of the antioxidant prenylated flavonoids from the roots of Sophora flavescens. *Biol. Pharm. Bull.* **2008**, *31*, 908–915. [CrossRef]
29. Jeong, T.S.; Ryu, Y.B.; Kim, H.Y.; Curtis-Long, M.J.; An, S.; Lee, J.H.; Lee, W.S.; Park, K.H. Low density lipoprotein (LDL)-antioxidant flavonoids from roots of Sophora flavescens. *Biol. Pharm. Bull.* **2008**, *31*, 2097–2102. [CrossRef]
30. Jeong, G.S.; Li, B.; Lee, D.S.; Byun, E.; An, R.B.; Pae, H.O.; Chung, H.T.; Youn, K.H.; Kim, Y.C. Lavandulyl flavanones from Sophora flavescens protect mouse hippocampal cells against glutamate-induced neurotoxicity via the induction of heme oxygenase-1. *Biol. Pharm. Bull.* **2008**, *31*, 1964–1967. [CrossRef]
31. Zuo, L.; Zhou, T.; Pannell, B.K.; Ziegler, A.C.; Best, T.M. Biological and physiological role of reactive oxygen species—The good, the bad and the ugly. *Acta Physiol.* **2015**, *214*, 329–348. [CrossRef] [PubMed]
32. Wojcik, P.; Gegotek, A.; Zarkovic, N.; Skrzydlewska, E. Oxidative Stress and Lipid Mediators Modulate Immune Cell Functions in Autoimmune Diseases. *Int. J. Mol. Sci.* **2021**, *22*, 723. [CrossRef] [PubMed]
33. Hashimoto, M. Th17 in Animal Models of Rheumatoid Arthritis. *J. Clin. Med.* **2017**, *6*, 73. [CrossRef] [PubMed]
34. Chen, H.L.; Lin, S.C.; Li, S.; Tang, K.T.; Lin, C.C. Alantolactone alleviates collagen-induced arthritis and inhibits Th17 cell differentiation through modulation of STAT3 signalling. *Pharm. Biol.* **2021**, *59*, 134–145. [CrossRef]
35. Zhang, J.; Hu, X.; Dong, X.; Chen, W.; Zhang, L.; Chang, Y.; Wu, Y.; Wei, W. Regulation of T Cell Activities in Rheumatoid Arthritis by the Novel Fusion Protein IgD-Fc-Ig. *Front. Immunol.* **2020**, *11*, 755. [CrossRef]
36. Miltenburg, A.M.; van Laar, J.M.; de Kuiper, R.; Daha, M.R.; Breedveld, F.C. T cells cloned from human rheumatoid synovial membrane functionally represent the Th1 subset. *Scand. J. Immunol.* **1992**, *35*, 603–610. [CrossRef]
37. Dolhain, R.J.; van der Heiden, A.N.; ter Haar, N.T.; Breedveld, F.C.; Miltenburg, A.M. Shift toward T lymphocytes with a T helper 1 cytokine-secretion profile in the joints of patients with rheumatoid arthritis. *Arthritis Rheum.* **1996**, *39*, 1961–1969. [CrossRef]
38. Dolhain, R.J.; ter Haar, N.T.; Hoefakker, S.; Tak, P.P.; de Ley, M.; Claassen, E.; Breedveld, F.C.; Miltenburg, A.M. Increased expression of interferon (IFN)-gamma together with IFN-gamma receptor in the rheumatoid synovial membrane compared with synovium of patients with osteoarthritis. *Rheumatology* **1996**, *35*, 24–32. [CrossRef]

39. Li, S.; Yin, H.; Zhang, K.; Wang, T.; Yang, Y.; Liu, X.; Chang, X.; Zhang, M.; Yan, X.; Ren, Y.; et al. Effector T helper cell populations are elevated in the bone marrow of rheumatoid arthritis patients and correlate with disease severity. *Sci. Rep.* **2017**, *7*, 4776. [CrossRef]
40. Shen, H.; Goodall, J.C.; Hill Gaston, J.S. Frequency and phenotype of peripheral blood Th17 cells in ankylosing spondylitis and rheumatoid arthritis. *Arthritis Rheum.* **2009**, *60*, 1647–1656. [CrossRef]
41. Dhaouadi, T.; Chahbi, M.; Haouami, Y.; Sfar, I.; Abdelmoula, L.; Ben Abdallah, T.; Gorgi, Y. IL-17A, IL-17RC polymorphisms and IL17 plasma levels in Tunisian patients with rheumatoid arthritis. *PLoS ONE* **2018**, *13*, e0194883. [CrossRef]
42. Kotake, S.; Udagawa, N.; Takahashi, N.; Matsuzaki, K.; Itoh, K.; Ishiyama, S.; Saito, S.; Inoue, K.; Kamatani, N.; Gillespie, M.T.; et al. IL-17 in synovial fluids from patients with rheumatoid arthritis is a potent stimulator of osteoclastogenesis. *J. Clin. Investig.* **1999**, *103*, 1345–1352. [CrossRef]
43. Ziolkowska, M.; Koc, A.; Luszczykiewicz, G.; Ksiezopolska-Pietrzak, K.; Klimczak, E.; Chwalinska-Sadowska, H.; Maslinski, W. High levels of IL-17 in rheumatoid arthritis patients: IL-15 triggers in vitro IL-17 production via cyclosporin A-sensitive mechanism. *J. Immunol.* **2000**, *164*, 2832–2838. [CrossRef]
44. Wang, X.; Zhen, L.; Zhang, G.; Wong, M.S.; Qin, L.; Yao, X. Osteogenic effects of flavonoid aglycones from an osteoprotective fraction of Drynaria fortunei—An in vitro efficacy study. *Phytomedicine* **2011**, *18*, 868–872. [CrossRef]
45. Kim, J.Y.; Kim, J.Y.; Kim, J.J.; Oh, J.; Kim, Y.C.; Lee, M.S. (2S)-2′-Methoxykurarinone inhibits osteoclastogenesis and bone resorption through down-regulation of RANKL signaling. *Biol. Pharm. Bull.* **2014**, *37*, 255–261. [CrossRef]
46. Yang, J.; Chen, H.; Wang, Q.; Deng, S.; Huang, M.; Ma, X.; Song, P.; Du, J.; Huang, Y.; Wen, Y.; et al. Inhibitory Effect of Kurarinone on Growth of Human Non-small Cell Lung Cancer: An Experimental Study Both in Vitro and in Vivo Studies. *Front. Pharmacol.* **2018**, *9*, 252. [CrossRef]
47. Yu, Q.; Cheng, N.; Ni, X. Identifying 2 prenylflavanones as potential hepatotoxic compounds in the ethanol extract of Sophora flavescens. *J. Food Sci.* **2013**, *78*, T1830–T1834. [CrossRef]
48. Jiang, P.; Zhang, X.; Huang, Y.; Cheng, N.; Ma, Y. Hepatotoxicity Induced by Sophora flavescens and Hepatic Accumulation of Kurarinone, a Major Hepatotoxic Constituent of Sophora flavescens in Rats. *Molecules* **2017**, *22*, 1809. [CrossRef]
49. Chuang, C.H.; Cheng, Y.-C.; Lin, S.-C.; Lehman, C.W.; Wang, S.-P.; Chen, D.-Y.; Tsai, S.-W.; Lin, C.-C. Atractylodin Suppresses Dendritic Cell Maturation and Ameliorates Collagen-Induced Arthritis in a Mouse Model. *J. Agric. Food Chem.* **2019**, *67*, 6773–6784. [CrossRef]
50. McCann, F.E.; Perocheau, D.P.; Ruspi, G.; Blazek, K.; Davies, M.L.; Feldmann, M.; Dean, J.L.; Stoop, A.A.; Williams, R.O. Selective tumor necrosis factor receptor I blockade is antiinflammatory and reveals immunoregulatory role of tumor necrosis factor receptor II in collagen-induced arthritis. *Arthritis Rheumatol.* **2014**, *66*, 2728–2738. [CrossRef]

International Journal of *Molecular Sciences*

MDPI

Article

Berberine Delays Onset of Collagen-Induced Arthritis through T Cell Suppression

Alexandra A. Vita [1], Hend Aljobaily [2], David O. Lyons [1] and Nicholas A. Pullen [1,*]

1 School of Biological Sciences, University of Northern Colorado, Greeley, CO 80639, USA; alexandra.vita@unco.edu (A.A.V.); david.lyons@unco.edu (D.O.L.)
2 Department of Applied Statistics and Research Methods, University of Northern Colorado, Greeley, CO 80639, USA; aljo5297@bears.unco.edu
* Correspondence: nicholas.pullen@unco.edu; Tel.: +1-(970)-351-1843; Fax: +1-(970)-351-2335

Abstract: There is evidence that berberine (BBR), a clinically relevant plant compound, ameliorates clinically apparent collagen-induced arthritis (CIA) in vivo. However, to date, there are no studies involving the use of BBR which explore its prophylactic potential in this model of rheumatoid arthritis (RA). The aim of this study was to determine if prophylactic BBR use during the preclinical phase of collagen-induced arthritis would delay arthritic symptom onset, and to characterize the cellular mechanism underlying such an effect. DBA/1J mice were injected with an emulsion of bovine type II collagen (CII) and complete Freund's adjuvant (day 0) and a booster injection of CII in incomplete Freund's adjuvant (day 18) to induce arthritis. Mice were then given i.p. injections of 1 mg/kg/day of BBR or PBS (vehicle with 0.01% DMSO) from days 0 to 28, were left untreated (CIA control), or were in a non-arthritic control group (n = 15 per group). Incidence of arthritis in BBR-treated mice was 50%, compared to 90% in both the CIA and PBS controls. Populations of B and T cells from the spleens and draining lymph nodes of mice were examined on day 14 (n = 5 per group) and day 28 (n = 10 per group). BBR-treated mice had significantly reduced populations of $CD4^{+}T_{h}$ and $CD4^{+}CXCR5^{+}$ T_{fh} cells, and an increased proportion of $Foxp3^{+}$ T_{reg} at days 14 and 28, as well as reduced expression of co-stimulatory molecules CD28 and CD154 at both endpoints. The effect seen on T cell populations and co-stimulatory molecule expression in BBR-treated mice was not mirrored in $CD19^{+}$ B cells. Additionally, BBR-treated mice experienced reduced anti-CII IgG2a and anti-CII total IgG serum concentrations. These results indicate a potential role for BBR as a prophylactic supplement for RA, and that its effect may be mediated specifically through T cell suppression. However, the cellular effector involved raises concern for BBR prophylactic use in the context of vaccine efficacy and other primary adaptive immune responses.

Keywords: arthritis; berberine; RA; autoimmune; T cell; T_{fh} cell

Citation: Vita, A.A.; Aljobaily, H.; Lyons, D.O.; Pullen, N.A. Berberine Delays Onset of Collagen-Induced Arthritis through T Cell Suppression. *Int. J. Mol. Sci.* **2021**, *22*, 3522. https://doi.org/10.3390/ijms22073522

Academic Editor: Chih-Hsin Tang

Received: 9 February 2021
Accepted: 22 March 2021
Published: 29 March 2021

1. Introduction

Rheumatoid arthritis (RA) is a systemic autoimmune disease typically characterized by chronic inflammation and deterioration within the joints. Extra-articular and systemic manifestations can also be present depending on the severity of the disease, and some individuals may experience damage to organs such as the heart, lungs, kidneys, and skin [1]. To date, there are a number of well-described treatments available for clinically apparent RA. Of these treatments, conventional disease-modifying antirheumatic drugs (DMARDs) and biological DMARDs, also known as biologics, are the most effective for long-term management of RA. However, the effectiveness of these treatments at managing disease progression varies among patients [1], and can be influenced by genetic factors [2,3] and the duration of symptoms prior to the first treatment [4–6]. Such interpatient variability in terms of response to medication can interfere with a patient's ability to achieve remission and/or the desired level of disease activity, and can also interfere with a patient's ability to adhere to a treatment regimen due to reasons of toxicity, lack of efficacy, and/or high cost [7–10].

Due to the large physiological and economic burden this disease places on its patients, research has become increasingly focused on ways to identify and develop effective preventative treatments targeting RA during the pre-clinical phase of the disease and thereby delay the onset of clinical RA [6,11–13]. The pre-clinical phase is commonly defined as the stage of the disease in which an individual experiences local or systemic autoimmunity, evidenced by serological abnormalities (e.g., high levels of CRP, TNF-α, etc.) and/or autoantibodies (e.g., anti-cyclic citrullinated peptide (ACPA), rheumatoid factor (RF), etc.) in the absence of clinical arthritis [13,14]. Targeting individuals in the pre-clinical phase of the disease with preventative therapies would provide the earliest initiation of treatment possible and could halt disease progression prior to significant joint damage. Furthermore, since the inflammatory load is far less in patients in the pre-clinical phase than in patients experiencing clinical arthritis, it presents an opportunity to potentially use lower-cost, broader spectrum complementary therapies that may be less affected by interpatient variability than conventional DMARDs and biologics, which act through specific, targeted pathways.

Berberine (BBR) is a plant-derived isoquinoline alkaloid found in the roots, rhizomes, and stem bark of plants among a variety of genera, such as *Berberis* (its namesake), *Mahonia*, *Hydrastis*, and *Coptis*, among others. BBR merits further exploration as a potential prophylactic therapy as it has already proved to be of importance for a variety of diseases through successful clinical trials [15–21]. As such, much is already known about the general toxicology and common side effects of BBR in humans, which are considered to be mild (e.g., diarrhea, flatulence, abdominal pain, and nausea), and do not occur in all patients [15,17,18,22]; there were no adverse effects observed on liver and kidney function [17,18,23]. Notably, amelioration of side effects in patients was reported once the dosage was lowered [18].

As an anti-inflammatory, BBR successfully suppresses the inflammatory responses involved in clinically apparent autoimmune diseases in vivo such as collagen-induced arthritis (CIA; a rodent model of RA) [24–27], type I diabetes mellitus [28], ulcerative colitis (UC) [29,30], and experimental autoimmune encephalomyelitis (EAE) [31]. In regard to RA specifically, BBR has been successful at treating clinically apparent CIA and other RA animal models in vivo through a number of suggested mechanisms, such as (**a**) dendritic cell apoptosis [24], (**b**) interference with MAPK signaling via inhibition of p-ERK, p-38, and p-JNK [25,32], (**c**) attenuation of T_h17 activity via inducing cortistatin in the gut [27], (**d**) restoration of the balance between T_{reg}/T_h17 cells [26], (**e**) the suppression of T_h17 differentiation/proliferation through inhibition of CD169 and the RORγt transcription factor, (**f**) induction of T_{reg} differentiation through aryl hydrocarbon receptor (AhR) activation [33], (**g**) and promotion of anti-inflammatory M2 macrophage polarization through upregulation of p-AMPK and inhibition of HIF1α [34]. A more detailed account of the anti-inflammatory actions of BBR in the context of rheumatoid arthritis can be found in the recent review by Shen et al. (2020) [35].

Despite evidence that BBR ameliorates clinically apparent CIA, to date there are no studies involving the use of BBR which explore its prophylactic, pre-clinical potential in a CIA mouse model. Thus, we examined such effects in a CIA mouse model with DBA/1J mice to determine whether or not BBR merits further exploratory analysis as a prophylactic treatment for patients in the pre-clinical phase of RA. The main highlights from this study are:

1. Berberine delays the onset of collagen-induced arthritis in DBA/1J mice.
2. Berberine treatment reduces splenic and lymph node CXCR5$^+$ follicular T helper (T_{fh}) cell populations.
3. Berberine polarizes splenic and lymph node T cells toward a CD25+ Foxp3+ regulatory (T_{reg}) phenotype.

2. Results

2.1. Berberine Treatment Delays Onset of CIA

To assess BBR's ability to delay the onset of clinical CIA, mice were observed daily for signs of redness and joint swelling as an indication of arthritis development, and severity of arthritis was scored on a scale of 0–16 as previously described. When mice were euthanized on day 28, we observed a significant reduction in absolute incidence of arthritis in the BBR group compared to the CIA and PBS controls (Figure 1A). About 90% of mice in both the CIA and PBS control groups developed arthritis, compared to 50% in the BBR group. In mice who developed arthritis, however, there was a trend but no significant difference in severity (Figure 1B).

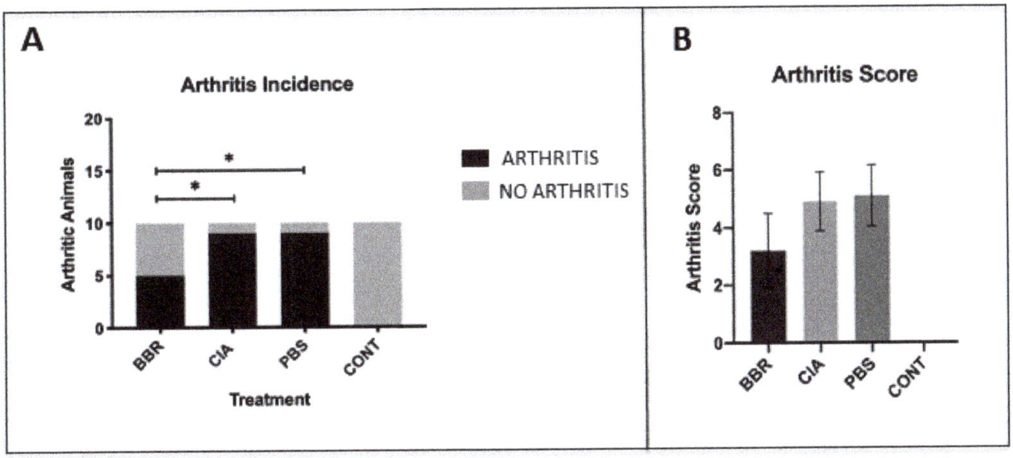

Figure 1. Assessment of collagen-induced arthritis (CIA) in DBA/1J mice in the context of berberine (BBR) treatment. (**A**) Absolute incidence of arthritis (proportions of animals with score ≥2) among treatment groups at day 28 compared using X^2 ($n = 10$ per group, * $p < 0.05$). Incidence proportions were BBR = 50%, CIA = 90%, PBS = 90%, and CONT = 0%. (**B**) Arthritis score, on a scale of 0–16 per manufacturer's protocol (as described in Materials and Methods), of mice at day 28 treated with BBR (1 mg/kg/day), volume-matched 1X PBS with 0.01% DMSO (PBS vehicle control), or no treatment (CIA control). Multiple comparisons conducted using the Kruskal–Wallis test with Dunn's multiple comparisons ($n = 10$ per group).

2.2. The Effect of Berberine on Circulating Anti-CII IgG in the CIA Model

To determine if BBR prophylactic treatment reduces autoantibody production, serum concentrations of anti-CII total IgG, anti-CII IgG1, and anti-CII IgG2a autoantibodies were measured at the day 28 endpoint. The BBR group saw significantly reduced serum concentrations of anti-CII IgG2a and anti-CII total compared to both CIA and PBS controls, although there was no significant difference in anti-CII IgG1 in BBR mice compared to CIA control mice (Figure 2A). To further examine if the aforementioned results were an artifact of including both arthritic and non-arthritic mice in the dataset, comparisons of just arthritic mice were performed. In this comparison, levels of anti-CII IgG2a among arthritic mice in the BBR group remained significantly reduced compared to CIA and PBS controls (Figure 2B). When comparing anti-CII IgG levels between arthritic and non-arthritic mice within the BBR group specifically, anti-CI IgG1, IgG2a, and total IgG were all significantly reduced in the non-arthritic mice compared to those who developed arthritis (Figure 2C). Additionally, there appeared to be a vehicle-specific effect on circulating anti-CII IgG in which the administration of PBS with 0.01% DMSO elicited elevated levels of anti-CII IgG1 and total IgG in vehicle control mice (Figure 2A,B).

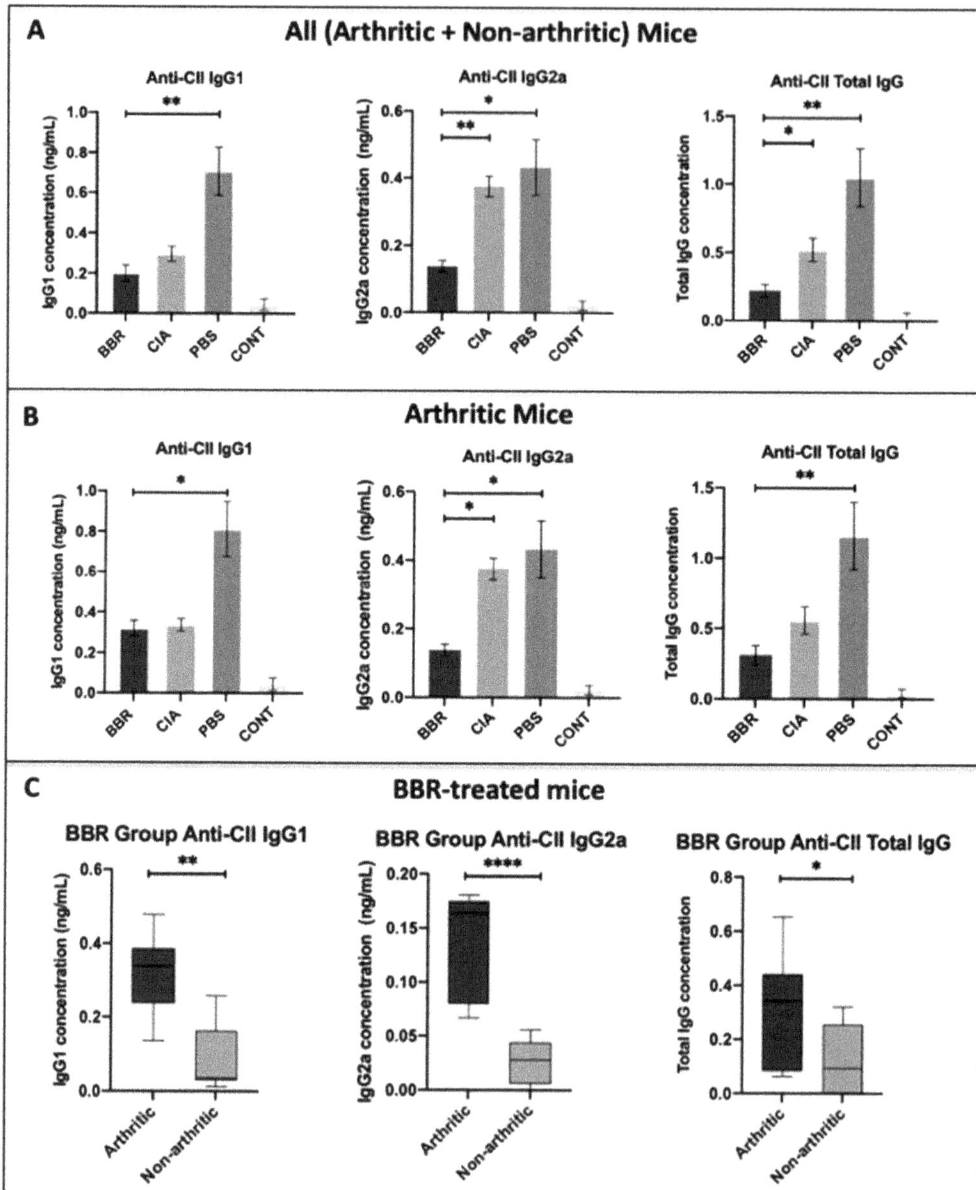

Figure 2. The effect of berberine on circulating anti-bovine type II collagen (CII) IgG in the CIA model. (**A**) Anti-CII IgG1, IgG2a, and total IgG at day 28 among all mice (arthritic and non-arthritic) within BBR, PBS (vehicle control), CIA (no treatment control), and non-CIA control animals (n = 10 per group). (**B**) Anti-CII IgG levels at day 28 compared among arthritic mice only (BBR n = 5; PBS n = 9; CIA n = 9). Statistical comparisons made with the Kruskal–Wallis test with Dunn's multiple comparisons. (**C**) Anti-CII IgG levels at day 28 compared among BBR-treated mice who developed arthritis ("arthritic") vs. those that did not ("non-arthritic"). Statistical comparisons made with the Mann–Whitney U test. For all statistical tests in Figure 2A–C, * $p < 0.05$, ** $p < 0.01$, **** $p < 0.0001$.

2.3. Key CD4⁺T Cell Population and Co-Stimulatory Molecule Characteristics in Response to Berberine Treatment

On day 14, we observed a significant reduction in populations of both $CD4^{+}$T cells and $CXCR5^{+}T_{fh}$ cells in the LNs and spleen of BBR-treated mice (Figure 3A,B), as well as a reduction in the expression of CD28 and CD154 on $CD4^{+}$T cells in the spleen and LNs of BBR-treated mice (Figure 4A,B). By the day 28 experimental endpoint, we continued to observe a significant reduction in $CD4^{+}$T cells and $CXCR5^{+}T_{fh}$ cells in the spleen and LNs of BBR-treated mice (Figure 3C,D), as well as decreased expression of CD28 and CD154 on the $CD4^{+}$T cells of BBR-treated mice (Figure 4C,D).

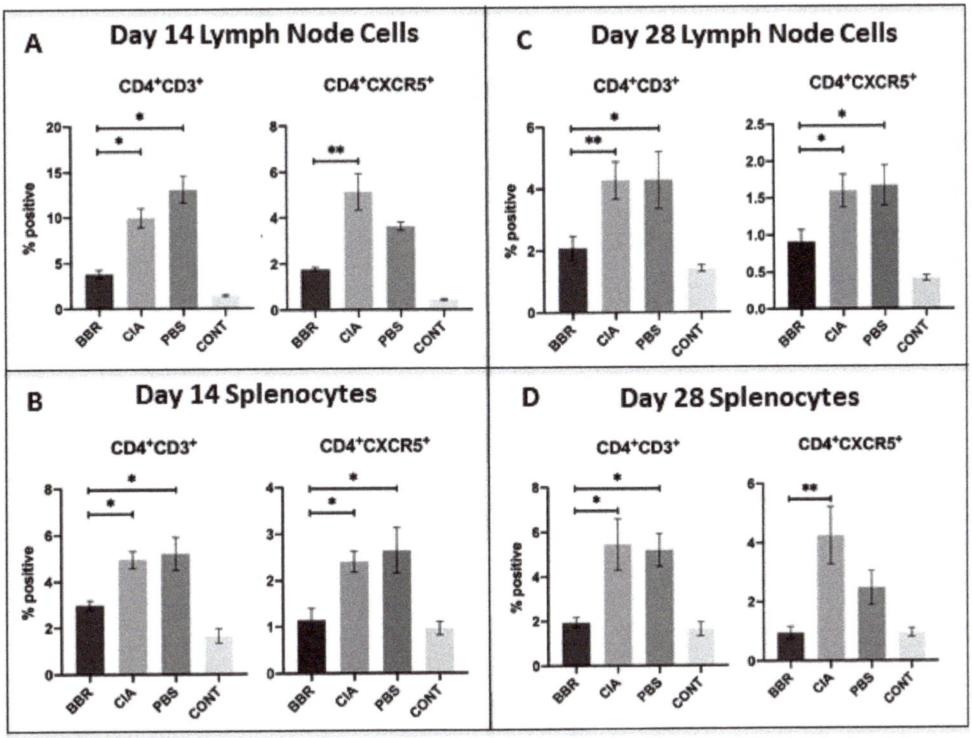

Figure 3. $CD4^{+}$ T cell populations during pre-clinical CIA (day 14) and at final day 28 endpoints. Cells compared were from the $CD4^{+}$ T cell population of lymph nodes (LNs) and spleen with further investigation into $CD4^{+}$ T cell populations expressing specific cell-surface markers. Shown are populations of $CD4^{+}$ T_h and $CXCR5^{+}$ T_{fh} cells of the LN (**A**) and spleen (**B**) at the day 14 endpoint (n = 5 per group), and of the LN (**C**) and spleen (**D**) at the day 28 experimental endpoint (n = 10 per group). Statistical comparisons made with the Kruskal–Wallis test with Dunn's multiple comparisons (* $p < 0.05$ and ** $p < 0.01$).

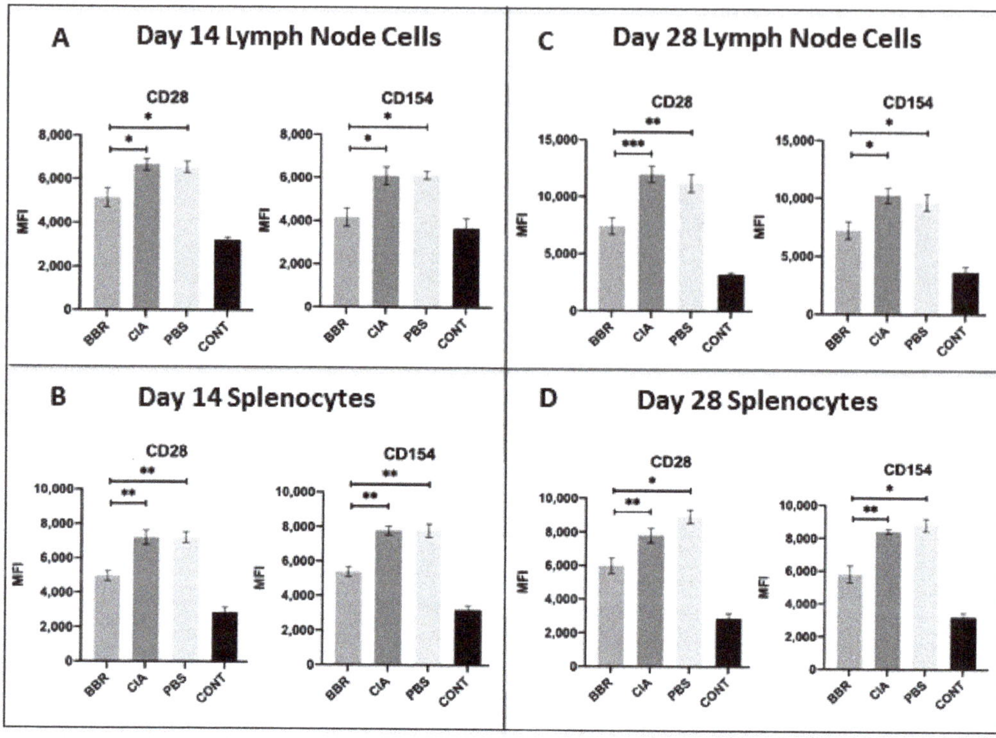

Figure 4. Expression of co-stimulatory molecules on CD4$^+$ T cells during pre-clinical CIA (day 14) and at final day 28 endpoints. Cells compared were from the CD4$^+$ T cell population of LN and spleen with further investigation into the expression of co-stimulatory molecules CD28 and CD154 on CD4$^+$ T cell populations. Shown are expression of CD28 and CD154 on CD4$^+$ T cells of the LN (**A**) and spleen (**B**) at the day 14 endpoint (n = 5 per group), and of the LN (**C**) and spleen (**D**) at the day 28 experimental endpoint (n = 10 per group). Statistical analysis of co-stimulatory molecule expression made with ANOVA and Tukey's multiple comparisons tests (* $p < 0.05$; ** $p < 0.01$, *** $p < 0.001$).

2.4. Berberine Treatment Leads to Increased Proportion of Foxp3$^+$CD4$^+$CD25$^+$ T Cells

To examine BBR's effect on T_{reg} populations, cells from the CD4$^+$ CD25$^+$ T population of LN or spleen were measured for the presence of the definitive T_{reg} transcription factor Foxp3. Out of this subset of cells, we observed an increased ratio of Foxp3$^+$:Foxp3$^-$ cells in the spleen and LNs of BBR-treated mice during the pre-clinical phase of CIA (day 14 endpoint) (Figure 5A). At the day 28 endpoint, BBR-treated mice had a significantly increased ratio of Foxp3$^+$:Foxp3$^-$ cells in the LNs, but not the spleen (Figure 5B). In order to determine whether or not the previously mentioned results were an artifact of including both arthritic and non-arthritic mice in the analysis, we compared this ratio between mice in the BBR group who developed arthritis and the mice who did not. There was no significant difference in the day 28 splenic Foxp3$^+$:Foxp3$^-$ T cell ratio between arthritic and non-arthritic mice in the BBR group. However, all non-arthritic BBR-treated mice had a larger percentage of Foxp3$^+$ cells compared to Foxp3$^-$ cells (ratio of >1) except for one outlier, whereas all arthritic BBR-treated mice had a smaller percentage of Foxp3$^+$ cells compared to Foxp3$^-$ cells (ratio of <1) (Figure 5C).

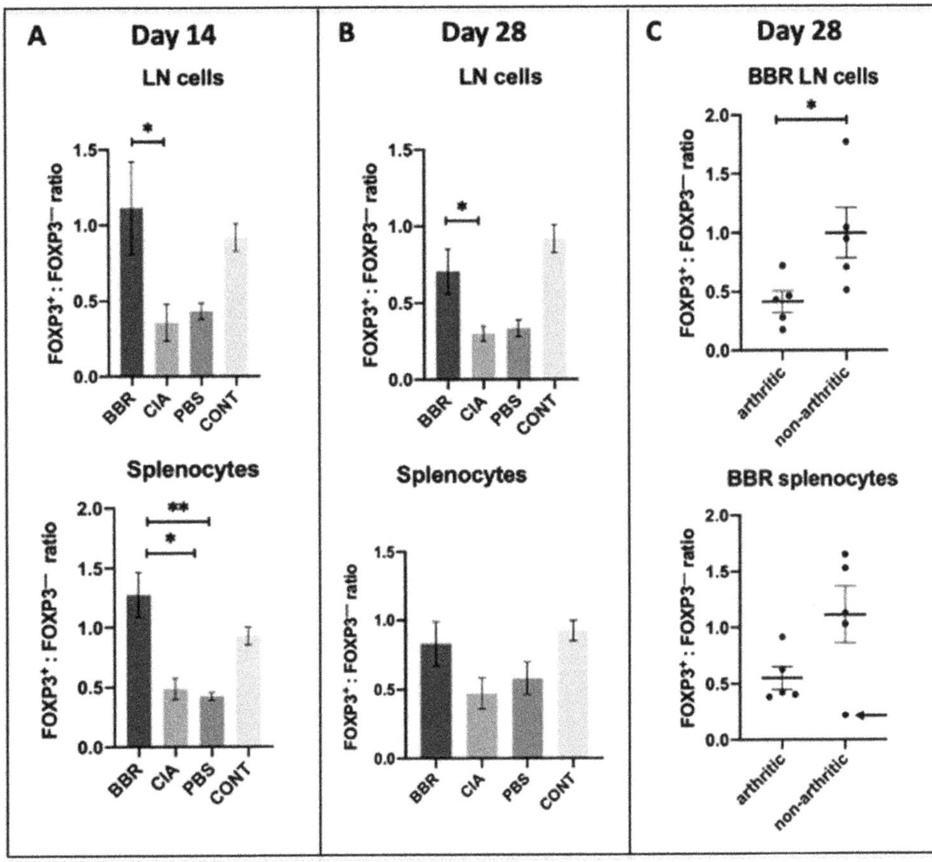

Figure 5. Berberine induces T_{reg} expansion in lymphoid tissue during CIA induction. Cells compared were from the CD4$^+$ CD25$^+$ T_h population of LN or spleen with further interrogation of the definitive T_{reg} transcription factor Foxp3. (**A**) The Foxp3$^+$:Foxp3$^-$ ratio during the pre-clinical phase of arthritis (day 14) ($n = 5$ per group, * $p < 0.05$). (**B**) The Foxp3$^+$:Foxp3$^-$ ratio at the day 28 experimental endpoint ($n = 10$ per group, * $p < 0.05$ and ** $p < 0.01$). (**C**) Comparisons of Foxp3$^+$:Foxp3$^-$ ratios from LN and spleen of the BBR treated group separated by status as arthritic or non-arthritic. Ratios compared using the Kruskal–Wallis test with Dunn's multiple comparisons. Arrow denotes outlier.

2.5. Key CD19$^+$B Cell Population and Co-Stimulatory Molecule Characteristics in Response to Berberine Treatment

Although there was a trend of reduced CD19$^+$ B cell populations in the spleen and LNs of BBR-treated mice during CIA development (day 14), this trend was non-significant. Additionally, BBR treatment did not reduce expression of the co-stimulatory molecules MHC II, CD40, and CD80/86 on CD19$^+$ B cells of the spleen and LNs at day 14 (Figure 6A,B).

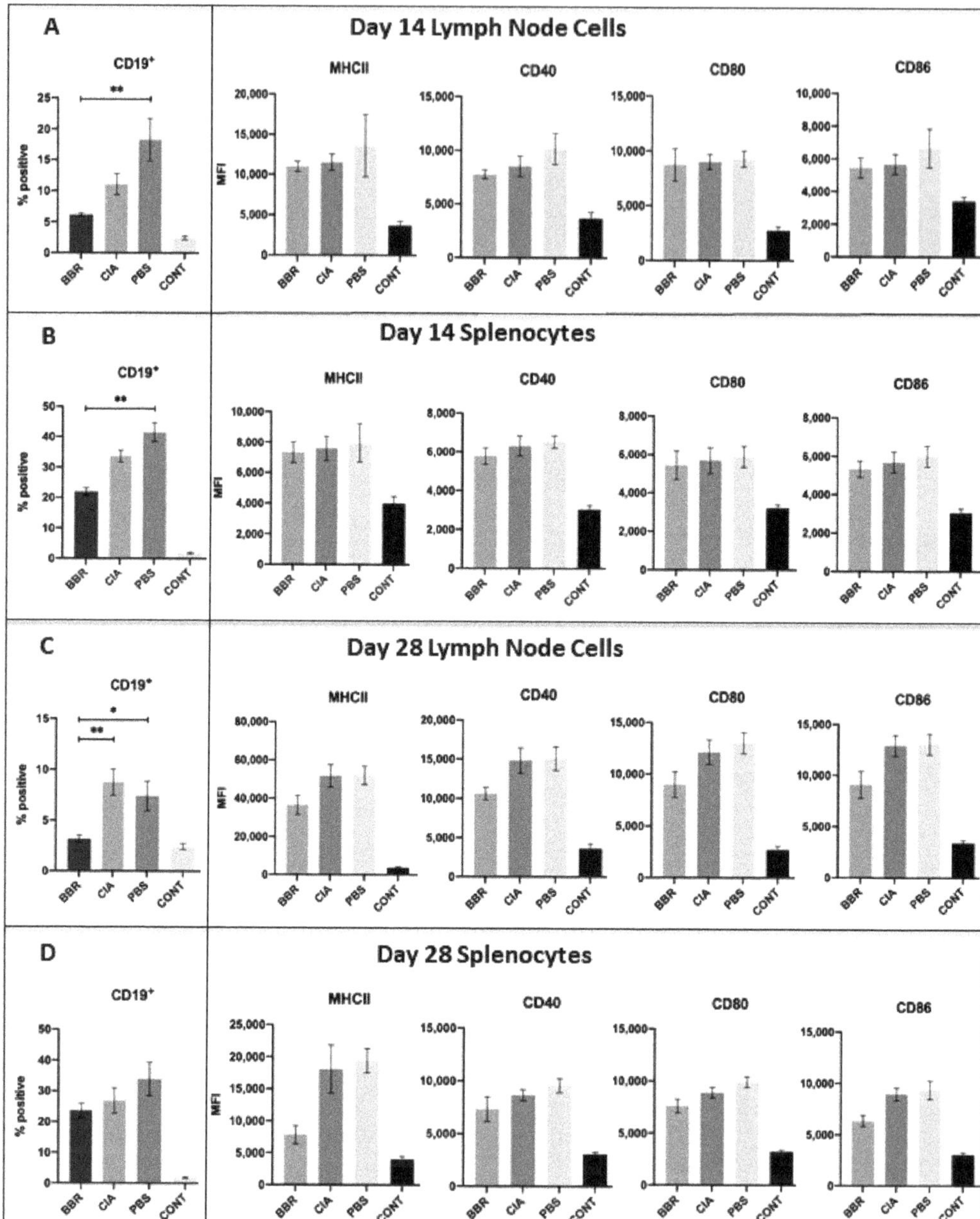

Figure 6. $CD19^+$ B cell populations and expression of co-stimulatory molecules during pre-clinical CIA (day 14) and at final day 28 endpoints. Cells compared were from the $CD19^+$ B cell population of LN and spleen with further investigation into $CD19^+$ cell populations expressing specific cell-surface markers. Shown are populations of $CD19^+$ B cells and expression of co-stimulatory molecules MHC Class II, CD40, CD80, and CD86 on $CD19^+$ B cells in the LN (**A**) and spleen (**B**) at the day 14 endpoint (n = 5), and of the LN (**C**) and spleen (**D**) at the day 28 experimental endpoint (n = 10). Statistical analysis of $CD19^+$ B cell populations made with the Kruskal–Wallis test with Dunn's multiple comparisons (* $p < 0.05$), and statistical analysis of co-stimulatory molecule expression made with ANOVA and Tukey's multiple comparisons tests (* $p < 0.05$ and ** $p < 0.01$).

By day 28, we observed a significant reduction in CD19$^+$B cells in the LNs, but not spleen, of BBR-treated mice (Figure 6C,D). While there was a trend of reduced expression of the co-stimulatory molecules MHC II, CD40, and CD80/86 on CD19$^+$ B cells in the spleen and LNs of BBR-treated mice at day 28, this trend was non-significant (Figure 6C,D).

We did, however, observe a vehicle-specific effect similar to that seen in the anti-CII IgG data. There were significantly larger CD19$^+$ B cell populations in both the spleen and LNs of the PBS control mice compared to the BBR-treated mice, and non-significant trends of increased co-stimulatory molecule expression (Figure 6A,D).

3. Discussion

Our results indicate that BBR treatment during the pre-clinical phase of CIA delayed the onset of CIA in DBA/1J mice, although mice in the BBR group who developed arthritis did not experience a significant decrease in clinical arthritis score compared to the CIA and PBS controls. Our results provide evidence at the cellular level that the mechanism underlying this protective effect is directly mediated through effector CD4$^+$ T$_h$ cell suppression, which subsequently influences activation, proliferation, and autoantibody production by B cells.

Our hypothesis that BBR is exerting its effect via CD4$^+$ T$_h$ cell suppression is supported by the observations that BBR-treated mice had significantly reduced populations of CD4$^+$ T cells and reduced expression of co-stimulatory molecules—effects which were not mirrored in CD19$^+$ B cells. While our CD4$^+$ T cell population data included all T cell subsets expressing CD4 (both T$_h$ and T$_{reg}$), we observed a higher ratio of Foxp3$^+$CD25$^+$CD4$^+$ T cells (representative of T$_{reg}$) to Foxp3$^-$ cells within the spleens and LNs of BBR-treated mice. This indicates that although the overall population of CD4$^+$ T cells was smaller in BBR-treated mice, they also had a higher proportion of T$_{reg}$ within the total CD4$^+$ T cell population. Additionally, a specific subset of the overall CD4$^+$ T cell population which plays a key role in T cell-dependent humoral responses, CD4$^+$CXCR5$^+$ T$_{fh}$ cells, was also decreased in BBR-treated mice. Together, these observations indicate a preference toward an immunosuppressive environment and specifically a reduced capacity to provide help in activating B cell autoantibody production.

A previous study by Moschovakis et al. (2017) [36] examining the role of CXCR5$^+$ T$_{fh}$ cells in RA showed that T cell-specific CXCR5 deficiency prevented RA development. Furthermore, an in vivo CIA study involving the use of hydroxychloroquine (HCQ) as a prophylactic (administered from day 0 of the experiment) noted a reduction in T$_{fh}$ cells, which corresponded to a decrease in both incidence and arthritis score in HCQ-treated mice [37]. Similar to this evidence, it is possible that our observation of reduced populations of CXCR5$^+$T$_{fh}$ cells seen in the BBR group compared to the CIA and PBS controls contributed to a lower incidence of arthritis as well. The reduction of CXCR5$^+$T$_{fh}$ cells we observed also likely contributed to the decreased generation of anti-CII total IgG and subtypes, as CXCR5$^+$T$_{fh}$ cells play a critical role in germinal center formation, B cell affinity maturation, isotype class switching, and subsequent autoantibody production [38]. As such, we propose the mediation of CXCR5$^+$T$_{fh}$ cell proliferation as a novel function of BBR, and we are unaware of any studies to date that specifically address the effect of BBR on CXCR5$^+$T$_{fh}$ cell populations.

Additionally, the reduced expression of co-stimulatory molecules CD28 and CD154 during CIA development (day 14) and at the day 28 endpoint in BBR-treated mice could be indicative of reduced activation and proliferation of CD4$^+$ T cells, thereby resulting in the lower CD4$^+$ T cell populations observed in the BBR-treated group. The blockade to CD4$^+$ T cell co-stimulation has proven to be an effective RA treatment and is the mechanism of action of abatacept, a biological immunotherapy used to treat clinically apparent RA [1,39]. CD28-CD80/86 interaction is an important therapeutic target as CD28 ligation leads not only to increased T cell proliferation and activation, but also to increased CD154 expression [40]; CD154 is a crucial ligand involved in the activation of B cells and other APCs, as well as affinity maturation and isotype class switching in B cells. We would also like to highlight that the reduced T cell populations and expression of co-stimulatory molecules was seen throughout the entirety of the experiment (day 14 and day 28). However, since BBR treatment occurred for the duration of the experiment, it is unknown whether the sustained reduction observed is due to the continual administration of BBR, or if ceasing BBR administration would have altered this outcome.

BBR's protective effect against CIA development is also likely mediated through its alteration of the Foxp3$^+$: Foxp3$^-$ CD4$^+$ T cell ratio. With the exception of the day 28 splenocytes whose data were skewed by one outlier, the BBR group saw a significantly higher proportion of Foxp3$^+$CD25$^+$CD4$^+$ T cells (T_{reg}) compared to CIA and PBS controls. Thus, while BBR treatment resulted in lower overall CD4$^+$ T cell populations, a higher percentage of cells within that reduced population were T_{reg}. Previous studies corroborate the protective effect of T_{reg} on CIA development; adoptive transfer of CD25$^+$ T_{reg} slowed disease progression of clinically apparent CIA [41], and the depletion of CD25$^+$ T_{reg} prior to immunization with bovine type II collagen (used to induce CIA) exacerbated arthritis [42]. Additionally, prior studies using BBR to ameliorate clinically apparent CIA resulted in a suppression of T_h17 activity alongside the activation/proliferation of T_{reg}, thereby resulting in an increased T_{reg}/T_h17 ratio in BBR-treated mice [26,33]. While a study by Yue et al. (2017) [27] provides opposing evidence in which BBR did not appear to have a significant effect on the frequency of T_{reg} in a CIA model despite seeing amelioration of clinically apparent CIA, their particular model used peripheral blood mononuclear cells to assess the T_{reg} population and Foxp3 expression, as opposed to our study which observed splenocytes and draining LN cells at the site of immune activation.

In regard to B cell-specific responses to BBR, during CIA development (day 14 end-point) the BBR-treated mice in our study did not see a significant reduction in overall CD19$^+$ B cell populations or expression of co-stimulatory molecules compared to the CIA control. However, by day 28 we observed a significant reduction in CD19$^+$ B cell populations in the draining LNs of BBR-treated mice compared to the CIA control, as well as a reduction in anti-CII IgG2a and total IgG. As such, we propose that the reduction in day 28 LN B cell populations and the subsequent lowering of anti-CII autoantibody production are largely due to BBR interfering with the T cell-mediated activation of B cells via T cell suppression, thereby contributing to decreased B cell activation. This interference could be due not only to the decreased CD4$^+$CXCR5$^+$ T_{fh} cell populations and enhanced proportion of T_{reg} seen throughout the experiment in BBR-treated mice, but also the decrease in the expression of CD28 and CD154 on T cells seen throughout the experiment. Both CD28–CD80/86 and CD154–CD40 interactions play an important role in B cell activation and proliferation, and CD154–CD40 ligation specifically provides key signaling for thymus-dependent humoral immunity responses, such as the isotype class-switching and affinity maturation required to generate high-affinity anti-CII IgG autoantibodies [43–45]. Furthermore, previous research has demonstrated that the disruption of CD28–CD80/86 and CD154–CD40 interactions results in reduced anti-CII autoantibody titers, prevention of disease development, and/or amelioration of disease in CIA and other autoimmune arthritis models [46–50]. In other words, pro-inflammatory T cell development and activation is inhibited by BBR early, which leads to a later reduction in B cells reactive to CII stimulus, and this timing fits with classical T cell-mediated B cell activity.

While there was no significant difference in anti-CII IgG1 observed between the BBR group and CIA control, we did observe a significant reduction in anti-CII IgG2a. Moreover, BBR-treated mice who experienced a delay in onset (remained non-arthritic by day 28, despite CIA induction) had significantly lower concentrations of anti-CII IgG1, anti-CII IgG2a, and anti-CII total IgG compared to BBR-treated mice who developed arthritis. In CIA, the IgG subtype that is thought to play the most direct role in inflammation and joint destruction is anti-CII IgG2a, which predominantly activates the complement cascade, although it can also bind Fcγ receptors (FcγR) on FcγR-bearing immune cells. High concentrations of anti-CII IgG1 are also typically present, however, IgG1 more readily binds to and activates FcγR-bearing immune cells and has a lower affinity for activating complement compared to IgG2a [51,52]. The important role of complement activation in CIA pathology is supported by studies that demonstrated amelioration of CIA in response to complement deficiency [53] and that C5-deficient mice were resistant to CIA development [54]. As IgG2a is a strong activator of complement in mice, IgG2a serum concentration has been shown to correlate to the degree of inflammation as well as cartilage and bone destruction in CIA models [55], and reduced serum concentrations of IgG2a were associated with delayed onset and reduced frequency of arthritis incidence [56,57]. However, a notable difference with our study is that while we observed significantly lower concentrations of IgG2a in BBR-treated mice compared to CIA and PBS controls, we did not see any significant difference in the degree of observable inflammation (arthritis scores). Additionally, as previous studies involving the use of BBR to treat clinically apparent CIA reported a significant reduction in anti-CII IgG1 in BBR-treated mice compared to both CIA and PBS controls [24,25], the lack of significant anti-CII IgG1 reduction in the BBR group compared to the CIA control in our own study was unexpected. It is notable, however, that when comparing arthritic and non-arthritic mice within the BBR group alone, the non-arthritic mice had significantly lower concentrations of both anti-CII IgG2a and anti-CII IgG1, indicating that the observed reduced incidence of arthritis is likely in part due to a reduction in circulating autoantibodies, as seen in other studies [56,57].

One major unexpected result regarding anti-CII autoantibody production involved a vehicle-specific effect in which the PBS control group saw the highest increase in autoantibody production in comparison to the CIA control and BBR group. Our solution of BBR dissolved in PBS and 0.01% DMSO was modeled in part after a previous CIA study that used BBR dissolved in a PBS/DMSO solution containing a slightly greater concentration DMSO than our own [25]; this previous study did not report elevated levels of anti-CII total IgG or anti-CII IgG subtypes in PBS control groups. However, DMSO has demonstrated the ability to stimulate antibody production in hybridoma cells, which are myeloma-B cell hybrids commonly used to generate large quantities of monoclonal antibodies in research and industry settings [58]. In light of this, it is possible we witnessed a B cell-specific response to the presence of DMSO, and furthermore that treatment of BBR was able to overcome this effect.

In addition to this unexpected vehicle-specific effect, our model also faced limitations. One major limitation was the final day 28 endpoint; prolonging the final endpoint past day 28 would provide more insight into the preventative capabilities of BBR. Due to the fact that our non-arthritic mice continued to have suppressed populations of $CD4^+$ T helper cells and $CXCR5^+$ T_{fh} cells, higher relative percentages of T_{reg}, and lower concentrations of circulating autoantibodies by day 28, we hypothesize that it is likely BBR treatment would at least continue to delay CIA development to a certain point. However, it is not known whether BBR would entirely prevent CIA development in those mice who remained non-arthritic by day 28, or if they would eventually develop symptoms of clinical arthritis at a later timepoint. Additionally, having equal sample sizes between the day 14 and day 28 endpoints would have allowed us to evaluate the progression of the immune response statistically, as opposed to just speculatively.

This model is further limited in that it assumes a mouse would be able to absorb the i.p. administered dose via oral administration, which is the preferred route of administration for human patients taking BBR dietary supplements. While estimates vary, it is widely known that BBR has an extremely low oral bioavailability (<1%) [59–61]. Thus, this model is not entirely reflective of how a human patient would ideally receive BBR as a treatment, nor of how a patient would absorb and distribute BBR as an orally delivered treatment. Finally, this model would have further benefited from a BBR control group, which would have involved receiving a BBR treatment but no CIA induction. This would have allowed us to examine the effects of BBR on the immune system under normal physiological conditions and could have provided us with additional insights into BBR's immunosuppressive capabilities.

4. Materials and Methods

4.1. General Reagents

DMSO (VWR, Radnor, PA, USA), isoflurane (VetOne, Boise, ID, USA), bovine type II collagen in complete Freund's adjuvant (Hooke Labs, Lawrence, MA, USA), 1X PBS, berberine hydrochloride (Sigma-Aldrich, St. Louis, MO, USA), ACK lysis buffer (Quality Biological, Gaithersburg, MD, USA), RPMI 1640 supplemented to 2 mM L-glutamine, 1% v/v penicillin/streptomycin, 1 mM sodium pyruvate, 10 mM HEPES (all from ThermoFisher, Waltham, MA, USA) 0.05 mM β-mercaptoethanol (Bio-Rad, Hercules, CA, USA), and 10% fetal bovine serum (VWR/Seradigm, Radnor, PA, USA).

4.2. Berberine Solution

A stock solution of 10 mM berberine dissolved in DMSO was stored at −20 °C when not in use. For all i.p. injections, this stock solution was diluted in PBS for a final DMSO concentration of 0.01% and a BBR concentration of 1 mg/kg when delivered to mice.

4.3. Antibodies

Brilliant Violet 421 anti-mouse CD4 (clone GK1.5), FITC anti-mouse CD3ε (clone 145-2C11), FITC anti-mouse CD19 (clone 1D3/CD19), APC anti-mouse CXCR5 (clone L138D7), Alexa Fluor 647 anti-mouse Foxp3 (clone MF-14), APC anti-mouse I-A/I-E (clone M5/114.15.2), PE anti-mouse I-A/I-E (clone M5/114.15.2), PE anti-mouse CD80 (clone 16-10A1), APC anti-mouse CD80 (clone 16-10A1), APC anti-mouse CD86 (clone GL-1), PE anti-mouse CD40 (clone 3/23), PE anti-mouse CD25 (clone 3C7), APC anti-mouse CD154 (clone MR1), PE anti-mouse CD28 (clone 37.51), and recommended isotype controls (all from BioLegend, San Diego, CA, USA). For interrogating the T_{reg} population, the manufacturer's protocol was followed for intracellular targets.

4.4. Mice

DBA/1J mice (6 weeks old) were purchased from Jackson Laboratories (Bar Harbor, ME, USA). Animals were acclimated to the housing facilities for one week prior to starting experiments and were housed 3 mice per cage in conditions that were in accordance with Institutional Animal Care and Use Committee (IACUC) guidelines to minimize distress. Mice were divided into four groups: Control (no CIA induction, no treatment), CIA (positive control), PBS (CIA induction, given volume-matched vehicle control of PBS with 0.01% DMSO), and BBR (CIA induction, given BBR treatment, 1 mg/kg per day). Before commencing the full experiment involving cellular analyses, a pilot study was performed to determine the efficacy of the CIA model (n = 3 per group). Treatments were administered via i.p. injections 5 times per week (5 days on/2 days off) and welfare-related assessments were made daily. In the full study (n = 15 per group; 60 animals total), five mice from each group were euthanized on day 14 (pre-clinical stage), with 10 mice from each group being euthanized on day 28. All mice were euthanized via CO_2 inhalation to effect in accordance with our approved IACUC protocol.

4.5. CIA Induction and Assessment

A pre-formulated emulsion of bovine type II collagen and complete Freund's adjuvant (Hooke Labs, Lawrence, MA, USA) was injected according to the manufacturer's instructions [62]. Briefly, 0.05 mL of the pre-formulated emulsion were injected subcutaneously near the base of the tail, about 7 to 10 mm distal to the body and at the space in between the ventral and lateral tail veins. This procedure was repeated with all mice in the CIA, CIA + BBR, and CIA + PBS groups, and was considered day 0 of the experiment. For mice undergoing full observation through day 28, on day 18 a booster injection of bovine type II collagen and incomplete Freund's adjuvant emulsion was given according to the manufacturer's instructions [62]. On day 28, mice were evaluated for the presence of arthritis, and scored on a scale of 0–16 as follows (per manufacturers' recommendation [62]): 0 = normal paw, 1 = one or two toes inflamed and swollen, 2 = more than two toes, but not entire paw inflamed and swollen OR mild swelling of entire paw without ankle swelling, 3 = entire paw inflamed and swollen (inclusion of ankle swelling), 4 = severely inflamed and swollen OR ankylosed paw; all paws were assessed for a total possible score of 16. Arthritis scoring was blinded to the researchers. Examples of mouse front and hind paws for each score category can be found in Supplemental Figure S1.

4.6. ELISA

Blood samples were collected by cardiac puncture immediately following euthanasia of mice on day 14 and 28. Whole blood samples were then centrifuged to separate plasma from cellular components. Serum concentrations of anti-collagen type II (anti-CII) total IgG (catalog # 1012T), anti-CII IgG1 (catalog # 20321T), and anti-CII IgG2a (catalog # 20322T) were measured by ELISA (Chondrex, Redmond, WA, USA) according to the manufacturer's instructions [63,64]. Optical densities were taken at 450 nm using a microplate reader.

4.7. Flow Cytometry

Single cell suspensions were made from spleens, inguinal lymph nodes (LNs), and axillary LNs of euthanized mice. Inguinal LNs were chosen in lieu of popliteal LNs because inguinal LNs are equidistant from the site of injection and the site of hind paw inflammation, and so are close enough to both sites to reflect the inflammatory responses of both the injection and the hind paw inflammatory events. To create single cell suspensions, briefly, spleens and LNs were separately ground, washed with 3 mL of ACK lysis buffer for 5 min, and then strained into 35 mL of complete RPMI 1640. Single cell suspensions were then stained with fluorescent antibodies specific for cell lineage markers: $CD3^+CD4^+Foxp3^-$ T helper (T_h) cells, $CD3^+CD4^+CXCR5^+$ T follicular helper (T_{fh}) cells, $CD3^+CD4^+Foxp3^+$ T regulatory cells (T_{reg}), and $CD19^+$ B cells were measured at day 14 and day 28. Spleen and LN cells were also stained with fluorescent antibodies specific for co-stimulatory molecules involved in T cell and B cell activation and differentiation: CD154 (CD40L) and CD28 on $CD3^+CD4^+Foxp3^-$ T_h cells, CD25 on $CD3^+CD4^+Foxp3^+$ T_{reg}, and MHC class II, CD40, and CD80/86 on $CD19^+$ B cells. The expression of these co-stimulatory molecules was measured by calculating the geometric mean fluorescence intensity (MFI) at day 14 and day 28. $CD3^+CD4^+$ staining was used as the parent gate for all the T cell subsets observed in this study. Example gating strategies can be found in Supplemental Figures S2 and S3.

4.8. Statistical Analysis

The assumption of normality was not met for cell population data but was met for co-stimulatory molecule expression data. A chi-square (X^2) test was used to compare absolute arthritic incidence (score ≥ 2) among control and treatment groups. For comparisons of non-normally distributed cell populations, the Kruskal–Wallis test with Dunn's multiple comparisons or Mann–Whitney *U* test were used. For comparisons of normally distributed co-stimulatory molecule expression data, the ANOVA test with Tukey's multiple comparisons test was used. All tests had an $\alpha = 0.05$. All analyses were performed using Prism version 8 (GraphPad, San Diego, CA, USA).

5. Concluding Remarks

In conclusion, BBR likely has protective effects against CIA development by directly suppressing $CD4^+$ T helper cell activity, including $CXCR5^+$ T_{fh} cells, thus having an indirect effect on B cell activation and autoantibody production. These T cell suppressive effects are evidenced by reduced expression of co-stimulatory molecules on $CD4^+$ T cells during CIA development (day 14) and at the final day 28 endpoint, as well as smaller populations of $CD4^+$ T cells (including $CXCR5^+$ T_{fh} cells), and higher percentages of T_{reg} in BBR-treated mice throughout the experiment. Although populations of $CD19^+$ B cells were reduced in the draining lymph nodes of BBR-treated mice by day 28, these suppressive effects are not reflected in other B cell populations throughout the experiment or the expression of co-stimulatory molecules on $CD19^+$ B cells of the spleen and LNs, indicating that reduced anti-CII auto-antibody production is likely due to decreased interaction of B cells with activated CXCR5$^+$ T$_{fh}$ cells. In the future, it is important to repeat this experiment with a later endpoint to better determine the duration of BBR's protective effects. Additionally, it is imperative to more closely examine BBR's influence on CXCR5$^+$ T$_{fh}$ cells, as these cells are crucial to the formation of germinal centers, high-affinity class-switched plasma cells, memory B cells, and the humoral immunological memory that is ultimately borne out of germinal center reactions. As such, BBR's suppressive effect on CXCR5$^+$ T$_{fh}$ cell populations, while potentially beneficial for autoimmune pathologies, also raises concern that prolonged use could impact a patient's ability to mount effective beneficial primary adaptive immune responses.

Supplementary Materials: The following are available online at https://www.mdpi.com/article/10.3390/ijms22073522/s1.

Author Contributions: Conceptualization, A.A.V. and N.A.P.; methodology, A.A.V., H.A., D.O.L. and N.A.P.; formal analysis A.A.V. and H.A.; investigation, A.A.V., D.O.L. and N.A.P.; resources, N.A.P.; data curation, A.A.V., D.O.L. and N.A.P.; writing—original draft preparation, A.A.V.; writing—review and editing, A.A.V. and N.A.P.; visualization, A.A.V.; supervision, N.A.P.; project administration, N.A.P.; funding acquisition, A.A.V. and N.A.P. All authors have read and agreed to the published version of the manuscript.

Funding: This research received no external funding.

Institutional Review Board Statement: All animal procedures were approved by the Institutional Animal Care and Use Committee (protocol # 1801BD-NP-M-21; approved March 10, 2018) and performed at the University of Northern Colorado in accordance with institutional and international guidelines.

Informed Consent Statement: Not applicable.

Data Availability Statement: All data generated or analyzed during this study are included in this manuscript.

Acknowledgments: The authors acknowledge the University of Northern Colorado Graduate Student Association and College of Natural and Health Sciences for generous graduate student support.

Conflicts of Interest: The authors declare no conflict of interest.

References

1. Smolen, J.S.; Aletaha, D.; McInnes, I.B. Rheumatoid arthritis. *Lancet* **2016**, *388*, 2023–2038. [CrossRef]
2. Gupta, V.; Katiyar, S.; Singh, A.; Misra, R.; Aggarwal, A. CD39 positive regulatory T cell frequency as a biomarker of treatment response to methotrexate in rheumatoid arthritis. *Int. J. Rheum. Dis.* **2018**, *21*, 1548–1556. [CrossRef]
3. Romão, V.C.; Vital, E.M.; Fonseca, J.E.; Buch, M.H. Right drug, right patient, right time: Aspiration or future promise for biologics in rheumatoid arthritis? *Arthritis Res. Ther.* **2017**, *19*, 239. [CrossRef] [PubMed]
4. Van Nies, J.A.B.; Tsonaka, R.; Gaujoux-Viala, C.; Fautrel, B.; Van Der Helm-Van Mil, A.H.M. Evaluating relationships between symptom duration and persistence of rheumatoid arthritis: Does a window of opportunity exist? Results on the Leiden Early Arthritis Clinic and ESPOIR cohorts. *Ann. Rheum. Dis.* **2015**, *74*, 806–812. [CrossRef]
5. Saevarsdottir, S.; Wallin, H.; Seddighzadeh, M.; Ernestam, S.; Geborek, P.; Petersson, I.F.; Bratt, J.; Van Vollenhoven, R.F. Predictors of response to methotrexate in early DMARD naïve rheumatoid arthritis: Results from the initial open-label phase of the SWEFOT trial. *Ann. Rheum. Dis.* **2011**, *70*, 469–475. [CrossRef]
6. Van Steenbergen, H.W.; Da Silva, J.A.P.; Huizinga, T.W.J.; Van Der Helm-Van Mil, A.H.M. Preventing progression from arthralgia to arthritis: Targeting the right patients. *Nat. Rev. Rheumatol.* **2018**, *14*, 32–41. [CrossRef]
7. Aletaha, D.; Smolen, J.S. Effectiveness profiles and dose dependent retention of traditional disease modifying antirheumatic drugs for rheumatoid arthritis. An observational study. *J. Rheumatol.* **2002**, *29*, 1631–1638. [PubMed]
8. Ebina, K.; Hashimoto, M.; Yamamoto, W.; Ohnishi, A.; Kabata, D.; Hirano, T.; Hara, R.; Katayama, M.; Yoshida, S.; Nagai, K.; et al. Drug retention and discontinuation reasons between seven biologics in patients with rheumatoid arthritis—The ANSWER cohort study. *PLoS ONE* **2018**, *13*, e0194130. [CrossRef] [PubMed]
9. Ebina, K.; Hashimoto, M.; Yamamoto, W.; Hirano, T.; Hara, R.; Katayama, M.; Onishi, A.; Nagai, K.; Son, Y.; Amuro, H.; et al. Correction to: Drug tolerability and reasons for discontinuation of seven biologics in 4466 treatment courses of rheumatoid arthritis—The ANSWER cohort study. *Arthritis Res. Ther.* **2019**, *21*, 114. [CrossRef]

10. Bonafede, M.; Johnson, B.H.; Tang, D.H.; Harrison, D.J.; Stolshek, B.S. Compliance and cost of biologic therapies for rheumatoid arthritis. *Am. J. Pharm. Benefits* **2017**, *9*, e1–e7.
11. Niewold, T.B.; Harrison, M.J.; Paget, S.A. Anti-CCP antibody testing as a diagnostic and prognostic tool in rheumatoid arthritis. *QJM Int. J. Med.* **2007**, *100*, 193–201. [CrossRef] [PubMed]
12. Deane, K.D.; Striebich, C.C.; Holers, V.M. Editorial: Prevention of rheumatoid arthritis: Now is the time, but how to proceed? *Arthritis Rheumatol.* **2017**, *69*, 873–877. [CrossRef] [PubMed]
13. Deane, K.D. Preclinical rheumatoid arthritis and rheumatoid arthritis prevention. *Curr. Rheumatol. Rep.* **2018**, *20*, 1–7. [CrossRef] [PubMed]
14. Deane, K.D.; Norris, J.M.; Holers, V.M. Preclinical rheumatoid arthritis: Identification, evaluation, and future directions for investigation. *Rheum. Dis. Clin. N. Am.* **2010**, *36*, 213–241. [CrossRef]
15. An, Y.; Sun, Z.; Zhang, Y.; Liu, B.; Guan, Y.; Lu, M. The use of berberine for women with polycystic ovary syndrome undergoing IVF treatment. *Clin. Endocrinol.* **2014**, *80*, 425–431. [CrossRef]
16. Li, Y.; Ma, H.; Zhang, Y.; Kuang, H.; Ng, E.H.Y.; Hou, L.; Wu, X. Effect of berberine on insulin resistance in women with polycystic ovary syndrome: Study protocol for a randomized multicenter controlled trial. *Trials* **2013**, *14*, 226. [CrossRef]
17. Zhang, H.; Wei, J.; Xue, R.; Wu, J.D.; Zhao, W.; Wang, Z.Z.; Wang, S.K.; Zhou, Z.X.; Song, D.Q.; Wang, Y.M.; et al. Berberine lowers blood glucose in type 2 diabetes mellitus patients through increasing insulin receptor expression. *Metabolism* **2010**, *59*, 285–292. [CrossRef] [PubMed]
18. Yin, J.; Xing, H.; Ye, J. Efficacy of berberine in patients with type 2 diabetes mellitus. *Metabolism* **2008**, *57*, 712–717. [CrossRef]
19. Chen, C.; Tao, C.; Liu, Z.; Lu, M.; Pan, Q.; Zheng, L.; Li, Q.; Song, Z.; Fichna, J. A Randomized clinical trial of berberine hydrochloride in patients with diarrhea-predominant irritable bowel syndrome. *Phyther. Res.* **2015**, *29*, 1822–1827. [CrossRef]
20. Janeczek, M.; Moy, L.; Lake, E.P.; Swan, J. Review of the efficacy and safety of topical mahonia aquifolium for the treatment of psoriasis and atopic dermatitis. *J. Clin. Aesthet. Dermatol.* **2018**, *11*, 42.
21. Oben, J.; Enonchong, E.; Kothari, S.; Chambliss, W.; Garrison, R.; Dolnick, D. Phellodendron and citrus extracts benefit joint health in osteoarthritis patients: A pilot, double-blind, placebo-controlled study. *Nutr. J.* **2009**, *8*, 38. [CrossRef] [PubMed]
22. Zeng, X.-H.; Zeng, X.-J.; Li, Y.-Y. Efficacy and safety of berberine for congestive heart failure secondary to ischemic or idiopathic dilated cardiomyopathy. *Am. J. Cardiol.* **2003**, *92*, 173–176. [CrossRef]
23. Yan, H.-M.; Xia, M.-F.; Wang, Y.; Chang, X.-X.; Yao, X.-Z.; Rao, S.-X.; Zeng, M.-S.; Tu, Y.-F.; Feng, R.; Jia, W.-P.; et al. Efficacy of berberine in patients with non-alcoholic fatty liver disease. *PLoS ONE* **2015**, *10*, e0134172. [CrossRef] [PubMed]
24. Hu, Z.; Jiao, Q.; Ding, J.; Liu, F.; Liu, R.; Shan, L.; Zeng, H.; Zhang, J.; Zhang, W. Berberine induces dendritic cell apoptosis and has therapeutic potential for rheumatoid arthritis. *Arthritis Rheum.* **2011**, *63*, 949–959. [CrossRef]
25. Wang, Z.; Chen, Z.; Yang, S.; Wang, Y.; Huang, Z.; Gao, J.; Tu, S.; Rao, Z. Berberine ameliorates collagen-induced arthritis in rats associated with anti-inflammatory and anti-angiogenic effects. *Inflammation* **2014**, *37*, 1789–1798. [CrossRef]
26. Wang, X.; He, X.; Zhang, C.-F.; Guo, C.-R.; Wang, C.-Z.; Yuan, C.-S. Anti-arthritic effect of berberine on adjuvant-induced rheumatoid arthritis in rats. *Biomed. Pharmacother.* **2017**, *89*, 887–893. [CrossRef]
27. Yue, M.; Xia, Y.; Shi, C.; Guan, C.; Li, Y.; Liu, R.; Wei, Z.; Dai, Y. Berberine ameliorates collagen-induced arthritis in rats by suppressing Th17 cell responses via inducing cortistatin in the gut. *FEBS J.* **2017**, *284*, 2786–2801. [CrossRef] [PubMed]
28. Li, Z.; Geng, Y.-N.; Jiang, J.-D.; Kong, W.-J. Antioxidant and Anti-inflammatory activities of berberine in the treatment of diabetes mellitus. *Evid. Based Complement. Altern. Med.* **2014**, *2014*, 289264. [CrossRef]
29. Yan, F.; Wang, L.; Shi, Y.; Cao, H.; Liu, L.; Washington, M.K.; Chaturvedi, R.; Israel, D.A.; Cao, H.; Wang, B.; et al. Berberine promotes recovery of colitis and inhibits inflammatory responses in colonic macrophages and epithelial cells in DSS-treated mice. *Am. J. Physiol. Liver Physiol.* **2012**, *302*, G504–G514. [CrossRef]
30. Li, Y.; Xiao, H.; Hu, D.; Fatima, S.; Lin, C.; Mu, H.; Lee, N.P.; Bian, Z. Berberine ameliorates chronic relapsing dextran sulfate sodium-induced colitis in C57BL/6 mice by suppressing Th17 responses. *Pharmacol. Res.* **2016**, *110*, 227–239. [CrossRef] [PubMed]
31. Jiang, Y.; Wu, A.; Zhu, C.; Pi, R.; Chen, S.; Liu, Y.; Ma, L.; Zhu, D.; Chen, X. The protective effect of berberine against neuronal damage by inhibiting matrix metalloproteinase-9 and laminin degradation in experimental autoimmune encephalomyelitis. *Neurol. Res.* **2013**, *35*, 360–368. [CrossRef] [PubMed]
32. Wang, H.; Tu, S.; Yang, S.; Shen, P.; Huang, Y.; Ba, X.; Lin, W.; Huang, Y.; Wang, Y.; Qin, K.; et al. Berberine modulates LPA function to inhibit the proliferation and inflammation of FLS-RA via p38/ERK MAPK pathway mediated by LPA1. *Evid. Based Complement. Altern. Med.* **2019**, *2019*. [CrossRef]
33. Dinesh, P.; Rasool, M.K. Berberine mitigates IL-21/IL-21R mediated autophagic influx in fibroblast-like synoviocytes and regulates Th17/Treg imbalance in rheumatoid arthritis. *Apoptosis* **2019**, *24*, 644–661. [CrossRef] [PubMed]
34. Yu, Y.; Cai, W.; Zhou, J.; Lu, H.; Wang, Y.; Song, Y.; He, R.; Pei, F.; Wang, X.; Zhang, R.; et al. Anti-arthritis effect of berberine associated with regulating energy metabolism of macrophages through AMPK/ HIF-1α pathway. *Int. Immunopharmacol.* **2020**, *87*, 106830. [CrossRef] [PubMed]
35. Shen, P.; Jiao, Y.; Miao, L.; Chen, J.-h.; Momtazi-Borojeni, A.A. Immunomodulatory effects of berberine on the inflamed joint reveal new therapeutic targets for rheumatoid arthritis management. *J. Cell. Mol. Med.* **2020**, *24*, 12234–12245. [CrossRef]
36. Moschovakis, G.L.; Bubke, A.; Friedrichsen, M.; Falk, C.S.; Feederle, R.; Förster, R. T cell specific Cxcr5 deficiency prevents rheumatoid arthritis. *Sci. Rep.* **2017**, *7*, 1–13. [CrossRef] [PubMed]

37. Han, J.; Zhou, Q.; Li, X.; He, J.; Han, Y.; Jie, H.; He, Y.; Sun, E. Novel function of hydroxychloroquine: Down regulation of T follicular helper cells in collagen-induced arthritis. *Biomed. Pharmacother.* **2018**, *97*, 838–843. [CrossRef]
38. Crotty, S. T follicular helper cell differentiation, function, and roles in disease. *Immunity* **2014**, *41*, 529–542. [CrossRef] [PubMed]
39. Dekkers, J.S.; Schoones, J.W.; Huizinga, T.W.; Toes, R.E.; Van Der Helm-Van Mil, A.H. Possibilities for preventive treatment in rheumatoid arthritis? Lessons from experimental animal models of arthritis: A systematic literature review and meta-analysis. *Ann. Rheum. Dis.* **2017**, *76*, 458–467. [CrossRef]
40. Podojil, J.R.; Miller, S.D. Molecular mechanisms of T-cell receptor and costimulatory molecule ligation/blockade in autoimmune disease therapy. *Immunol. Rev.* **2009**, *229*, 337–355. [CrossRef]
41. Morgan, M.E.; Flierman, R.; Van Duivenvoorde, L.M.; Witteveen, H.J.; Van Ewijk, W.; Van Laar, J.M.; De Vries, R.R.P.; Toes, R.E.M. Effective treatment of collagen-induced arthritis by adoptive transfer of CD25+ regulatory T cells. *Arthritis Rheum.* **2005**, *52*, 2212–2221. [CrossRef]
42. Morgan, M.E.; Sutmuller, R.P.M.; Witteveen, H.J.; van Duivenvoorde, L.M.; Zanelli, E.; Melief, C.J.M.; Snijders, A.; Offringa, R.; de Vries, R.R.P.; Toes, R.E.M. CD25+ cell depletion hastens the onset of severe disease in collagen-induced arthritis. *Arthritis Rheum.* **2003**, *48*, 1452–1460. [CrossRef]
43. Gray, D.; Siepmann, K.; Wohlleben, G. CD40 ligation in B cell activation, isotype switching and memory development. *Semin. Immunol.* **1994**, *6*, 303–310. [CrossRef] [PubMed]
44. Bishop, G.A.; Hostager, B.S. The CD40–CD154 interaction in B cell–T cell liaisons. *Cytokine Growth Factor Rev.* **2003**, *14*, 297–309. [CrossRef]
45. Durie, F.H.; Foy, T.M.; Masters, S.R.; Laman, J.D.; Noelle, R.J. The role of CD40 in the regulation of humoral and cell-mediated immunity. *Immunol. Today* **1994**, *15*, 406–411. [CrossRef]
46. Durie, F.; Fava, R.; Foy, T.; Aruffo, A.; Ledbetter, J.; Noelle, R. Prevention of collagen-induced arthritis with an antibody to gp39, the ligand for CD40. *Science* **1993**, *261*, 1328–1330. [CrossRef]
47. Webb, L.M.C.; Walmsley, M.J.; Feldmann, M. Prevention and amelioration of collagen-induced arthritis by blockade of the CD28 co-stimulatory pathway: Requirement for both B7-1 and B7-2. *Eur. J. Immunol.* **1996**, *26*, 2320–2328. [CrossRef]
48. Tellander, A.C.; Pettersson, U.; Runström, A.; Andersson, M.; Michaëlsson, E. Interference with CD28, CD80, CD86 or CD152 in collagen-induced arthritis. Limited role of IFN-γ in Anti-B7-mediated suppression of disease. *J. Autoimmun.* **2001**, *17*, 39–50. [CrossRef]
49. Choi, E.W.; Lee, K.W.; Park, H.; Kim, H.; Lee, J.H.; Song, J.W.; Yang, J.; Kwon, Y.; Kim, T.M.; Park, J.B.; et al. Therapeutic effects of anti-CD154 antibody in cynomolgus monkeys with advanced rheumatoid arthritis. *Sci. Rep.* **2018**, *8*, 2135. [CrossRef]
50. Vierboom, M.P.M.; Breedveld, E.; Kap, Y.S.; Mary, C.; Poirier, N.; 't Hart, B.A.; Vanhove, B. Clinical efficacy of a new CD28-targeting antagonist of T cell co-stimulation in a non-human primate model of collagen-induced arthritis. *Clin. Exp. Immunol.* **2016**, *183*, 405–418. [CrossRef]
51. Cho, Y.-G.; Cho, M.-L.; Min, S.-Y.; Kim, H.-Y. Type II collagen autoimmunity in a mouse model of human rheumatoid arthritis. *Autoimmun. Rev.* **2007**, *7*, 65–70. [CrossRef]
52. Strait, R.T.; Thornton, S.; Finkelman, F.D. Cγ1 deficiency exacerbates collagen-induced arthritis. *Arthritis Rheumatol.* **2016**, *68*, 1780–1787. [CrossRef] [PubMed]
53. Hietala, M.A.; Jonsson, I.-M.; Tarkowski, A.; Kleinau, S.; Pekna, M. Complement deficiency ameliorates collagen-induced arthritis in mice. *J. Immunol.* **2002**, *169*, 454–459. [CrossRef] [PubMed]
54. Wang, Y.; Kristan, J.; Hao, L.; Lenkoski, C.S.; Shen, Y.; Matis, L.A. A role for complement in antibody-mediated inflammation: C5-Deficient DBA/1 mice are resistant to collagen-induced arthritis. *J. Immunol.* **2000**, *164*, 4340–4347. [CrossRef] [PubMed]
55. Seeuws, S.; Jacques, P.; Van Praet, J.; Drennan, M.; Coudenys, J.; Decruy, T.; Deschepper, E.; Lepescheux, L.; Pujuguet, P.; Oste, L.; et al. A multiparameter approach to monitor disease activity in collagen-induced arthritis. *Arthritis Res. Ther.* **2010**, *12*, R160. [CrossRef] [PubMed]
56. Mikulowska, A.; Metz, C.N.; Bucala, R.; Holmdahl, R. Macrophage migration inhibitory factor is involved in the pathogenesis of collagen type II-induced arthritis in mice. *J. Immunol.* **1997**, *158*, 5514–5517.
57. McIntyre, K.W.; Shuster, D.J.; Gillooly, K.M.; Warrier, R.R.; Connaughton, S.E.; Hall, L.B.; Arp, L.H.; Gately, M.K.; Magram, J. Reduced incidence and severity of collagen-induced arthritis in interleukin-12-deficient mice. *Eur. J. Immunol.* **1996**, *26*, 2933–2938. [CrossRef]
58. Ling, W.L.W.; Deng, L.; Lepore, J.; Cutler, C.; Cannon-Carlson, S.; Wang, Y.; Voloch, M. Improvement of monoclonal antibody production in hybridoma cells by dimethyl sulfoxide. *Biotechnol. Prog.* **2003**, *19*, 158–162. [CrossRef]
59. Chen, W.; Miao, Y.-Q.; Fan, D.-J.; Yang, S.-S.; Lin, X.; Meng, L.-K.; Tang, X. Bioavailability study of berberine and the enhancing effects of TPGS on intestinal absorption in rats. *AAPS PharmSciTech* **2011**, *12*, 705–711. [CrossRef]
60. Liu, Y.-T.; Hao, H.-P.; Xie, H.-G.; Lai, L.; Wang, Q.; Liu, C.-X.; Wang, G.-J. Extensive intestinal first-pass elimination and predominant hepatic distribution of berberine explain its low plasma levels in rats. *Drug Metab. Dispos.* **2010**, *38*, 1779–1784. [CrossRef]
61. Liu, C.-S.; Zheng, Y.-R.; Zhang, Y.-F.; Long, X.-Y. Research progress on berberine with a special focus on its oral bioavailability. *Fitoterapia* **2016**, *109*, 274–282. [CrossRef] [PubMed]

62. Hooke Laboratories. CIA Induction in DBA/1 Mice. Available online: https://hookelabs.com/protocols/ciaInduction_DBA1.html (accessed on 20 May 2019).
63. Chondrex Inc. *Mouse Anti-Type I and Type II Collagen IgG Assay Kit with TMB Standard ELISA Kit*; Chondrex Inc.: Woodinville, WA, USA, 2011; pp. 8–10.
64. Chondrex Inc. Mouse Anti-Type II Collagen IgG Subtype Antibody Assay Kit with TMB. Available online: https://www.chondrex.com/documents/MouseELISASubtypeTMB.pdf (accessed on 1 November 2019).

International Journal of
Molecular Sciences

MDPI

Article

Increased Serum Levels of Brain-Derived Neurotrophic Factor Contribute to Inflammatory Responses in Patients with Rheumatoid Arthritis

Ning-Sheng Lai [1,2,†], Hui-Chun Yu [1,†], Hsien-Yu Huang Tseng [1], Chia-Wen Hsu [1], Hsien-Bin Huang [3] and Ming-Chi Lu [1,2,*]

1 Division of Allergy, Immunology and Rheumatology, Dalin Tzu Chi Hospital, Buddhist Tzu Chi Medical Foundation, Dalin, Chiayi 62247, Taiwan; Q12015@tzuchi.com.tw (N.-S.L.); junvsusagi@gmail.com (H.-C.Y.); dm248871@tzuchi.com.tw (H.-Y.H.T.); dl50299@tzuchi.com.tw (C.-W.H.)
2 School of Medicine, Tzu Chi University, Hualien City 97071, Taiwan
3 Department of Life Science and Institute of Molecular Biology, National Chung Cheng University, Minxiong, Chiayi 62130, Taiwan; biohbh@ccu.edu.tw
* Correspondence: e360187@yahoo.com.tw
† These authors contributed equally to this work.

Abstract: The aim of this study is to investigate the role of brain-derived neurotrophic factor (BDNF) in the inflammatory responses in patients with rheumatoid arthritis (RA). Serum levels of BDNF and the precursor form of BDNF (proBDNF) from 625 RA patients and 40 controls were analyzed using enzyme-linked immunosorbent assay. Effects of BDNF on the mitogen-activated protein kinase pathway were analyzed by Western blotting. Microarray analysis was conducted to search BDNF regulated gene expression in Jurkat cells, and the differentially expressed genes were validated using T cells from patients with RA and controls. Serum BDNF levels were significantly elevated in patients with RA compared with the controls. Low serum BDNF levels were found in RA patients with anxiety or receiving biologics treatment. BDNF (20 ng/mL) enhanced the phosphorylation of ERK, JNK, and c-Jun, but suppressed the phosphorylation of p38, whereas BDNF (200 ng/mL) enhanced the phosphorylation of ERK and p38. After validation, the expression of *CAMK2A*, *MASP2*, *GNG13*, and *MUC5AC*, regulated by BDNF and one of its receptors, *NGFR*, was increased in RA T cells. BDNF increased the *IL-2*, *IL-17*, and *IFN-γ* expression in Jurkat cells and IL-2 and IFN-γ secretion in activated peripheral blood mononuclear cells.

Keywords: BDNF; rheumatoid arthritis; JNK; T cells; anxiety; proinflammatory cytokines

Citation: Lai, N.-S.; Yu, H.-C.; Huang Tseng, H.-Y.; Hsu, C.-W.; Huang, H.-B.; Lu, M.-C. Increased Serum Levels of Brain-Derived Neurotrophic Factor Contribute to Inflammatory Responses in Patients with Rheumatoid Arthritis. *Int. J. Mol. Sci.* **2021**, *22*, 1841. https://doi.org/10.3390/ijms22041841

Academic Editor: Chih-Hsin Tang
Received: 28 January 2021
Accepted: 10 February 2021
Published: 12 February 2021

1. Introduction

Rheumatoid arthritis (RA) is a chronic systemic disease characterized by persisting joint inflammation. In addition to articular manifestations, patients with RA have an increased incidence of developing depression, which is itself a risk factor for developing RA [1]. Decreased brain-derived neurotrophic factor (BDNF) expression is well-known to play a critical role in the pathogenesis of depression [2]. BDNF is initially synthesized as the precursor form of BDNF (proBDNF) in neurons and glia, which is cleaved to mature BDNF intracellularly or extracellularly to release mature BDNF [3].

Previous research suggested that the increased serum levels of proBDNF or decreased BDNF/proBDNF ratio could be a serum marker for depression [4,5]. However, few studies have investigated the serum levels of BDNF in patients with RA, and the results were conflicting. Low serum BDNF levels were observed in RA patients with depression compared to RA patients without depression [6]. Grimsholm et al. found that serum BDNF was elevated in 18 patients with RA compared with controls, and their BDNF levels were declined after receiving anti-TNF treatment [7]. Whether patients with RA have elevated serum BDNF levels remains to be elucidated. Furthermore, there were no data available for serum proBDNF levels and BDNF/proBDNF ratio in patients with RA.

Recent evidence suggested that there are close interactions and communications between the immune system and the nervous system. For example, melatonin, which is secreted by the pineal gland, could suppress inflammation in preclinical models of RA [8,9]. We speculated that BDNF and it's signaling pathway could play a role in the inflammatory response of RA. Therefore, the aim of this study was to investigate the serum levels of BDNF, proBDNF and their ratio in RA patients compared with controls and to search for significant clinical manifestations associated with BDNF. We also searched for the expression of genes that are regulated by BDNF and clarified the potential roles of BDNF in the inflammatory response using T cells and its respective cell line, Jurkat cells.

2. Results

2.1. Serum BDNF, proBDNF Levels, and proBDNF/BDNF Ratio in Patients with RA and Controls

A total of 625 patients (78.2% female) with RA aged 62.0 ± 13.5 years and 40 controls (67.5% female) aged 62.2 ± 14.1 years were enrolled in this study. The demographic, clinical, and psychological variables of study patients with RA are presented in our earlier study [10]. Ninety-six subjects (15.4%) were classified as having depression, and 65 subjects (10.4%) were classified as having anxiety. Patients with RA had significantly elevated serum BDNF levels compared with those of the controls (17.9 ± 4.2 ng/mL vs. 16.4 ± 5.3 ng/mL, $p = 0.032$). There were no statistically significant differences between the serum proBDNF levels (464 ± 583 pg/mL vs. 372 ± 487 pg/mL; $p = 0.328$) and proBDNF/BDNF ratio (0.03 ± 0.05 vs. 0.04 ± 0.09; $p = 0.370$) between patients with RA and controls (Figure 1). After adjusting for age and sex, the serum BDNF levels remained significantly ($p = 0.033$) elevated in patients with RA compared with the controls.

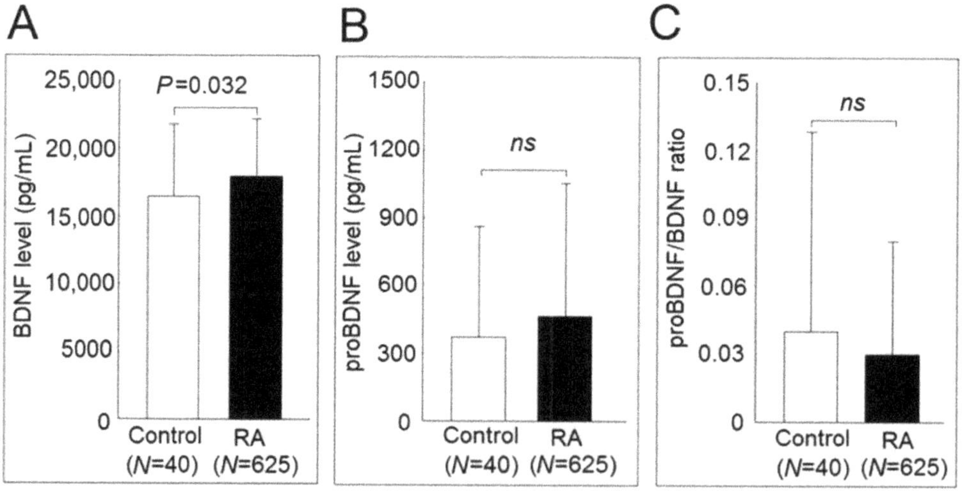

Figure 1. Serum brain-derived neurotrophic factor (BDNF), the precursor form of BDNF (proBDNF) concentration, and proBDNF/BDNF ratio in healthy controls and patients with rheumatoid arthritis. Serum levels of (**A**) BDNF, and (**B**) proBDNF concentration and (**C**) proBDNF/BDNF ratio in 40 healthy controls and 625 patients with rheumatoid arthritis. Serum levels of BDNF and proBDNF were measured by enzyme-linked immunosorbent assay (ELISA). After adjusting for age and sex in the multiple linear regression analysis, the BDNF levels remained significantly ($p = 0.033$) elevated in serum from patients with rheumatoid arthritis compared with those from controls. (*ns* not significant; * $p < 0.05$).

2.2. Correlation of Clinical Parameters with Serum BDNF Levels in Patients with RA

The association of various clinical parameters and serum levels of BDNF in patients with RA was analyzed in Table 1. In the univariate analysis, serum BDNF levels were inversely associated with an increased swollen joint count over 28 joints ($p = 0.023$) and age ($p = 0.015$). RA patients with anxiety ($p = 0.003$), receiving biologics (including etanercept, adalimumab, golimumab, abatacept, tocilizumab, tofacitinib, and rituximab) ($p = 0.01$), retired ($p = 0.006$), and had a disease duration of more than 5 years showed significantly lower serum level of BDNF. In the multiple regression analysis, only RA patients with anxiety ($p = 0.002$) and receiving biologics ($p = 0.020$) were significantly associated with lower serum levels of BDNF.

Table 1. Univariate and multiple linear analyses of clinical parameters associated with serum levels of BDNF in patients with rheumatoid arthritis (RA) ($N = 625$).

Variable	Univariate Regression Analysis			Multiple Regression Analysis		
	B	(95% CI)	*p*	B	(95% CI)	*p*
Depression (yes/no)	167.23	(−743.59, 1078.05)	0.719			
Anxiety (yes/no)	−1633.44	(−2701.60, −565.28)	0.003	−1660.31	(−2719.44, −601.18)	0.002
DAS-28	−222.15	(−467.34, 23.04)	0.076			
TJC 28	−22.19	(−74.37, 29.98)	0.404			
SJC 28	−91.32	(−169.83, −12.82)	0.023	−52.64	(−131.60, 30.25)	0.220
ESR (mm per h)	−3.66	(−24.65, 17.32)	0.732			
PGA	−8.56	(−21.28, 4.15)	0.187			
CRP (mg/dL)	−158.45	(−426.45, 109.56)	0.247			
Biologics (yes/no)	−920.07	(−1620.78, −219.36)	0.010	−827.25	(−1548.76, −147.37)	0.018
csDMARD (yes/no)	12.08	(−1299.53, 1323.70)	0.986			
Steroid (yes/no)	−312.66	(−1088.67, 463.34)	0.430	−241.91	(−1014.94, 531.11))	0.540
Female	−84.11	(−880.21, 712.00)	0.836			
Age (year)	−30.08	(−54.31, −5.86)	0.015	−12.34	(−47.50, 21.04)	0.449
Educational level						
Below high school	Ref					
High school or above	−33.33	(−713.61, 646.94)	0.923			
Marital status						
Single	Ref					
Married	−728.57	(−1864.78, 407.64)	0.209			
Widowed, divorced or separated	−1144.96	(−2430.36, 140.44)	0.081			
Employment status						
Being employed	Ref					
Unemployed	−601.33	(−1522.66, 320.01)	0.201	−310.42	(−1214.69, 647.55)	0.551
Retired	−1072.76	(−1830.40, −315.12)	0.006	−564.53	(−1554.66, 515.62)	0.325
Income						
High	Ref					
Median	309.26	(−413.22, 1031.73)	0.401			
Low	−147.90	(−1170.72, 874.92)	0.777			
Religious belief (yes/no)	−78.16	(−1568.03, 1411.70)	0.918			
Disease duration ≥5 years (yes/no)	−939.35	(−1767.40, −111.29)	0.026	−626.75	(−1469.76, 218.40)	0.146
Comorbidities	−453.24	(−1153.14, 246.66)	0.204			

CI: confidence interval; CRP: C-reactive protein; DAS28: disease activity score 28; csDMARD: conventional synthetic disease-modifying anti-rheumatic drug; ESR: erythrocyte sedimentation rate; PGA: patient global assessment; RA: rheumatoid arthritis; SJC28: swollen joint count over 28 joints; TJC28: tender joint count over 28 joints. Biologics include etanercept, adalimumab, golimumab, abatacept, tocilizumab, tofacitinib, and rituximab.

2.3. Expression of BDNF Receptors and Effects of BDNF in Mitogen-Activated Protein Kinase Phosphorylation and Cell Proliferation

We confirmed that two BDNF receptors-NTRK2 and NGFR were expressed on T cells from patients with RA and controls and Jurkat cells (Figure 2).

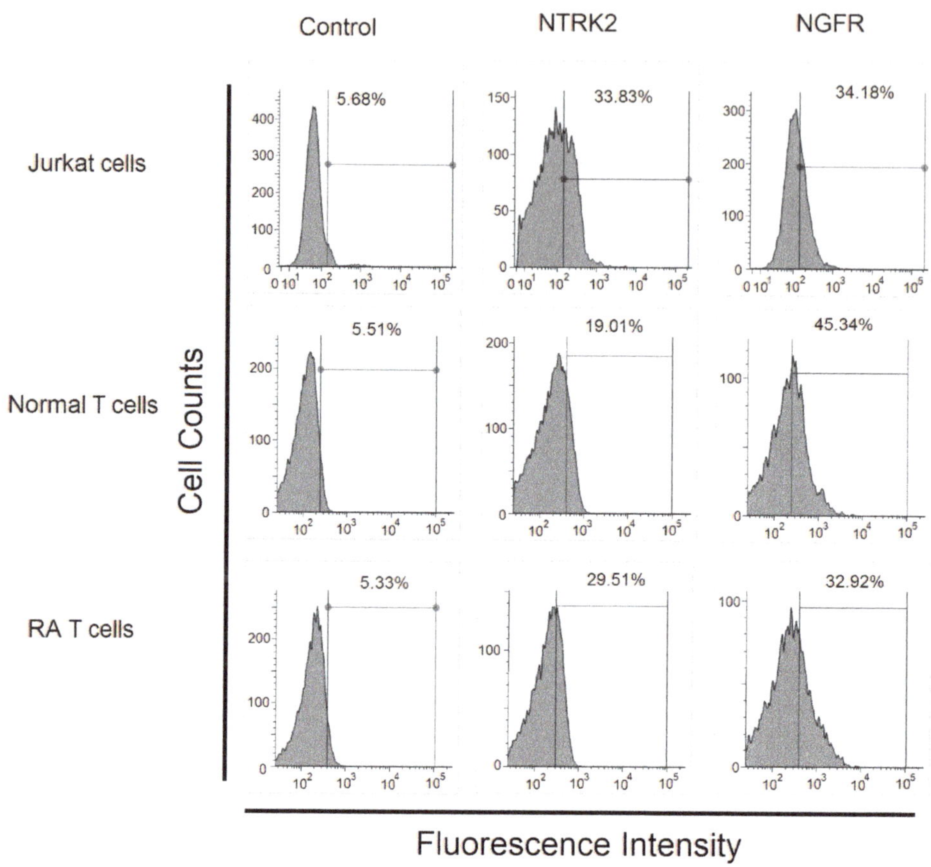

Figure 2. Expression of BDNF receptor in Jurkat cells and T cells from healthy controls and patients with rheumatoid arthritis. The expression of BDNF receptors, including neurotrophic receptor tyrosine kinase 2 (NTRK2) and nerve growth factor receptor (NGFR) in Jurkat cells, T cells from healthy controls and patients with rheumatoid arthritis analyzed using flow cytometry.

We further investigated the downstream signaling pathway of BDNF. The phosphorylated ratio of ERK, p38, and JNK in Jurkat cells after culturing with a high concentration of BDNF (200 ng/mL), low concentration of BDNF (20 ng/mL) for 48 h or culture medium only as the control group was measured (Figure 3A,B). We found that BDNF could increase the phosphorylation of ERK in a dose-dependent manner. The phosphorylated ratio of p38 was decreased significantly in Jurkat cells cocultured with a low concentration of BDNF compared with the controls ($p = 0.006$). The phosphorylated ratio of p38 was elevated in Jurkat cells cocultured with a high concentration of BDNF compared with the controls ($p = 0.013$) or low concentration BDNF group ($p = 0.002$). Finally, the phosphorylation ratio of JNK was found to be significantly elevated in the Jurkat cells cocultured with a low concentration BDNF compared with the controls ($p = 0.041$) or a high concentration BDNF group ($p = 0.025$). There were no differences in the phosphorylation ratio of JNK between the high concentration BDNF group and the controls. For the possible effect of ERK activation, we found that the addition of a low or high concentration BDNF did not affect the Jurkat cell viability and proliferation (Figure 3C). We also confirmed that the activation of JNK led to the increased phosphorylation of c-Jun, a downstream molecule of the JNK signaling pathway in the low concentration BDNF group (Figure 3D).

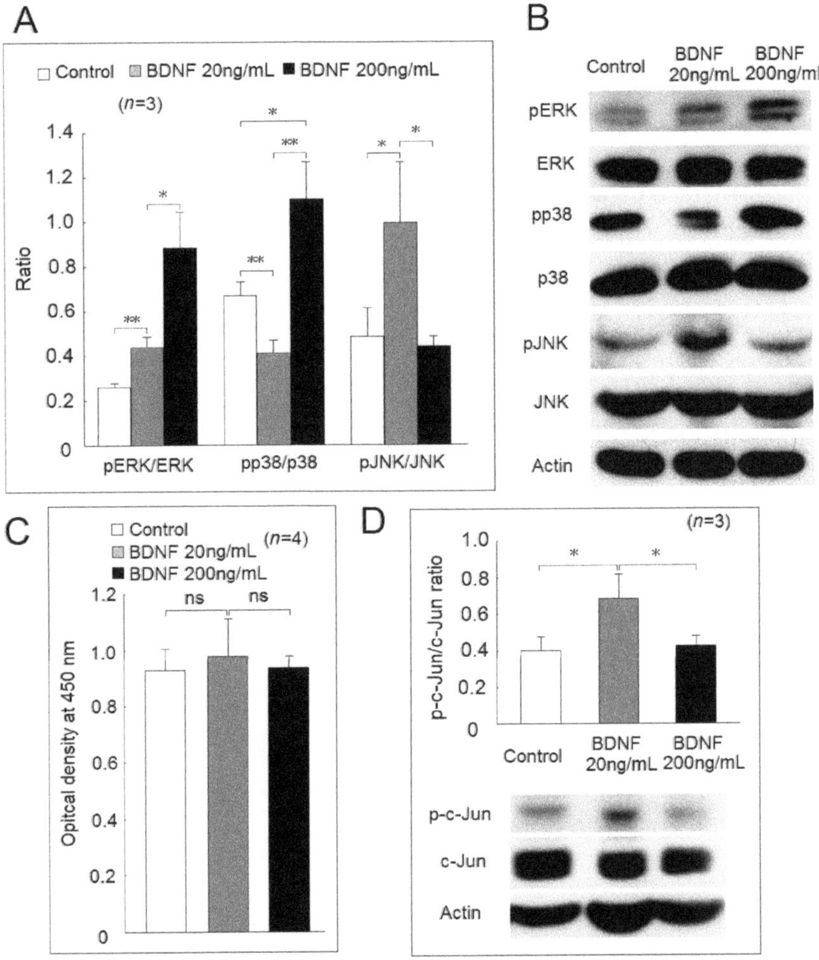

Figure 3. Effect of different concentrations of BDNF in mitogen-activated protein kinase (MAPK) phosphorylation and cell proliferation. (**A**) The phosphorylation ratio of p38, extracellular signal-regulated kinases (ERK), and c-Jun N-terminal kinases (JNK) in Jurkat cells after cocultured in culture medium with a low concentration BDNF (20 ng/mL) or a high concentration BDNF (200 ng/mL) for 48 h. (**B**) a representative case. (**C**) The viability and proliferation of Jurkat cells after cocultured in culture medium with a low and a high concentration of BDNF for 48 h analyzed by WST-1 cell proliferation assay. (**D**) The phosphorylation ratio of c-Jun in Jurkat cells after cocultured in culture medium with a low and a high concentration BDNF for 48 h (*ns*, not significant; * $p < 0.05$; ** $p < 0.01$).

2.4. Investigation of the BDNF-Regulated Gene Focusing on Inflammation-Related Proteins and Their Expression in Patients with RA

After microarray analysis, we found that the expression of 77 protein-coding genes was significantly decreased, and 142 protein-coding genes were significantly increased in Jurkat cells after cocultured with BDNF 200 ng/mL for 48 h compared with the controls (Figure 4A). We selected genes that could potentially involve in inflammatory responses and validated them using real-time PCR. We found that the expression of *Cluster of differentiation 40 (CD40), Calcium/Calmodulin-Dependent Protein Kinase II Alpha (CAMK2A), StAR Related Lipid Transfer Domain-Containing 13 (STARD13), Mannan-binding lectin serine protease 2 (MASP2), G Protein Subunit Gamma 13 (GNG13)* and *Mucin 5AC, Oligomeric Mucus/Gel-*

Forming (MUC5AC) were significantly higher after validation (Figure 4B). The gene expression of *NTRK2* and *NGFR* did not differ in the microarray analysis; we checked their expression levels in the validation step by real-time PCR. As expected, their expression was not different in Jurkat cells after cocultured with BDNF 200 ng/mL for 48 h compared with the controls. We then obtained T cells from an additional 40 patients with RA and 20 healthy controls. The demographic and clinical data of the patients with RA and controls are shown in Table 2. There were no differences in age or sex between the two groups. Among the BDNF-regulated genes, we found that the expression of *CD40, CAMK2A, MASP2, GNG13*, and *MUC5AC* was significantly increased in T cells from patients with RA compared with the controls. Of the BDNF receptors, the expression of *NGFR* was significantly increased in T cells from patients with RA (Figure 4C). After adjusting for sex and age, the expression of *CAMK2A* ($p < 0.001$), *MASP2* ($p < 0.001$), *GNG13* ($p < 0.001$), *MUC5AC* ($p < 0.001$), and *NGFR* ($p = 0.035$) was significantly increased in T cells from patient with RA compared with the controls.

Table 2. Comparison of demographics and clinical data between patients with rheumatoid arthritis and healthy volunteers.

Variable	Healthy Volunteers (N = 20)	Patients with Rheumatoid Arthritis (N = 40)	p
Age (mean years ± SD)	48.0 ± 6.8	50.6 ± 10.2	0.144
Sex (F:M)	15:5	31:9	>0.999
RF positivity	-	65.7% (26/40)	
ACPA positivity	-	65.7% (23/35)	
DAS28-ESR		3.19 ± 1.05	
CRP (mg/dL)	-	0.56 ± 0.79	
Medication			
Corticosteroids	-	87.5% (35/40)	
Salazopyrine	-	72.5% (29/40)	
MTX	-	80.0% (32/40)	
Leflunomide	-	10.0% (4/40)	
Biologics	-	67.5% (27/40)	

ACPA, anti-citrullinated protein antibody; CRP, C-reactive protein; MTX, methotrexate; RF, rheumatoid factor; SD, standard deviation, - not available; biologics including etanercept, adalimumab, golimumab, tocilizumab, tofacitinib, and rituximab.

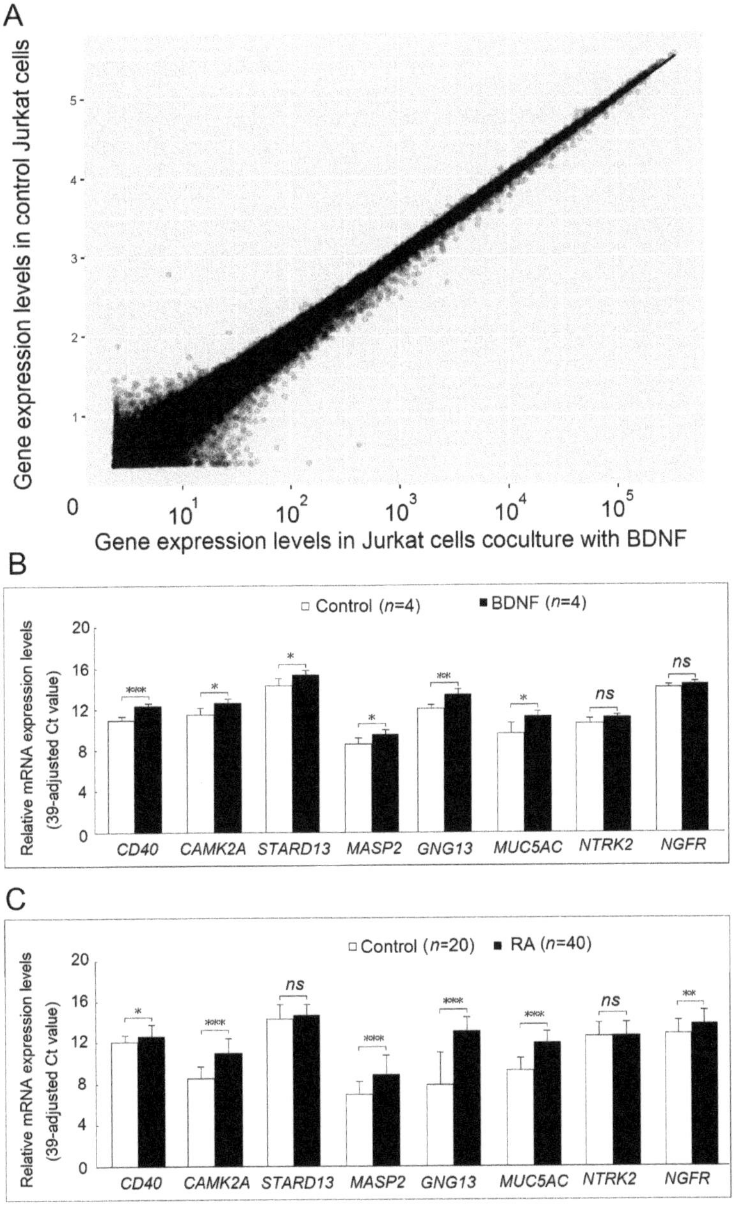

Figure 4. Identification and validation of BDNF regulated gene and its expression levels in T cells from patients with rheumatoid arthritis and healthy controls. (**A**) Expression profiles of mRNAs in Jurkat cells cocultured with BDNF 200 ng/mL or culture medium for 48 h were evaluated using microarray analysis. Each scatter spot represents the mean raw signal of mRNA in three repeats of each treatment. (**B**) Six genes, including *CD40, CAMK2A, STARD13, MASP2, GNG13,* and *MUC5AC,* which are related to the inflammatory pathway, were validated using real-time PCR. The expression levels of the BDNF receptors: *NTRK2* and *NGFR* were compared in Jurkat cells cocultured with BDNF 200 ng/mL or culture medium for 48 hours. (**C**) The expressed levels of *CD40, CAMK2A, STARD13, MASP2, GNG13, MUC5AC, NTRK2,* and *NGFR* were compared in T cells from healthy controls and patients with rheumatoid arthritis. (*ns*, not significant; * $p < 0.05$; ** $p < 0.01$; *** $p < 0.001$).

2.5. Correlation of Clinical Parameters with Expression Level of BDNF-Regulated Genes or BDNF Receptor-NGFR in T Cells from Patients with RA

We analyzed the expression levels of BDNF-regulated genes, including *CAMK2A*, *MASP2*, *GNG13*, and *MUC5AC* or BDNF receptor-*NGFR* in T cells from patients with RA by linear regression analyses. In the simple linear regression analysis, we found that the expression of *GNG3* (p = 0.007) and *NGFR* (p = 0.012) was positively associated with increasing age in patients with RA. In the multiple linear regression analysis, adjusting for age and sex, RA patients with each 10 year increment of age had a significant 1.45-fold increase (p = 0.009; 95% confidence interval (CI) = 1.11–1.91) in *GNG13* expression and 1.40-fold increase (p = 0.015; 95% CI = 1.07–1.84) in *NGFR* expression (Table 3).

Table 3. Simple and multiple linear regression analyses for assessing the correlations among different clinical parameters, and expression levels of brain-derived neurotrophic factor (BDNF) regulated genes in T cells of patients with rheumatoid arthritis.

	CAMK2A	*MASP2*	*GNG13*	*MUC5A*	*NGFR*
Sex (F/M)	0.144 (0.791)	0.581 (0.414)	−0.380 (0.458)	0.081 (0.841)	0.493 (0.299)
Age (per 10 years)	0.409 (0.064)	0.427 (0.144)	0.549 (0.007) *	0.029 (0.077)	0.504 (0.012) *
Positivity of RF (yes/no)	0.293 (0.538)	0.648 (0.297)	0.616 (0.165)	−0.077 (0.827)	0.013 (0.977)
CRP (per 1 mg/dL)	−0.071 (0.807)	0.037 (0.922)	−0.140 (0.610)	0.082 (0.703)	−0.114 (0.672)
DAS28-ESR	−0.031 (0.887)	0.035 (0.902)	0.109 (0.597)	0.011 (0.946)	0.064 (0.753)
Biologic (yes/no)	−0.209 (0.666)	−0.248 (0.696)	0.236 (0.606)	−0.143 (0.690)	−0.012 (0.979)

DAS28-ESR, Disease Activity Score 28-erythrocyte sedimentation rate; CRP, C-reactive protein; RF, rheumatoid factor. Values are correlation coefficients and (p values) from simple linear regression analyses. * After adjusting for age and sex, each 10-year increment of age was significantly associated with a 1.45-fold increase (p = 0.009; 95% confidence interval (CI) = 1.11–1.91) in *GNG13* expression and 1.40-fold increase (p = 0.015; 95% confidence interval (CI) = 1.07–1.84) in *NGFR* expression among patients with rheumatoid arthritis.

2.6. Functional Studies of BDNF and Its Receptor in Jurkat Cells and Normal PBMCs

In Jurkat cells, we found that the mRNA expression of *IL-2* and *IFN-γ*, but not *IL-17*, was significantly elevated in those cocultured with a low concentration of BDNF compared with the controls. The mRNA expression of *IL-2, IL-17*, and *IFN-γ* were all significantly elevated in those cocultured with a high concentration of BDNF compared with the controls (Figure 5A). In stimulated Jurkat cells, we found that the mRNA expression of *IL-2, IL-17*, and *IFN-γ* was significantly elevated in those cocultured with a low concentration of BDNF compared with the controls. The mRNA expression of *IL-2* and *IL-17*, but not *IFN-γ*, was significantly elevated in those cocultured with high concentrations of BDNF compared with the controls in stimulated Jurkat cells (Figure 5B). In anti-CD3+anti-CD28 activated PBMCs, we found that low concentrations of BDNF increased IL-2, but neither IL-17 nor IFN-γ secretion. High concentrations of BDNF could increase IL-2 and IFN-γ, but not IL-17 secretion (Figure 5C). There were no differences in *NTRK2* and *NGFR* expression between the stimulated Jurkat cells or controls (Figure 5D). We also noted that Jurkat cells did not secrete BDNF either upon activation or not (Figure 5E).

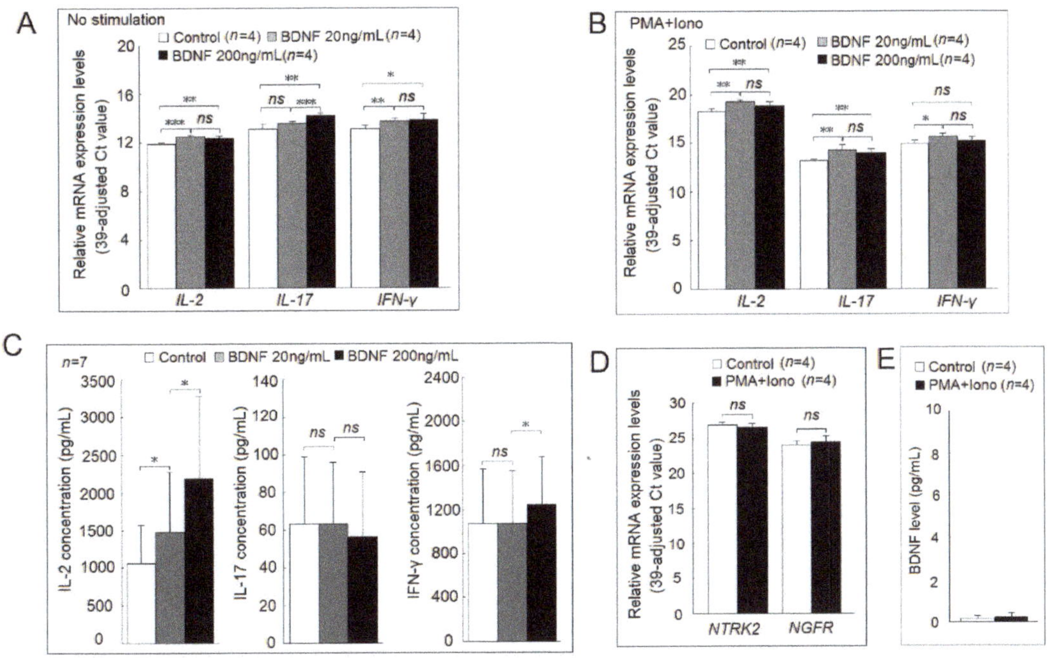

Figure 5. Functional studies of BDNF and its receptors in Jurkat cells and normal peripheral blood mononuclear cells (PBMCs). (**A**) The mRNA expression of *IL-2*, *IL-17* and *IFN-γ* in Jurkat cells with BDNF (0, 20 or 200 ng/mL) for 4 hours. (**B**) The mRNA expression of *IL-2*, *IL-17*, and *IFN-γ* in Jurkat stimulated with phorbol 12-myristate 13-acetate (PMA; 20 ng/mL) + ionomycin (Iono; 1000 ng/mL) plus BDNF (0, 20 or 200 ng/mL) for 4 h. (**C**) Normal PBMCs (1×10^6/mL) were stimulated with 1 μg/mL anti-human CD3 and 1 μg/mL anti-human CD28 plus different concentrations of BDNF (0, 20 or 200 ng/mL) for 24 h. (**D**) The mRNA expression of *NTRK2* and *NGFR* in Jurkat cells after stimulated with PMA and ionomycin for 4 h. (**E**) The concentration of BDNF in culture soup of Jurkat cells after cocultured with culture medium or PMA (20 ng/mL) + Iono (1000 ng/mL) for 24 h (*ns*, not significant; * $p < 0.05$; ** $p < 0.01$; *** $p < 0.001$).

3. Discussion

The development of depression in patients with RA is common and is associated with poor treatment response. BDNF is a key mediator of depression. However, few studies have investigated the BDNF levels in patients with RA. Our study showed that serum BDNF levels were higher in patients with RA. Clinically, patients with anxiety, but not depression, and those using biologics were associated with lower BDNF levels. Cheon et al. observed that BDNF was lower in RA patients with depression using serum samples from 154 RA patients with depression and 320 RA patients without depression [6]. However, in our cohort, 96 RA patients suffered from possible depression (HADS-D score ≥ 8), the number of probable depression was only 38. We did not find a significant association between depression and BDNF levels. On the other hand, Suliman et al. found that the serum level of BDNF was reduced in patients with anxiety in a meta-analysis of eight studies with a total of 1179 participants [11]. We did find RA patients with anxiety had lower serum levels of BDNF compared to those without anxiety symptoms. As the symptoms of anxiety and depression are often overlapping, further studies are needed to clarify this issue. The higher serum level of BDNF in patients with RA and the association with biologics used as well as the lack of association between serum BDNF levels and DAS-28 in RA patients, are consistent with a previous study [7]. Steroids or sex hormones could affect the BDNF expression and function [12,13]. We found that 76.6% of the patients with

RA were currently using steroids. There was no statistically significant difference in serum BDNF levels between those using steroids or not (17.8 ± 4.3 ng/mL vs. 18.2 ± 3.9 ng/mL, $p = 0.431$). Moreover, the use of steroids was not statistically significantly associated with the serum BDNF levels in the univariate and multiple linear analyses. The impaired hypothalamic-pituitary-adrenal axis in patients with RA might affect the result [14]. Due to the fact that the prevalence of RA is three times more frequent in women than men, up to 78.2% of the RA patients were female in this study. Females also suffered from a higher prevalence of depression. In our study, the percentage of females was comparable in patients with RA and controls (78.2% vs. 67.5%; $p = 0.114$) and the serum BDNF levels remained significantly ($p = 0.033$) elevated in patients with RA compared with the controls after adjusting for age and sex. The result was consistent with a previous report [15]. More studies are needed to clarify this complex issue.

Current evidence showed that there is a close interaction between the immune and nervous systems [8,9]. Several reports have indicated that neurotrophins were involved in the inflammation response of chronic arthritis, including RA [16–18]. Neurotrophins, especially BDNF, are known to participate in the pathogenesis of depression [19]. In the immune systems, human T cells, B cells, and monocytes were able to produce BDNF upon activation [20]), and BDNF has been shown to involve in the pathogenesis of experimental autoimmune encephalomyelitis and multiple sclerosis through regulating the survival of autoreactive T cells [21]. With respect to RA, Barthel et al. showed that the two BDNF receptors: *NTRK2* and *NGFR*, were overexpressed in synovial tissue from patients with RA [22]. We found that the mRNA expression of *NGFR*, but not *NTRK2*, was significantly higher in T cells from patients with RA compared with the controls. We further found that patients with RA had elevated serum levels of BDNF, and different concentrations of BDNF had different effects on the phosphorylation of MAPKs. In fact, BDNF binds two receptors; one is the high-affinity receptor NTRK2, also called TrkB, a transmembrane protein that mediates most of its biological functions in neurons. The other one is a low-affinity receptor NGFR, also call p75NTR, for neurite growth and apoptosis [23]. The low concentration of BDNF (20 ng/mL) would affect the Jurkat cells through binding to the high-affinity BDNF receptor, NTRK2, resulting in increased phosphorylation of JNK and ERK and a decreased phosphorylation of p38. The increased phosphorylation of ERK and decreased phosphorylation of p38 in Jurkat cells were consistent with previous reports [24,25]. Increased phosphorylation of JNK could lead to increased phosphorylation of c-Jun. A high concentration of BDNF (200 ng/mL) would affect the functions of Jurkat cells through binding to both NTRK2 and NGFR, resulting in enhanced ERK and p38 phosphorylation in Jurkat cells. However, NGFR binds not only to BDNF but also to NGF, neurotrophin-3 (NT-3), and neurotrophin-4 (NT-4) [26]. NGF is well-known to participate in the immunopathogenesis of RA [16,22,27]. However, the serum levels of BDNF were at least 30-fold higher than NGF, NT-3, or NT-4 [28,29]. We demonstrated that several genes involving inflammation responses, including *CAMK2A, MASP2, GNG13,* and *MUC5AC,* were upregulated in Jurkat cells after cocultured with BDNF as well as T cells from patients with RA. The most important is that BDNF could enhance the mRNA expression of proinflammatory cytokines including *IL-2, IL-17,* and *IFN-γ* in resting or stimulated Jurkat cells and increased IL-2 and IFN-γ secretion in activated PBMCs. This finding was consistent with previous studies, which demonstrated that blocking NTRK2 or NGFR could attenuate inflammatory responses [30,31]. We believed this finding could support that increased BDNF levels and differential expression of its receptor in patients with RA could enhance inflammation responses.

The relationship between mood disorder and serum BDNF levels is complex in patients with RA. Patients with depression had lower serum levels of BDNF [32]. Patients with RA also have a high prevalence of depression. However, we were surprised to find that the serum BDNF levels were elevated in patients with RA in our study. Fauchais et al. found that serum levels of BDNF in primary Sjögren's syndrome patients were significantly higher than those in healthy controls, and the levels were correlated directly with disease activity [33]. Patients with primary Sjögren's syndrome patients also had a higher risk of depression [34]. We proposed that the local expression and the effect of BDNF in the brain could be critical for the development of depression and anxiety [35]. The effect of increased serum levels of BDNF in patients with systemic autoimmune diseases, such as RA or primary Sjögren's syndrome, worth further investigation.

4. Materials and Methods

4.1. Study Subjects

All participants signed informed consent under a study protocol approved by the institutional review board of Dalin Tzu Chi Hospital, Buddhist Tzu Chi Medical Foundation (No. B10603008). The study was performed in accordance with the Declaration of Helsinki. Patients with RA, aged 20 years and above, fulfilled the 2010 American College of Rheumatology (ACR)/European League Against Rheumatism (EULAR) criteria [36] from the outpatient department of rheumatology at the Buddhist Dalin Tzu Chi Hospital were enrolled. The demographic data, medication, and disease activity of patients with RA were recorded. The anxiety and depressive symptoms were recorded with the disease activity score using the hospital anxiety and depression scale (HADS), and we defined depression and anxiety using a cutoff point of 8 in this study [37,38]. In addition, 40 patients with RA and 20 healthy individuals served as a control group for the collection of T cells. Blood samples were collected at least 12 h after the last dose of immunosuppressants to minimize their effects. T cells were purified using anti-human CD3-coated magnetic beads (IMag Cell separation system, BD Bioscience, Franklin Lakes, NJ, USA) according to the method described previously [39].

4.2. Flow Cytometry Analysis

The surface expression of two BDNF receptors-neurotrophic receptor tyrosine kinase 2 (NTRK2; also named tropomyosin-related kinase B, TrkB) and nerve growth factor receptor 2 (NGFR, also named neurotrophin receptor, p75NTR) was determined by stained phycoerythrin-conjugated mouse monoclonal antibody against human NTRK2 (BioLegend, San Diego, California, U.S.), rabbit polyclonal antibodies against NGFR followed by fluorescein isothiocyanate conjugate polyclonal goat-anti-rabbit antibodies (BD Biosciences, Franklin Lakes, NJ, USA) or isotype control (BD Biosciences) analyzing by flow cytometry (FACSMelody, Becton Dickinson, Franklin Lakes, NJ, USA) using FACSChorus software.

4.3. Enzyme-Linked Immunosorbent Assay (ELISA)

The concentration of BDNF or proBDNF in the culture supernatants or serum was determined using an ELISA kit (Biosensis, Adelaide, Australia) according to the manufacturer specification. Because the serum levels of proBDNF in some RA patients were undetectable, we used the proBDNF/BDNF ratio instead.

4.4. Western Blot Analysis

Western blot analysis was performed as previously described [40]. In brief, the cell lysate was electrophoresed and transferred to a polyvinylidene difluoride (PVDF) sheet (Sigma-Aldrich), then the membranes were nonspecifically blocked in 1% skim milk solution and incubated with the primary antibodies followed by respective HRP-conjugated secondary antibodies. The antibodies used for Western blotting were rabbit monoclonal antibodies against extracellular signal-regulated kinases (ERK)1/2, phospho-ERK1/2 (Thr202/Tyr204), anti-p38, phospho-p38 (Thr180/Tyr182), c-Jun N-terminal kinases (JNK), phospho-JNK (Thr183/Tyr185), anti-c-Jun, anti-phospho-c-Jun (Ser63), and goat-anti-rabbit IgG conjugated with horseradish peroxidase (Cell Signaling Technology, Danvers, MA, USA). Anti-β-actin antibody was used as an internal control (Sigma-Aldrich, St. Louis, MO, USA). Blots were visualized by chemiluminescence reaction (ECL; GE Healthcare, Little Chalfont, UK), and band intensities were measured using Image J (version 1.42; http://rsb.info.nih.gov/ij).

4.5. Cell Viability and Proliferation Using the Mitochondrial Dehydrogenase Cleavage Assay

The WST-1 assay was performed according to the method described previously with modifications [41]. After initial treatment, 10 µL WST-1 (Roche Applied Science, Basel, Switzerland) was added to each well, and the plate was incubated for 2 h. The intensity of color formation was detected at OD_{450nm} using an ELISA microplate reader (Anthos Zenyth 3100, Cambridge, UK).

4.6. Microarray Analysis

The expression profiles of mRNAs in Jurkat cells cocultured with culture medium or BDNF 200 ng/mL for 48 h were evaluated using microarray analysis. The microarray analysis was performed by Welgene Biotech (Taipei, Taiwan) as in our previous study [38]. In brief, total RNA was extracted by TRIzol reagent (Invitrogen, Carlsbad, CA, USA), then quantified at OD_{260nm} by an ND-1000 spectrophotometer (Thermo Scientific, Wilmington, DE, USA) and quantified using a Bioanalyzer 2100 (Agilent Technology, USA) with an RNA 6000 lab chip kit (Agilent Technologies, Santa Clara, CA, USA). Total RNA was labeled with cyanine 3 (Cy3; Agilent Technologies) dye and hybridized to Agilent SurePrint G3 human V2 GE 8 × 60 K microarray (Agilent Technologies). Microarrays were scanned with an Agilent microarray scanner (Agilent Technologies), and the scanned images were analyzed by Feature extraction 10.5.1.1 software (Agilent Technologies, USA); image analysis and normalization software were used to quantify signal and background intensity for each feature. Raw signal data were normalized by quantile normalization for differential expressed genes discovering.

4.7. Measurement of mRNA Expression Levels by Real-Time Reverse Transcription–Polymerase Chain Reaction (RT–PCR)

Jurkat cells or Jurkat cells after activation by phorbol 12-myristate 13-acetate (PMA; 20 ng/mL) + ionomycin (Iono; 1000 ng/mL) were cocultured with BDNF (0, 20 ng/mL or 200 ng/mL) for 4 h. Total RNA was extracted from cells using the Quick-RNA MiniPrep kit (Zymo Research, Irvine, CA, USA) according to the manufacturer's protocol. RNA concentration was quantified using a spectrophotometer (NanoDrop 1000, Thermo Fisher Scientific, Waltham, MA, USA). Subsequently, mRNA expression levels were quantified by real-time RT–PCR using a one-step RT–PCR kit (TaKaRa, Shiga, Japan) with an ABI Prism 7500 Fast Real-Time PCR system (Applied Biosystems, Waltham, MA, USA) according to the conditions described previously [42]. The relative expression levels of mRNA were defined by the following equation: (39– threshold cycle (Ct) after adjustment based on the expression of 18S ribosomal RNA).

4.8. Effect of BDNF on Proinflammatory Cytokines Secretion in Activated Peripheral Blood Mononuclear Cells (PBMCs) from Healthy Individuals

In brief, heparinized venous blood obtained from healthy volunteers was mixed with a 2% dextran solution (mol. wt. 464,000 daltons; Sigma-Aldrich Chemical Company, St. Louis, MO, USA) at a ratio of four parts blood to one part dextran, and the mixture was incubated at room temperature for 30 min. A leukocyte-enriched supernatant was collected and layered over a Ficoll–Hypaque density gradient solution (specific gravity 1.077; Pharmacia Biotech, Uppsala, Sweden). After centrifugation at 250× g for 25 min, PBMCs were aspirated from the interface. Then PBMCs (1 × 10^6/mL) were stimulated with 1 µg/mL anti-human CD3 and 1 µg/mL anti-human CD28 (BioLegend, San Diego, CA, USA) plus different concentrations of BDNF (0, 20, or 200 ng/mL) at 37 °C in 5% CO_2 for 24 h. After culture, cells were pelleted by centrifugation at 300× g, and the supernatant was concomitantly collected and stored at −80 °C for the measurement of cytokines.

4.9. Statistical Analysis

Results are represented as the mean ± standard deviation (SD) or n (%), as appropriate. Simple and multiple linear regression analyses were performed to obtain correlation coefficients between clinical parameters and serum levels of BDNF, or expression levels of genes in patients with RA. Mann–Whitney U test, Wilcoxon signed-rank test, or Student's *t*-test was used, as appropriate, to compare different parameters in patients with RA and controls. A p value < 0.05 was considered statistically significant. All statistical analyses were conducted using the Stata software (StataCorp, College Station, TX, USA).

5. Conclusions

We found that the serum levels of BDNF and T-cell expression of its receptor NGFR were elevated in patients with RA, and decreased serum BDNF levels were correlated with anxiety and biologics used in patients with RA. BDNF promoted inflammatory responses by enhancing the JNK and c-Jun phosphorylation and increased gene expression of *CAMK2A*, *MASP2*, *GNG13*, and *MUC5AC*, in T cells from patients with RA. BDNF could promote the expression of *IL-2*, *IL-17*, and *IFN-γ* in resting or activated Jurkat cells and enhanced IL-2 and IFN-γ secretion in activated normal PBMCs. Targeting BDNF and its signaling pathway may be a novel treatment strategy for RA.

Author Contributions: Conceptualization, N.-S.L., H.-C.Y., H.-B.H., and M.-C.L.; data curation, N.-S.L., H.-Y.H.T., and M.-C.L.; formal analysis, H.-C.Y., H.-Y.H.T., C.-W.H. and M.-C.L.; funding acquisition, M.-C.L.; investigation, H.-C.Y. and H.-Y.H.T.; methodology, H.-C.Y., H.-Y.H.T., C.-W.H. and H.-B.H.; supervision, N.-S.L. and H.-B.H.; writing—original draft, C.-W.H. and M.-C.L.; writing—review and editing, M.-C.L.. All authors revising the manuscript critically for important intellectual content. All authors have read and agreed to the published version of the manuscript.

Funding: This work was supported by grants from Dalin Tzu Chi Hospital, Buddhist Tzu Chi Medical Foundation (No: DTCRD107-I-03) and Buddhist Tzu Chi Medical Foundation (TCMF-A 108-05), Taiwan.

Institutional Review Board Statement: Ethics approval and consent to participate: This study was conducted in accordance with the Declaration of Helsinki and was approved by the institutional review board of Buddhist Dalin Tzu Chi Hospital, Taiwan (No. B10603008, 22 September 2017).

Informed Consent Statement: Informed consent was obtained from all subjects involved in the study.

Data Availability Statement: The datasets analyzed during the current study are available from the corresponding author on reasonable request.

Acknowledgments: We thank Malcolm Koo for providing statistical advice and language editing.

Conflicts of Interest: The authors declare no conflict of interest. The funders had no role in the design of the study; in the collection, analyses, or interpretation of data; in the writing of the manuscript, or in the decision to publish the results.

Abbreviations

BDNF	Brain-derived neurotrophic factor
CAMK2A	Calcium/calmodulin-dependent protein kinase II alpha
CD40	Cluster of differentiation 40
ELISA	Enzyme-linked immunosorbent assay
ERK	Extracellular signal-regulated kinase
GNG13	G protein subunit gamma 13
IFN-γ	Interferon-gamma
IL	Interleukin
Iono	Ionomycin
JNK	c-Jun N-terminal kinase
MASP2	Mannan-binding lectin serine protease 2
MUC5AC	Oligomeric mucus/gel-forming
NGFR	Nerve growth factor receptor
NTRK2	Neurotrophic receptor tyrosine kinase 2
PBMCs	Peripheral blood mononuclear cells
PMA	Phorbol 12-myristate 13-acetate

PVDF	Polyvinylidene difluoride
RA	Rheumatoid arthritis
RT–PCR	Real-time reverse transcription–polymerase chain reaction
STARD13	Star-related lipid transfer domain-containing 13

References

1. Lu, M.-C.; Guo, H.-R.; Lin, M.-C.; Livneh, H.; Lai, N.-S.; Tsai, T.-Y. Bidirectional associations between rheumatoid arthritis and depression: A nationwide longitudinal study. *Sci. Rep.* **2016**, *6*, 20647. [CrossRef]
2. Malhi, G.S.; Mann, J.J. Depression. *Lancet* **2018**, *392*, 2299–2312. [CrossRef]
3. Yang, J.; Siao, C.-J.; Nagappan, G.; Marinic, T.; Jing, D.; McGrath, K.; Chen, Z.-Y.; Mark, W.; Tessarollo, L.; Lee, F.-S.; et al. Neuronal release of proBDNF. *Nat. Neurosci.* **2009**, *12*, 113–115. [CrossRef] [PubMed]
4. Zhao, G.; Zhang, C.; Chen, J.; Su, Y.; Zhou, R.; Wang, F.; Xia, W.; Huang, J.; Wang, Z.; Hu, Y.; et al. Ratio of mBDNF to proBDNF for differential diagnosis of major depressive disorder and bipolar depression. *Mol. Neurobiol.* **2017**, *54*, 5573–5582. [CrossRef] [PubMed]
5. Zhou, L.; Xiong, J.; Lim, Y.; Ruan, Y.; Huang, C.; Zhu, Y.; Zhong, J.-H.; Xiao, Z.; Zhou, X.F. Upregulation of blood proBDNF and its receptors in major depression. *J. Affect. Disord.* **2013**, *150*, 776–784. [CrossRef]
6. Cheon, Y.-H.; Lee, S.-G.; Kim, M.; Kim, H.-O.; Suh, Y.S.; Park, K.-S.; Kim, R.-B.; Yang, H.-S.; Kim, J.-M.; Son, C.-N.; et al. The association of disease activity, pro-inflammatory cytokines, and neurotrophic factors with depression in patients with rheumatoid arthritis. *Brain Behav. Immun.* **2018**, *73*, 274–281. [CrossRef] [PubMed]
7. Grimsholm, O.; Rantapää-Dahlqvist, S.; Dalén, T.; Forsgren, S. BDNF in RA: Downregulated in plasma following anti-TNF treatment but no correlation with inflammatory parameters. *Clin. Rheumatol.* **2008**, *27*, 1289–1297. [CrossRef]
8. Huang, C.-C.; Chiou, C.-H.; Liu, S.-C.; Hu, S.-L.; Su, C.-M.; Tsai, C.-H.; Tang, C.-H. Melatonin attenuates TNF-α and IL-1β expression in synovial fibroblasts and diminishes cartilage degradation: Implications for the treatment of rheumatoid arthritis. *J. Pineal Res.* **2019**, *66*, e12560. [CrossRef]
9. MacDonald, I.J.; Huang, C.-C.; Liu, S.-C.; Tang, C.-H. Reconsidering the role of melatonin in rheumatoid arthritis. *Int. J. Mol. Sci.* **2020**, *21*, 2877. [CrossRef] [PubMed]
10. Ng, K.-J.; Huang, K.-Y.; Tung, C.-H.; Hsu, B.-B.; Wu, C.-H.; Lu, M.-C.; Lai, N.-S. Risk factors, including different biologics, associated with depression and anxiety in patients with rheumatoid arthritis: A cross-sectional observational study. *Clin. Rheumatol.* **2020**, *39*, 737–746. [CrossRef]
11. Suliman, S.; Hemmings, S.M.; Seedat, S. Brain-Derived neurotrophic factor (BDNF) protein levels in anxiety disorders: Systematic review and meta-regression analysis. *Front. Integr. Neurosci.* **2013**, *7*, 55. [CrossRef]
12. Pluchino, N.; Russo, M.; Santoro, A.N.; Litta, P.; Cela, V.; Genazzani, A.R. Steroid hormones and BDNF. *Neuroscience* **2013**, *239*, 271–279. [CrossRef] [PubMed]
13. Chen, H.; Lombès, M.; Le Menuet, D. Glucocorticoid receptor represses brain-derived neurotrophic factor expression in neuron-like cells. *Mol. Brain* **2017**, *10*, 12. [CrossRef] [PubMed]
14. Alten, R.; Wiebe, E. Hypothalamic-pituitary-adrenal axis function in patients with rheumatoid arthritis treated with different glucocorticoid approaches. *Neuroimmunomodulation* **2015**, *22*, 83–88. [CrossRef]
15. Katoh-Semba, R.; Wakako, R.; Komori, T.; Shigemi, H.; Miyazaki, N.; Ito, H.; Kumagai, T.; Tsuzuki, M.; Shigemi, K.; Yoshida, F.; et al. Age-Related changes in BDNF protein levels in human serum: Differences between autism cases and normal controls. *Int. J. Dev. Neurosci.* **2007**, *25*, 367–372. [CrossRef]
16. Raychaudhuri, S.P.; Raychaudhuri, S.K.; Atkuri, K.R.; Herzenberg, L.A. Nerve growth factor: A key local regulator in the pathogenesis of inflammatory arthritis. *Arthritis Rheum.* **2011**, *63*, 3243–3252. [CrossRef]
17. Aloe, L.; Tuveri, M.A.; Carcassi, U.; Levi-Montalcini, R. Nerve growth factor in the synovial fluid of patients with chronic arthritis. *Arthritis Rheum.* **1992**, *35*, 351–355. [CrossRef]
18. Manni, L.; Lundeberg, T.; Fiorito, S.; Bonini, S.; Vigneti, E.; Aloe, L. Nerve growth factor release by human synovial fibroblasts prior to and following exposure to tumor necrosis factor-alpha, interleukin-1 beta and cholecystokinin-8: The possible role of NGF in the inflammatory response. *Clin. Exp. Rheumatol.* **2003**, *21*, 617–624.
19. Hashimoto, K.; Shimizu, E.; Iyo, M. Critical role of brain-derived neurotrophic factor in mood disorders. *Brain Res. Rev.* **2004**, *45*, 104–114. [CrossRef]
20. Kerschensteiner, M.; Gallmeier, E.; Behrens, L.; Leal, V.V.; Misgeld, T.; Klinkert, W.E.; Kolbeck, R.; Hoppe, E.; Oropeza-Wekerle, R.L.; Bartke, I.; et al. Activated human T cells, B cells, and monocytes produce brain-derived neurotrophic factor in vitro and in inflammatory brain lesions: A neuroprotective role of inflammation? *J. Exp. Med.* **1999**, *189*, 865–870. [CrossRef] [PubMed]
21. De Santi, L.; Annunziata, P.; Sessa, E.; Bramanti, P. Brain-Derived neurotrophic factor and TrkB receptor in experimental autoimmune encephalomyelitis and multiple sclerosis. *J. Neurol. Sci.* **2009**, *287*, 17–26. [CrossRef]
22. Barthel, C.; Yeremenko, N.; Jacobs, R.; Schmidt, R.E.; Bernateck, M.; Zeidler, H.; Tak, P.P.; Baeten, D.; Rihl, M. Nerve growth factor and receptor expression in rheumatoid arthritis and spondyloarthritis. *Arthritis Res. Ther.* **2009**, *11*, R82. [CrossRef] [PubMed]
23. Tejeda, G.S.; Díaz-Guerra, M. Integral characterization of defective BDNF/TrkB signalling in neurological and psychiatric disorders leads the way to new therapies. *Int. J. Mol. Sci.* **2017**, *18*, 268. [CrossRef]

24. Liang, J.; Deng, G.; Huang, H. The activation of BDNF reduced inflammation in a spinal cord injury model by TrkB/p38 MAPK signaling. *Exp. Ther. Med.* **2019**, *17*, 1688–1696. [CrossRef]
25. Numakawa, T.; Suzuki, S.; Kumamaru, E.; Adachi, N.; Richards, M.; Kunugi, H. BDNF function and intracellular signaling in neurons. *Histol. Histopathol.* **2010**, *25*, 237–258. [PubMed]
26. Bothwell, M. Recent advances in understanding context-dependent mechanisms controlling neurotrophin signaling and function. *F1000Research* **2019**, *8*. [CrossRef]
27. Raychaudhuri, S.P.; Raychaudhuri, S.K. The regulatory role of nerve growth factor and its receptor system in fibroblast-like synovial cells. *Scand. J. Rheumatol.* **2009**, *38*, 207–215. [CrossRef]
28. del Porto, F.; Aloe, L.; Laganà, B.; Triaca, V.; Nofroni, I.; D'Amelio, R. Nerve growth factor and brain-derived neurotrophic factor levels in patients with rheumatoid arthritis treated with TNF-alpha blockers. *Ann. N. Y. Acad. Sci.* **2006**, *1069*, 438–443. [CrossRef] [PubMed]
29. Mishra, B.R.; Maiti, R.; Nath, S.; Sahoo, P.; Jena, M.; Mishra, A. Effect of sertraline, dosulepin, and venlafaxine on Non-BDNF neurotrophins in patients with depression: A cohort study. *J. Clin. Psychopharmacol.* **2019**, *39*, 220–225. [CrossRef] [PubMed]
30. Jin, M.; Sheng, W.; Han, L.; He, Q.; Ji, X.; Liu, K. Activation of BDNF-TrkB signaling pathway-regulated brain inflammation in pentylenetetrazole-induced seizures in zebrafish. *Fish Shellfish Immunol.* **2018**, *83*, 26–36. [CrossRef] [PubMed]
31. Lee, S.; Mattingly, A.; Lin, A.; Sacramento, J.; Mannent, L.; Castel, M.N.; Canolle, B.; Delbary-Gossart, S.; Ferzaz, B.; Morganti, J.M.; et al. A novel antagonist of p75NTR reduces peripheral expansion and CNS trafficking of pro-inflammatory monocytes and spares function after traumatic brain injury. *J. Neuroinflamm.* **2016**, *13*, 88. [CrossRef]
32. Jin, Y.; Sun, L.-H.; Yang, W.; Cui, R.-J.; Xu, S.-B. The role of BDNF in the neuroimmune axis regulation of mood disorders. *Front. Neurol.* **2019**, *10*, 515. [CrossRef]
33. Fauchais, A.L.; Boumediene, A.; Lalloue, F.; Gondran, G.; Loustaud-Ratti, V.; Vidal, E.; Jauberteau, M.O. Brain-Derived neurotrophic factor and nerve growth factor correlate with T-cell activation in primary Sjogren's syndrome. *Scand. J. Rheumatol.* **2009**, *38*, 50–57. [CrossRef]
34. Hsieh, M.-C.; Hsu, C.-W.; Lu, M.-C.; Koo, M. Increased risks of psychiatric disorders in patients with primary Sjogren's syndrome-a secondary cohort analysis of nationwide, population-based health claim data. *Clin. Rheumatol.* **2019**, *38*, 3195–3203. [CrossRef] [PubMed]
35. Yu, H.; Chen, Z.-Y. The role of BDNF in depression on the basis of its location in the neural circuitry. *Acta Pharmacol. Sin.* **2011**, *32*, 3–11. [CrossRef] [PubMed]
36. Aletaha, D.; Neogi, T.; Silman, A.J.; Funovits, J.; Felson, D.T.; Bingham, C.O., 3rd; Birnbaum, N.S.; Burmester, G.R.; Bykerk, V.P.; Cohen, M.D.; et al. 2010 rheumatoid arthritis classification criteria: An American College of Rheumatology/European league against rheumatism collaborative initiative. *Ann. Rheum. Dis.* **2010**, *69*, 1580–1588. [CrossRef] [PubMed]
37. Ng, K.-J.; Huang, K.-Y.; Tung, C.-H.; Hsu, B.-B.; Wu, C.-H.; Koo, M.; Hsu, C.-W.; Lu, M.-C.; Lai, N.-S. Modified rheumatoid arthritis impact of disease (RAID) score, a potential tool for depression and anxiety screening for rheumatoid arthritis. *Jt. Bone Spine* **2019**, *86*, 805–807. [CrossRef]
38. Zigmond, A.S.; Snaith, R.P. The hospital anxiety and depression scale. *Acta Psychiatr. Scand.* **1983**, *67*, 361–370. [CrossRef]
39. Lu, M.-C.; Lai, N.-S.; Chen, H.-C.; Yu, H.-C.; Huang, K.-Y.; Tung, C.-H.; Huang, H.-B.; Yu, C.-L. Decreased microRNA(miR)-145 and increased miR-224 expression in T cells from patients with systemic lupus erythematosus involved in lupus immunopathogenesis. *Clin. Exp. Immunol.* **2013**, *171*, 91–99. [CrossRef]
40. Lu, M.-C.; Lai, N.-S.; Yin, W.-Y.; Yu, H.-C.; Huang, H.-B.; Tung, C.-H.; Huang, K.-Y.; Yu, C.-L. Anti-Citrullinated protein antibodies activated ERK1/2 and JNK mitogen-activated protein kinases via binding to surface-expressed citrullinated GRP78 on mononuclear cells. *J. Clin. Immunol.* **2013**, *33*, 558–566. [CrossRef]
41. Lai, N.-S.; Yu, C.-L.; Yin, W.-Y.; Yu, H.-C.; Huang, H.-B.; Tung, C.-H.; Lu, M.-C. Combination of nifedipine and subtherapeutic dose of cyclosporin additively suppresses mononuclear cells activation of patients with rheumatoid arthritis and normal individuals via Ca(2+)-calcineurin-nuclear factor of activated T cells pathway. *Clin. Exp. Immunol.* **2012**, *168*, 78–86. [CrossRef] [PubMed]
42. Lai, N.-S.; Yu, H.-C.; Huang, K.-Y.; Tung, C.-H.; Huang, H.-B.; Lu, M.-C. Decreased T cell expression of H/ACA box small nucleolar RNA 12 promotes lupus pathogenesis in patients with systemic lupus erythematosus. *Lupus* **2018**, *27*, 1499–1508. [CrossRef] [PubMed]

International Journal of *Molecular Sciences*

MDPI

Article

Expression Pattern of iNOS, BCL-2 and MMP-9 in the Hip Synovium Tissue of Patients with Osteoarthritis

Davor Caric [1], Sandra Zekic Tomas [2], Natalija Filipovic [3], Violeta Soljic [4], Benjamin Benzon [3], Sandro Glumac [5], Ivan Rakovac [6] and Katarina Vukojevic [3,4,*]

1 Department of Orthopaedics and Traumatology, University Hospital in Split, Spinciceva 1, 21000 Split, Croatia; caric.davor@gmail.com
2 Department of Pathology, Forensic Medicine and Cytology, University Hospital in Split, Spinciceva 1, 21000 Split, Croatia; szekic@mefst.hr
3 Department of Anatomy, Histology and Embryology, School of Medicine, University of Split, Soltanska 2, 21000 Split, Croatia; natalija.filipovic@mefst.hr (N.F.); benjamin.benzon@mefst.hr (B.B.)
4 Department of Histology and Embryology, School of Medicine, University of Mostar, Kralja Petra Kresimira IV, 88000 Mostar, Bosnia and Herzegovina; violeta.soljic@mef.sum.ba
5 Department of Anesthesiology and Intensive Care, University Hospital in Split, Spinciceva 1, 21000 Split, Croatia; sandro.glumac@gmail.com
6 Department of Natural and Health Sciences, Juraj Dobrila University of Pula, Pula, Zagrebačka ul. 30, 52100 Pula, Croatia; ivan.rakovac@gmail.com
* Correspondence: katarina.vukojevic@mefst.hr

Citation: Caric, D.; Zekic Tomas, S.; Filipovic, N.; Soljic, V.; Benzon, B.; Glumac, S.; Rakovac, I.; Vukojevic, K. Expression Pattern of iNOS, BCL-2 and MMP-9 in the Hip Synovium Tissue of Patients with Osteoarthritis. *Int. J. Mol. Sci.* **2021**, *22*, 1489. https://doi.org/10.3390/ijms22031489

Academic Editor: Chih-Hsin Tang
Received: 11 January 2021
Accepted: 27 January 2021
Published: 2 February 2021

Abstract: Hip osteoarthritis (HOA) is characterized by degradation of the cartilage and synovitis. However, the pathohistological effects of synovial tissue inflammation on HOA are not clear. The aim of this study was to evaluate the expression of iNOS, BCL-2 and MMP-9 markers in different synovial cell populations. A total of 32 patients were evaluated retrospectively. Age, sex, height, weight, body mass index were recorded and lymphocyte, fibrocytes and macrophages were analysed in tissue sections. Osteoarthritis cartilage histopathology assessment system (OARSI), Western Ontario and McMaster Universities Osteoarthritis Index (WOMAC), Krenn score, Harris Hip Score (HHS) and Kellgren–Lawrence (K-L) grading of the hip joints were performed. Total hip arthroplasty was performed on 32 patients and controls. Patients were divided into two groups according to their disease severity. The tissues were immunohistochemically analysed. K-L grade and Krenn score differ between all three groups, but also between moderate and severe OA. Synovial lining cell layer, resident cells in stroma and especially inflammatory infiltration were increasing with severity of OA. iNOS expression in both intima and subintima was positively correlated with Krenn score in moderate and severe osteoarthritis (OA) groups. Expression of BCL-2 in intima of severe OA patients was positively correlated with Krenn score. In conclusion, iNOS, BCL-2 and MMP-9 are involved in the regulation of HOA. Our study indicates a relationship between the pathohistological features, the synovial inflammation and the cartilage condition at the time of hip replacement due to OA or femoral neck fracture.

Keywords: osteoarthritis; Hip; iNOS; BCL-2; MMP-9; cartilage; subchondral tissue; synovia

1. Introduction

Osteoarthritis is a degenerative joint disease that causes progressive damage to articular cartilage and surrounding structures and is a common cause of pain and disability among older adults [1–3]. Among all osteoarthritis, hip osteoarthritis (HOA) has a huge impact on quality of life as well as significant negative economic impact due to reduced work capacity of the working population and treatment costs [4,5]. Prevalence of symptomatic HOA is 9.2% in the population older than 45 years [6]. Osteoarthritis OA is defined as a degenerative joint disorder affecting not only a cartilage and subchondral bone but whole joint including ligaments, menisci and synovial membrane and leads to cartilage degradation, inflammation of the synovial membrane, subchondral bone sclerosation, degeneration of ligaments and menisci and osteophytes formation [1,2]. Primarily the process appears to take place in the cartilage due to disturbed homeostasis of the extracellular matrix (ECM) with increase in water content, decrease in proteoglycans content of the ECM and changes in collagen type II production [7,8]. An inflammatory process or damage after trauma increases enzymatic activity and activates macrophages whose breakdown products affects chondrocytes by secreting proteolytic enzymes [9,10]. Macrophages, predominantly from the synovial membrane, phagocytize degradation products of collagen and proteoglycans causing production and release of proinflammatory cytokines: interleukin (IL)-1, IL-2, IL-6, IL-12, TNF-α and cyclooxygenase-2 (COX-2) [9,10]. Cytokines bind to chondrocyte receptors which is followed by increased synthesis and release of matrix metalloproteinases (MMPs) and change in production of collagen type II [11]. The synovial membrane in HOA shows thickening, increased vascularization and monocyte and lymphocyte infiltration [12]. The synovial membrane is composed of two layers: intima and subintima [13] and contains macrophages, Fibroblast Like Synoviocytes (FLS), endothelium of blood vessels, smooth muscles, lymphocytes and plasma cells [14–16]. Cytokines, adipokines, MMPs, COX-2, Inducible Nitric Oxide Synthase (iNOS) are secreted by synovial cells, as well as chondrocytes, so the synovial membrane has an important role in OA pathogenesis [17–20]. Considering presence of pro-inflammatory factors in synovial fluid and histological changes occurring predominantly in the synovial membrane, it has been proposed that OA is an inflammatory disease [21]. In the last few years there has been growing evidence that the FLS mediate inflammatory synovitis in OA by producing cytokines, NO and prostaglandin E_2 [22]. In OA, cartilage and the synovial membrane produce large quantities of nitric oxide (NO) [19]. NO in OA mediates the expression of inflammatory factors, inhibits synthesis of collagen and proteoglycan synthesis, and induces chondrocyte apoptosis and pain [23,24]. MMPs are the family of enzymes involved in the ECM breakdown [25]. MMPs are produced by both synoviocytes and chondrocytes and their activation causes irreversible tissue destruction, targeting collagens (types II, IX, and XI) and proteoglycans [25,26] as main components of the ECM. Contrary to inflammation, antiapoptotic factors maintain tissue homeostasis through the anti-apoptotic BCL-2 protein that controls mitochondrial apoptotic signaling by preventing mitochondrial permeabilization and release of cytochrome c [27]. Fibroblast-like synoviocytes survival is dependent of apoptosis and over-expression of BCL-2 protects them from programmed cell death [28].

To our knowledge, there are no studies that analyze distribution patterns of iNOS, MMP-9 and BCL-2 in the synovial membrane of severe HOA. The aim of the study was to establish a correlation between of iNOS, BCL-2 and MMP-9 synovial membrane distribution patterns and radiological grades, histological grades and patient clinical scores as well. The differences in the expression pattern of these markers in different synovial membrane cell populations could be the target of a new pharmacologic agent that can relieve the symptoms of HOA.

2. Results

In total there were 32 patients (9 men; 23 women). There was no statistical difference between groups according to age and BMI ($p = 0.884$ and $p = 0.055$, respectively) (Table 1). Symptoms average duration was 2.5 years in moderate OA and 3 years in severe OA. Although the osteoarthritis cartilage histopathology assessment system (OARSI) score differs significantly between all three groups, when we compare only moderate and severe OA, there are no significant differences (Figures 1 and 2, Table 1). Similarly, the Harris Hip Score (HHS), visual analogue scale (VAS) and The Western Ontario and McMaster Universities Osteoarthritis Index (WOMAC) score showed no difference as well. On the other hand, the Kellgren–Lawrence (K-L) grade and Krenn score differ between all three groups, but also between moderate and severe OA (Table 1).

Table 1. Clinical, radiological and pathohistological characteristics of the examined groups.

	Controls	Moderate OA	Severe OA	* p Value
Age (median ± IQR, years)	73 (72.25–76.75)	72 (63.5–75.5)	72 (67–77)	0.884
BMI (median ± IQR, kg/m^2)	25.67 (23.83–26.8)	24.9 (23.28–25.88)	26.9 (25.4–29.53)	0.055
K-L grade (median ± IQR)	0.5 (0–1)	2 (2–2)	4 (3–4)	<0.0001
Krenn score (median ± IQR)	0 (0–0)	6.5 (5.7–9)	9 (7–9)	<0.0001
OARSI (median ± IQR)	1 (0.25–1)	3 (1.5–4.5)	2.5 (2–4.7)	0.0005
HHS (median ± IQR)	–	48.9 (43.8–56.9)	41 (33.18–49.7)	0.271
VAS (median ± IQR)	–	6 (4.5–6.7)	6 (5–7)	0.781
Total WOMAC (median ± IQR)	–	46.1 (40–57.4)	47.3 (36.1–55.3)	0.917

IQR (interquartile range), OA (osteoarthritis), BMI (body mass index), K-L grade (Kellgren–Lawrence grading scale), OARSI (osteoarthritis cartilage histopathology assessment system), HHS (Harris Hip Score), VAS (visual analogue scale), WOMAC (The Western Ontario and McMaster Universities Osteoarthritis Index) * $p < 0.05$, Kruskal–Wallace test.

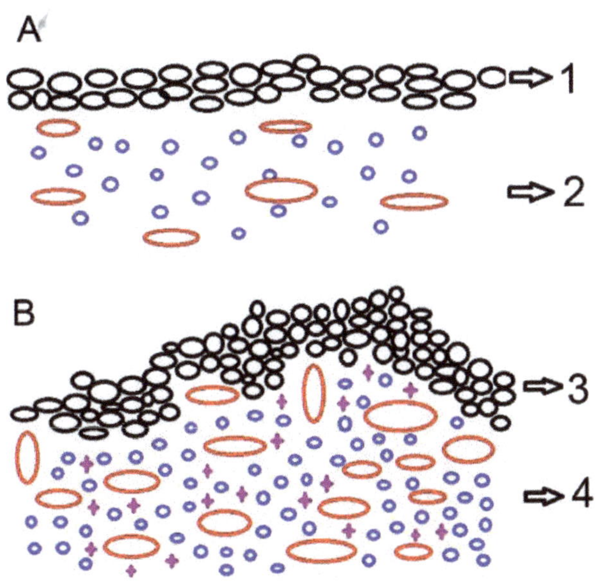

Figure 1. Schematic drawing of synovial membrane of patients with moderate (**A**), and severe (**B**) hip osteoarthritis (HOA). The epithelial lining (black circles) represents intima and stroma underneath represent subintima; 1—synovial surface lined by moderate hyperplasia of synovial cells (black circles); 2—underlying stroma with moderate amount of lymphocytes (blue circles) and blood vessel proliferation (red circles); 3—severe hyperplasia of synovial cells (black circles) in a papillary pattern; 4—underlying stroma with abundant lymphocytes (blue circles), macrophages (violet crosses) and pronounced blood vessel proliferation (red circles).

Synovial lining cell layer, resident cells in the stroma and especially inflammatory infiltration increased with severity of OA. Additionally, lymphoid aggregates in the synovium were not seen in normal tissue and only rarely in moderate OA but were present in a quarter of severe OA synovial membranes.

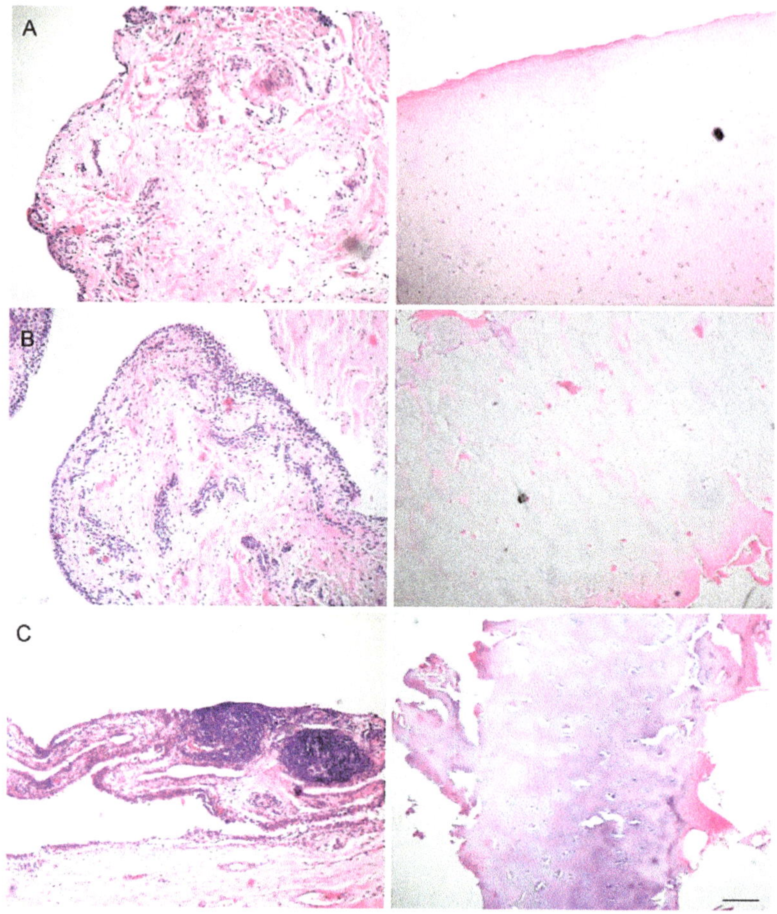

Figure 2. Synovial membrane (first column) and cartilage (second column) of control patients (**A**), and patients with moderate (**B**) and severe (**C**) hip osteoarthritis (HOA). Hematoxylin and Eosin staining. Magnification ×40, scale bar = 40 μm.

iNOS expression in the intima showed a parabolic trend with the highest level of 6899 ± 940.8 positive cells/mm^2 in moderate OA (Figure 3). Similar results were noted in subintima. BCL-2 expression was similar in intima of moderate and severe OA, however when compared to control, BCL-2 expression was higher in the latter groups. However, BCL-2 expression in subintima showed a linear trend of increasing expression with severity of disease. When examining expression of MMP-9 in intima, a linear trend was observed between disease severity and MMP-9 levels. On the other hand, expression of MMP-9 in subintima had parabolic trend with the peak level of 3301 ± 101.6 positive cells/mm^2 in mild OA (Figure 3).

iNOS expression in both intima and subintima was positively correlated with Krenn score in moderate and severe OA groups. Expression of BCL-2 in intima of severe OA patients positively correlated with Krenn score. However, expression of BCL-2 in the subintima and expression of MMP-9 in both intima and subintima showed no correlation with Krenn score (Table 2).

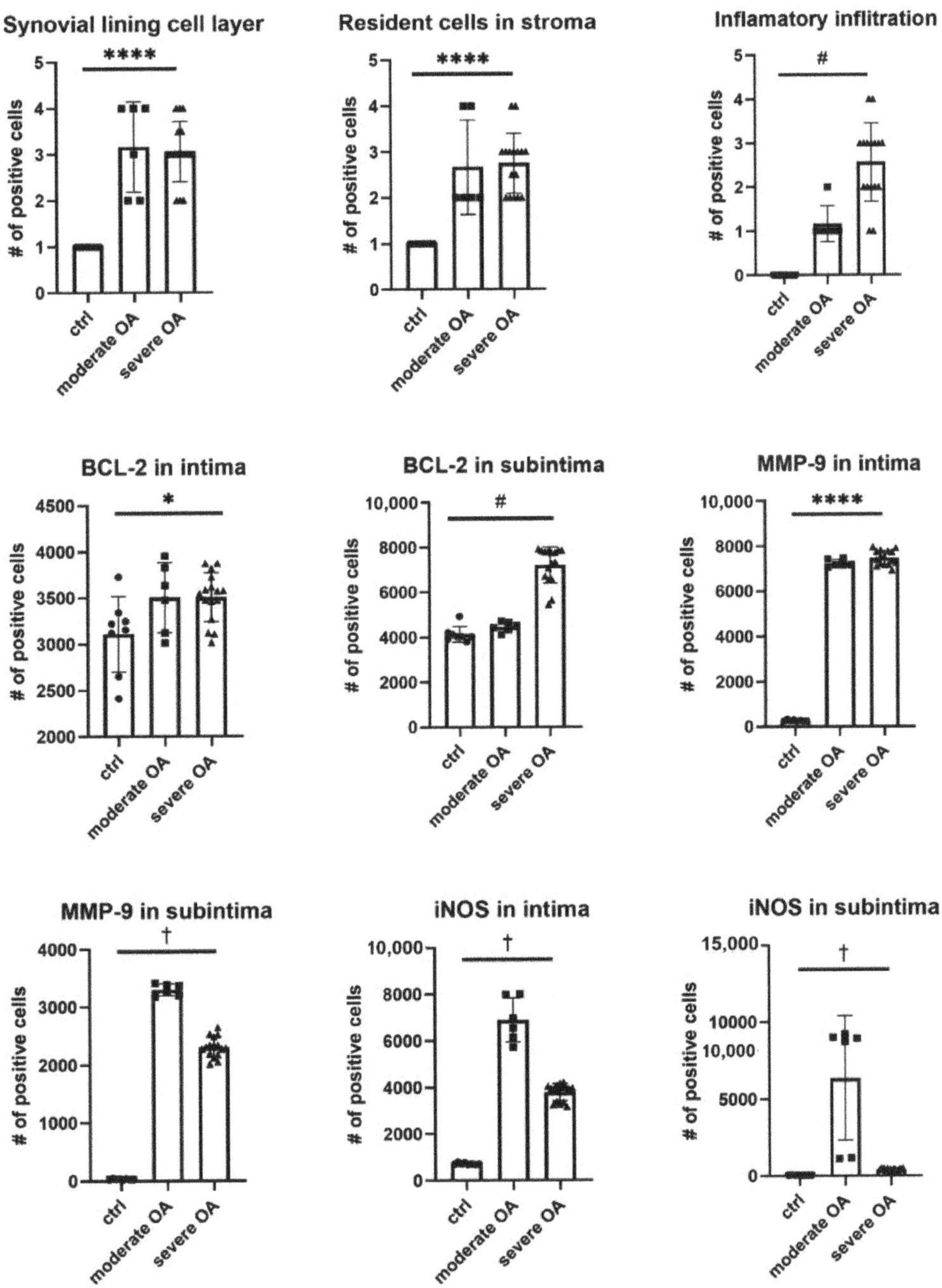

Figure 3. Pathological characteristics and expression of BCL-2, MMP-9 and iNOS in intima and subintima of hip OA patients. Legend: ctrl (control), osteoarthritis (OA); * $p < 0.05$, ****, $p < 0.0001$ for ANOVA; #, $p < 0.05$ for the test for linear trend; † $p < 0.05$ for the test for parabolic (quadratic) trend.

Table 2. Correlation of disease severity (β) and Krenn score (α) with expression of iNOS, BCL-2 and MMP-9 in intima and subintima of OA patients.

	Disease Severity								
	Control			Moderate OA			Severe OA		
	α	β	R^2	α	β	R^2	α	β	R^2
Age (years)									
iNOS intima	0	727.3 (692.9–761.6)	0	556.6 (446.2–667)	3003 (2212–3793)	98% *	372.7 (319.3–426.1)	670.2 (220–1120)	94% *
iNOS subintima	0	59 (49.3–68.7)	0	supplementary Figure S1	7464 (7023–7904)	99% *	67.45 (53.85–81.04)	−154.9 (−269.5–0)	89% *
BCL-2 intima	0	3110 (2769–3451)	0	0	3504 (3108–3900)	0	177.2 (56.26–298.1)	2022 (1003–3041)	41% *
BCL-2 subintima	0	4134 (3845–4423)	0	0	4460 (4230–4689)	0	0	7194 (6762–7626)	0
MMP-9 intima	0	261 (234–288)	0	0	7223 (7043–7404)	0	0	7465 (7292–7638)	0
MMP-9 subintima	0	33.88 (23.42–44.33)	0	0	3252 (2652–3852)	0	0	2184 (1304–3065)	0

* ANOVA p value for model < 0.0001; α–slope; β–intercept. Data in the brackets indicate 95% CI of model parameter. Number of examined iNOS, BCL-2 and MMP-9 positive cells are expressed as number of cells/mm^2.

According to staining intensity to specific antibodies in moderate OA, severe OA and control, we observed the strongest staining intensity in of iNOS in moderate OA, BCL-2 in severe OA and MMP-9 in both moderate and severe OA (Table 3, Figures 4 and 5). All of these markers co-localized with tissue specific cells (i.e., angiogenic cells, fibroblasts, macrophages and T-lymphocytes) (Figures 4 and 5).

Table 3. Staining intensity to specific antibodies in moderate OA, severe OA and control.

Antibodies	Diagnosis		
	Moderate OA	Severe OA	Control
iNOS	+++	++	+
BCL-2	++	+++	++
MMP-9	+++	+++	+

Three pluses indicate strong reactivity; two pluses indicate moderate reactivity; one plus indicates mild reactivity; minus indicates no reactivity.

In order to study potential angiogenesis in synovial tissue we observed numbers of cells which co-localized iNOS, BCL-2 and MMP-9 with different angiogenic markers (Figure 4). VEGFR1+/iNOS+ cells in intima and subintima showed a parabolic trend with peak expression of 975.3 ± 10.27 and 279.3 ± 10.01 positive cells/mm^2, respectively, in moderate OA (Figure 6). We need to point out that the level of VEGFR1+/iNOS+ expression in subintima was almost 12 times higher in moderate OA than in control. Numbers of CD31+/iNOS+ as well as actin+/iNOS+ cells in both intima and subintima had linear trend with severity of disease. The highest level of CD31+/iNOS+ cells was observed in severe OA (75.75 ± 6.2 positive cells/mm^2).

In order to examine fibroblast-like cells biology in context of antiapoptotic activity and EMC remodeling in both intima and subintima, we calculated the numbers of vimentin+/BCL-2+ cells that had a linear trend, while vimentin+/MMP-9+ had a parabolic trend (i.e., with the peak of 194 ± 2.82 in the moderate OA) with severity of disease. On the other hand, considering possible macrophages (i.e., CD68+ cells) in the same contexts, it was obvious that CD68+ cells were more prominent in antiapoptotic process (especially in severe OA intima), than in the EMC remodeling in both intima and subintima. Similarly, considering possible T-lymphocytes (i.e., CD3+ cells), which co-express BCL-2, there is parabolic trend in subintima, while T-lymphocytes that co-express MMP-9 showed linear increase with disease severity (Figure 6).

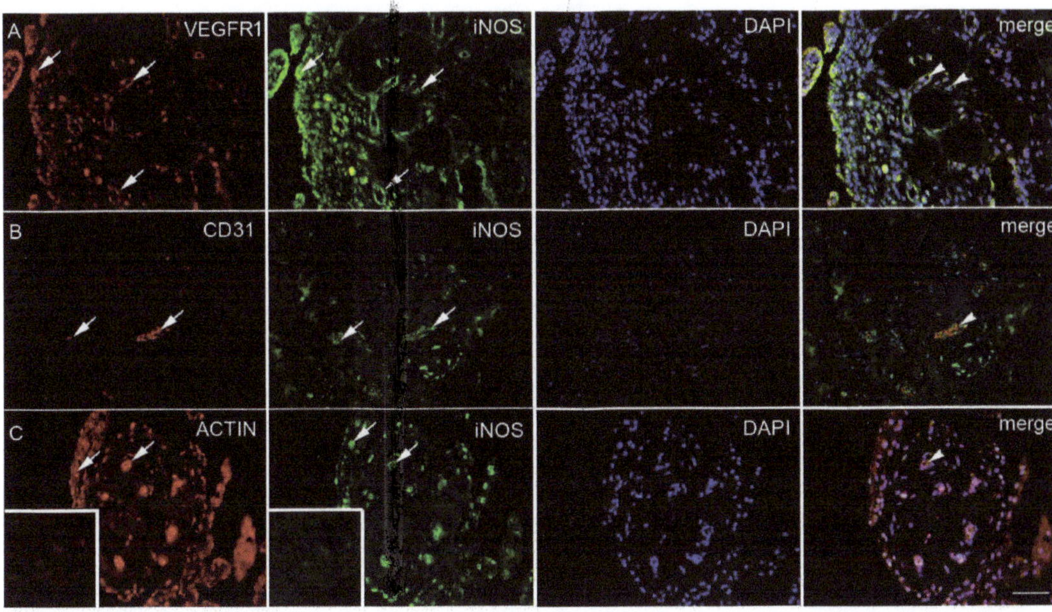

Figure 4. Synovial membrane of patients with hip osteoarthritis (HOA). VEGFR1 (vascular endothelial growth factor receptor 1) positive cells (red) in the synovial intima and subintima (first left arrow) and the blood vessels (arrows); iNOS positive cells (green) in the blood vessels and surrounding synovial intima and subintima (arrows); 4′,6-diamidino-2-phenylindole (DAPI) (blue) nuclear staining. Co-localization of VEGFR1 and iNOS merged with DAPI nuclear staining (arrowheads) is displayed in the far-right column (merge); moderate HOA (**A**). CD31 positive cells (red) in the blood vessels (arrows); iNOS positive cells (green) in the blood vessels within surrounding synovial subintima and superficial intima (arrows); DAPI (blue) nuclear staining; co-localization of CD31 and iNOS merged with DAPI nuclear staining (arrowheads) is displayed in the far-right column (merge); severe HOA (**B**). ACTIN smooth muscle (red) positive cells in in synovial intima and blood vessels (arrows); iNOS (green) positive cells in the blood vessels, synovial intima (arrows) and surrounding synovial subintima; DAPI (blue) nuclear staining; co-localization of ACTIN and iNOS merged with DAPI nuclear staining is displayed in the intima and blood vessels (arrowheads) in the far right column (merge); severe HOA (**C**). Inset: negative control of the synovial membrane. Magnification ×40, scale bar = 80 μm.

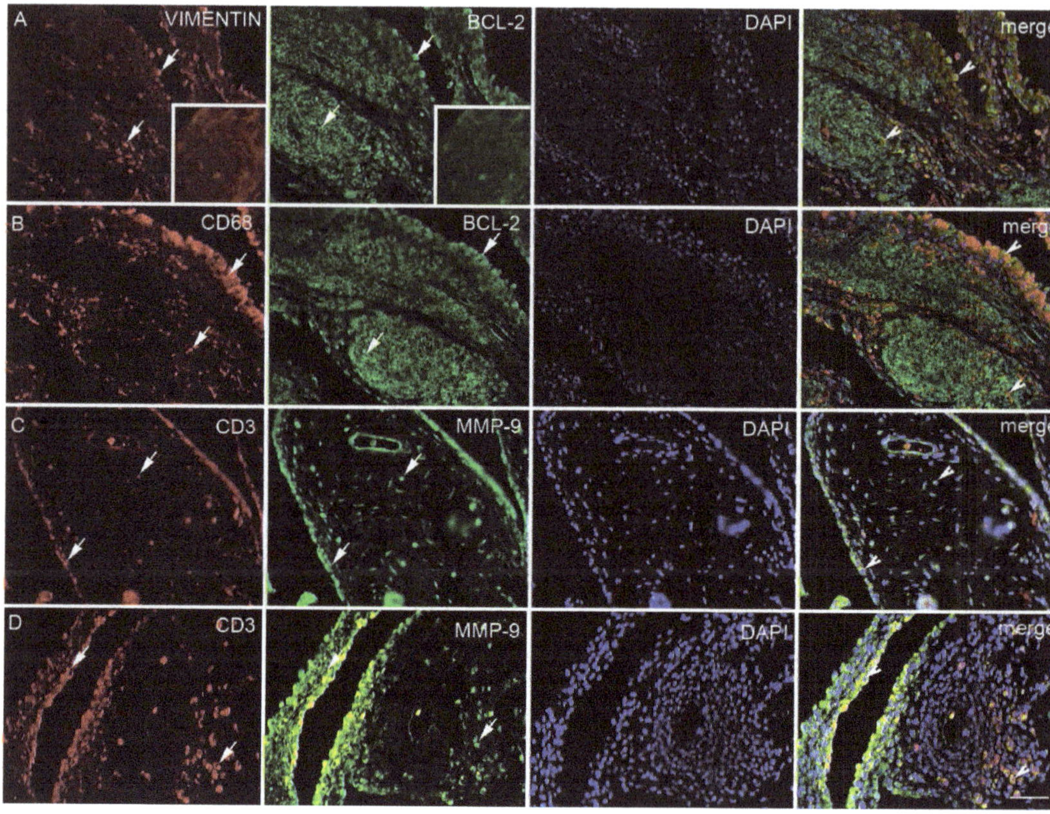

Figure 5. Synovial membrane of patients with hip osteoarthritis (HOA). Vimentin (red) fibroblasts and BCL-2 (green) positive cells in the intima and subintima (arrows); DAPI (blue) nuclear staining; co-localization of VIMENTIN and BCL-2 merged with DAPI nuclear staining is displayed in the intima and lymph node (arrowheads) in the far-right column (merge); severe HOA (**A**). CD68 (red) macrophages and BCL-2 (green) positive cells in the intima and subintima (arrows); DAPI (blue) nuclear staining; Co-localization of CD68 and BCL-2 merged with DAPI nuclear staining are displayed in the intima and lymph node (arrowheads) in the far-right column (merge); severe HOA (**B**). CD3 (red) and MMP-9 (green) positive cells in the intima and subintima (arrows); DAPI (blue) nuclear staining; co-localization of CD3 and MMP-9 merged with DAPI nuclear staining is displayed in the intima and subintima (arrowheads) in the far-right column (merge) in the moderate HOA (**C**). CD3 (red) and MMP-9 (green) positive cells in the intima and subintima (arrows); DAPI (blue) nuclear staining; co-localization of CD3 and MMP-9 merged with DAPI nuclear staining is displayed in the intima and lymph node (arrowheads) in the far-right column (merge) in the severe HOA (**D**). Inset: negative control of the lymph node. Magnification ×40, scale bar = 80 μm.

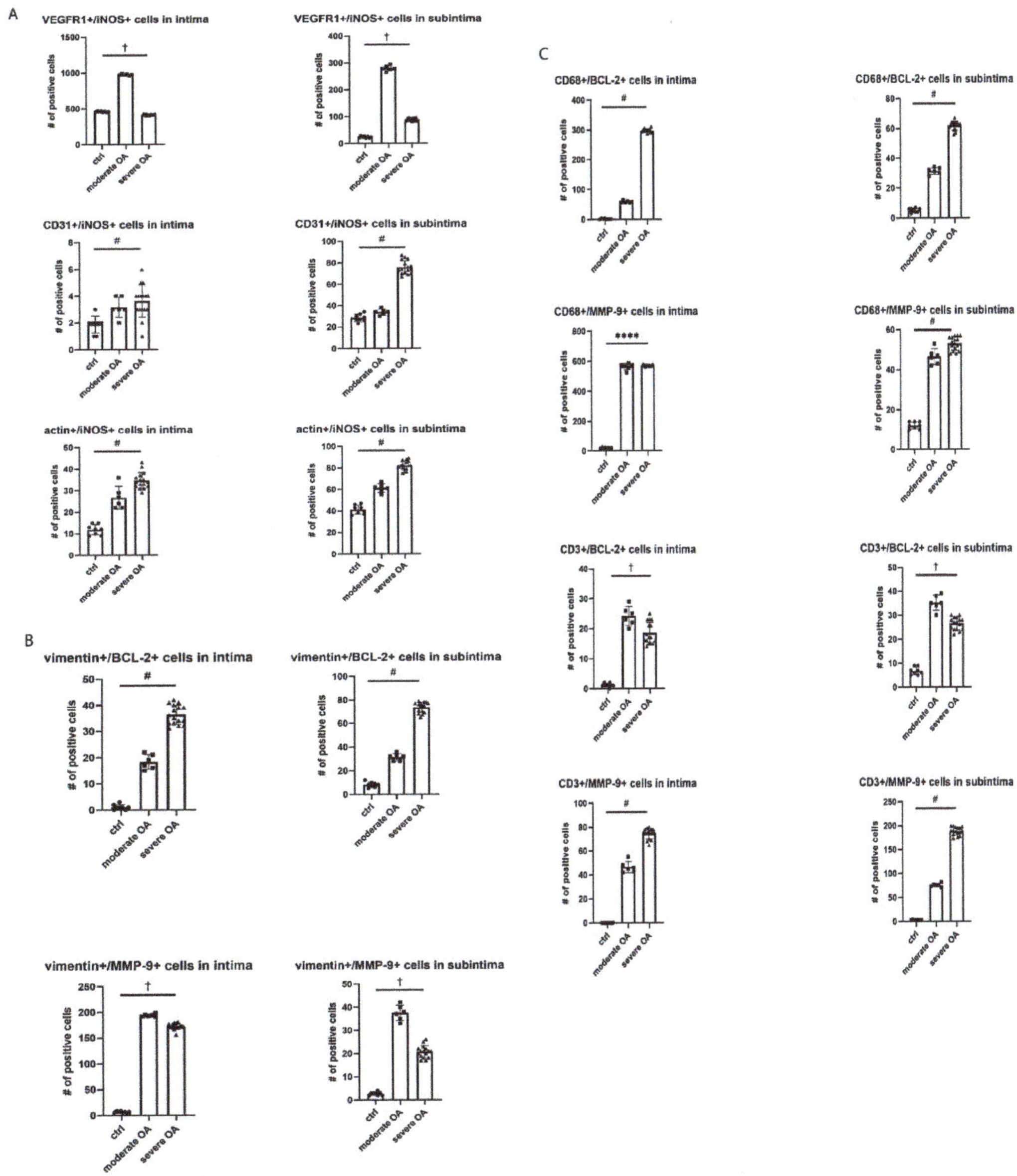

Figure 6. Expression of VEGFR1, CD31, BCL2 and MMP-9 in vascular cells (**A**), fibroblast like cells (**B**) and macrophages and T cells (**C**) in synovial tissue of OA patients. Legend: osteoarthritis (OA); ****, $p < 0.0001$ for ANOVA; #, $p < 0.05$ for the test for linear trend; † $p < 0.05$ for the test for parabolic (quadratic) trend.

3. Discussion

OA has elements of inflammatory events, which are triggered by macrophages from the synovium. Studies of the knee OA have shown correlation of synovial inflammation and progression of disease [29] and correlation of synovial inflammation and sensation of pain expressed in a visual–analogue scale as well [30]. Macrophages and FLS from the synovium also secrete MMPs [31]. Given the important proinflammatory role of the synovial macrophages, FLS and T cells [32] in the pathogenesis of OA, in this paper we decided to investigate their co-localization with BCL-2, MMP-9 and iNOS in order to achieve a better insight into the inflammatory changes of the synovial membrane in HOA. Our results point to inflammation, remodeling and survival process in the synovial membrane of HOA patients. By analyzing BCL-2 (survival of inflammatory tissue), iNOS (important proinflammatory and an angiogenic molecule) and MMP-9 (tissue degradation and angiogenesis) in hip synovial membrane, we wanted to establish a correlation between their expression with histological changes of hip synovium during HOA. We found no differences between moderate and severe HOA groups according to Krenn score and K-L grade in HHS, WOMAC and VAS. HHS and WOMAC assess range of motion, difficulties in activities of daily living and pain. Activities of daily living are influenced by both, joint stiffness and pain. Therefore, it can be speculated that Krenn score does not influence on joint stiffness or sensation of pain. Since those scores are dependent on several components it is difficult to conclude whether Krenn score has influence on some of the HHS and WOMAC components. We found no correlation to VAS either. In the later stages of HOA, joint stiffness is probably caused by marked osteophytosis and joint capsule contraction, while, in moderate OA, decrease in HHS and WOMAC compared to healthy individuals may be caused by pain due to synovitis.

Our work showed that the numbers of synovial lining cell layers, resident cells in stroma and inflammatory infiltrate were increasing along with the severity of HOA according to Krenn score and K-L grade, probably due to more chronic inflammation. The limitation of this study is that we did not have an early OA group since specimens were taken during joint replacement surgery. Previous studies confirmed the existence of lymphoid infiltrate in OA synovia. In the study of knee OA, it was found in five out of twenty synovial membranes [33], while in the study investigating hip and knee OA, CD3+ aggregates were found in 65% of synovial membranes [34]. We found one quarter of synovial membranes in the severe OA group that showed the presence of lymphoid aggregates. Lymphoid aggregates are present only in advanced OA. Results may vary because of the different influences from surrounding tissues i.e., synovial membrane in the knee may be influenced by the infrapatellar fat pad as a source of pro-inflammatory cytokines [35]. T cells are the major represented cells in OA lymphoid infiltrate [36] while they represent about 22% of the immune cells that the infiltrate OA synovial membrane. Macrophages are the most represented immune cell of the inflamed synovial membrane in OA and make about 65% of infiltrate [37]. Those studies were conducted on the knee OA synovial membrane. Our study confirms that the most abundant cells in hip OA synovia were presumably macrophages according to the high number of CD68+/MMP-9+ and CD68+/BCL-2+ cells. However, although using surface marker to distinguish cell type is common, clarifying the cell type with only marker is risky and, therefore, these results should be carefully interpreted. Additionally, another limitation is that this study is an observational study and did not include the functional role of each marker. Therefore, the changes of these markers may not play a dominant role in the progression of OA.

The inflammation process is influenced by iNOS [38]. Ostojic et al. reported higher expression of iNOS in an early radiological knee OA then in advanced OA [24]. Although we did not have an early OA group, our results were in line with that, considering that moderate OA had higher levels of iNOS, but a lower synovitis score than severe. It is possible that higher levels of iNOS expression precede a higher Krenn score in the severe OA group. Additionally, positive correlation with Krenn score is established between the control and both HOA groups. Krenn score is based on enlargement of lining cell layers, cellular density of synovial stroma and leukocytic infiltrate [39]. BCL-2 expression was increased in both HOA groups with a linear trend in the severe HOA group in the subintima, emphasizing the importance of the antiapoptotic mechanism in the synovial inflammatory cells and fibroblast-like synoviocytes that contribute to inflammation. In line with the fact that inflammation process is influenced by iNOS is our observation of the most prominent co-localization of iNOS and VEGFR1 positive cells, especially in the subintima of moderate OA patients. Vascular endothelial growth factor (VEGF) is produced by inflamed synovium during OA and may promote angiogenesis [40]. Angiogenesis may be present in all stages of OA and is associated with chronic synovitis [41]. Contrarily, severe OA has shown more co-localization of iNOS with maturated blood vessels i.e., CD31 and actin positive cells.

Based on vimentin+/MMP-9 co-localization among the groups it seems that matrix remodeling is most intensive in moderate OA, while the survival ability of fibroblast-like cells increases with severity of OA. Increased BCL-2 expression in the synovial fibroblasts is documented in the RA (rheumatoid arthritis) synovial membrane where it contributes to inflammation [42] and is more pronounced than in OA synovial fibroblasts. Little is known about the same process in OA. We observed a similar but less intense process in HOA. Fibroblasts protection from apoptosis may contribute to synovial inflammation.

Considering possible macrophages in the same contexts, they were more prominent in severe OA intima, implying their long life potential. They showed strong co-expression with MMP-9 in both HOA groups which was anticipated given their role in OA pathogenesis [9]. T-lymphocytes have their helper role in the subintima of moderate OA while co-localizing BCL-2 and contributing to the remodeling process in severe OA.

In conclusion, matrix remodeling and angiogenesis might play more a prominent role in moderate OA, whereas severe OA seems to be marked by fibrosis and completed angiogenesis; the latter is accompanied by increased long living macrophages infiltration.

4. Materials and Methods

4.1. Study Population

This cross-sectional study was approved by The Ethics Committee of the University Hospital in Split in accordance with the 1964 Helsinki declaration. Thirty-two patients were included in this study. There were three groups of patients: displaced femoral neck fracture in ambulatory patients older than 65 years (control group, No 8), moderate osteoarthritis group (No 6), and severe osteoarthritis group (No 18). In the OA group only patients with a diagnosis of primary HOA were included. Exclusion criteria for HOA groups were hip dysplasia, history of hip fracture or infection and history of rheumatic conditions. Osteoarthritis groups were scored according to the Harris Hip Score (HHS), Western Ontario and McMaster Universities Arthritis Index (WOMAC), visual analogue scale (VAS) and the radiologic Kellgren–Lawrence (K-L) grading scale. HHS, WOMAC and VAS were obtained for osteoarthritis groups within 1 month before surgery by the same orthopedic surgeon. The HHS and WOMAC and were not assessed in patients with a femoral neck fracture since these two scores assess the range of motion. VAS was obtained only for OA groups. In order to be put in the group of severe OA patients had to reach a K-L grade of at least 3, and a Krenn score at least 7. The patients used as control all had K-L grades of 0 or 1. Standard anteroposterior hip radiographs for OA group were taken no more than 6 months prior to a surgery. HOA diagnosis was established according to the American College of Rheumatology criteria for the classification and reporting of osteoarthritis of the hip [43]. Indication for surgery in HOA patients was failed conservative treatment with persistence of pain and functional limitations. The written informed consent form was signed by each patient prior to surgery, after the procedure was explained by an orthopedic surgeon. Age, gender, body mass index (BMI), symptoms duration, and the radiological stage of the disease were documented.

4.2. Tissue Collection and Basic Staining Procedures

All patients underwent total hip arthroplasty (Pinnacle Acetabular Cup System and Corail Hip System by Depuy, Warsaw, IN, USA) at the Department of Orthopaedics and Traumatology of University Hospital in Split. Total hip arthroplasty was performed through posterolateral hip approach with posterior capsule incision. Tendons of m. piriformis, m. obturator internus and both mm. gemellis were divided. After luxation of the hip, femoral neck was osteotomized by a 1.3 mm saw (Trauma Reckon System by Synthes, Switzerland)

and femoral head together with a part of femoral neck was extracted. In trauma cases there was no need for hip luxation, but femoral head was removed by a corkscrew after femoral neck osteotomy followed by partial femoral neck extraction. Then, a sample from the weight bearing area of the femoral head was taken by a sew in triangular manner. Samples were taken adjacent to the most damaged part of the weight bearing area but still containing a cartilage. Synovial tissue from inferior part of the femoral neck adjacent to the femoral head was taken.

The tissue samples were collected in the period of 2017 to 2020. Samples were put into formalin solution and sent to the Department of Anatomy, Histology and Embryology of the University of Split School of Medicine for histological analysis. Cartilage and subchondral degeneration was assessed using the OARSI grading system, while the synovial membrane was assessed according to Krenn score with 0 to 1 corresponding to no synovitis (inflammatory grade = 0), 2 to 3 to a slight synovitis (inflammatory grade 1), 4 to 6 to a moderate synovitis (inflammatory grade 2), and 7 to 9 to a strong synovitis (inflammatory grade 3). Tissues were formalin fixed, decalcified with 14% ethylenediaminetetraacetic acid (EDTA) solution (four months), paraffin embedded and cut to 5-μm thick sections. Each 10th section was stained with hematoxylin and eosin.

4.3. Double Immunofluorescence

After deparaffinization, sections for immunohistochemistry were rehydrated in decreased ethanol grades as we described previously [44–47]. Briefly, the slides were heated in citrate buffer (pH 6.0) in a microwave oven for 12 min. After cooling off at room temperature the slides were rinsed with Phosphate-Buffered Saline (PBS). Block protein was then put on the tissue sections for 30 min following overnight incubation with appropriate primary antibodies mixture (Table 4). On the next day, the slides were rinsed with PBS and an appropriate combination of secondary antibodies was applied (Table 4). The nuclei were stained with 4′,6-diamidino-2-phenylindole (DAPI) and slides were mounted in Immu-mont and cover slipped. Slides were examined using an Olympus (Tokyo, Japan) BX51 microscope equipped with a Nikon DS-Ri1 camera (Nikon Corporation, Tokyo, Japan). Images were assembled using Adobe Photoshop (Adobe Systems, MI, USA). Ten non overlapping fields were taken using 40× objective magnification. Double immunofluorescence with primary antibodies to iNOS, BCL-2 and MMP-9 was used in a combination of different specific cell type markers (Table 4), to determine the number of positive cells in the surface layer of cells (intima) and the underlying tissue (subintima) of the synovial membrane. We counted only cells that displayed both markers in the same cell (red or green signal) in the nucleus or cytoplasm. The cell count was performed using ImageJ software (National Institutes of Health, Bethesda, MD, USA). The total number of VEGFR1+/iNOS+, CD31+/iNOS+, actin+/iNOS+, vimentin+/BCL-2+, CD68+/BCL-2+, CD3+/BCL-2+, vimentin+/MMP-9+, CD68+/MMP-9+, CD3+/MMP-9+ positive cells were calculated as the number of cells per mm2 in the intima and subintima of the synovial membrane. The final total number per patient was the mean of 20 sections that were calculated and compared between groups (control, moderate and severe OA).

4.4. Statistical Analysis

Data analysis was conducted with GraphPad Prism (GraphPad Software, La Jolla, CA, USA). Nominal variables are presented as fraction, ordinal and continuous variables are presented as the median and interquartile range or mean and standard deviation. To test for differences and trends between groups ANOVA, a Kruskal–Wallace test and tests for linear or parabolic (quadratic) trends were used. For modelling relationships between different variables, linear regression was used. Statistical evidence is presented as R2 and p values. p values were interpreted according to the American Statistical Association Statement on p values.

Table 4. Primary and secondary antibodies used.

Antibodies	Host	Dilution	Structures Identified by Antibodies	Source
ab59348 (polyclonal antibody)	Rabbit	1:500	BCL-2	Abcam (UK)
sc-651 (monoclonal antibody)	Rabbit	1:200	iNOS	Santacruz Biotechnology (Santa Cruz, CA, USA)
A0150 (polyclonal antibody)	Rabbit	1:100	MMP-9	DAKO (Gloustrup, Denmark)
M0823 (monoclonal antibody)	Mouse	1:20	CD31 (endothelial cells of blood vessels)	DAKO (Gloustrup, Denmark)
M0851 (monoclonal antibody)	Mouse	1:40	Actin (smooth muscle cells of blood vessels)	DAKO (Gloustrup, Denmark)
ab212369 (monoclonal antibody)	Mouse		VEGFR1	Abcam (UK)
M0725 (monoclonal antibody)	Mouse	1:50	Vimentin (fibroblasts)	DAKO (Gloustrup, Denmark)
M0876 (monoclonal antibody)	Mouse	1:75	CD68 (macrophages)	DAKO (Gloustrup, Denmark)
M7254 (monoclonal antibody)	Mouse	1:50	CD3 (lymphocytes)	DAKO (Gloustrup, Denmark)
Rhodamine Goat AP124R	Mouse	1:100	Secondary antibody	MerckMillipore (Billerica, MA, USA)
Fluorescein Goat AP132F	Rabbit	1:100	Secondary antibody	MerckMillipore (Billerica, MA, USA)

Supplementary Materials: The following are available online at https://www.mdpi.com/1422-0067/22/3/1489/s1, Figure S1: Relationship between Krenn score and iNOS expression in subintima of OA patients.

Author Contributions: Conceptualization, D.C., S.Z.T., N.F., V.S., B.B., S.G., I.R. and K.V.; formal analysis, D.C., S.Z.T., N.F., V.S., B.B., S.G., I.R. and K.V.; methodology, D.C., S.Z.T., N.F., V.S., B.B., S.G., I.R. and K.V.; writing—original draft, D.C., S.Z.T., N.F., V.S., B.B., S.G., I.R. and K.V.; writing—review and editing, D.C., S.Z.T., N.F., V.S., B.B., S.G., I.R. and K.V. All authors have read and agreed to the published version of the manuscript.

Funding: This research received no external funding.

Institutional Review Board Statement: The study was conducted according to the guidelines of the Declaration of Helsinki and approved by the Institutional Review Board (or Ethics Committee) of The Ethics Committee of the University Hospital in Split Class 500-03/17-01/75, No. 2181-147-01/06/M.S.-17-2. Issued in Split on 25 October 2017.

Informed Consent Statement: Informed consent was obtained from all subjects involved in the study.

Data Availability Statement: The data presented in this study are available on request from the corresponding author.

Conflicts of Interest: The authors declare no conflict of interest.

References

1. Chen, D.; Shen, J.; Zhao, W.; Wang, T.; Han, L.; Hamilton, J.L.; Im, H.-J. Osteoarthritis: Toward a comprehensive understanding of pathological mechanism. *Bone Res.* **2017**, *5*, 16044. [CrossRef]
2. Loeser, R.F.; Goldring, S.R.; Scanzello, C.R.; Goldring, M.B. Osteoarthritis: A disease of the joint as an organ. *Arthritis Rheum.* **2012**, *64*, 1697–1707. [CrossRef]

3. Lawrence, R.C.; Felson, D.T.; Helmick, C.G.; Arnold, L.M.; Choi, H.; Deyo, R.A.; Gabriel, S.; Hirsch, R.; Hochberg, M.C.; Hunder, G.G.; et al. Estimates of the prevalence of arthritis and other rheumatic conditions in the United States: Part II. *Arthritis Rheum.* **2007**, *58*, 26–35. [CrossRef]
4. Salmon, J.; Rat, A.-C.; Sellam, J.; Michel, M.; Eschard, J.; Guillemin, F.; Jolly, D.; Fautrel, B. Economic impact of lower-limb osteoarthritis worldwide: A systematic review of cost-of-illness studies. *Osteoarthr. Cartil.* **2016**, *24*, 1500–1508. [CrossRef]
5. Solignac, M. COART France 2003 report on new socioeconomic data on osteoarthritis in France. *Presse Médicale* **2004**, *33*, 4–6.
6. Jordan, J.M.; Helmick, C.G.; Renner, J.B.; Luta, G.; Dragomir, A.D.; Woodard, J.; Fang, F.; Schwartz, T.A.; Nelson, A.E.; Abbate, L.M.; et al. Prevalence of Hip Symptoms and Radiographic and Symptomatic Hip Osteoarthritis in African Americans and Caucasians: The Johnston County Osteoarthritis Project. *J. Rheumatol.* **2009**, *36*, 809–815. [CrossRef]
7. Lahm, A.; Mrosek, E.; Spank, H.; Erggelet, C.; Kasch, R.; Esser, J.; Merk, H. Changes in content and synthesis of collagen types and proteoglycans in osteoarthritis of the knee joint and comparison of quantitative analysis with Photoshop-based image analysis. *Arch. Orthop. Trauma Surg.* **2009**, *130*, 557–564. [CrossRef] [PubMed]
8. Buckwalter, J.A.; Mankin, H.J.; Grodzinsky, A.J. Articular cartilage and osteoarthritis. *Instr. Course Lect.* **2005**, *54*, 465–480. [PubMed]
9. Zhang, H.; Cai, D.; Bai, X.-C. Macrophages regulate the progression of osteoarthritis. *Osteoarthr. Cartil.* **2020**, *28*, 555–561. [CrossRef] [PubMed]
10. Man, G.S.; Mologhianu, G. Osteoarthritis pathogenesis—A complex process that involves the entire joint. *J. Med. Life* **2014**, *7*, 37–41. [PubMed]
11. Goldring, M.B.; Otero, M.; Tsuchimochi, K.; Ijiri, K.; Li, Y. Defining the roles of inflammatory and anabolic cytokines in cartilage metabolism. *Ann. Rheum. Dis.* **2008**, *67*, iii75–iii82. [CrossRef] [PubMed]
12. De Lange-Brokaar, B.; Ioan-Facsinay, A.; Van Osch, G.; Zuurmond, A.-M.; Schoones, J.; Toes, R.; Huizinga, T.W.J.; Kloppenburg, M. Synovial inflammation, immune cells and their cytokines in osteoarthritis: A review. *Osteoarthr. Cartil.* **2012**, *20*, 1484–1499. [CrossRef] [PubMed]
13. Smith, M.D. The Normal Synovium. *Open Rheumatol. J.* **2011**, *5*, 100–106. [CrossRef] [PubMed]
14. Castrogiovanni, P.; Di Rosa, M.; Ravalli, S.; Castorina, A.; Guglielmino, C.; Imbesi, R.; Vecchio, M.; Drago, F.; Szychlinska, M.A.; Musumeci, G. Moderate Physical Activity as a Prevention Method for Knee Osteoarthritis and the Role of Synoviocytes as Biological Key. *Int. J. Mol. Sci.* **2019**, *20*, 511. [CrossRef]
15. O'Brien, K.; Tailor, P.; Leonard, C.; DiFrancesco, L.M.; Hart, D.A.; Matyas, J.; Frank, C.B.; Krawetz, R. Enumeration and Localization of Mesenchymal Progenitor Cells and Macrophages in Synovium from Normal Individuals and Patients with Pre-Osteoarthritis or Clinically Diagnosed Osteoarthritis. *Int. J. Mol. Sci.* **2017**, *18*, 774. [CrossRef]
16. Zhang, H.; Lin, C.; Zeng, C.; Wang, Z.; Wang, H.; Lu, J.; Liu, X.; Shao, Y.; Zhao, C.; Pan, J.; et al. Synovial macrophage M1 polarisation exacerbates experimental osteoarthritis partially through R-spondin-2. *Ann. Rheum. Dis.* **2018**, *77*, 1524–1534. [CrossRef]
17. Sellam, J.; Berenbaum, F. The role of synovitis in pathophysiology and clinical symptoms of osteoarthritis. *Nat. Rev. Rheumatol.* **2010**, *6*, 625–635. [CrossRef]
18. Presle, N.; Pottie, P.; Dumond, H.; Guillaumé, C.; Lapicque, F.; Pallu, S.; Mainard, D.; Netter, P.; Terlain, B. Differential distribution of adipokines between serum and synovial fluid in patients with osteoarthritis. Contribution of joint tissues to their articular production. *Osteoarthr. Cartil.* **2006**, *14*, 690–695. [CrossRef]
19. Abramson, S.B. Osteoarthritis and nitric oxide. *Osteoarthr. Cartil.* **2008**, *16*, S15–S20. [CrossRef]
20. Loeuille, D.; Chary-Valckenaere, I.; Champigneulle, J.; Rat, A.-C.; Toussaint, F.; Pinzano-Watrin, A.; Goebel, J.C.; Mainard, D.; Blum, A.; Pourel, J.; et al. Macroscopic and microscopic features of synovial membrane inflammation in the osteoarthritic knee: Correlating magnetic resonance imaging findings with disease severity. *Arthritis Rheum.* **2005**, *52*, 3492–3501. [CrossRef]
21. Berenbaum, F. Osteoarthritis as an inflammatory disease (osteoarthritis is not osteoarthrosis!). *Osteoarthr. Cartil.* **2013**, *21*, 16–21. [CrossRef] [PubMed]
22. Han, D.; Fang, Y.; Tan, X.; Jiang, H.; Gong, X.; Wang, X.; Hong, W.; Tu, J.; Wei, W. The emerging role of fibroblast-like synoviocytes-mediated synovitis in osteoarthritis: An update. *J. Cell. Mol. Med.* **2020**, *24*, 9518–9532. [CrossRef]
23. Pelletier, J.-P.; Martel-Pelletier, J.; Abramson, S.B. Osteoarthritis, an inflammatory disease: Potential implication for the selection of new therapeutic targets. *Arthritis Rheum.* **2001**, *44*, 1237–1247. [CrossRef]
24. Ostojic, M.; Soljic, V.; Vukojević, K.; Dapic, T. Immunohistochemical characterization of early and advanced knee osteoarthritis by NF-κB and iNOS expression. *J. Orthop. Res.* **2017**, *35*, 1990–1997. [CrossRef]
25. Rose, B.J.; Kooyman, D.L. A Tale of Two Joints: The Role of Matrix Metalloproteases in Cartilage Biology. *Dis. Markers* **2016**, *2016*, 1–7. [CrossRef] [PubMed]
26. Maldonado, M.; Nam, J. The Role of Changes in Extracellular Matrix of Cartilage in the Presence of Inflammation on the Pathology of Osteoarthritis. *BioMed Res. Int.* **2013**, *2013*, 1–10. [CrossRef] [PubMed]
27. Cheleschi, S.; Gallo, I.; Barbarino, M.; Giannotti, S.; Mondanelli, N.; Giordano, A.; Tenti, S.; Fioravanti, A. MicroRNA Mediate Visfatin and Resistin Induction of Oxidative Stress in Human Osteoarthritic Synovial Fibroblasts Via NF-kappaB Pathway. *Int. J. Mol. Sci.* **2019**, *20*, 5200. [CrossRef]
28. Hwang, H.S.; Kim, H.A. Chondrocyte Apoptosis in the Pathogenesis of Osteoarthritis. *Int. J. Mol. Sci.* **2015**, *16*, 26035–26054. [CrossRef]

29. Ayral, X.; Pickering, E.; Woodworth, T.; MacKillop, N.; Dougados, M. Synovitis: A potential predictive factor of structural progression of medial tibiofemoral knee osteoarthritis—Results of a 1 year longitudinal arthroscopic study in 422 patients. *Osteoarthr. Cartil.* **2005**, *13*, 361–367. [CrossRef]
30. Torres, L.; Dunlop, D.; Peterfy, C.; Guermazi, A.; Prasad, P.; Hayes, K.; Song, J.; Cahue, S.; Chang, A.; Marshall, M.; et al. The relationship between specific tissue lesions and pain severity in persons with knee osteoarthritis. *Osteoarthr. Cartil.* **2006**, *14*, 1033–1040. [CrossRef]
31. Fuchs, S.; Skwara, A.; Bloch, M.; Dankbar, B. Differential induction and regulation of matrix metalloproteinases in osteoarthritic tissue and fluid synovial fibroblasts. *Osteoarthr. Cartil.* **2004**, *12*, 409–418. [CrossRef] [PubMed]
32. Li, Y.-S.; Luo, W.; Zhu, S.-A.; Lei, G. T Cells in Osteoarthritis: Alterations and Beyond. *Front. Immunol.* **2017**, *8*, 356. [CrossRef] [PubMed]
33. Revell, P.A.; Mayston, V.; Lalor, P.; Mapp, P. The synovial membrane in osteoarthritis: A histological study including the characterisation of the cellular infiltrate present in inflammatory osteoarthritis using monoclonal antibodies. *Ann. Rheum. Dis.* **1988**, *47*, 300–307. [CrossRef] [PubMed]
34. Sakkas, L.I.; Scanzello, C.; Johanson, N.; Burkholder, J.; Mitra, A.; Salgame, P.; Katsetos, C.D.; Platsoucas, C.D. T Cells and T-Cell Cytokine Transcripts in the Synovial Membrane in Patients with Osteoarthritis. *Clin. Diagn. Lab. Immunol.* **1998**, *5*, 430–437. [CrossRef] [PubMed]
35. Favero, M.; El-Hadi, H.; Belluzzi, E.; Granzotto, M.; Porzionato, A.; Sarasin, G.; Rambaldo, A.; Iacobellis, C.; Cigolotti, A.; Fontanella, C.G.; et al. Infrapatellar fat pad features in osteoarthritis: A histopathological and molecular study. *Rheumatology* **2017**, *56*, 1784–1793. [CrossRef]
36. Haynes, M.K.; Hume, E.L.; Smith, J.B. Phenotypic Characterization of Inflammatory Cells from Osteoarthritic Synovium and Synovial Fluids. *Clin. Immunol.* **2002**, *105*, 315–325. [CrossRef]
37. Pessler, F.; Chen, L.X.; Dai, L.; Gomez-Vaquero, C.; Diaz-Torné, C.; Paessler, M.E.; Scanzello, C.; Cakir, N.; Einhorn, E.; Schumacher, H.R. A histomorphometric analysis of synovial biopsies from individuals with Gulf War Veterans' Illness and joint pain compared to normal and osteoarthritis synovium. *Clin. Rheumatol.* **2008**, *27*, 1127–1134. [CrossRef]
38. Mapp, P.I.; Walsh, D.A. Mechanisms and targets of angiogenesis and nerve growth in osteoarthritis. *Nat. Rev. Rheumatol.* **2012**, *8*, 390–398. [CrossRef]
39. Krenn, V.; Morawietz, L.; Häupl, T.; Neidel, J.; Petersen, I.; König, A. Grading of Chronic Synovitis—A Histopathological Grading System for Molecular and Diagnostic Pathology. *Pathol.-Res. Pr.* **2002**, *198*, 317–325. [CrossRef]
40. Haywood, L.; McWilliams, D.F.; Pearson, C.I.; Gill, S.E.; Ganesan, A.; Wilson, D.; Walsh, D.A. Inflammation and angiogenesis in osteoarthritis. *Arthritis Rheum.* **2003**, *48*, 2173–2177. [CrossRef]
41. Sakkas, L.I.; Platsoucas, C.D. The role of T cells in the pathogenesis of osteoarthritis. *Arthritis Rheum.* **2007**, *56*, 409–424. [CrossRef] [PubMed]
42. Perlman, H.; Georganas, C.; Pagliari, L.J.; Koch, A.E.; Haines, K.; Pope, R.M. Bcl-2 expression in synovial fibroblasts is essential for maintaining mitochondrial homeostasis and cell viability. *J. Immunol.* **2000**, *164*, 5227–5235. [CrossRef] [PubMed]
43. Altman, R.; Alarcón, G.; Appelrouth, D.; Bloch, D.; Borenstein, D.; Brandt, K.; Brown, C.; Cooke, T.D.; Daniel, W.; Feldman, D.; et al. The American College of Rheumatology criteria for the classification and reporting of osteoarthritis of the hip. *Arthritis Rheum.* **1991**, *34*, 505–514. [CrossRef] [PubMed]
44. Vukojevic, K.; Skobic, H.; Saraga-Babic, M. Proliferation and differentiation of glial and neuronal progenitors in the development of human spinal ganglia. *Differentiation* **2009**, *78*, 91–98. [CrossRef] [PubMed]
45. Jurić, M.; Zeitler, J.; Vukojević, K.; Bočina, I.; Grobe, M.; Kretzschmar, G.; Saraga-Babić, M.; Filipović, N. Expression of Connexins 37, 43 and 45 in Developing Human Spinal Cord and Ganglia. *Int. J. Mol. Sci.* **2020**, *21*, 9356. [CrossRef]
46. Kosovic, I.; Filipović, N.; Benzon, B.; Bočina, I.; Durdov, M.G.; Vukojević, K.; Saraga, M.; Saraga-Babić, M. Connexin Signaling in the Juxtaglomerular Apparatus (JGA) of Developing, Postnatal Healthy and Nephrotic Human Kidneys. *Int. J. Mol. Sci.* **2020**, *21*, 8349. [CrossRef]
47. Urlić, M.; Urlić, I.; Urlić, H.; Mašek, T.; Benzon, B.; Vitlov Uljević, M.; Vukojevic, K.; Filipovic, N. Effects of Different n6/n3 PUFAs Dietary Ratio on Cardiac Diabetic Neuropathy. *Nutrients* **2020**, *12*, 2761. [CrossRef]

International Journal of
Molecular Sciences

MDPI

Article

Anti-Rheumatic Effect of Antisense Oligonucleotide Cytos-11 Targeting TNF-α Expression

Tatyana P. Makalish [1], Ilya O. Golovkin [1,*], Volodymyr V. Oberemok [2,3,*], Kateryna V. Laikova [2,4], Zenure Z. Temirova [1], Olesya A. Serdyukova [2], Ilya A. Novikov [2,4], Roman A. Rosovskyi [2], Andrey I. Gordienko [1], Evgeniya Yu. Zyablitskaya [1], Elvina A. Gafarova [1], Kseniya A. Yurchenko [1], Iryna I. Fomochkina [1] and Anatoly V. Kubyshkin [1]

1 Medical Academy Named after S.I. Georgievsky, V.I. Vernadsky Crimean Federal University, Lenin Boulevard 5/7, 295051 Simferopol, Russia; makalisht@mail.ru (T.P.M.); wwwzzznnn333@gmail.com (Z.Z.T.); uu4jey@mail.ru (A.I.G.); evgu79@mail.ru (E.Y.Z.); gafarova.elvina@inbox.ru (E.A.G.); yurchenkokseniya28@gmail.com (K.A.Y.); fomochkina_i@mail.ru (I.I.F.); kubyshkin_av@mail.ru (A.V.K.)

2 Taurida Academy, V.I. Vernadsky Crimean Federal University, Vernadsky Av. 4, 295007 Simferopol, Russia; botan_icus@mail.ru (K.V.L.); aliss.serdyuckova@yandex.ru (O.A.S.); i.nowikow2012@mail.ru (I.A.N.); roman.rosovsky@yahoo.com (R.A.R.);

3 Nikita Botanical Gardens—National Scientific Centre Russian Academy of Sciences, 298648 Simferopol, Russia

4 Research Institute of Agriculture of Crimea, 295005 Simferopol, Russia

* Correspondence: golovkin.io.1996@gmail.com (I.O.G); genepcr@mail.ru (V.V.O.); Tel.: +7-978-814-68-66 (V.V.O.)

Citation: Makalish, T.P.; Golovkin, I.O.; Oberemok, V.V.; Laikova, K.V.; Temirova, Z.Z.; Serdyukova, O.A.; Novikov, I.A.; Rosovskyi, R.A.; Gordienko, A.I.; Zyablitskaya, E.Y.; et al. Anti-Rheumatic Effect of Antisense Oligonucleotide Cytos-11 Targeting TNF-α Expression. *Int. J. Mol. Sci.* **2021**, *22*, 1022. https://doi.org/10.3390/ijms22031022

Academic Editor: Chih-Hsin Tang

Received: 19 December 2020
Accepted: 19 January 2021
Published: 20 January 2021

Abstract: The urgency of the search for inexpensive and effective drugs with localized action for the treatment of rheumatoid arthritis continues unabated. In this study, for the first time we investigated the Cytos-11 antisense oligonucleotide suppression of TNF-α gene expression in a rat model of rheumatoid arthritis induced by complete Freund's adjuvant. Cytos-11 has been shown to effectively reduce peripheral blood concentrations of TNF-α, reduce joint inflammation, and reduce pannus development. The results achieved following treatment with the antisense oligonucleotide Cytos-11 were similar to those of adalimumab (Humira®); they also compared favorably with those results, which provides evidence of the promise of drugs based on antisense technologies in the treatment of this disease.

Keywords: rheumatoid arthritis; antisense technologies; TNF-α; Humira®; phosphorothioate oligonucleotides; inflammation

1. Introduction

Currently, rheumatoid arthritis is one of the most common chronic joint inflammation conditions worldwide, with an incidence of 0.5–2% among all ethnic groups [1–3]. No specific cause for the development of this disease has been established, but it is believed to be a combination of genetic predisposition and an interaction with environmental factors [4,5]. The disease process is accompanied by a decrease in the quality of life, beginning with pain and stiffness in the joints, sleep disturbances and depression, increased fatigue, and decreased labor productivity [6–9]. In the absence of treatment, it ends in early disability and complete immobilization of the affected joints [2]. The economic burden of rheumatoid arthritis is significant both for people with the disease and for health care facilities and is associated with high medical costs and a loss of performance among patients [6,10]. It should also be noted that the juvenile form of the disease is a serious problem in children. This disease, which ranks first among inflammatory diseases of the joints, is characterized by the involvement of vital organs in some children, complications and side effects of basic therapy, and a decreased quality of life [11,12].

Today, several groups of drugs are used to treat rheumatoid arthritis. Non-steroidal anti-inflammatory drugs quickly and effectively relieve the symptoms of the disease, such as pain and swelling of the joints, but have a limited effect on the destructive processes in the joints. Steroid drugs effectively suppress both destructive processes and the inflammatory response [13,14] but have many unwanted side effects, such as growth retardation, hyperglycemia, and allergic reactions, among others [15,16]. A revolution in the treatment of rheumatoid arthritis occurred when drugs aimed at inhibiting pro-inflammatory cytokines were introduced, especially those targeting tumor necrosis factor alpha (TNF-α), which is involved in most of the studied inflammatory processes. Based on determination of the amount of TNF-α in the peripheral blood, it is possible to assess the severity of the course of rheumatoid arthritis [17].

Adalimumab (Humira®) is currently the gold standard for treatment. Compared to its predecessor analogs, such as infliximab or etanercept, it is less immunogenic and less likely to cause allergic reactions [13]. Within an hour of taking infliximab, it is not uncommon for patients to experience headache, fever, hypotension, or vomiting. In about 20% of patients, depending on the dose, antibodies against the drug are produced; in these patients, the frequency of infusion reactions reaches up to 60% [18,19]. Etanercept causes fewer reactions after drug administration, the most frequent of which are local reactions at the injection site [20]. Since it is a chimeric protein created from the TNF-α receptor and human IgG1 [21], antibodies against it are produced less often, unlike infliximab, which is the combination of an Fc-fragment of human IgG1 and a mouse Fab-region [22]. Adalimumab, on the other hand, is a human monoclonal antibody against TNF-α, identical to IgG1, which binds in peripheral blood or on cell membranes with high efficiency and low immunogenicity [23]. The use of adalimumab in combination with drugs from other groups significantly increases the effectiveness of treatment and avoids irreversible damage to the joints [24,25]. However, adalimumab is rather expensive and, like infliximab and etanercept, has side effects associated with its systemic action, which limits its use. The most common adverse event associated with use of adalimumab is an increased risk of developing serious infectious diseases such as pneumonia, tuberculosis, and other pulmonary diseases [26–28]; according to some data, the frequency of developing serious infections may be increased by 1.5- to 2-fold [28,29].

Since adalimumab and similar drugs have immunosuppressive potential, attention should be focused of the need for more detailed research on how these drugs affect the risk of developing infections and the severity of those infections, including viral disease. It is now known that taking TNF-α inhibitors can affect the rate of reactivation of hepatitis B virus [30] or herpes virus [31]. However, although few studies have been done on viral respiratory infections, one study reported that patients taking TNF-α inhibitors were about 10% more likely to develop influenza-like illnesses [32]. Thus, the quest to find safe and effective drugs for the treatment of rheumatoid arthritis, with an efficacy similar to that of adalimumab, but a lower frequency of adverse reactions and a more localized effect, as well as a greater market availability, remains relevant.

In our opinion, the highest potential lies in drugs developed using antisense oligonucleotides (ASOs). Antisense technologies are based on the specific inhibition of unwanted gene expression by blocking or destroying mRNA activity [33,34]. They have several advantages over traditional drug therapies, such as the rapid and relatively affordable production of targeted oligonucleotides. In addition, the hydrogen bonds between the oligonucleotide and the complementary target mRNA are stronger than the bonds between different proteins; therefore, inhibition of gene expression leads to a longer lasting clinical effect [35]. As of 2020, more than 50 drugs based on antisense technologies are undergoing clinical trials, some of which are in Phase 2 and Phase 3 [33]. Currently, several drugs approved for treatment have been developed based on antisense technologies [36,37]; among these, nusinersen has shown very high efficacy in the treatment of spinal muscular atrophy without causing serious side effects [38]. The low frequency of side effects is associated with the structure of ASO-based drugs. Compared to typical biological drugs such as antibodies,

ASOs are relatively small and have fewer potential epitopes; in addition, nucleic acids are considered relatively non-immunogenic, and a properly selected ASO sequence will affect only the target region, making its possible effects easy to predict [33,39]. Thus, the research and production of drugs based on antisense technologies is a promising area in medicine, with a real possibility of creating affordable drugs with high efficacy and low side effects.

Previous studies have been conducted on the effects of ASOs aimed at various targets to suppress the inflammation of the joints caused by rheumatoid arthritis. When ASOs aimed at a highly sensitive C-reactive protein (hs-CRP) were studied, they were found to have selectively reduced hs-CRP levels with a frequency of adverse reactions equal to that of the placebo group, but its utility as therapy in rheumatoid arthritis (RA) remains unclear [40]. In another study, the effect of an ASO aimed at proliferating cell nuclear antigen (PCNA) was studied, which was shown to be effective in suppressing the proliferation of synovitis in a cell model [41]. It is worth noting that one company developing drugs based on antisense technologies tested an ASO aimed at suppressing TNF-α expression, similar to our study presented in this article; however, in that study, a 20-mer methoxyethyl-modified ASO was used, whereas our 11-mer-modified ASO was without methoxyethyl protection. Their study showed that the ASO had an efficacy comparable to that of monoclonal antibodies against TNF-α and was well tolerated when tested in mice and in the first phase of clinical trials, but they stopped further research in 2005 in favor of other projects [42,43].

Reducing TNF-α activity has proven efficacy in the treatment of rheumatoid arthritis, and as antisense technologies are now an actively developing industry, the development of an ASO aimed at inhibiting TNF-α is both promising and timely. In our study, we synthesized an 11-mer phosphorothioate ASO aimed at inhibiting TNF-α and compared its effects on the dynamics of the course of rheumatoid arthritis in rats to the effects of adalimumab.

2. Results

According to the results of organometry carried out at the beginning of the experiment, there were no significant differences in the lengths of the thigh, lower leg, or foot among the different groups. Over the course of the experiment, there was a trend towards an increase in the vertical and transverse proportions of the foot in animals from the control group, while the use of Humira® or Cytos-11 had a positive effect on reducing joint swelling. There was also a more pronounced swelling of the joints in the Humira group. There were no significant differences between the effects of the different drugs, not were there differences between the treatment groups and the Sham group (Figure 1).

2.1. Morphological Examination

At the beginning of the experiment, during morphological examination of the metatarsophalangeal joints, it was found that their condition corresponded to arthritis of 1–2 degrees of severity. Hyperplasia of synovitis and the development of the pannus were observed, containing, in addition to fibroblasts, lymphoid cells and macrophages. In the joint space of the individual joints, lymphoid infiltration was present, and the articular cartilage near the pannus was significantly thinned and had a fringed edge (Table 1).

In the group without treatment, we observed that the pannus developed faster than in the treatment groups during the experiment, the condition of the articular cartilage had worsened, and in some cases, bone tissue erosion had occurred. By Day 21, most of the animals in the control group had grade 3 arthritis (Figure 2b,c).

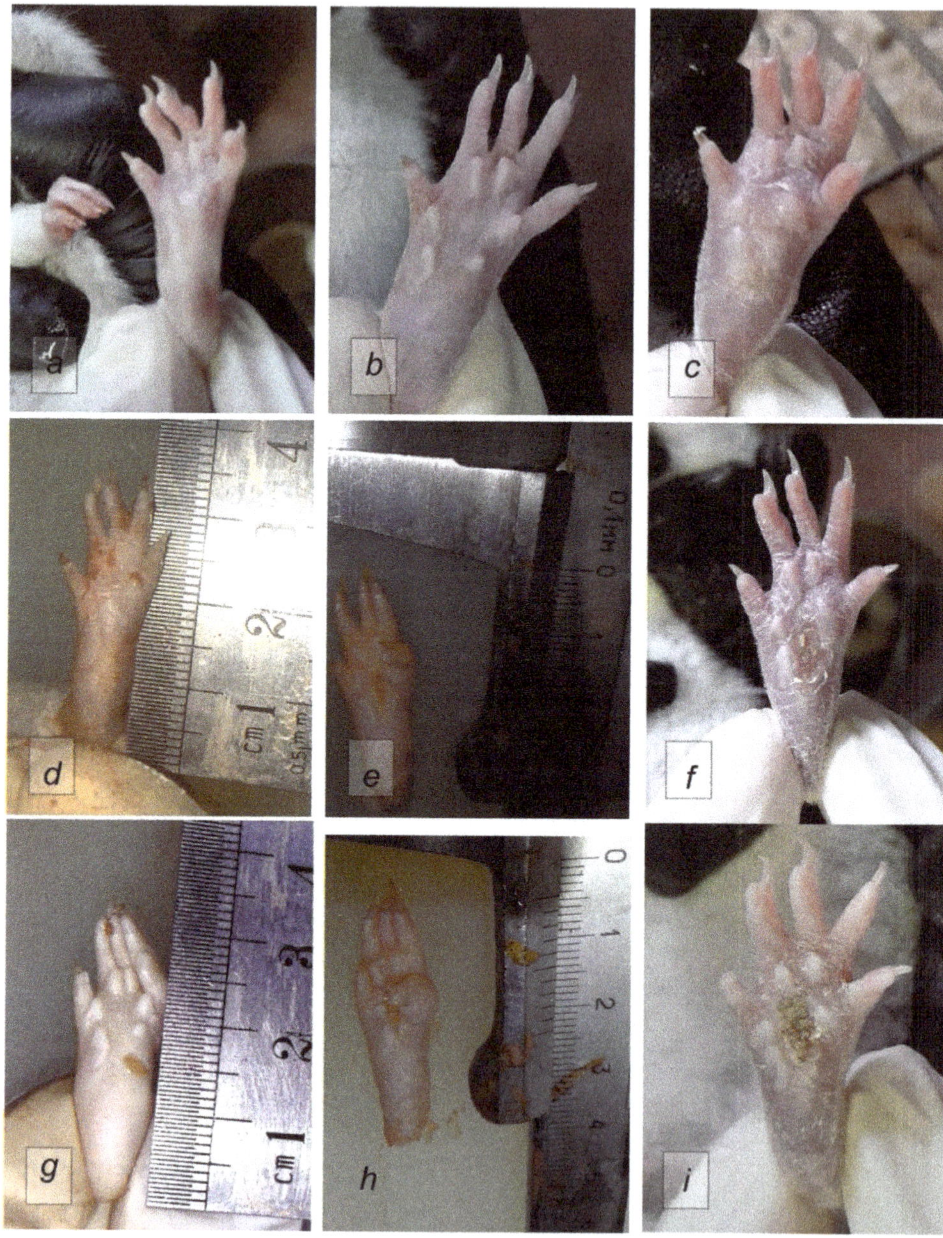

Figure 1. Left hind paws of rats. (**a**) Sham; (**b**,**c**) control after 7 and 21 days, respectively; (**d**–**f**) 7, 14, and 21 days after treatment with Cytos-11, respectively; (**g**–**i**) 7, 14, and 21 days after treatment with Humira, respectively.

Table 1. Evaluation of the degree of destruction of joint elements in rats in the experiment (Median [1Q;3Q]).

	Days	Infiltration (0–5)	Bone Changes (0–3)	Synovial Hyperplasia (0–3)	Severity of Pannus (0–5)	Destruction of Cartilage Tissue (0–3)	Total Points
Sham		0.0 [0.0;0.0]	0.0 [0.0;0.0]	0.0 [0.0;0.0]	0.0 [0.0;0.0]	0.0 [0.0;0.0]	0.0 [0.0;0.0]
Start of treatment		1.0 [1.0;2.0]	1.0 [0.0;1.0]	1.0 [1.0;1.0]	2.0 [1.0;2.0]	1.0 [1.0;1.0]	6.0 [4.0;7.0]
Control	7	2.0 [1.0;2.0]	1.0 [0.0;1.0]	1.0 [1.0;1.0]	2.0 [1.0;2.0]	1.0 [1.0;1.0]	7.0 [5.0;7.0]
	14	**2.5 [2.0;3.0]**	1.0 [1.0;1.0]	2.0 [2.0;2.0]	3.0 [3.0;3.0]	**2.0 [2.0;2.0]**	**11.0 [10.0;11.0]**
	21	**3.0 [3.0;3.0]**	**1.0 [1.0;1.5]**	**2.5 [2.0;3.0]**	**3.0 [2.5;3.0]**	**2.0 [2.0;2.5]**	**11.5 [11.0;12.5]**
Humira	7	**2.0 [1.0;3.0]**	**1.0 [1.0;1.0]**	**1.0 [1.0;2.0]**	**3.0 [2.0;3.0]**	1.0 [0.0;1.0]	**8.0 [7.0;9.0]**
	14	**2.0 [1.0;3.0]**	**1.0 [1.0;2.0]**	**2.5 [2.0;3.0]**	**3.0 [3.0;3.0]**	1.0 [1.0;1.0]	**9.5 [8.0;11;0]**
	21	**2.0 [1.0;2.0]**	1.0 [0.0;1.0]	**1.0 [1.0;1.0]**	**2.0 [1.0;2.0]**	1.0 [0.;1.0]	**7.0 [5.0;7.0]**
Cytos-11	7	**2.0 [2.0;2.0]**	**1.0 [1.0;2.0]**	**2.0 [2.0;2.0]**	**2.0 [2.0;2.0]**	1.0 [1.0;1.0]	**8.0 [8.0;10.0]**
	14	1.5 [1.0;2.0]	**1.0 [1.0;2.0]**	**2.0 [2.0;3.0]**	**4.5 [3.0;5.0]**	1.0 [0.5;1.5]	**10.0 [8.0;11.0]**
	21	1.0 [1.0;2.0]	1.0 [0.0;1.0]	0.0 [0.0;1.0] *	1.5 [0.0;2.0]	1.0 [1.0;1.0]	5.5 [3.0;7.0]

Boldface indicates values that have significant differences from the sham group ($p < 0.05$). * Significant differences in experimental groups vs. the control group.

In the treatment groups on Day 7, an increase in the level of leukocyte infiltration in the pannus was observed ($p < 0.05$). We also observed synovial hyperplasia ($p < 0.05$) accompanied by the growing pannus ($p < 0.05$) (Figure 2d,g). However, the state of the cartilage tissue did not differ from that of the sham group, and there was no damage to the bone tissues, except for mild erosion of the tibia in the Humira group ($p < 0.05$).

By Day 14, pannus leukocyte infiltration remained ($p < 0.05$) in the control and Humira groups. The condition of the bone tissue had deteriorated in the Humira and Cytos-11 groups ($p < 0.05$), accompanied by synovial hyperplasia ($p < 0.05$), and an increase in the severity of the pannus ($p < 0.05$) (Figure 2e,h). Observations of the thickness of the articular cartilage on Day 14 revealed that it did not differ significantly among the groups, apart from the control group.

At the end of the experiment, on Day 21, there were no significant differences from the healthy animals in the treatment groups, apart from synovial hyperplasia in the Humira group ($p < 0.05$) (Figure 2f,i).

Multivariate analysis showed that the method of treatment had the strongest influence on the joint condition. This effect was most pronounced on indicators such as infiltration ($F = 10.35$; $p < 0.05$), the degree of pannus development ($F = 10.97$; $p < 0.05$), and synoviocyte hyperplasia ($F = 10.79$; $p < 0.05$).

In the control group, the joint cavity was occupied by the pannus, which had a border of hyperplastic synovitis with a tendency to increase over the course of the experiment; the arrow indicates bone erosion (Figure 2c).

2.2. Immunohistochemical Analysis

Immunohistochemical staining of tissues for the presence of TNF-α revealed that in the sham group, synoviocytes did not express this cytokine, while in the surrounding tissues, single cells of the myeloid series, mainly macrophages, showed cytoplasmic staining of moderate intensity (Figure 3a). In the control group, there was an increase in the expression of TNF-α by cells of the lymphoid series in the tissues surrounding the joint during the experiment from 2 units on Day 7 to 3 units on Day 21; in addition, TNF-α is synthesized by synoviocytes with the progression of the disease, the staining intensity of which was estimated at an average of 2.5 units by the last day of the experiment (Figure 3b,c). Administration of the drug directly into the region of the joint had a positive effect on the joint, which was reflected by reduced expression of TNF-α synoviocytes and lymphocytes after 14 days of the experiment to 1 unit in the Cytos-11 group and an average of 0.5 units in the Humira group. After 21 days, there were no significant differences between the treatment groups and the sham group (Figure 3d–f).

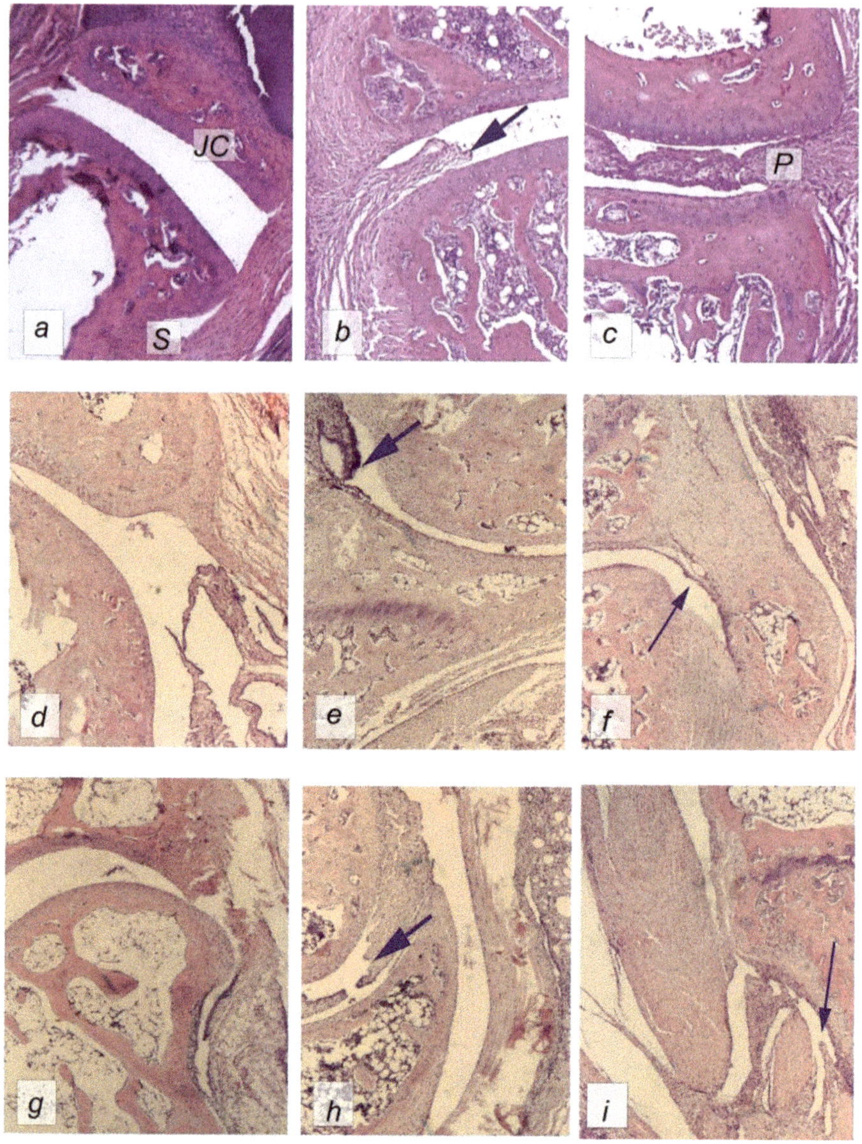

Figure 2. Hematoxylin–eosin-stained rat metatarsophalangeal joints from different periods during the experiment (used 5× lens); (**a**) sham; (**b**,**c**) control after 7 and 21 days, respectively; (**d**–**f**) 7, 14, and 21 days after treatment with Cytos-11, respectively; (**g**–**i**) 7, 14, and 21 days after treatment with Humira, respectively. Thick arrows indicate destructive changes in the joints and synovial hyperplasia. Thin arrows show the restoration of the normal structure of the synovium. P—pannus, S—synovial membrane, JC—joint cartilage.

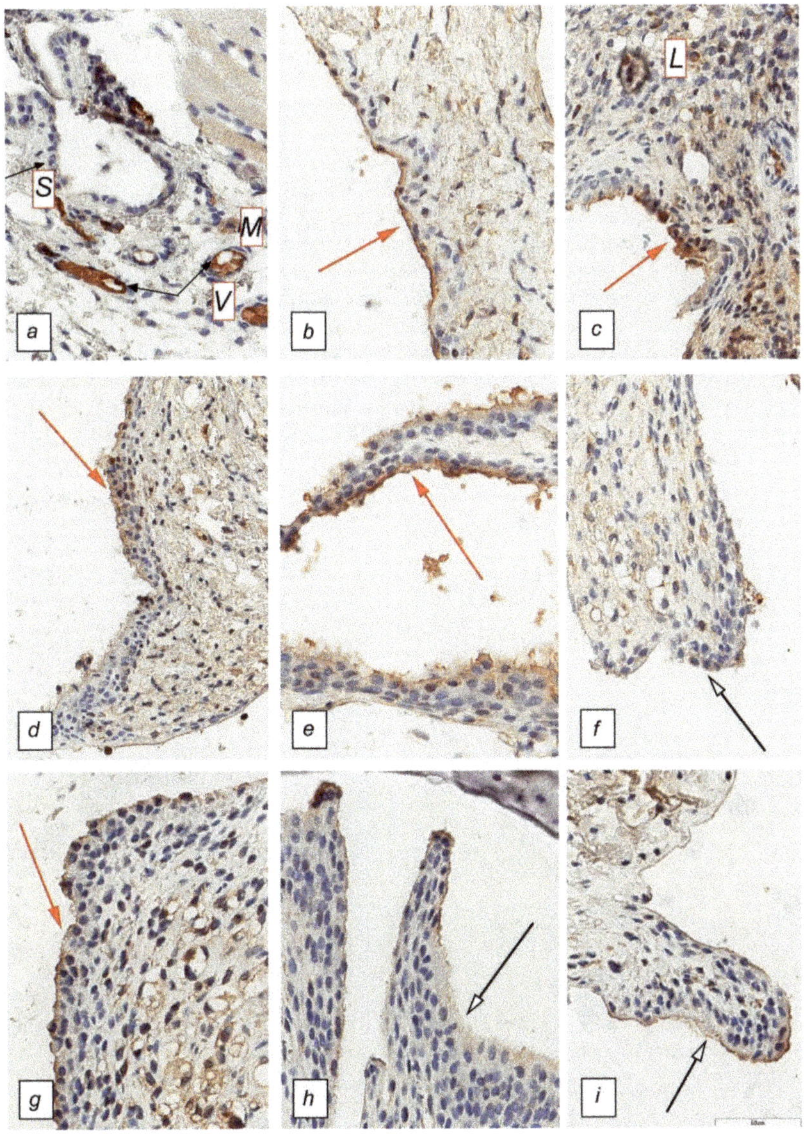

Figure 3. Synovial membrane of the metatarsophalangeal joints. Immunohistochemical staining with antibodies against TNF-α. Magnification 40×. (**a**) Sham; (**b**,**c**) control after 7 and 21 days; (**d**–**f**) 7, 14, and 21 days after treatment with Cytos-11; (**g**–**i**) 7, 14, and 21 days after treatment with Humira. L—lymphocytes, M—macrophages, S—synoviocytes, V—vascular endothelium. Red arrows indicate high TNF-α expression in untreated groups as well as early treatment with Cytos-11 and Humira. White arrows indicate a decrease in TNF-α expression.

In the sham group there was no positive staining of synoviocytes. Both single macrophages and vascular endothelium demonstrated moderate cytoplasmic color. In the control group, hyperplastic synoviocytes were expressed with a bright staining of the cytoplasm. Staining was also present in lymphocytes (Figure 3).

2.3. Linked Immunosorbent Assay

The concentration of TNF-α in the peripheral blood correlated with the results of immunohistochemical analysis and corresponded to the dynamics of the inflammatory process. At the beginning of the experiment, before dividing the rats into treatment groups, the mean concentration of TNF-α in the sham group was 30.3 pg/mL, and in the group with RA 31.6 pg/mL. On the 7th day of the experiment, there were no differences in the concentration of TNF-α among the groups, and the concentration of TNF-α was approximately 31 ± 2.1 pg/mL for all groups (Figure 4). On the 14th day, an increase in the concentrations of TNF-α was observed in animals with RA: 48.01 ± 11.73 pg/mL for the Humira group, 94.12 ± 9.69 pg/mL for the Cytos-11 group, and 86.15 ± 5.9 pg/mL for the control group. At the same time, there was an almost significant difference in indicators between the Humira group and the control group (p = 0.06). On the 21st day, the concentration of TNF-α had decreased in the treatment groups: 46.68 ± 7.67 pg/mL for the Humira group and 41.77 ± 7.8 pg/mL for the Cytos-11 group. This was significantly different from the group without treatment ($p < 0.05$), in which the concentration continued to increase to 129.8 pg/mL (±8.34).

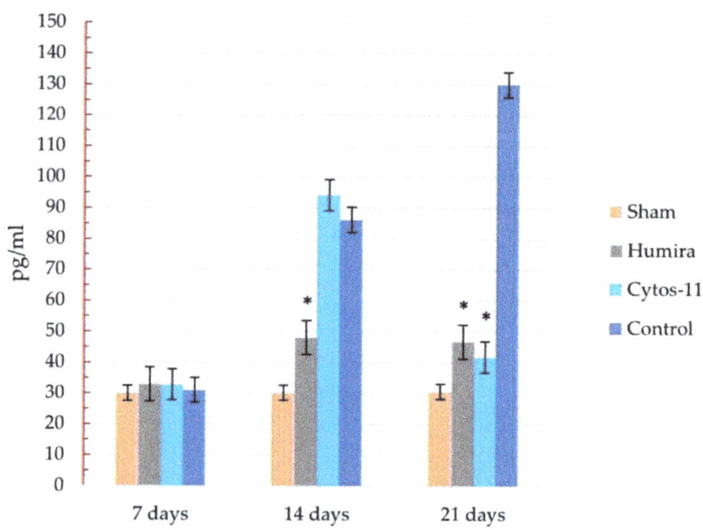

Figure 4. Dynamics of changes in the concentration of TNF-α in peripheral blood in different groups of the experiment. * Significant differences compared to the control group. I—error of the mean.

3. Discussion

The great advantage of antisense strategies is their specificity. This makes the use of antisense technologies attractive in clinical practice. The ability of ASOs to selectively block the expression of target genes means that studying the pathogenesis of diseases and their underlying molecular pathways opens up many targets for therapeutic intervention using antisense technologies. This is especially desirable because in addition to causing selective effects on target genes, ASOs do not induce immunological factors [44]. ASOs such as Cytos-11 are a valuable addition to biologic and standard antirheumatic drugs, particularly adalimumab, making use of ASO technology, a promising method in the development of treatment for rheumatoid arthritis.

In rat models of RA (induced by Freund's complete adjuvant), Cytos-11 was shown to reduce signs of joint inflammation. There was a decrease in edema around the affected joints, a decrease in morphological signs of the disease, and a decrease in TNF-α expression on cell membranes and in the peripheral blood. Comparison with adalimumab showed that Cytos-11 has a similar efficacy and that both drugs showed a major effect after 14 days of treatment. However, while organometric indices and morphological examination showed similar results on the same day, there were differences in immunohistochemical analysis and the concentrations of TNF-α. While Cytos-11 showed more significant results on the 21st day of treatment, it also had higher concentrations of TNF-α on the 14th day. Adalimumab selectively binds to TNF-α and neutralizes its biological functions; it is probable that the mechanism of action of this drug explains the low degree of immunohistochemical staining and levels of TNF-α in peripheral blood in our experiment, since the antigen is bound, making it inaccessible for detection when stained with antibodies during enzyme immunoassay analysis. Additionally, due to some inertness in the regulatory mechanisms of TNF-α synthesis associated with chromatin rearrangement and the synthesis of intermediate signaling molecules, the effect of ASO treatment on the genome manifests later than effects seen after treatment with adalimumab. This was accompanied by a higher level of staining in the micropreparation and the levels of TNF-α in the peripheral blood, which were comparable to those of the control group with RA on the 7th and 14th days, but led to values similar to those of adalimumab by the 21st day.

Several studies have investigated a specific ASO targeting TNF-α used to treat a collagen-induced RA model in mice [42,45]. This substance, analogue of ASO ISIS 104838 directed against human TNF-α [43], showed a strong dose–effect relationship with activity comparable to anti-TNF-α antibodies. The pharmacokinetics of the drug was studied in mice, rats, dogs, and monkeys in the preclinical stage of the study. However, it is impossible to accurately assess the results of the experiment and compare them with ours, because the internal data from the experiments have not been published. However, since in addition to the treatment of RA, monoclonal antibodies have been shown to be effective in treating Crohn's disease, psoriasis, and other diseases associated with TNF-α overexpression, it is possible to compare the results of ASO testing against TNF-α in a model of chronic colitis. One study, which used a specific ASO against murine TNF-α (ISIS 25302) at doses of 0.25, 2.5, and 12.5 mg/kg injected subcutaneously, reported a dose-dependent decrease in TNF-α mRNA expression in the colon and a decrease in the severity of chronic colitis. A decrease in the severity of chronic colitis was also observed with intravenous administration of the drug at a dose of 1 mg/kg and was demonstrated to be comparable to a similar dose of antibodies against TNF-α (0.03 mg/mouse) [46,47]. It is difficult to compare both the dose of ISIS 25302 used to treat chronic colitis with the dose of Cytos-11 used to treat RA, and the effects of each drug, because they were administered differently and different animal models were used. However, for comparison, in the treatment of colitis, 0.005 to 0.23 mg of the substance was administered via one subcutaneous injection every 2 days for 8 days, with results comparable to the administration of 0.03 mg of an anti-TNF-α antibody. Cytos-11 was administered via subplantar injections using 0.175 mg of the substance twice a week and had a positive effect in the treatment of RA. Again, it is worth noting that the differences in animal models and diseases means that we can only speculate, not confirm, the similarities and differences in the effects of the ASO data. However, as the data from even disparate ASO experiments accumulate, it is important to review them for similarities that could reveal useful trends and patterns.

In another study, researchers investigated a 20-mer-modified ASO with methoxyethyl protection (ISIS 104838), which showed high efficacy, good tolerance, and drug stability during Stage 1 clinical trials. Assessment of its pharmacological effect revealed a dose-dependent, linear, specific decrease in the synthesis of TNF-α by leukocytes in peripheral blood after stimulation with lipopolysaccharide ex vivo; in addition, the maximum concentration of ASO in the plasma proportionally and predictably corresponded to the dose [43]. In our past research with insects, 11-mer ASOs were found to be the most effective and produced optimal effects [44–50], which is why we used 11-mer phosphorothioate-modified Cytos-11 without methoxyethyl protection. To study its effects, it was administered twice a week for 21 days in a volume of 0.05 mL (3.5 mg/mL) via subplantar injection, followed by evaluation of the effects on the state of the joint and the concentration of TNF-α. This was comparable with the methods used in another study; in one group, ISIS 104838 was injected intravenously at a dose of 0.1, 0.5, 1, 2, 4, or 6 mg/mL on days 1, 8, 10, and 12 of the experiment; in a separate group, it was injected subcutaneously at a concentration of 25, 50, 100, or 200 mg/mL. It was found that ISIS 104838 selectively suppressed TNF-α mRNA expression, reducing its production in keratinocytes and lipopolysaccharide-activated leukocytes. However, the drawback to this study is that the effect of the drug was studied in healthy subjects, so it can only be assumed, not proven, that the drug will have a positive effect on joints affected by RA. In addition, the assessment of TNF-α expression occurred only on the first day (Day 1) and the last day (Day 13) of the experiment. Thus, this work for the first time analyzed the effect of antisense oligonucleotides on the condition of the rheumatic joints.

Comparing these data, we expect that Cytos-11 will have sufficient stability, specificity, and tolerance, as well as linear and dose-dependent drug effects. We plan to confirm this in future studies, as well as searching for possible side effects and non-invasive methods of drug administration. Our experiments showed the effectiveness of the drug in the treatment of RA, demonstrated by the decrease in signs of inflammation, both external and internal edema of the joints, as well as a decrease in lymphocytic infiltration of joint tissues, a decrease in the pannus, and decreases in the levels of TNF-α in the peripheral blood.

4. Materials and Methods

4.1. Rheumatoid Arthritis Models

Arthritis modeled on human rheumatoid arthritis (RA) was induced by subplantar injection of complete Freund's adjuvant at a dose of 0.04 mL every third day for 21 days into the left hind paw. After 21 days of injections, the model was allowed to mature for 10 days. An increase in the size of the foot and deformity of the metatarsophalangeal joints served as a signal to begin treatment. The results of the morphological examination showed that by the time the experiment started, the state of the joints corresponded to arthritis with a severity of 1–2 degrees.

4.2. Animals and Treatments

A simple, blinded, prospective randomized comparative study was carried out on 30-day-old white Wistar rats. The animals were randomized using the block method [51] and were divided into four groups, each of which had 6 males and 6 females, apart from the control group, where there were 4 more animals. The first group (sham) consisted of non-arthritic animals. The second group (control) consisted of animals treated with 0.9% sodium chloride. Animals in the third group were treated with the drug Humira® at a dose of 0.04 mL once a week via subplantar injection (Humira). Animals in the fourth group were injected with the phosphorothioate antisense oligonucleotide Cytos-11 (sequence 5′-TCC-GTG-CTC-AT-3′), which inhibits the synthesis of TNF-α, at a dose of 0.05 (3.5 mg/mL) ml twice a week for 21 days (Cytos-11). The animals were sequentially withdrawn from the experiment on days 7, 14, and 21 by 4 animals from each group to determine the time of the onset of the therapeutic effect. An additional 4 animals from control group were withdraw on the first day of drug administration.

All manipulations with animals were carried out in accordance with the European Convention for the Protection of Vertebrate Animals Used for Experiments and Other Scientific Purposes and approved by the ethical committee of the Crimean Federal University (Protocol № 10 from 12 November 2020).

4.3. Morphology Examination

At the end of treatment, the animals were decapitated under ether anesthesia. A caliper was used to measure the linear dimensions of the thigh, lower leg, foot (foot length, width at the base of the toes, and width at the ankle joint, as well as thickness in the largest dimension). The foot, cleaned of skin, was fixed in formalin for a day and then placed in an acid-free decalcifying solution for 10 days with daily fluid replacement. After that, the feet were dehydrated and soaked in paraffin on an automatic histological processor (Myelstone;

Sorisole, Italy). Pieces of foot embedded in paraffin blocks were cut on a Leica RM 2255 microtome (Leica, Nussloch, Germany) into slices with a thickness of 4 μm and stained with hematoxylin and eosin. The preparations were examined and photographed on a DM 2000 microscope (Leica, Wetzlar, Germany) with a digital camera and Plan 5×, Plan 10×, and Plan 40× objectives.

The assessment of the degree of inflammation was carried out according to the scale developed by us using the following criteria:

Leukocyte infiltration rate (1 to 5: 1—single immune cells in the field of view, 2—up to 5% of leukocyte infiltration of the total number of cells in the field of view, 2—6 to 10%, 3—11 to 20%, 4—21 to 50%, 5—more than 50%).

Bone changes (0 to 3: 0—no changes, 1—single changes, 2—pronounced changes, 3—very pronounced changes in the form of tissue structure disturbance, "pitted edge").

Synovial hyperplasia (0 to 3: 0—absent, 1—weak, 2—medium, 3—strong).

Pannus severity (0 to 5: 0—pannus is absent, 1—small, un-infiltrated, 2—small, infiltrated, 3—medium infiltrated, 4—creeps into the joint cavity, 5—erodes the cartilage).

The degree of destruction of cartilage tissue (0 to 3: 0—no changes, 1—slight changes—fistonic edge, 2—strong changes—about half of the surface is damaged, 3—complete replacement of cartilage with fibrous tissue).

Provisional points were assigned to each animal for each of the criteria. The absence of these signs was assessed as 0 points and the maximum severity of the sign as 3 or 5 points, respectively.

Determination of the thickness of the articular cartilage was carried out using the Image J program with the calibration of the scale using photographs of the reference standard (Stage Micrometer TS-M1 PN 106011) taken with the same camera with similar objectives.

4.4. Immunohistochemical Analysis

Immunohistochemistry was used to determine the level of TNF-α in the joint tissues. Paraffin sections were stained with antibodies to TNF-α (Abcam TNFA/1172, clone ab220210, concentration 1:200). Staining was performed in a BondMax semi-automatic immunohistostainer (Leica, Melbourne, Australia). The staining protocol included glass dewaxing, high-temperature unmasking with Bond Epitope Retrieval 2 unmasking solution (pH = 9) for 20 min at 96 °C, peroxidase block, incubation with antibody for 15 min at room temperature, and visualization with the Bond Polymer Refine Detection system.

The staining on the images of the preparations was assessed by scanning them with the Aperio CS2 scanner into the Aperio Image Scope program. Lymphoid cells, synoviocytes, and fibroblasts with distinct membrane, and/or cytoplasmic staining were considered positively stained. Each specimen was assessed in 10 visual fields at three locations: pannus (if any), synovitis, and surrounding soft tissue infiltration. In each case, points were assigned using the following scale:

0—staining of less than 1% of cells or its absence
1—staining of 2–10% of cells
2—staining of 11–30% of cells
3—staining of 31–50% of cells
4—staining of more than 51% of cells.

4.5. Linked Immunosorbent Assay

Every 7 days, 1 mL blood was collected from the venous plexus of the floor of the oral cavity into tubes with EDTA. The resulting blood was centrifuged for 5 min at 3000 rpm. The plasma was removed and frozen at −20 °C. After the end of the experiment, the analytes were examined for the content of TNF-α in the peripheral blood using the BMS622 Rat TNF alpha test system on a Multiskan FC plate spectrophotometer (ThermoFisher, Shanghai, China) according to the protocol of the test system manufacturer.

4.6. Statistical Analysis

All data obtained as a result of the study were subjected to statistical processing using the STATISTICA 10.0 program. The normality of the trait distribution was assessed using the Kolmogorov–Smirnov method. Using descriptive statistics methods, the median, mean value of the trait, standard deviation, error of the mean, and upper and lower quartiles was obtained. For comparison between groups, the Mann–Whitney test was used. Differences were considered significant if the error probability was $p < 0.05$.

All studies were carried out using equipment at the Center for Collective Use "Molecular Biology" of the Medical Academy named after S. I. Georgievsky (structural unit) and equipment of the Laboratory on Cell Technologies and Elaboration of DNA Medicines of the Taurida Academy (structural unit) of FGAOU VO "Crimean Federal University named after V. I. Vernadsky".

5. Conclusions

In this study, ASO Cytos-11 selectively reduced levels of TNF-α in the peripheral blood and cell membranes and reduced joint swelling in rats with rheumatoid arthritis with an efficacy similar to that of adalimumab. By analogy with the results for an ASO used for the treatment of other diseases, Cytos-11 showed a low frequency of immunological reactions, was well tolerated by the rats, and demonstrated the possibility of being used in combination with other drugs. Therefore, it is important to continue studying Cytos-11 to discover any possible undesirable side effects, its potential impact on other markers of inflammation, and the possibility of using it in medical practice.

Author Contributions: Conceptualization, V.V.O.; Data curation, T.P.M. and V.V.O.; Formal analysis, T.P.M. and I.O.G.; Funding acquisition, I.I.F. and A.V.K.; Investigation, K.V.L., Z.Z.T., O.A.S., and K.A.Y.; Methodology, T.P.M. and A.I.G.; Project administration, T.P.M., V.V.O., and E.Y.Z.; Resources, I.A.N. and R.A.R.; Software, R.A.R.; Supervision, V.V.O.; Validation, I.I.F. and A.V.K.; Visualization, T.P.M. and E.A.G.; Writing—original draft, T.P.M., I.O.G., and V.V.O.; Writing—review and editing, T.P.M., I.O.G., and V.V.O. All authors have read and agreed to the published version of the manuscript.

Funding: This research was funded by university development programs, grant number AAAA-A19-119122390041-9 from 23 December 2019.

Institutional Review Board Statement: All manipulations with animals were carried out in accordance with the European Convention for the Protection of Vertebrate Animals Used for Experiments and Other Scientific Purposes and approved by the ethical committee of the Crimean Federal University (Protocol № 10 from 12 November 2020).

Informed Consent Statement: Not applicable.

Data Availability Statement: Data is contained within the article.

Acknowledgments: We thank our families for the opportunity to conduct scientific research.

Conflicts of Interest: The authors declare no conflict of interest. The funders had no role in the design of the study; in the collection, analyses, or interpretation of data; in the writing of the manuscript; or in the decision to publish the results.

References

1. Crane, M.M.; Juneja, M.; Allen, J.; Kurrasch, R.H.; Chu, M.E.; Quattrocchi, E.; Manson, S.C.; Chang, D.J. Epidemiology and treatment of new-onset and established rheumatoid arthritis in an insured US population. *Arthritis Care Res.* **2015**, *67*, 1646–1655. [CrossRef] [PubMed]
2. Van der Woude, D.; Annette, H.M.; van der Helm-van, M. Update on the epidemiology, risk factors, and disease outcomes of rheumatoid arthritis. *Best Pract. Res. Clin. Rheumatol.* **2018**, *32*, 174–187. [CrossRef] [PubMed]
3. Lawrence, R.C.; Felson, D.T.; Helmick, C.G.; Arnold, L.M.; Choi, H.; Deyo, R.A.; Gabriel, S.; Hirsch, R.; Hochberg, M.C.; Hunder, G.G.; et al. Estimates of the prevalence of arthritis and other rheumatic conditions in the United States: Part II. *Arthritis Rheum.* **2008**, *58*, 26–35. [CrossRef] [PubMed]
4. Firestein, G.S.; McInnes, I.B. Immunopathogenesis of rheumatoid arthritis. *Immunity* **2017**, *46*, 183–196. [CrossRef]

5. Croia, C.; Bursi, R.; Sutera, D.; Petrelli, F.; Alunno, A.; Puxeddu, I. One year in review 2019: Pathogenesis of rheumatoid arthritis. *Clin. Exp. Rheumatol.* **2019**, *37*, 347–357, PMID: 31111823. [PubMed]
6. Cooper, N.J. Economic burden of rheumatoid arthritis: A systematic review. *Rheumatology* **2000**, *39*, 28–33. [CrossRef]
7. Nikiphorou, E.; Norton, S.; Young, A.; Dixey, J.; Walsh, D.; Helliwell, H.; Kiely, P. Early rheumatoid arthritis study and the early rheumatoid arthritis network, the association of obesity with disease activity, functional ability and quality of life in early rheumatoid arthritis: Data from the early rheumatoid arthritis study/early rheumatoid arthritis network UK prospective cohorts. *Rheumatology* **2018**, *57*, 1194–1202. [CrossRef]
8. van Vilsteren, M.; Boot, C.R.; Knol, D.L.; van Schaardenburg, D.; Voskuyl, A.E.; Steenbeek, R.; Anema, J.R. Productivity at work and quality of life in patients with rheumatoid arthritis. *BMC Musculoskelet Disord.* **2015**, *16*, 107. [CrossRef]
9. Purabdollah, M.; Lakdizaji, S.; Rahmani, A.; Hajalilu, M.; Ansarin, K. Relationship between sleep disorders, pain and quality of life in patients with rheumatoid arthritis. *J. Caring Sci.* **2015**, *4*, 233–241. [CrossRef]
10. Fazal, S.A.; Khan, M.; Nishi, S.E.; Alam, F.; Zarin, N.; Bari, M.T.; Ashraf, G. A clinical update and global economic burden of rheumatoid arthritis. *Endocr. Metab. Immune Disord. Drug Targets* **2018**, *18*. [CrossRef]
11. Kwon, H.; Kim, Y.L.; Lee, S.M. Relation between functional ability and health-related quality of life of children with juvenile rheumatoid arthritis. *J. Phys. Ther. Sci.* **2015**, *27*, 837–840. [CrossRef] [PubMed]
12. Hefti, F. Juvenile rheumatoid arthritis. In *Pediatric Orthopedics in Practice*; Springer: Berlin/Heidelberg, Germany, 2015; pp. 661–665. [CrossRef]
13. Kasapçopur, Ö.; Barut, K. Treatment in juvenile rheumatoid arthritis and new treatment options. *Turk Pediatri Ars.* **2015**, *50*, 1–10. [CrossRef] [PubMed]
14. Chaudhari, K.; Rizvi, S.; Syed, B. Rheumatoid arthritis: Current and future trends. *Nat. Rev. Drug Discov.* **2016**, *15*, 305–306. [CrossRef] [PubMed]
15. Coondoo, A.; Phiske, M.; Verma, S.; Lahiri, K. Side-effects of topical steroids: A long overdue revisit. *Indian Derm. Online J.* **2014**, *5*, 416–425. [CrossRef] [PubMed]
16. Dhar, S.; Seth, J.; Parikh, D. Systemic side-effects of topical corticosteroids. *Indian J. Derm.* **2014**, *59*, 460–464. [CrossRef]
17. Edrees, A.F.; Misra, S.N.; Abdou, N.I. Anti-tumor necrosis factor (TNF) therapy in rheumatoid arthritis: Correlation of TNF-alpha serum level with clinical response and benefit from changing dose or frequency of infliximab infusions. *Clin. Exp. Rheumatol.* **2005**, *23*, 469–474.
18. Ruperto, N.; Lovell, D.J.; Cuttica, R.; Wilkinson, N.; Woo, P.; Espada, G.; Wouters, C.; Silverman, E.D.; Paediatric Rheumatology International Trials Organisation; Pediatric Rheumatology Collaborative Study Group. A randomized, placebo-controlled trial of infliximab plus methotrexate for the treatment of polyarticular-course juvenile rheumatoid arthritis. *Arthritis Rheum.* **2007**, *56*, 3096–3106. [CrossRef] [PubMed]
19. Markham, A.; Lamb, H.M. Infliximab. *Drugs* **2000**, *59*, 1341–1359. [CrossRef]
20. Kreiner, F.; Galbo, H. Effect of etanercept in polymyalgia rheumatica: A randomized controlled trial. *Arthritis Res. Ther.* **2010**, *12*, R176. [CrossRef]
21. Jarvis, B.; Faulds, D. Etanercept. *Drugs* **1999**, *57*, 945–966. [CrossRef]
22. Khanna, R.; Feagan, B.G. Safety of infliximab for the treatment of inflammatory bowel disease: Current understanding of the potential for serious adverse events. *Expert Opin. Drug Saf.* **2015**, *14*, 987–997. [CrossRef] [PubMed]
23. Bang, L.M.; Keating, G.M. Adalimumab. *BioDrugs* **2004**, *18*, 121–139. [CrossRef] [PubMed]
24. Aletaha, D.; Smolen, J.S. Diagnosis and management of rheumatoid arthritis: A review. *JAMA* **2018**, *320*, 1360–1372. [CrossRef] [PubMed]
25. Guo, Q.; Wang, Y.; Xu, D.; Nossent, J.; Pavlos, N.J.; Xu, J. Rheumatoid arthritis: Pathological mechanisms and modern pharmacologic therapies. *Bone Res.* **2018**, *6*, 15. [CrossRef] [PubMed]
26. Downey, C. Serious infection during etanercept, infliximab and adalimumab therapy for rheumatoid arthritis: A literature review. *Int. J. Rheum. Dis.* **2016**, *19*, 536–550. [CrossRef]
27. Schiff, M.H.; Burmester, G.R.; Kent, J.D.; Pangan, A.L.; Kupper, H.; Fitzpatrick, S.B.; Donovan, C. Safety analyses of adalimumab (HUMIRA) in global clinical trials and US postmarketing surveillance of patients with rheumatoid arthritis. *Ann. Rheum. Dis.* **2006**, *65*, 889–894. [CrossRef]
28. Singh, J.A.; Cameron, C.; Noorbaloochi, S.; Cullis, T.; Tucker, M.; Christensen, R.; Ghogomu, E.T.; Coyle, D.; Clifford, T.; Tugwell, P.; et al. Risk of serious infection in biological treatment of patients with rheumatoid arthritis: A systematic review and meta-analysis. *Lancet* **2015**, *386*, 258–265. [CrossRef]
29. Dixon, W.G. Rheumatoid arthritis: Biological drugs and risk of infection. *Lancet* **2015**, *386*, 224–225. [CrossRef]
30. Nard, F.D.; Todoerti, M.; Grosso, V.; Monti, S.; Breda, S.; Rossi, S.; Montecucco, C.; Caporali, R. Risk of hepatitis B virus reactivation in rheumatoid arthritis patients undergoing biologic treatment: Extending perspective from old to newer drugs. *World J. Hepatol.* **2015**, *7*, 344–361. [CrossRef]
31. Pappas, D.A.; Hooper, M.M.; Kremer, J.M.; Reed, G.; Shan, Y.; Wenkert, D.; Greenberg, J.D.; Curtis, J.R. Herpes zoster reactivation in patients with rheumatoid arthritis: Analysis of disease characteristics and disease-modifying antirheumatic drugs. *Arthritis Care Res.* **2015**, *67*, 1671–1678. [CrossRef]

32. Bello, S.; Serafino, L.; Bonali, C.; Terlizzi, N.; Fanizza, C.; Anecchino, C.; Lapaldula, G. Incidence of influenza-like illness into a cohort of patients affected by chronic inflammatory rheumatism and treated with biological agents. *Reumatismo* **2012**, *64*, 299–306. [CrossRef] [PubMed]
33. Shen, X.; Corey, D.R. Chemistry, mechanism and clinical status of antisense oligonucleotides and duplex RNAs. *Nucleic Acids Res.* **2018**, *46*, 1584–1600. [CrossRef] [PubMed]
34. Mallory, A.; Havens, M.L. Hastings, splice-switching antisense oligonucleotides as therapeutic drugs. *Nucleic Acids Res.* **2016**, *44*, 6549–6563. [CrossRef]
35. Singh, J.; Kaur, H.; Kaushik, A.; Peer, S. A review of antisense therapeutic interventions for molecular biological targets in various diseases. *Int. J. Pharmacol.* **2011**, *7*, 294–315. [CrossRef]
36. Oberemok, V.V.; Laikova, K.V.; Repetskaya, A.I.; Kenyo, I.M.; Gorlov, M.V.; Kasich, I.N.; Krasnodubets, A.M.; Gal'chinsky, N.V.; Fomochkina, I.I.; Zaitsev, A.S.; et al. A half-century history of applications of antisense oligonucleotides in medicine, agriculture and forestry: We should continue the journey. *Molecules* **2018**, *23*, 1302. [CrossRef]
37. Bennett, C.F. Therapeutic antisense oligonucleotides are coming of age. *Annu. Rev. Med.* **2019**, *70*, 307–321. [CrossRef]
38. Gidaro, T.; Servais, L. Nusinersen treatment of spinal muscular atrophy: Current knowledge and existing gaps. *Dev. Med. Child Neurol.* **2019**, *61*, 19–24. [CrossRef] [PubMed]
39. Stebbins, C.C.; Petrillo, M.; Stevenson, L.F. Immunogenicity for antisense oligonucleotides: A risk-based assessment. *Bioanalysis* **2019**, *11*, 1913–1916. [CrossRef] [PubMed]
40. Warren, M.S.; Hughes, S.G.; Singleton, W.; Yamashita, M.; Genovese, M.C. Results of a proof of concept, double-blind, randomized trial of a second generation antisense oligonucleotide targeting high-sensitivity C-reactive protein (hs-CRP) in rheumatoid arthritis. *Arthritis Res Ther.* **2015**, *17*, 80. [CrossRef]
41. Morita, Y.; Kashihara, N.; Yamamura, M.; Okamoto, H.; Harada, S.; Maeshima, Y.; Okamoto, K.; Makino, H. Inhibition of rheumatoid synovial fibroblast proliferation by antisense oligonucleotides targeting proliferating cell nuclear antigen messenger RNA. *Arthritis Rheum.* **1997**, *40*, 1292–1297. [CrossRef]
42. Holmlund, J.T. Applying antisense technology. *Ann. N. Y. Acad. Sci.* **2003**, *1002*, 244–251. [CrossRef] [PubMed]
43. Sewell, K.L.; Geary, R.S.; Baker, B.F.; Glover, J.M.; Mant, T.G.K.; Yu, R.Z.; Tami, J.A.; Dorr, F.A. Phase I Trial of ISIS 104838, a 2′-methoxyethyl modified antisense oligonucleotide targeting tumor necrosis factor-α. *J. Pharmacol. Exp. Ther.* **2002**, *303*, 1334–1343. [CrossRef] [PubMed]
44. Jason, T.L.; Koropatnick, J.; Berg, R.W. Toxicology of antisense therapeutics. *Toxicol. Appl. Pharmacol.* **2004**, *201*, 66–83. [CrossRef] [PubMed]
45. Richard, S.G.; Rosie, Z.Y.; Watanabe, T.; Scott, P.H.; Greg, E.; Hardee, A.C.; Matson, J.; Sasmor, H.; Cummins, L.; Levin, A.A. Pharmacokinetics of a tumor necrosis factor-α prhosphorothioate 2′-O-(2-metoxyethyl) modified antisense oligonucleotide: Comparison across species. *Drug Metab. Dispos.* **2003**, *31*, 1419–1428. [CrossRef]
46. Baker, B.F.; Murthy, S.; Flanigan, A.M.; Siwkowski, A.M.; Butler, M.; Dean, N.M. Dose-dependent reduction of chronic dextran sulfate sodium (DSS)-induced colitis in mice treated with TNF-A antisense oligonucleotide (ISIS 25302). *Gastroenterology* **2000**, *118*, 571. [CrossRef]
47. Gareb, B.; Otten, A.T.; Frijlink, H.W.; Dijkstra, G.; Kosterink, J.G.W. Review: Local tumor necrosis factor-α inhibition in inflammatory bowel disease. *Pharmaceutics* **2020**, *12*, 539. [CrossRef]
48. Oberemok, V.V.; Laikova, K.V.; Gal'chinsky, N.V.; Useinov, R.Z.; Novikov, I.A.; Temirova, Z.Z.; Shumskykh, M.N.; Krasnodubets, A.M.; Repetskaya, A.I.; Dyadichev, V.V.; et al. DNA insecticide developed from the *Lymantria dispar* 5.8S ribosomal RNA gene provides a novel biotechnology for plant protection. *Sci. Rep.* **2019**, *9*, 6197. [CrossRef]
49. Gal'chinsky, N.; Useinov, R.; Yatskova, E.; Laikova, K.; Novikov, I.; Gorlov, M.; Trikoz, N.; Sharmagiy, A.; Plugatar, Y.; Oberemok, V. A breakthrough in the efficiency of contact DNA insecticides: Rapid high mortality rates in the sap-sucking insects dynaspidiotusbritannicus comstock and unaspiseuonymi newstead. *J. Plant Prot. Res.* **2020**, *60*, 220–223. [CrossRef]
50. Useinov, R.Z.; Gal'chinsky, N.; Yatskova, E.; Novikov, I.; Puzanova, Y.; Trikoz, N.; Sharmagiy, A.; Plugatar, Y.; Laikova, K.; Oberemok, V. To bee or not to bee: Creating DNA insecticides to replace non-selective organophosphate insecticides for use against the soft scale insect Ceroplastes japonicus Green. *J. Plant Prot. Res.* **2020**. [CrossRef]
51. Festing, M.F.; Altman, D.G. Guidelines for the design and statistical analysis of experiments using laboratory animals. *ILAR J.* **2005**, *46*, 320. [CrossRef]

International Journal of
Molecular Sciences

MDPI

Review

A 2022 Systematic Review and Meta-Analysis of Enriched Therapeutic Diets and Nutraceuticals in Canine and Feline Osteoarthritis

Maude Barbeau-Grégoire [1], Colombe Otis [1], Antoine Cournoyer [1], Maxim Moreau [1], Bertrand Lussier [1,2] and Eric Troncy [1,2,*]

1 Groupe de Recherche en Pharmacologie Animale du Québec (GREPAQ), Département de Biomédecine Vétérinaire, Faculté de Médecine Vétérinaire, Université de Montréal, Saint-Hyacinthe, QC J2S 7C6, Canada

2 Unité de Recherche en Arthrose, Centre de Recherche du Centre Hospitalier Universitaire de L'Université de Montréal, Montréal, QC H2X 0A9, Canada

* Correspondence: eric.troncy@umontreal.ca

Abstract: With osteoarthritis being the most common degenerative disease in pet animals, a very broad panel of natural health products is available on the market for its management. The aim of this systematic review and meta-analysis, registered on PROSPERO (CRD42021279368), was to test for the evidence of clinical analgesia efficacy of fortified foods and nutraceuticals administered in dogs and cats affected by osteoarthritis. In four electronic bibliographic databases, 1578 publications were retrieved plus 20 additional publications from internal sources. Fifty-seven articles were included, comprising 72 trials divided into nine different categories of natural health compound. The efficacy assessment, associated to the level of quality of each trial, presented an evident clinical analgesic efficacy for omega-3-enriched diets, omega-3 supplements and cannabidiol (to a lesser degree). Our analyses showed a weak efficacy of collagen and a very marked non-effect of chondroitin-glucosamine nutraceuticals, which leads us to recommend that the latter products should no longer be recommended for pain management in canine and feline osteoarthritis.

Keywords: osteoarthritis; nutraceuticals; enriched diets; pain; animal; methodological quality; scientific evidence; metrological validation

Citation: Barbeau-Grégoire, M.; Otis, C.; Cournoyer, A.; Moreau, M.; Lussier, B.; Troncy, E. A 2022 Systematic Review and Meta-Analysis of Enriched Therapeutic Diets and Nutraceuticals in Canine and Feline Osteoarthritis. *Int. J. Mol. Sci.* **2022**, *23*, 10384. https://doi.org/10.3390/ijms231810384

Academic Editor: Chih-Hsin Tang

Received: 1 August 2022
Accepted: 4 September 2022
Published: 8 September 2022

1. Introduction

Osteoarthritis (OA) is a widespread musculoskeletal disorder in pets [1]. In the absence of a curative treatment, veterinarians attempt to control the symptoms of pain. Therapeutic goals therefore focus on reducing joint pain and improving motor function to increase the quality of life of the affected animals. The most recommended drugs are non-steroidal anti-inflammatory drugs (NSAIDs) based on their efficacy [2,3]. However, compliance with this treatment is difficult due to repeated (often daily) administration; side effects are not uncommon (mainly gastrointestinal irritation, nephrotoxicity, hepatotoxicity); and the benefits of long-term management on the longevity and quality of life remain limited [4].

To the best of the authors' knowledge, no therapeutic approach has any indication of a delayed effect on the progression of OA. Thus, the terms "chondroprotective", "structure-modulator" or "disease-modifying" do not yet apply to the therapeutic approaches available in pet OA, with all therapeutic indications revolving around an improvement in the behavioural or physiologic signs associated with OA pain.

The lack of alternatives in OA therapy would benefit from an evidence-based statement on the different approaches available and their potential benefits for OA-affected animals. Fortified diets and nutraceuticals have gained popularity among the veterinary community in recent decades. Indeed, the field of nutraceuticals has experienced a rapid and substantial economic growth. The increase in the consumption of natural substances is mainly associated with the rise of owners' awareness of their health and lifestyle beliefs, which they transpose to the care of their animals as well [5,6]. The global veterinary dietary supplements market was valued at USD 1.6 billion in 2020 and is expected to continue growing with an estimated annual growth rate of 8.2% by 2028 [7]. Within the veterinary recommendations of nutraceuticals use, OA and degenerative joint disorder are the diseases for which veterinary practitioners most commonly emit a recommendation [8,9]. However, regulatory assessments of these compounds primarily focused on the absence of side effects (safety), quality and nutrition but did not require proof in therapeutic efficacy [10,11].

This review focused on fortified therapeutic diets as well as nutraceuticals, i.e., products made from food substances, available in a wide variety of formulations such as tablets, capsules, drops, powders, treats or other medicinal forms usually not associated with food, which have been shown to have a possible beneficial or protective pharmacological effect against chronic diseases.

Three previous systematic reviews on the treatment of animal OA revealed a disappointing quantity and quality of scientific evidence regarding fortified therapeutic diets and nutraceuticals [12–14]. The evidence from these three systematic reviews on the use of these products was not strong enough to adopt or support meaningful recommendations.

The aim of this systematic review and meta-analysis was to examine the evidence for analgesic efficacy of fortified therapeutic diets and nutraceuticals to build up solid research evidence (evidence-based medicine) and to properly disseminate findings on the efficacy of the therapeutic potential in dogs and cats affected by OA. This project, therefore, benefits from the addition of an objective and quantitative assessment of quality and efficacy, which allows conclusions to be drawn that are supported by good scientific evidence. Our hypothesis was that, in 2022, we have sufficient evidence to support, or not, the use of therapeutic diets or nutraceuticals in the management of canine and feline OA.

2. Methods

2.1. Literature Search and Inclusion of Studies

Four electronic databases (CAB-Abstract, Embase, Global-Health and Pubmed) were searched for articles published from 1980 to 10 October 2021. A systematic search was performed using the following predefined terms: (arthrosis OR osteoarthr* OR "degenerative joint disease") AND (cat OR cats OR feline) AND (dog OR dogs OR canine) AND ("disease modifying agent" OR nutrient* OR nutritional OR "nutritional medicinal product" OR "nutritional supplements" OR nutraceutical* OR "botanical drugs" OR "botanical food supplements" OR "herbal health nutritionals" OR "herbal health nutritional" OR "herbal medicine" OR "fortified food" OR "food additive" OR "food additives" OR diet OR "dietary supplements" OR "dietary supplement" OR dietary OR "geriatric diet" OR "natural product" OR "natural products" OR phytotherapy OR "complementary medicines" OR "complementary medicine" OR homeopathy OR antioxidant OR "food derived products" OR "food derived product" OR "mineral supplements" OR "mineral supplement" OR supplement OR supplements). All duplicates present between the different databases were removed in the selection of articles (Figure 1). A few articles from complementary internal sources were also added ($N = 20$). The references were then all transferred to the EndNoteTM X9 platform (Clarivate Analytics, Philadelphia, PA, USA).

All articles were then assessed for inclusion. Briefly, the selected studies had to test the effect of nutraceuticals, or therapeutic diets, on canine or feline OA pain. Induced OA models were also included. If a research article had multiple treatment arms (i.e., multiple compounds or doses under study), each trial was assessed and independently analysed. The data from the included studies were extracted using a standardised format for the assessment of trial quality and analgesic efficacy. Two reviewers (M.B.-G., A.C.) independently extracted the data; discrepancies were identified and resolved by discussion with a third reviewer (C.O.), if necessary.

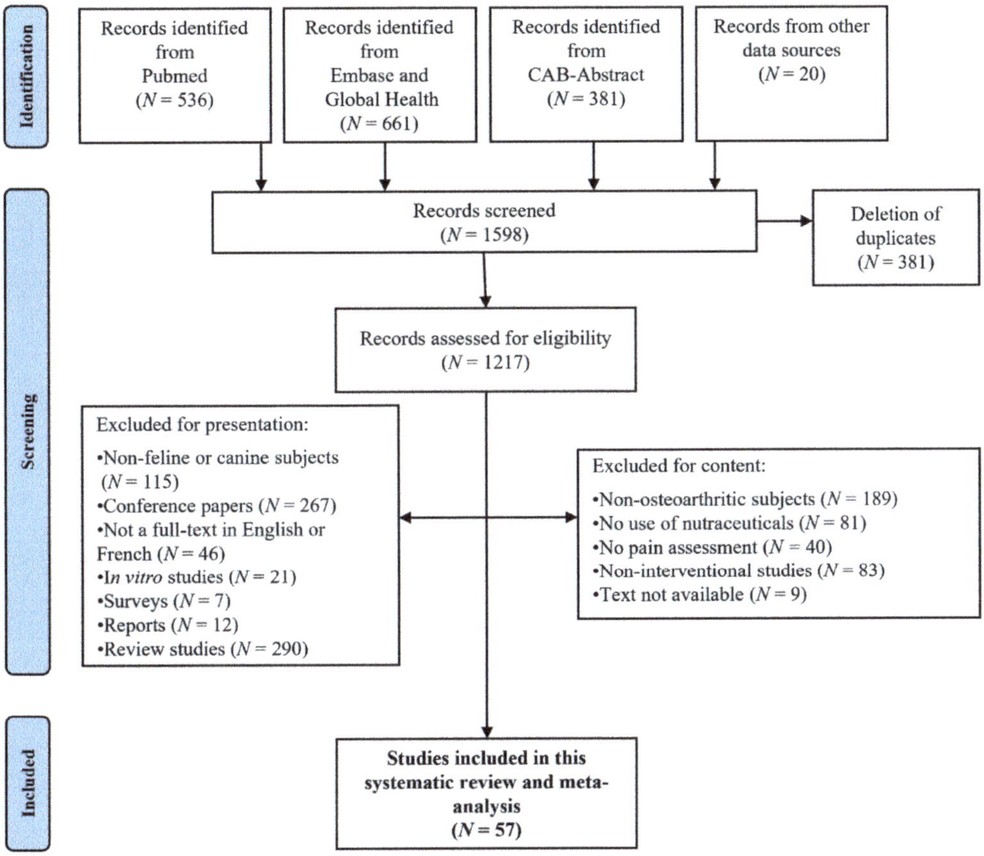

Figure 1. PRISMA flowchart of publications on use of nutraceuticals and therapeutic diets in canine and feline OA.

2.2. Selection of Articles

Figure 1 shows the PRISMA flowchart of the identified studies.

While 57 articles on canine and feline OA were selected, a total of 72 trials, due to the different arms tested in many studies, and 38 different compounds were evaluated. Whereas 69 of these trials used a canine model, only 3 were tested in cats.

2.3. Meta-Analysis: Construction and Validation of Analysis Scales for Data Extracted from Publications

A "quality of the trial" meta-analysis scale was developed, based on three evaluation criteria, in order to assess each therapeutic trial in a systematic, independent and quantitative manner. A meta-analysis scale "analgesic efficacy" was also constructed in the form of a simple categorisation (see below) of the effect of the treated group vs. control group, temporal (within-group) improvement and non-effect. The assessment grids were developed based on the models used in three previous systematic reviews [12–14], in compliance with ARRIVE recommendations (Animal Research: Reporting In Vivo Experiments; [15]), CONSORT (Consolidated Standards of Reporting Trials; [16]) and CAMARADES (Collaborative Approach to Meta Analysis and Review of Animal Data from Experimental Studies; [17,18]). Finally, the study was registered on the international prospective register of systematic reviews PROSPERO (www.crd.york.ac.uk/prospero/; accessed on 4 February

2022, CRD42021279368) whose educational tools guide the systematic review process. The report of the information collected followed the PRISMA guide (Preferred Reporting Items for Systematic reviews and Meta-Analyses; [19,20]).

After the primary construction of the quality of trial scale, it was subjected to a series of validation (face validation, internal and external content validation) by several independent evaluators, as well as construct validation. Once the development of the grids was fully completed (Table 1), all the articles selected (with the different product and dose trials) were evaluated and scored by three independent investigators considered to have different levels of expertise (M.B.-G., C.O. and E.T.). The values assigned by each evaluator were compared for each trial tested, and the single final score, used for the statistical analyses, was systematically obtained by consensus.

Table 1. Quality assessment scale.

Criterion	Sub-Criteria (Score)
Risk of bias	1. Randomisation: Non-randomised (0), Not mentioned (0) or Randomised (2) 2. Type of study: Single cohort (0), Cross-over (1) or Parallel (2) 3. Controlled study: No control group (0), Positive control (1*) or Placebo (1*) 4. Blinding procedure: Non-blinded (0), Single-blinded (1) or Double-blinded (2)
Methodological quality	5. Inclusion criteria: None (0), Other (1*), Experimental induction of OA in healthy animals (2), Owner-reported lameness (2*), Veterinary orthopaedic examination (2*), Inclusion grid (2*) or X-rays (2*) 6. Non-inclusion criteria: None (0), Weaning period too short (1*), Adequate weaning period (2*) or Description of non-inclusion criteria (2*) 7. Exclusion criteria: None (0) or Description of exclusion criteria (2) 8. Control of possible bias: Non-randomised, or non-blinded, study with subjective assessment (0), Non-randomised, or non-blinded, study with objective assessments (1*), Research hypotheses and objectives clearly stated (0.5/each*), Ethics committee approval indicated (1*), Manuscript edited according to ARRIVE or CONSORT criteria (1*), Declaration of any conflict of interest (1*), Randomised, blinded study (2*) or No indication of the dose used (−5*) 9. Data collection and analysis: No information (0), Electronic collection, or methods already used (1), Quality assurance control (2*), Statistical analyses clearly described (1 or 2*)
Strengths of the scientific evidence	10. Sample size: <10 per group (0), Between 10 and 20 per group (2) or >20 per group (4) 11. Nature of data: Non-validated subjective (0*), Validated subjective (2*), Non-validated objective (1*) or Validated objective (4*) outcomes 12. Repetition of results obtained (according to the level of risk of bias): Only one study carried out (except if [A]) (0), Several studies [C] or [D] (1), One study [A] (2), Several studies [B or less] (3), Several studies [A and/or less] (4) or Several studies of level [A] (6)

[A] = Prospective, randomised, controlled, blinded study; [B] = prospective, randomised, observational cohort; [C] = non-randomised, controlled interventional trial (historical or prospective); [D] = cross-sectional study, or clinical case, or interventional trial, non-randomised, non-controlled. Scores followed by an asterisk (*) are cumulative and were therefore not exclusive.

2.4. *Quality of Trials Assessment Scale (Table 1)*

The assessment grid consisted of three sections, seeking to test three fundamental criteria: risk of bias, methodological quality and strength of scientific evidence. The quality total score was obtained by adding the scores of the three constituent criteria, and all trials were classified into four quality levels based on the distribution of the totals obtained.

2.5. *Efficacy Assessment Scale*

The evidence of efficacy, or non-effect, of the compound tested was supplemented by a simple categorisation: (1) trials with "analgesic effect" represented an improvement in the condition of the animal with the treatment, over time and compared with a control group. This is, therefore, an inter-group temporal comparison. (2) Trials with "improvement" represented within-group improvement in condition over time. Animals are, therefore, only temporally evaluated. Considering that chronic conditions, such as OA, are subject to changes over time, this effectiveness was less than the previous one. (3) Finally, the trials with a "non-effect" did not represent any improvement, neither over time within the same group nor between the groups. This assessment was also systematically carried out by consensus of the three assessors.

2.6. Statistical Analyses

All trials were grouped into nine categories as shown in Table 2: 1. omega-3-enriched therapeutic diets (N = 10); 2. omega-3-based nutraceuticals (fish oil, green mussels, etc.) (N = 10); 3. collagen-based nutraceuticals (N = 11); 4. nutraceuticals based on chondroitin–glucosamine (N = 9); 5. cannabinoid-based nutraceuticals (N = 7); 6. nutraceuticals based on hydroxycitric acid (N = 3); 7. nutraceuticals based on calcium fructoborate (N = 3); 8. composite nutraceuticals (N = 3); and 9. others (N = 16). Only categories (ctg.) 1 to 5 were kept for comparison of quality and efficacy, as the others (ctg. 6 to 9) did not present a sufficiently large number of trials ($N \leq 3$).

Table 2. Presentation, by category, of clinical trials on therapeutic nutrition and nutraceuticals in canine and feline osteoarthritis.

Categories and Compounds Tested	References
Category 1. Omega-3-enriched therapeutic diets	
Green-lipped mussels	[21–24]
Fish oil	[25–29]
Category 2. Omega-3-based nutraceuticals	
Green-lipped mussels	[21,30–34]
Fish oil	[35–37]
Category 3. Collagen-based nutraceuticals	
Collagen	[38–41]
Collagen, glucosamine hydrochloride and chondroitin sulphate	[40,42]
Collagen-derived gelatine	[43]
NEM®	[44]
Ovopet®	[45]
Movoflex™	[46]
Category 4. Nutraceuticals with chondroitin-glucosamine	
Chondroitin sulphate	[30]
Glucosamine hydrochloride, chondroitin sulphate and manganese	[47]
Glucosamine hydrochloride and chondroitin sulphate	[40,42,48]
Glucosamine hydrochloride, chondroitin sulphate, N-acetyl-D-glucosamine, ascorbic acid and zinc sulphate	[49,50]
Glucosamine hydrochloride, chondroitin sulphate and hyaluronic acid	[51]
Glucosamine hydrochloride, chondroitin sulphate and avocado and soya unsaponifiables	[52]
Category 5. Cannabinoid-based nutraceuticals	
Cannabidiol	[53–57]
Category 6. Nutraceuticals based on hydroxycitric acid	
Hydroxycitric acid	[39]
Hydroxycitric acid and chromemate	[39]
Hydroxycitric acid, chromemate and collagen	[39]
Category 7. Nutraceuticals based on calcium fructoborate	
Calcium fructoborate	[58]
Calcium fructoborate, glucosamine hydrochloride and chondroitin sulphate	[58]
Category 8. Composite Nutraceuticals	
Flexodol®/Flexxil®	[59]
Dinamic™	[60]
Curcuvet®-boswellic acid-glucosamine-chondroitin-omega-3-Vit. C, E-*Saccharomyces cerevisiae*	[61]

Table 2. *Cont.*

Categories and Compounds Tested	References
Category 9. Others	
Special protein milk concentrate	[62]
Curcumoids	[63]
Elk velvet antler	[64]
Boswellia serrata extracts	[65]
Avocado and soybean unsaponifiables	[66]
Yeast (Beta-1.3/1.6 glucans)	[67]
Brachystemma calycinum D don extracts	[68,69]
STA-LITE® polydextrose	[70]
S-adenosyl L-methionine (SAMe)	[71]
Crominex 3+ ® (chrome trivalent, *Phyllanthus emblica*, shilajit)	[72]
Shilajit (*Asphaltum punjabianum*)	[73]
Vitamin E	[74]
Terminalia chebula (Indian myrobolan)	[75]
Diets enriched with curcumoid extract, hydrolysed collagen and green tea extract	[76]
4CYTE™ Epiitalis® Forte (*Biota orientalis*)	[77]

The null hypothesis was that no statistically significant difference existed between the scores of the five categories for trial quality or analgesic efficacy. For statistical analyses, we used R® software (Version 4.0.3, R Foundation for Statistical Computing, Vienna, Austria) with an alpha threshold of 0.05 for the significance of the results.

2.6.1. Quality of Trials

In the process of the construct validation of the grid, we tested the correlation links between the three constituent criteria as well as the links between these criteria and the quality total using linear mixed models (LMMs), integrating the trial identifier as a random factor to control for pseudo-replication bias. Finally, an LMM with the trial identifier as a random factor tested the effect of the category (1 to 5) on the quality total. Tukey's post hoc tests without correction for multiple comparisons were then performed, in an exploratory manner, to identify the pairs that were significantly different between categories. These analyses only considered publications with canine subjects as we did not want to combine species in the analyses, and dogs represented most of the trials listed.

2.6.2. Analgesic Efficacy

The descriptive analyses initially focused on all the trials included in categories 1 to 5, without considering their quality, indicating the level of efficacy in the percentage of effect, improvement and non- effect. A weighing method (Table 3) was then applied to give more weight to the efficacy results obtained on the better-quality trials.

Table 3. Weighing of efficacy scores in function of quality of each trial.

Quality of Trial	Level	Effect	Improvement	Non-Effect
Very high	A	+5	+3	−5
Good	B	+4	+2	−4
Medium	C	+2	+1	−2
Low	D	+1	+1	−1

Generalised linear models (GLMs) tested the effect of each category (1 to 5) on efficiency in the interaction with quality total, again only using the canine publications. Here, the dependent variable efficacy was considered in two different ways: first, when there was an effect only and, second, when there was an effect or improvement. With the dependent variable being, in both cases, binomial, we used a logit link in the GLMs. A mixed proportional odds (POM) model finally identified the differences between categories on effectiveness, if any.

2.6.3. Complementary Analyses

The effects of follow-up duration, dose used in each trial and quality total on efficacy were analysed for the dog trials of categories 1 to 5 as the dosage and duration varied according to the species, and most of the trials focused on dogs. A POM model was again used. The effect size was also calculated for these same 5 categories, this time including all trials, for the efficacy data using SPSS software (Version 27.0; IBM Corp. SPSS Statistics for Windows, Armonk, NY, USA). The measure chosen was Cohen's d with the global variance as the normaliser. First, the efficacy scores of the different categories were compared with the scores of the negative controls of these same trials, which were then scored as inversely described above for the test article.

Secondly, the 5 product categories were also compared with each other, again based on their effectiveness score. The interpretation of the results was made because of the benchmarks suggested by Cohen [78].

3. Results

3.1. Validation of the "Quality of Trial" Scale

The statistical validation of the scale was carried out considering only the publications in the canine OA, but the publications on cats revealed the same tendencies. The criteria "methodological quality" and "strength of scientific evidence" were significantly associated (LMM: $F = 13.29$; $CI^{95\%} = [0.15; 0.49]$). Neither of the other two relationships tested between the constituent criteria was significant. In addition, all three constituent criteria of the scale had a positive and significant link with the "quality total", with the most associated criterion ($R^2 = 0.81$) being "methodological quality". This indicated that each criterion was significantly involved in the composition of the quality of trial scale and justified the use of the quality total as a variable reflecting the quality of each trial.

3.2. Quality Assessment

3.2.1. Descriptive Distribution of Quality

Following the classification of the quality total into four levels, the number of trials per quality level was balanced. Thus, there were 38 high-quality trials (grouping levels A "very high" and B "good") and 34 trials of mediocre quality (levels C "medium" and D "low quality").

For compound categories 1 to 5 (see Table 2 for details), similar proportions were also observed: 28 high-quality trials (levels A and B) and 19 mediocre-quality trials (levels C and D). However, this distribution was not homogeneous between the five categories as shown in Figure 2.

Collagen-based (ctg. 3) and chondroitin-glucosamine-based (ctg. 4) nutraceuticals stand out with a higher presence of lower-quality trials. The quality level ratios (the number of AB/CD level trials) were 0.6 and 0.8, respectively, for these two categories. Conversely, omega-3-enriched therapeutic diets (ctg. 1), omega-3-based nutraceuticals (ctg. 2) and cannabinoids (ctg. 5) had more high-quality trials as evidenced by the quality level ratios of 4.0, 2.3 and 2.5, respectively.

For the remaining categories, the quality level of the trials varied between them. Hydroxycitric acid nutraceuticals (ctg. 6) had three low-quality trials (level D). Calcium fructoborate nutraceuticals (ctg. 7) had three very high-quality trials (level A). Composite nutraceuticals (ctg. 8) included one very high-quality trial (level A) [59] and two medium-quality trials (level C).

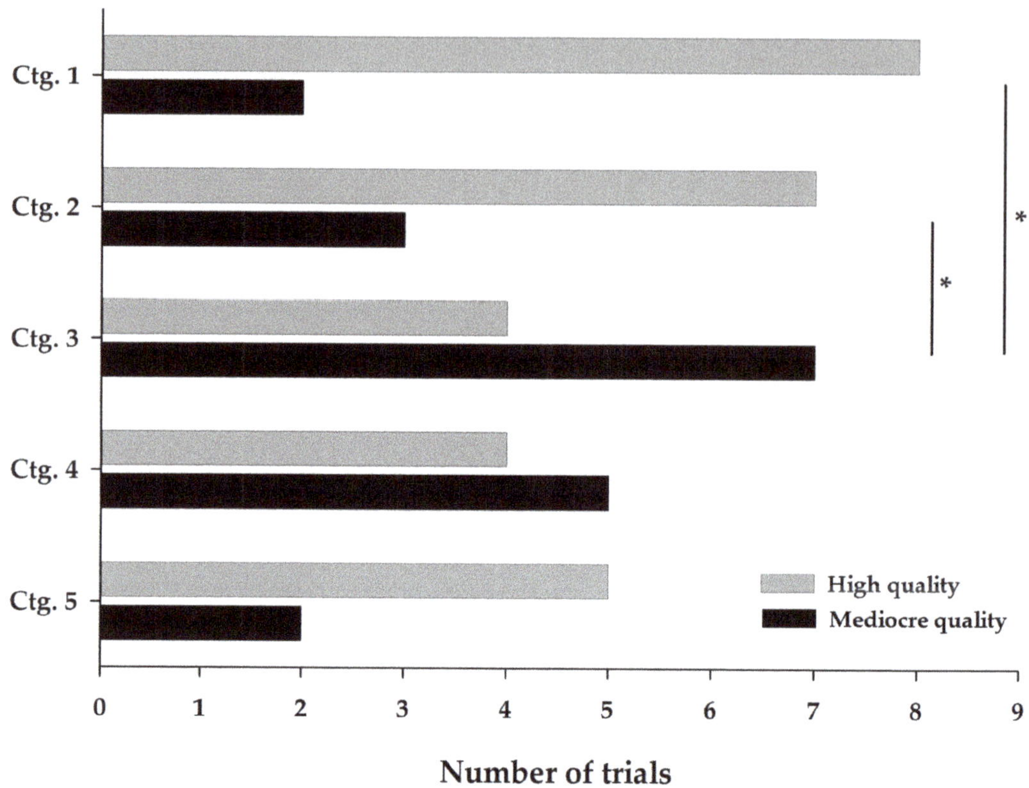

Figure 2. Distribution of quality levels of compound categories 1 to 5. A high-quality trial is represented by levels A and B, while a mediocre-quality trial is represented by levels C and D. Ctg. 1 (omega-3-enriched therapeutic diets), ctg. 2 (omega-3-based nutraceuticals), ctg. 3 (collagen-based nutraceuticals), ctg. 4 (chondroitin-glucosamine-based nutraceuticals) and ctg. 5 (cannabinoid-based nutraceuticals). Ctg., category. * indicates a significant difference ($p < 0.05$) between categories.

Finally, in the category of other products (ctg. 9), out of the 16 trials selected, there were three very high-quality (level A) [63,69,76], three good-quality (level B) [64,68,71], seven medium-quality (level C) and three low-quality (level D) trials [67,70,75].

3.2.2. Effect of the Category on the Quality Total

The descriptive differences observed in Figure 2 were confirmed by statistically significant differences between the trials on canine OA. Collagen-based nutraceuticals (ctg. 3) showed a lower quality total (median 18.5 [min = 13.0; max = 32.0]) than omega-3-enriched therapeutic diets (ctg. 1) (31.5 [13.5; 38.0], $p = 0.043$) and omega-3-based nutraceuticals (ctg. 2) (33.0 [14.0; 44.0], $p = 0.026$). The quality total of the other categories lied between these two extremes, namely chondroitin-glucosamine nutraceuticals (ctg. 4) (23.0 [16.0; 40.0]) and cannabinoid nutraceuticals (ctg. 5) (26.0 [18.5; 37.5]).

Regarding the three trials on feline OA, they all showed a good quality level. The trial presenting omega-3-enriched therapeutic diets (ctg. 1) was of very high quality [23], while the other two on omega-3-based (ctg. 2) and chondroitin-glucosamine nutraceuticals (ctg. 4) were of good quality [36,50].

3.3. Analgesic Efficacy Assessment

3.3.1. Descriptive Distribution of Efficacy

Figure 3 shows the distribution of efficacy, i.e., effect (compared with a control group), improvement (within-time) and non-effect for all trials included in categories 1 to 5. It was observed that omega-3 nutraceuticals (ctg. 2) stand out in terms of effect, while chondroitin-glucosamine nutraceuticals (ctg. 4) stand out for their lack of efficacy with 88.9% non-effect and 0% effect. The other categories showed a reduced percentage of non-effect: from 10.0% for omega-3-enriched therapeutic diets (ctg. 1) and omega-3-based nutraceuticals (ctg. 2) to 18.2% for collagen-based nutraceuticals (ctg. 3) and 14.3% for cannabinoid-based nutraceuticals (ctg. 5).

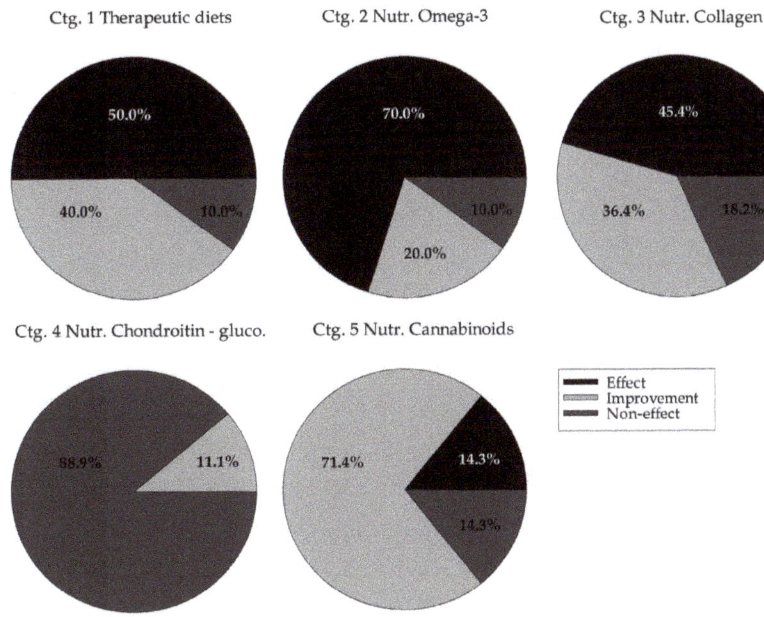

Figure 3. Distribution of efficacy levels of compound categories 1 to 5. On the total number of trials included in each category, expressed are the percentages of trials classified as an analgesic effect (vs. a control group), an improvement over time of the treatment group or a non-effect of the treatment. Ctg. 1 (omega-3-enriched therapeutic diets), ctg. 2 (omega-3-based nutraceuticals), ctg. 3 (collagen-based nutraceuticals), ctg. 4 (chondroitin-glucosamine-based nutraceuticals) and ctg. 5 (cannabinoid-based nutraceuticals). Ctg., category.

For categories 6 to 8 ($N = 3$, each), as for the quality level, the efficacy was also variable. Hydroxycitric acid (ctg. 6) used alone had no effect and only showed improvement when combined with chromemate, alone or with collagen as well [39]. None of the three trials of calcium fructoborate nutraceuticals (ctg. 7) had any effect, whether used alone or in combination with chondroitin-glucosamine [58]. For composite nutraceuticals (ctg. 8), the combination of phytotherapeutic extracts with omega-3, chondroitin-glucosamine, vitamins, etc. showed an analgesic effect [59,60] and a non-effect [61].

Finally, of the 16 trials of other products (ctg. 9), four detected an analgesic effect with special protein milk concentrate [62], elk velvet antler [64], avocado and soy unsaponifiables [66] and vitamin E [74]; nine detected a simple improvement; and three detected a non-effect for turmeric [63], STA-LITE polydextrose [70] and S-adenosyl L-methionine [71] compounds.

3.3.2. Effect of Category on Trial Efficacy

In both the GLMs tested on the canine trials, category had a significant effect on analgesic effectiveness, whether restricted to effect alone (goodness-of-fit = 0.248, LRT 2 = 12.74, df = 4, $p = 0.013$) or when combining effect + improvement (goodness-of-fit = 0.500, LRT 2 = 16.31, df = 4, $p = 0.003$). The results of the subsequent analysis of the quality-adjusted efficacy scores also showed that the level of efficacy of the chondroitin-glucosamine nutraceuticals (ctg. 4) was significantly lower than those of the other four categories (estimated = 3.96 (1.06), Z = 3.72, $p < 0.001$) as shown in Figure 4.

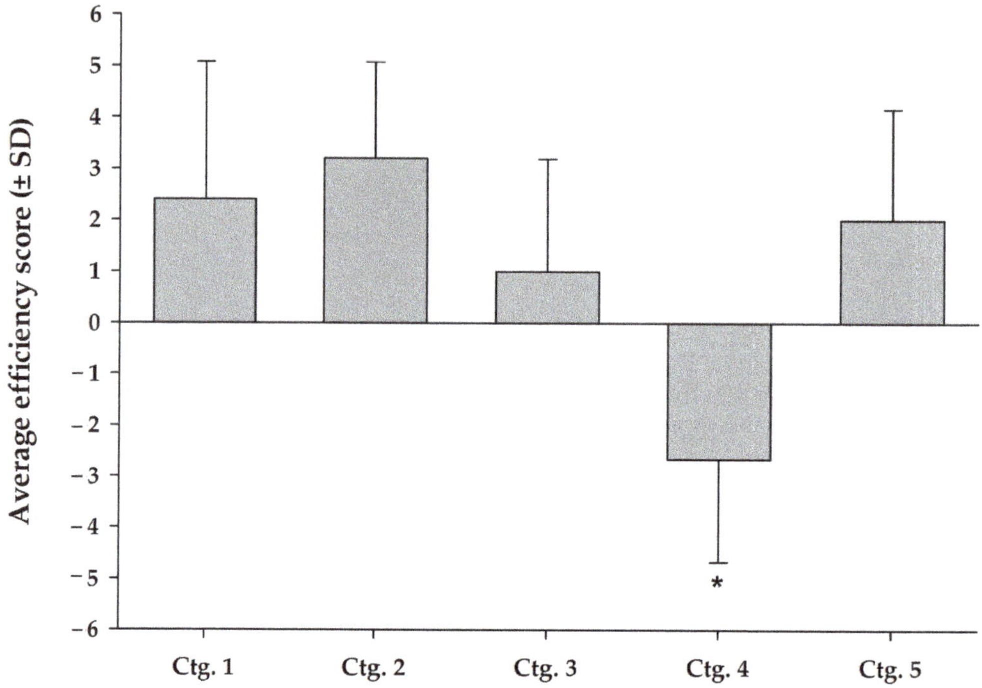

Figure 4. Average score (with standard deviation) of efficacy weighed for the quality level of categories 1 to 5. Weighted average efficacy score is plotted along with standard deviation of the score for each category. Ctg. 1 (omega-3-enriched therapeutic diets), ctg. 2 (omega-3-based nutraceuticals), ctg. 3 (collagen-based nutraceuticals), ctg. 4 (chondroitin-glucosamine-based nutraceuticals) and ctg. 5 (cannabinoid-based nutraceuticals). Ctg., category. * indicates significant difference ($p < 0.001$) vs. other categories.

Figure 4 shows, without significance, that omega-3-based nutraceuticals (ctg. 2) had the highest level of efficacy (mean 3.3 ± 1.9), followed by omega-3-enriched therapeutic diets (ctg. 1) (2.4 ± 2.7) and cannabinoid nutraceuticals (ctg. 5) (2.0 ± 2.2). Collagen-based nutraceuticals (ctg. 3) (1.0 ± 2.2) showed the lowest efficacy, while chondroitin-glucosamine nutraceuticals (ctg. 4) (-2.7 ± 2.0) were ineffective.

3.3.3. Complementary Analyses

Complementary analyses were conducted only on canine articles as the duration and dosage could not be compared between species, and the sample on canine OA was much larger. No significant effect of treatment duration, dose and quality total of the trials was noted on efficacy in any of the five categories tested. The follow-up duration greatly varied for all categories, with the range varying between 28 and 180 days. Overall, the treatment dose had no significant effect on the level of efficacy, with doses being fairly consistent within each category. It should be noted, however, that for cannabinoid-based nutraceuticals (ctg. 5), one trial used a much lower dose (0.5 mg/kg/d), and this was the only one to show a non-effect [56].

Effect size calculations show a medium to large effect of enriched therapeutic diets (d = 0.58) (ctg. 1) and omega-3-based nutraceuticals (d = 1.19) (ctg. 2) compared with the score of controls in these same categories. A large effect was also observed, this time favouring the efficacy score of the negative control, for the collagen-based nutraceuticals (d = −1.57) (ctg. 3) and chondroitin-glucosamine-based nutraceuticals (d = −1.39) (ctg. 4) categories. Finally, no effect could be noted for cannabinoid-based products (d = 0) (ctg. 5).

The comparison between categories revealed a large effect of all categories (ctg. 1: d = 2.13; ctg. 2: d = 3.03; ctg. 3: d = 1.74; ctg. 5: d = 2.25) compared with the chondroitin-glucosamine nutraceuticals category (ctg. 4). Collagen-based nutraceuticals (ctg. 3) also appeared to have a smaller effect than omega-3-enriched therapeutic diets (d = 0.58) (ctg. 1), omega-3-based nutraceuticals (d = 1.08) (ctg. 2) and cannabinoid-based nutraceuticals (d = 0.46) (ctg. 5).

4. Discussion

4.1. Review of the Work

This systematic review and meta-analysis assessed the efficacy of 38 compounds in the treatment of clinical signs of OA. A total of 57 articles, comprising 72 trials, were analysed.

Of the 57 articles identified, we obtained 54 articles on canine OA, while only 3 articles on the use of nutraceuticals in the context of feline OA could be found by our searches. This lack of literature on cats can perhaps be explained by the challenge in their pain evaluation. Cats are known to be less expressive, and since the domestication of cats has historically been very different from dogs, humans tend to have poorer skills in recognising painful behaviour [79]. This phenomenon is very unfortunate since these animals are as affected by OA as dogs, even though their condition is, by far, much less studied.

4.2. Evaluation Scales: Trial Quality and Analgesic Efficacy

Both scales were established following the review of methodologies presented in previous articles, including three systematic reviews assessing the benefits of enriched therapeutic diets and nutraceuticals in canine OA [12–14] (Materials and Methods). They were subsequently successful for face, content and construct validity. The latter justified the single use of the quality total in our statistical analyses. This validation assures that our meta-analysis results from systematic, independent and quantitative measures in quality and efficacy [80].

In contrast to our work, the assessment methods of the three previous systematic reviews were rather based on qualitative scales; only the review by Vanderweerd et al. [14] added an assessment of quality attributed in percentages. The enrichment of the quality of trials scale, therefore, was mainly the addition of this quantitative aspect that was missing in the previous works and follows the present rules of evidence-based medicine. In addition, several sub-criteria were developed and detailed in the construction of our evaluation scales to extract a maximum of information from each trial. This evaluation also included a test of intra-observer repeatability and inter-observer reproducibility.

The analgesic efficacy scale was simpler to establish as it had only three levels: statistically significant effect of the treatment tested vs. a control group, improvement only of the treated group over time and non-effect. It should be noted that this assessment of analgesic efficacy was based on the methods, results and statistical analyses used in each trial. Following the PROSPERO procedures helps to standardise the collection of data in the systematic review and therefore its quality. Finally, all trials were assessed and scored in a consensual manner by three observers with different levels of expertise for both grids.

4.3. Combination of Quality of Trials and Analgesic Efficacy (Ctg. 1–5)

Regarding the results of our analyses on categories 1–5 ($N > 3$ trials), the assessment of quality tended to be significantly impacted by the product category, while efficacy was significantly influenced by the category.

Combining the results of the quality (Figure 2) and efficacy (Figure 4) assessments allowed us to support the efficacy, associated to the quality of trials, of omega-3 nutraceuticals in supplement form (ctg. 2) or omega-3-enriched therapeutic diets (ctg. 1) and cannabinoid nutraceuticals (ctg. 5) (respectively from the most to least effective). Our analyses also showed, with studies of lesser quality, a weak efficacy of collagen-based nutraceuticals (ctg. 3) and a very marked non-effect of chondroitin-glucosamine-based products (ctg. 4). The quality of the latter studies is disappointing in terms of concluding on the use of these products, and the total lack of efficacy of chondroitin-glucosamine nutraceuticals (ctg. 4) stands out in comparison with the other categories, and therefore indicates that these products should no longer be recommended in cases of canine or feline OA.

4.4. Enriched Therapeutic Diets (Ctg. 1) and Nutraceuticals (Ctg. 2) Based on Omega-3

For omega-3-based compounds, i.e., categories 1 and 2, the results of all previous reviews support our inferences with a high level of comfort that these products are highly effective [12–14]. The one difficulty encountered by previous reviews, and the present one, is the lack of objective data available in studies of these products. However, there is a preponderance of high-quality trials within these two categories. The complexity of efficacy assessment in the studies of therapeutic diets in canine OA has already been raised [81]. Compared with other therapeutic modalities (e.g., NSAID), the rate of negative responders (using objective kinetic podobarometric assessment) to the introduction of a therapeutic diet is three times higher, while, conversely, the rate of positive responders to a placebo-control diet is up to two times higher. A therapeutic diet role is to primarily meet the dog nutritional needs while providing active ingredients susceptible to modify the condition. The contribution of a balanced diet may, therefore, have less impact on dogs recruited into a clinical trial because they are already well-nourished, while, on the other hand, the condition of dogs receiving the control diet will improve [81]. Moreover, the variability in the diet ingestion compared with that of supplements could also explain a variation in the exposure to the active ingredients, and thus in the expression of their expected benefits, not to mention inter-individual perturbations on the gut microbiota [81].

Regarding the efficacy of omega-3 products, only 2 [25,30] of the 20 trials on them were non-effective, which underlines the analgesic potential of these products. The same finding was also true concerning the feline OA trials that provided good-quality studies and both showed an analgesic effect [23,36]. Only one trial of omega-3-enriched therapeutic diets (ctg. 1) [25] showing no improvement in the OA condition of the dogs was a dose titration study, and this trial tested the lowest dose.

This meta-analysis supports the use of omega-3 supplementation for the management of canine and feline OA. The incorporation of omega-3 into a therapeutic diet offers the ease of administration of adapted doses of omega-3, and the diets also facilitate, through their nutritional quality, the maintenance of digestive and renal functions that are often affected in these geriatric patients, while theoretically favouring excess weight loss.

4.5. Cannabinoid Nutraceuticals (Ctg. 5)

Trials with cannabidiol in dogs also indicated high-quality studies and good evidence of efficacy. It is interesting to note that these studies are recent (published between 2018 and 2021) and more in line with international recommendations. The efficacy of cannabidiol in the treatment of chronic pain, mainly neuropathic in nature, has already been reported in rodent models [82] and in human patients [83]. Seven trials testing cannabidiol in the management of OA pain in dogs were evaluated. All showed an improvement in the condition with the exception of a single trial conducted by Verrico et al. [56]. In this trial, the authors tested a low dose (0.5 mg/kg/day) compared with a higher dose

(1.2 mg/kg/day). Interestingly, in the same study, a trial of a liposomal formulation at the same low dose (0.5 mg/kg/day) was effective. Liposomal encapsulation has already shown, in humans and mice, a better bioavailability [56]. The results of this meta-analysis are promising, but further investigation is needed to determine the efficacy, doses, formulations and combinations recommended for the treatment of canine OA pain. Further studies will also be necessary to conclude on the use of cannabinoids in cats since none have been carried out to this day.

4.6. Collagen-Based Nutraceuticals (Ctg. 3)

The scientific evidence for the efficacy of collagen (ctg. 3) in its UC-II (undenatured type II collagen) formulation, alone or combined most often with chondroitin-glucosamine, or in the formulation derived from an eggshell membrane [44–46] was the lowest of the four categories with a positive efficacy score. The main reason for this relates to the poor quality of the trials that evaluated it: small sample size (N = 5 dogs per group [38,39,42], N = 7–10 per group [40] and N = 9 [46]); assessment using non-validated subjective tools without observer guidance [38–40,42,43] with a visibly non-adapted statistical methodology; and a limited (often single) number of assessment times in the follow-up period [38,41,44,46]. In addition, one study investigated a therapeutic diet with green tea extract, turmeric and hydrolysed collagen as active ingredients, and while the subjective assessments were positive, the objective podobarometric assessment (kinetic analysis of ground reaction forces) was inconclusive [76]. It, therefore, appears impossible to rule, at the present time, on an indication for collagen in canine OA based on the results of this meta-analysis.

4.7. Chondroitin-Glucosamine Nutraceuticals (Ctg. 4)

The systematic review of the literature included nine trials that evaluated, mostly in combination, glucosamine hydrochloride and chondroitin sulphate. Chondroitin-glucosamine nutraceuticals (ctg. 4) showed strong evidence of non-effect and a significant statistical difference in efficacy from the other categories (ctg. 1, 2, 3 and 5) in the meta-analysis. Of the nine trials assessed in this review, only one [49] showed an improvement in the condition of the animals assessed, but this was using a non-validated subjective tool and for only one assessment time (at day 70), a difference not present before (day 14 or 42) or after (day 90). It should be noted that dosing was reduced by one third between days 42 and 70 and stopped after day 70, while the authors concluded that there was non-inferiority of the nutraceuticals vs. a positive control using carprofen in their OA dogs [49].

In the human literature, there are several criticisms of its use in OA, and a meta-analysis similarly found no effect on OA pain compared with the placebo [84]. A veterinary systematic review on the use of chondroitin-glucosamine was also inconclusive in dogs [85]. Like these previous reviews, the results of the present meta-analysis led to the conclusion that chondroitin-glucosamine nutraceuticals should not be prescribed in canine or feline OA.

4.8. Nutraceuticals Based on Hydroxycitric Acid (Ctg. 6), Calcium Fructoborate (Ctg. 7) and Composite Nutraceuticals (Ctg. 8)

The results of the hydroxycitric acid (ctg. 6) or fructoborate (ctg. 7) products were not conclusive. The low quality of the hydroxycitric acid trials and the lack of efficacy of the fructoborate trials did not allow one to definitively conclude on the use of these products. However, for both types of products, all trials were obtained from the same article [39,58], which could potentially bias our conclusions. Regarding composite nutraceuticals (ctg. 8), they do seem to be of interest as two of the trials showed an effect * in [59], ψ in [60]. The composition of the two composite nutraceuticals is based on a combination of herbal medicine (*Harpagophytum procumbens*, *Boswellia serrata*, *Ribes nigrum*, *Salix alba**, *Tanacetum parthenium**, *Ananas comosus**, *Lentinus edodes*$^{\psi}$, *Equisetum arvense*$^{\psi}$ and *Curcuma longa*), omega-3s, chondroitin-glucosamine, methylsulphonylmethane*, L-glutamine* and hyaluronic acid*. Both studies were characterised by a remarkable safety profile in

$N = 16$ [59] and $N = 10$ [60] dogs treated over 2 and 3 months, respectively. The results of the Canadian study were impressive as they incorporated objective assessments (podobarometric gait analysis and actimetry), but it is regrettable that the products are not marketed [59]. In any case, more high-quality studies are needed to properly assess these products.

4.9. Other (Ctg. 9)

Finally, all the other nutraceuticals evaluated did not present sufficient evidence of efficacy to decide on their indication. However, some of these compounds seemed promising, with high-quality studies, such as elk velvet antler [64] or *Brachystemma calycinum* D don extracts [68,69]. The results with turmeric were conflicting, being either negative [63], ambiguous [61,76] or positive [59,60]. Although turmeric seems to benefit from a composite synergistic approach, evidence of efficacy remains to be confirmed with further studies.

4.10. Effect Sizes

The calculated effect sizes, in comparison with negative controls, supported the evidence of efficacy of omega-3-enriched diets (ctg. 1) and omega-3-based nutraceuticals (ctg. 2). This indicates a clinically important effect of these products.

For collagen-based nutraceuticals (ctg. 3), this comparison highlighted the uncertainty about the efficacy of these products. The calculation of the effect size took into account the level of not only efficacy but also quality for the trials. For ctg. 3, quality had a huge influence on the scores obtained. The measures collected, therefore, indicated that we cannot conclude to an effect of collagen and that further studies of high quality would be required.

The effect size obtained for the chondroitin-glucosamine nutraceuticals (ctg. 4) clearly showed the lack of efficacy of these products, with the negative controls showing even a higher averaged efficacy than the product trials. Furthermore, the comparison of the efficacy with the other categories showed a strong non-effect of these nutraceuticals.

Finally, the results obtained for the cannabinoid-based nutraceuticals (ctg. 5) did not support a definitive conclusion on the use of these products, and further studies would, again, be necessary.

Interpretation of these effect sizes must be performed with caution as this is not a comparison of the data obtained from the evaluations of these trials but a comparison of the scores assigned. These scores tend to favour the effects, and, therefore, the evaluation of negative controls is tricky. The use of control was also not present in all the included trials, so they could not be counted in the averaged efficacy level of the categories. The lack of follow-up over time for these control groups was another constraint that was often encountered. The assessment of the efficacy level of the controls was therefore sometimes solely based on an interpretation of the results presented without the support of the statistical analyses presented in the trials.

4.11. Potential Mechanism of Nutraceuticals Action

Nutraceuticals' precise mechanisms of action are still not well-determined in any target species [86,87]. Moreover, the poor application of consistency and standardisation in the nutraceuticals composition makes it difficult to conclude on the mechanisms of action underlying a single product [88,89]. Regarding OA, the favourite molecular targets focus on anti-inflammatory, anti-oxidative and anti-catabolic actions, thus sustaining the global attention to cytokine (tumour necrosis factor—TNF, interleukins—IL, etc.) implication in inflammation and degradative proteases [90].

Historically, with nutraceuticals being related to the natural components of the cartilage matrix (e.g., collagen, glucosamine and chondroitin), the study of their mechanism of action focused on structural (cartilage) effects [87].

Glucosamine and chondroitin are often used in combination. The primary interest of these products in osteoarthritic pain is their supposed anti-inflammatory properties. In fact, many in vitro and preclinical studies have shown their interaction in the nuclear factor-kappa B and p38 mitogen-activated protein kinase inflammatory pathways, as well as their involvement in the regulation of pro- and anti -inflammatory cytokines [91–93]. Glucosamine and chondroitin tend to stimulate, in in vitro and in vivo tests (mice and rat models), the expression of anti-inflammatory interleukins (IL-2, IL-10), reduce that of pro-inflammatory molecules (IL-1B, IL-6, TNF-α) and downregulate the production and expression of prostaglandin E_2 synthetase and inducible cyclooxygenase (COX-2) or nitric oxide synthase (iNOS) [91,92,94–96]. Some antioxidant claims have also been made following in vitro results [97,98]. Finally, glucosamine and chondroitin are believed to modulate the expression and activity of certain catabolic enzymes implicated in the OA pathology. The results of different in vitro studies revealed, indeed, a decrease in the transcription and expression of degradative enzymes such as aggrecanases and matrix metalloproteinases (MMP-3, MMP-13) [92,94,99,100].

Collagen, especially in its hydrolysate form, will have the ability to prevent the destruction of cartilage through the production of macromolecules and suppression of catabolic enzymes. Many in vitro and preclinical studies have pointed to increased collagen type II synthesis, an important matrix component [101–103] and anti-inflammatory effects [104]. Another role, specific to collagen, is the oral tolerance phenomenon. It involves the intervention of the immune system and regulatory T cells (Tregs). The Tregs get activated by the collagen and are suspected to secrete many anti-inflammatory mediators upon meeting an articular cartilage (IL-4, IL-10, transforming growth factor-β) [105,106]. This modulation of the natural immune reaction is an important support for the anti-inflammatory activity and provides an environment conducive to cartilage repair. Moreover, it could be involved in the occurrence of adverse effects, which was elevated in human studies [107].

Omega-3s have evident anti-inflammatory properties through the reduction of IL-1α, IL-1β and TNF-α levels and the release of anti-inflammatory molecules [108,109]. In fact, the production of endogenous special proresolving mediators (SPMs) derived from these fatty acids helps to ease the inflammatory response in part responsible for osteoarthritic pain with even long-lasting effect shown [109,110]. Due to the competition for enzymes between omega-3 and omega-6 fatty acids, it has been suggested to promote the intake of high n-3/n-6 ratio diets to support the production of anti-inflammatory molecules and minimise the conversion of omega-6 in prostaglandins, leukotrienes and other pro-inflammatory lipoxygenase or COX by-products [111]. Omega-3s also seem to have anti-catabolic effects. Indeed, through in vitro and in vivo preclinical studies, the expressions of catabolic enzymes such as MMP-3, MMP-13 and ADAMTS-4/5 (a disintegrin and metalloproteinase with thrombospondin motifs) were downregulated [108,112,113]. More recently, the transient receptor potential vanilloid 1 (TRPV1) and the modulation of glial cells, both involved in pathologic pain, have been linked as a new target of omega-3 [114–116].

Many other nutraceuticals presented in vitro demonstration of anti-inflammatory, anti-oxidative and anti-catabolic properties. This was the case of hydroxycitric acid (extract from *Garcinia indica*) and other phytochemicals (*Boswellia serrata, Harpagophytum procumbens, Ribes nigrum, Salix alba, Brachystemma calycinum*, etc.). In recent years, the focus was on their anti-nociceptive properties, such as with cannabidiol. Cannabinoid pain-relieving effects are linked to various interactions and modulation of the endocannabinoid, inflammatory and nociceptive systems [117], with cannabidiol presenting high affinity for cannabinoid CB1 and CB2 receptors (antagonist), G-protein-coupled receptor 55 (antagonist) and many TRPV receptors (agonist) as well as peroxisome proliferator-activated receptor gamma [118], the latter two being largely recognised for their role in chronic pain and OA-related joint degradation [119]. Cannabinoids have shown great promises in animal models with acute and chronic pain [120–122].

Despite the importance of the data obtained and accumulated on these different mechanisms over the years, the application of this information remains limited. Most of the studies conducted on the mechanisms of action critically lacked about model and essay validity for the targeted OA pathology, as well as pharmacokinetics assessments.

Several models of acute (inflammatory) pain have been used to represent OA, although this disease is much more complex, entangling chronic and degenerative conditions of many components, not just chondrocytes (in cell culture) [123]. These in vitro studies should be only kept producing precise mechanistic evidence of a chemical entity and then transposed into more complete models [124]. It has also been suggested that the use of models with naturally occurring disease provides the most valid models [125]. As for pharmacokinetics, the evaluation of the degree of systemic absorption and organ distribution is particularly lacking in nutraceuticals research. In fact, many products show very little systemic absorption, which inevitably translates to low efficacy. Is this the case of oral products based on glucosamine and chondroitin that showed relatively poor bioavailability in dogs (approximately 12% and 5% after a single dosing, respectively) [126]? Collagen-based products in rats, on the other hand, presented an absolute bioavailability of 58%, which is quite good [127].

4.12. General Discussions and Conclusions

Overall, previous systematic reviews support our findings [12–14]. However, a major difference between our systematic review and the previous ones is the number of articles identified. The most recent of these publications [14] was already from 2012; only 16 total publications were included, and their conclusions were based on the analysis of only one to four trials per nutraceutical. Surprisingly, 31 (out of 57) of the articles in our systematic review are dated from 2012 to the present, which is not consistent with previous review searches.

The quality of the studies we identified is often impoverished by the use of subjective and/or non-validated measurement tools. These tools, often carried out by owners who are not trained to complete them, are too susceptible to experimental bias and are not recommended in pain assessment according to recent professional guidelines [128,129]. In our assessments, we predetermined the degrees of reliability of the measurement tools. We prioritised objective pain quantification with kinetic or actimetric assessment methods, as these results are recognised as more valid and reliable (reference standard). Conversely, the subjective quantification of pain, very often estimated by the owner or veterinarian, shows less valid results and is more sensitive to the placebo effect [130] than objective methods [81].

Finally, several variables can influence the efficacy of nutraceuticals and thus affect the data that were evaluated. Among all the studies, we observed a wide variety of formulations (capsules, powdered food supplements, therapeutic diets, etc.). The mode of administration of nutraceuticals may affect the bioavailability of the nutraceuticals in the system and thus affect the physiological response observed [131]. Dosage, frequency and duration are also factors influencing the receipt of treatment. The studies analysed in this review had very variable treatment durations, ranging from about 1 to 6 months. As OA is a progressive disease, the duration of treatment is a key factor in the observation of pain clinical signs in pets [132]. Some lower-dose trials have shown a lack of effect probably due to dosage [25,56]. However, our results on the analysis of duration and dose on efficacy could not confirm the influence of these factors. This is probably due to the lack of power of analysis, related to the small sample size and huge variability in each category.

In addition, although some trials provide the same feeding bases as others, the content of each ingredient remains variable between studies and trials. For example, for two trials based on omega-3 polyunsaturated fatty acid supplementation, the content of eicosapentaenoic and docosahexaenoic acids may vary [133]. This example highlights the need for requirements on origin, standardised extraction and preparation methods. The content of the active ingredient and synergistic effects with other components of the formulation can also be a source of variability in expected results.

The studies in this systematic review and meta-analysis greatly vary in their methodology. The development of clear norms and requirements that establish a standardisation of future clinical studies [85,134,135] will increase the quality and strength of evidence of efficacy and seek consensus on the true benefits of different nutraceuticals.

5. Conclusions

Our rigorous approach to meta-analysis allowed us to conclude with certainty that the use of omega-3 products beneficially modulates the painful condition of OA dogs and cats, while the intake of chondroitin-glucosamine has no analgesic effect. Further studies will be necessary to be able to state on the potential effects of collagen, cannabidiol and composite nutraceuticals, but these products seem promising.

Author Contributions: Conceptualisation, B.L. and E.T.; methodology, M.B.-G., C.O. and E.T.; validation, C.O., M.M., B.L. and E.T.; formal analysis, M.B.-G., C.O. and E.T.; investigation, M.B.-G. and A.C.; resources, M.M., B.L. and E.T.; data curation, M.B.-G., C.O. and E.T.; writing—original draft preparation, M.B.-G. and E.T.; writing—review and editing, M.B.-G., A.C., C.O., M.M., B.L. and E.T.; visualisation, M.B.-G. and C.O.; supervision, B.L. and E.T.; project administration, E.T.; funding acquisition, E.T. All authors have read and agreed to the published version of the manuscript.

Funding: There was no proprietary interest or funding directly provided for this project or to any of the authors. This work was indirectly supported (E.T.) by a Discovery Grant (#RGPIN 441651-2013, and #RGPIN 05512-2020) and a Collaborative Research and Development Grant (#RDCPJ 491953-2016) supporting operations and salaries from the Natural Sciences and Engineering Research Council of Canada (NSERC). M.B.-G. and A.C. were recipients of an NSERC Undergraduate Student Research Award (USRA). C.O. was the recipient of a MITACS Canada Postdoctoral Fellowship Elevation (#IT 11643).

Institutional Review Board Statement: This is not applicable as this project did not involve humans or animals.

Informed Consent Statement: Not applicable.

Data Availability Statement: Not applicable.

Acknowledgments: The authors would like to thank Tristan Juette, Statistical Advisor to the Faculty of Veterinary Medicine, Université de Montréal, for his assistance with the statistical analyses and review of the manuscript.

Conflicts of Interest: The authors report having conducted work in canine osteoarthritis for the following companies: Biotanika, Inc; Boehringer-Ingelheim Animal Health, Inc; Centrexion Therapeutics, Corp; Ceva Santé Animale, S.A.; Elanco, Ltd.; Intervet, Corp; Merck Animal Health, Inc; Midwest Health Technologies, L.L.C.; Nestlé Purina Petcare, S.A.; Royal-Canin, Inc, a division of Mars Petcare; Vétoquinol, S.A.; Vita Green Health Products Co, Ltd.; and Zoetis, L.L.C.; many of which have led to publications that are included in this systematic review and meta-analysis. The authors declare no conflict of interest directly related to the conduct of this review.

References

1. Shearer, P. Epidemiology of orthopedic disease. In *Orthopedic Conditions in Cats and Dogs*; McNeill, E., Ed.; Royal Canin: Aimargues, France, 2011; Volume 21, pp. 24–25.
2. Engelhardt, G.; Bögel, R.; Schnitzler, C.; Utzmann, R. Meloxicam: Influence on arachidonic acid metabolism: Part II. *In vivo* findings. *Biochem. Pharmacol.* **1996**, *51*, 29–38. [CrossRef]
3. Serni, U.; Mannoni, A.; Benucci, M. Is there preliminary in-vivo evidence for an influence of nonsteroidal antiinflammatory drugs on progression in osteoarthritis? Part II-evidence from animal models. *Osteoarthr. Cartil.* **1999**, *7*, 351–352. [CrossRef] [PubMed]
4. Mabry, K.; Hill, T.; Tolbert, M.K. Prevalence of gastrointestinal lesions in dogs chronically treated with nonsteroidal anti-inflammatory drugs. *J. Vet. Intern. Med.* **2021**, *35*, 853–859. [CrossRef] [PubMed]
5. Astin, J.A. Why Patients Use Alternative Medicine Results of a National Study. *JAMA* **1998**, *279*, 1548–1553. [CrossRef] [PubMed]
6. Chopra, A.S.; Lordan, R.; Horbańczuk, O.K.; Atanasov, A.G.; Chopra, I.; Horbańczuk, J.O.; Jóźwik, A.; Huang, L.; Pirgozliev, V.; Banach, M.; et al. The current use and evolving landscape of nutraceuticals. *Pharmacol. Res.* **2022**, *175*, 106001. [CrossRef]
7. Grand View Research. Available online: https://www.grandviewresearch.com/industry-analysis/veterinary-dietary-supplements-market-report (accessed on 20 August 2022).
8. Elrod, S.M.; Hofmeister, E.H. Veterinarians' attitudes towards use of nutraceuticals. *Can. J. Vet. Res.* **2019**, *83*, 291–297.
9. Finno, C.J. Veterinary Pet Supplements and Nutraceuticals. *Nutr. Today* **2020**, *55*, 97–101. [CrossRef]
10. Taylor, C.L. Regulatory frameworks for functional foods and dietary supplements. *Nutr. Rev.* **2004**, *62*, 55–59. [CrossRef]

11. Zeisel, S.H. Regulation of "nutraceuticals". *Science* **1999**, *285*, 1853–1855. [CrossRef]
12. Aragon, C.L.; Hofmeister, E.H.; Budsberg, S.C. Systematic review of clinical trials of treatments for osteoarthritis in dogs. *J. Am. Vet. Med. Assoc.* **2007**, *230*, 514–521. [CrossRef]
13. Sanderson, R.O.; Beata, C.; Flipo, R.M.; Genevois, J.P.; Macias, C.; Tacke, S.; Vezzoni, A.; Innes, J.F. Systematic review of the management of canine osteoarthritis. *Vet. Rec.* **2009**, *164*, 418–424. [CrossRef] [PubMed]
14. Vandeweerd, J.M.; Coisnon, C.; Clegg, P.; Cambier, C.; Pierson, A.; Hontoir, F.; Saegerman, C.; Gustin, P.; Buczinski, S. Systematic review of efficacy of nutraceuticals to alleviate clinical signs of osteoarthritis. *J. Vet. Intern. Med.* **2012**, *26*, 448–456. [CrossRef] [PubMed]
15. Kilkenny, C.; Browne, W.J.; Cuthill, I.C.; Emerson, M.; Altman, D.G. Improving Bioscience Research Reporting: The ARRIVE Guidelines for Reporting Animal Research. *Animals* **2014**, *4*, 35–44. [CrossRef]
16. Schulz, K.F.; Altman, D.G.; Moher, D. CONSORT 2010 statement: Updated guidelines for reporting parallel group randomised trials. *BMJ* **2010**, *340*, c332. [CrossRef]
17. Sena, E.; van der Worp, H.B.; Howells, D.; Macleod, M. How can we improve the pre-clinical development of drugs for stroke? *Trends Neurosci.* **2007**, *30*, 433–439. [CrossRef]
18. Suokas, A.K.; Sagar, D.R.; Mapp, P.I.; Chapman, V.; Walsh, D.A. Design, study quality and evidence of analgesic efficacy in studies of drugs in models of OA pain: A systematic review and a meta-analysis. *Osteoarthr. Cartil.* **2014**, *22*, 1207–1223. [CrossRef]
19. Moher, D.; Liberati, A.; Tetzlaff, J.; Altman, D.G. Preferred reporting items for systematic reviews and meta-analyses: The PRISMA statement. *PLoS Med.* **2009**, *6*, e1000097. [CrossRef]
20. Page, M.J.; McKenzie, J.E.; Bossuyt, P.M.; Boutron, I.; Hoffmann, T.C.; Mulrow, C.D.; Shamseer, L.; Tetzlaff, J.M.; Akl, E.A.; Brennan, S.E.; et al. The PRISMA 2020 statement: An updated guideline for reporting systematic reviews. *BMJ* **2021**, *372*, n71. [CrossRef]
21. Bierer, T.L.; Bui, L.M. Improvement of arthritic signs in dogs fed green-lipped mussel (*Perna canaliculus*). *J. Nutr.* **2002**, *132*, 1634S–1636S. [CrossRef]
22. Servet, E.; Biourge, V.; Marniquet, P. Dietary Intervention Can Improve Clinical Signs in Osteoarthritic Dogs. *J. Nutr.* **2006**, *136*, 1995S–1997S. [CrossRef]
23. Lascelles, B.D.X.; DePuy, V.; Thomson, A.; Hansen, B.; Marcellin-Little, D.J.; Biourge, V.; Bauer, J.E. Evaluation of a therapeutic diet for feline degenerative joint disease. *J. Vet. Intern. Med.* **2010**, *24*, 487–495. [CrossRef] [PubMed]
24. Rialland, P.; Bichot, S.; Lussier, B.; Moreau, M.; Beaudry, F.; del Castillo, J.R.E.; Gauvin, D.; Troncy, E. Effect of a diet enriched with green-lipped mussel on pain behavior and functioning in dogs with clinical osteoarthritis. *Can. J. Vet. Res.* **2013**, *77*, 66–74. [PubMed]
25. Fritsch, D.; Allen, T.A.; Dodd, C.E.; Jewell, D.E.; Sixby, K.A.; Leventhal, P.S.; Hahn, K.A. Dose-Titration effects of fish oil in Osteoarthritic dogs. *J. Vet. Intern. Med.* **2010**, *24*, 1020–1026. [CrossRef] [PubMed]
26. Fritsch, D.A.; Allen, T.A.; Dodd, C.E.; Jewell, D.E.; Sixby, K.A.; Leventhal, P.S.; Brejda, J.; Hahn, K.A. A multicenter study of the effect of dietary supplementation with fish oil omega-3 fatty acids on carprofen dosage in dogs with osteoarthritis. *J. Am. Vet. Med. Assoc.* **2010**, *236*, 535–539. [CrossRef]
27. Roush, J.K.; Cross, A.R.; Renberg, W.C.; Dodd, C.E.; Sixby, K.A.; Fritsch, D.A.; Allen, T.A.; Jewell, D.E.; Richardson, D.C.; Leventhal, P.S.; et al. Evaluation of the effects of dietary supplementation with fish oil omega-3 fatty acids on weight bearing in dogs with osteoarthritis. *J. Am. Vet. Med. Assoc.* **2010**, *236*, 67–73. [CrossRef] [PubMed]
28. Roush, J.K.; Dodd, C.E.; Fritsch, D.A.; Allen, T.A.; Jewell, D.E.; Schoenherr, W.D.; Richardson, D.C.; Leventhal, P.S.; Hahn, K.A. Multicenter veterinary practice assessment of the effects of omega-3 fatty acids on osteoarthritis in dogs. *J. Am. Vet. Med. Assoc.* **2010**, *236*, 59–65. [CrossRef] [PubMed]
29. Moreau, M.; Troncy, E.; Del Castillo, J.R.E.; Bedard, C.; Gauvin, D.; Lussier, B. Effects of feeding a high omega-3 fatty acids diet in dogs with naturally occurring osteoarthritis. *J. Anim. Physiol. Anim. Nutr.* **2013**, *97*, 830–837. [CrossRef] [PubMed]
30. Dobenecker, B.; Beetz, Y.; Kienzle, E. A placebo-controlled double-blind study on the effect of nutraceuticals (chondroitin sulfate and mussel extract) in dogs with joint diseases as perceived by their owners. *J. Nutr.* **2002**, *132*, 1690S–1691S. [CrossRef]
31. Pollard, B.; Guilford, W.G.; Ankenbauer-Perkins, K.L.; Hedderley, D. Clinical efficacy and tolerance of an extract of green-lipped mussel (Perna canaliculus) in dogs presumptively diagnosed with degenerative joint disease. *N. Z. Vet. J.* **2006**, *54*, 114–118. [CrossRef]
32. Hielm-Björkman, A.; Tulamo, R.-M.; Salonen, H.; Raekallio, M. Evaluating Complementary Therapies for Canine Osteoarthritis Part I: Green-lipped Mussel (Perna canaliculus). *Evid.-Based Complement. Altern. Med. eCAM* **2009**, *6*, 365–373. [CrossRef]
33. Soontornvipart, K.; Mongkhon, N.; Nganvongpanit, K.; Kongtawelert, P. Effect of PCSO-524 on OA biomarkers and weight-bearing properties in canine shoulder and coxofemeral osteoarthritis. *Thai J. Vet. Med.* **2015**, *45*, 157–165.
34. Vijarnsorn, M.; Kwananocha, I.; Kashemsant, N.; Jarudecha, T.; Lekcharoensuk, C.; Beale, B.; Peirone, B.; Lascelles, B.D.X. The effectiveness of marine based fatty acid compound (PCSO-524) and firocoxib in the treatment of canine osteoarthritis. *BMC Vet. Res.* **2019**, *15*, 349. [CrossRef] [PubMed]
35. Hielm-Bjorkman, A.; Roine, J.; Elo, K.; Lappalainen, A.; Junnila, J.; Laitinen-Vapaavuori, O. An un-commissioned randomized, placebo-controlled double-blind study to test the effect of deep sea fish oil as a pain reliever for dogs suffering from canine OA. *BMC Vet. Res.* **2012**, *8*, 157. [CrossRef] [PubMed]

36. Corbee, R.J.; Barnier, M.M.C.; Van de Lest, C.H.A.; Hazewinkel, H.A.W. The effect of dietary long-chain omega-3 fatty acid supplementation on owner's perception of behaviour and locomotion in cats with naturally occurring osteoarthritis. *J. Anim. Physiol. Anim. Nutr.* **2013**, *97*, 846–853. [CrossRef] [PubMed]
37. Mehler, S.J.; May, L.R.; King, C.; Harris, W.S.; Shah, Z. A prospective, randomized, double blind, placebo-controlled evaluation of the effects of eicosapentaenoic acid and docosahexaenoic acid on the clinical signs and erythrocyte membrane polyunsaturated fatty acid concentrations in dogs with osteoarthritis. *Prostaglandins Leukot. Essent. Fat. Acids* **2016**, *109*, 1–7. [CrossRef]
38. Deparle, L.A.; Gupta, R.C.; Canerdy, T.D.; Goad, J.T.; D'Altilio, M.; Bagchi, M.; Bagchi, D. Efficacy and safety of glycosylated undenatured type-II collagen (UC-II) in therapy of arthritic dogs. *J. Vet. Pharmacol. Ther.* **2005**, *28*, 385–390. [CrossRef]
39. Peal, A.; D'Altilio, M.; Simms, C.; Alvey, M.; Gupta, R.C.; Goad, J.T.; Canerdy, T.D.; Bagchi, M.; Bagchi, D. Therapeutic efficacy and safety of undenatured type-II collagen (UC-II) alone or in combination with (-)-hydroxycitric acid and chromemate in arthritic dogs. *J. Vet. Pharmacol. Ther.* **2007**, *30*, 275–278. [CrossRef]
40. Gupta, R.C.; Canerdy, T.D.; Lindley, J.; Konemann, M.; Minniear, J.; Carroll, B.A.; Hendrick, C.; Goad, J.T.; Rohde, K.; Doss, R.; et al. Comparative therapeutic efficacy and safety of type-II collagen (UC-II), glucosamine and chondroitin in arthritic dogs: Pain evaluation by ground force plate. *J. Anim. Physiol. Anim. Nutr.* **2012**, *96*, 770–777. [CrossRef]
41. Stabile, M.; Samarelli, R.; Trerotoli, P.; Fracassi, L.; Lacitignola, L.; Crovace, A.; Staffieri, F. Evaluation of the Effects of Undenatured Type II Collagen (UC-II) as Compared to Robenacoxib on the Mobility Impairment Induced by Osteoarthritis in Dogs. *Vet. Sci.* **2019**, *6*, 72. [CrossRef]
42. D'Altilio, M.; Peal, A.; Alvey, M.; Simms, C.; Curtsinger, A.; Gupta, R.C.; Canerdy, T.D.; Goad, J.T.; Bagchi, M.; Bagchi, D. Therapeutic Efficacy and Safety of Undenatured Type II Collagen Singly or in Combination with Glucosamine and Chondroitin in Arthritic Dogs. *Toxicol. Mech. Methods* **2007**, *17*, 189–196. [CrossRef]
43. Beynen, A.C.; van Geene, H.W.; Grim, H.V.; Jacobs, P.; Van der Vlerk, T. Oral administration of gelatin hydrolysate reduces clinical signs of canine osteoarthritis in a double-blind, placebo-controlled trial. *Am. J. Anim. Vet. Sci.* **2010**, *5*, 102–106. [CrossRef]
44. Ruff, K.J.; Kopp, K.J.; Von Behrens, P.; Lux, M.; Mahn, M.; Back, M. Effectiveness of NEM(®) brand eggshell membrane in the treatment of suboptimal joint function in dogs: A multicenter, randomized, double-blind, placebo-controlled study. *Vet. Med.* **2016**, *7*, 113–121. [CrossRef] [PubMed]
45. Aguirre, A.; Gil-Quintana, E.; Fenaux, M.; Sanchez, N.; Torre, C. The efficacy of Ovopet®in the treatment of hip dysplasia in dogs. *J. Vet. Med. Anim. Health* **2018**, *10*, 198–207. [CrossRef]
46. Muller, C.; Enomoto, M.; Buono, A.; Steiner, J.M.; Lascelles, B.D.X. Placebo-controlled pilot study of the effects of an eggshell membrane-based supplement on mobility and serum biomarkers in dogs with osteoarthritis. *Vet. J.* **2019**, *253*, 105379. [CrossRef] [PubMed]
47. Moreau, M.; Dupuis, J.; Bonneau, N.H.; Desnoyers, M. Clinical evaluation of a nutraceutical, carprofen and meloxicam for the treatment of dogs with osteoarthritis. *Vet. Rec.* **2003**, *152*, 323–329. [CrossRef] [PubMed]
48. Maihasap, P.; Soontornwipart, K.; Techaarpornkul, N. Clinical effect of glucosamine and chondroitin contained nutraceutical on osteoarthritis in dogs after anterior cruciate ligament rupture surgical repair. *Thai J. Vet. Med.* **2014**, *44*, 67–73.
49. McCarthy, G.; O'Donovan, J.; Jones, B.; McAllister, H.; Seed, M.; Mooney, C. Randomised double-blind, positive-controlled trial to assess the efficacy of glucosamine/chondroitin sulfate for the treatment of dogs with osteoarthritis. *Vet. J.* **2007**, *174*, 54–61. [CrossRef]
50. Sul, R.M.; Chase, D.; Parkin, T.; Bennett, D. Comparison of meloxicam and a glucosamine-chondroitin supplement in management of feline osteoarthritis: A double-blind randomised, placebo-controlled, prospective trial. *Vet. Comp. Orthop. Traumatol.* **2014**, *27*, 20–26. [CrossRef]
51. Alves, J.C.; Santos, A.M.; Jorge, P.I. Effect of an Oral Joint Supplement When Compared to Carprofen in the Management of Hip Osteoarthritis in Working Dogs. *Top. Companion Anim. Med.* **2017**, *32*, 126–129. [CrossRef]
52. Scott, R.M.; Evans, R.; Conzemius, M.G. Efficacy of an oral nutraceutical for the treatment of canine osteoarthritis. A double-blind, randomized, placebo-controlled prospective clinical trial. Vet. Comp. *Orthop. Traumatol.* **2017**, *30*, 318–323. [CrossRef]
53. Gamble, L.J.; Boesch, J.M.; Frye, C.W.; Schwark, W.S.; Mann, S.; Wolfe, L.; Brown, H.; Berthelsen, E.S.; Wakshlag, J.J. Pharmacokinetics, safety, and clinical efficacy of cannabidiol treatment in osteoarthritic dogs. *Front. Vet. Sci.* **2018**, *5*, 165. [CrossRef] [PubMed]
54. Brioschi, F.A.; Di Cesare, F.; Gioeni, D.; Rabbogliatti, V.; Ferrari, F.; D'Urso, E.S.; Amari, M.; Ravasio, G. Oral Transmucosal Cannabidiol Oil Formulation as Part of a Multimodal Analgesic Regimen: Effects on Pain Relief and Quality of Life Improvement in Dogs Affected by Spontaneous Osteoarthritis. *Animals* **2020**, *10*, 1505. [CrossRef] [PubMed]
55. Kogan, L.; Hellyer, P.; Downing, R. The Use of Cannabidiol-Rich Hemp Oil Extract to Treat Canine Osteoarthritis-Related Pain: A Pilot Study. *AHVMA J.* **2020**, *58*, 1–10.
56. Verrico, C.D.; Wesson, S.; Konduri, V.; Hofferek, C.J.; Vazquez-Perez, J.; Blair, E.; Dunner, K., Jr.; Salimpour, P.; Decker, W.K.; Halpert, M.M. A randomized, double-blind, placebo-controlled study of daily cannabidiol for the treatment of canine osteoarthritis pain. *Pain* **2020**, *161*, 2191–2202. [CrossRef]
57. Mejia, S.; Duerr, F.M.; Griffenhagen, G.; McGrath, S. Evaluation of the effect of cannabidiol on naturally occuring osteoarthritis-associated pain: A pilot study in dogs. *J. Am. Anim. Hosp. Assoc.* **2021**, *57*, 81–90. [CrossRef] [PubMed]

58. Price, A.K.; de Godoy, M.R.C.; Harper, T.A.; Knap, K.E.; Joslyn, S.; Pietrzkowski, Z.; Cross, B.K.; Detweiler, K.B.; Swanson, K.S. Effects of dietary calcium fructoborate supplementation on joint comfort and flexibility and serum inflammatory markers in dogs with osteoarthritis. *J. Anim. Sci.* **2017**, *95*, 2907–2916. [CrossRef]
59. Moreau, M.; Lussier, B.; Pelletier, J.P.; Martel-Pelletier, J.; Bédard, C.; Gauvin, D.; Troncy, E. A medicinal herb-based natural health product improves the condition of a canine natural osteoarthritis model: A randomized placebo-controlled trial. *Res. Vet. Sci.* **2014**, *97*, 574–581. [CrossRef]
60. Musco, N.; Vassalotti, G.; Mastellone, V.; Cortese, L.; Della Rocca, G.; Molinari, M.L.; Calabro, S.; Tudisco, R.; Cutrignelli, M.I.; Lombardi, P. Effects of a nutritional supplement in dogs affected by osteoarthritis. *Vet. Med. Sci.* **2019**, *5*, 325–335. [CrossRef]
61. Caterino, C.; Aragosa, F.; Della Valle, G.; Costanza, D.; Lamagna, F.; Piscitelli, A.; Nieddu, A.; Fatone, G. Clinical efficacy of Curcuvet and Boswellic acid combined with conventional nutraceutical product: An aid to canine osteoarthritis. *PLoS ONE* **2021**, *16*, e0252279. [CrossRef]
62. Gingerich, D.A.; Strobel, J.D. Use of client-specific outcome measures to assess treatment effects in geriatric, arthritic dogs: Controlled clinical evaluation of a nutraceutical. *Vet. Ther.* **2003**, *4*, 56–66.
63. Innes, J.F.; Fuller, C.J.; Grover, E.R.; Kelly, A.L.; Burn, J.F. Randomised, double-blind, placebo-controlled parallel group study of P54FP for the treatment of dogs with osteoarthritis. *Vet. Rec.* **2003**, *152*, 457–460. [CrossRef] [PubMed]
64. Moreau, M.; Dupuis, J.; Bonneau, N.H.; Lécuyer, M. Clinical evaluation of a powder of quality elk velvet antler for the treatment of osteoarthrosis in dogs. *Can. Vet. J.* **2004**, *45*, 133–139.
65. Reichling, J.; Schmokel, H.; Fitzi, J.; Bucher, S.; Saller, R. Dietary support with Boswellia resin in canine inflammatory joint and spinal disease. *Schweiz. Arch. Fur Tierheilkd.* **2004**, *146*, 71–79. [CrossRef]
66. Boileau, C.; Martel-Pelletier, J.; Caron, J.; Msika, P.; Guillou, G.B.; Baudouin, C.; Pelletier, J.P. Protective effects of total fraction of avocado/soybean unsaponifiables on the structural changes in experimental dog osteoarthritis: Inhibition of nitric oxide synthase and matrix metalloproteinase-13. *Arthritis Res. Ther.* **2009**, *11*, R41. [CrossRef]
67. Beynen, A.C.; Legerstee, E. Influence of dietary beta-1,3/1,6-glucans on clinical signs of canine osteoarthritis in a double-blind, placebo-controlled trial. *Am. J. Anim. Vet. Sci.* **2010**, *5*, 97–101. [CrossRef]
68. Boileau, C.; Martel-Pelletier, J.; Caron, J.; Paré, F.; Troncy, E.; Moreau, M.; Pelletier, J.P. Oral treatment with a Brachystemma calycinum D don plant extract reduces disease symptoms and the development of cartilage lesions in experimental dog osteoarthritis: Inhibition of protease-activated receptor 2. *Ann. Rheum. Dis.* **2010**, *69*, 1179–1184. [CrossRef]
69. Moreau, M.; Lussier, B.; Pelletier, J.P.; Martel-Pelletier, J.; Bédard, C.; Gauvin, D.; Troncy, E. Brachystemma calycinum D. Don Effectively Reduces the Locomotor Disability in Dogs with Naturally Occurring Osteoarthritis: A Randomized Placebo-Controlled Trial. *Evid.-Based Complement. Altern. Med.* **2012**, *2012*, 646191. [CrossRef]
70. Beynen, A.C.; Saris, D.H.J.; De Jong, L.; Staats, M.; Einerhand, A.W.C. Impact of dietary polydextrose on clinical signs of canine osteoarthritis. *Am. J. Anim. Vet. Sci.* **2011**, *6*, 93–99. [CrossRef]
71. Imhoff, D.J.; Gordon-Evans, W.J.; Evans, R.B.; Johnson, A.L.; Griffon, D.J.; Swanson, K.S. Evaluation of S-adenosyl l-methionine in a double-blinded, randomized, placebo-controlled, clinical trial for treatment of presumptive osteoarthritis in the dog. *Vet. Surg.* **2011**, *40*, 228–232. [CrossRef]
72. Fleck, A.; Gupta, R.C.; Goad, J.T.; Lasher, M.A.; Canerdy, T.D.; Kalidindi, S.R. Anti-Arthritic Efficacy And Safety Of Crominex®3+ (Trivalent Chromium, Phyllanthus emblica Extract, And Shilajit) In Moderately Arthritic Dogs. *J. Vet. Sci. Anim. Husb.* **2014**, *2*, 101. [CrossRef]
73. Lawley, S.; Gupta, R.C.; Goad, J.T.; Canerdy, T.D.; Kalidindi, S.R. Anti-Inflammatory and Anti-Arthritic Efficacy and Safety of Purified Shilajit in Moderately Arthritic Dogs. *J. Vet. Sci. Anim. Husb.* **2013**, *1*, 302. [CrossRef]
74. Rhouma, M.; de Oliveira El-Warrak, A.; Troncy, E.; Beaudry, F.; Chorfi, Y. Anti-inflammatory response of dietary vitamin E and its effects on pain and joint structures during early stages of surgically induced osteoarthritis in dogs. *Can. J. Vet. Res.* **2013**, *77*, 191–198.
75. Murdock, N.; Gupta, R.C.; Vega, N.; Kotora, K.; Miller, J.; Goad, T.J.; Lasher, A.M.; Canerdy, D.T.; Kalidindi, S.R. Evaluation of Terminalia chebula extract for anti-arthritic efficacy and safety in osteoarthritic dogs. *J. Vet. Sci. Technol.* **2016**, *7*, 1. [CrossRef]
76. Comblain, F.; Barthélémy, N.; Lefèbvre, M.; Schwartz, C.; Lesponne, I.; Serisier, S.; Feugier, A.; Balligand, M.; Henrotin, Y. A randomized, double-blind, prospective, placebo-controlled study of the efficacy of a diet supplemented with curcuminoids extract, hydrolyzed collagen and green tea extract in owner's dogs with osteoarthritis. *BMC Vet. Res.* **2017**, *13*, 395. [CrossRef] [PubMed]
77. Beths, T.; Munn, R.; Bauquier, S.H.; Mitchell, P.; Whittem, T. A pilot study of 4CYTETM Epiitalis Forte, a novel nutraceutical, in the management of naturally occurring osteoarthritis in dogs. *Aust. Vet. J.* **2020**, *98*, 591–595. [CrossRef] [PubMed]
78. Cohen, J. *Statistical Power Analysis for the Behavioral Sciences*, 2nd ed.; Routledge Academic: New York, NY, USA, 1988.
79. Steagall, P.V. Analgesia: What Makes Cats Different/Challenging and What Is Critical for Cats? *Vet. Clin. Small Anim. Pract.* **2020**, *50*, 749–767. [CrossRef]
80. Roberts, P.; Priest, H. Reliability and validity in research. *Nurs. Stand* **2006**, *20*, 41–45. [CrossRef]
81. Gagnon, A.; Brown, D.; Moreau, M.; Lussier, B.; Otis, C.; Troncy, E. Therapeutic response analysis in dogs with naturally occurring osteoarthritis. *Vet. Anaesth. Analg.* **2017**, *44*, 1373–1381. [CrossRef]
82. Mitchell, V.A.; Harley, J.; Casey, S.L.; Vaughan, A.C.; Winters, B.L.; Vaughan, C.W. Oral efficacy of Δ(9)-tetrahydrocannabinol and cannabidiol in a mouse neuropathic pain model. *Neuropharmacology* **2021**, *189*, 108529. [CrossRef]

83. Urits, I.; Gress, K.; Charipova, K.; Habib, K.; Lee, D.; Lee, C.; Jung, J.W.; Kassem, H.; Cornett, E.; Paladini, A.; et al. Use of cannabidiol (CBD) for the treatment of chronic pain. *Best Pract. Res. Clin. Anaesthesiol.* **2020**, *34*, 463–477. [CrossRef]
84. Wandel, S.; Jüni, P.; Tendal, B.; Nüesch, E.; Villiger, P.M.; Welton, N.J.; Reichenbach, S.; Trelle, S. Effects of glucosamine, chondroitin, or placebo in patients with osteoarthritis of hip or knee: Network meta-analysis. *BMJ* **2010**, *341*, c4675. [CrossRef] [PubMed]
85. Bhathal, A.; Spryszak, M.; Louizos, C.; Frankel, G. Glucosamine and chondroitin use in canines for osteoarthritis: A review. *Open Vet. J.* **2017**, *7*, 36–49. [CrossRef] [PubMed]
86. Wang, A.; Leong, D.J.; Cardoso, L.; Sun, H.B. Nutraceuticals and osteoarthritis pain. *Pharmacol. Ther.* **2018**, *187*, 167–179. [CrossRef] [PubMed]
87. Colletti, A.; Cicero, A.F.G. Nutraceutical Approach to Chronic Osteoarthritis: From Molecular Research to Clinical Evidence. *Int. J. Mol. Sci.* **2021**, *22*, 12920. [CrossRef] [PubMed]
88. Bernal del Nozal, J.; Mendiola, J.; Ibáñez, E.; Cifuentes, A. Advanced analysis of nutraceuticals. *J. Pharm. Biomed. Anal.* **2010**, *55*, 758–774. [CrossRef]
89. Grundmann, O.; Kumar, P.; Rogge, M.; Committee, A.P.P. Regulation of Dietary Supplements and Nutraceutical Products in the United States: An Argument for Greater Oversight and Uniform Standards. *J. Clin. Pharmacol.* **2022**, *62*, 14–16. [CrossRef]
90. Leong, D.J.; Choudhury, M.; Hirsh, D.M.; Hardin, J.A.; Cobelli, N.J.; Sun, H.B. Nutraceuticals: Potential for chondroprotection and molecular targeting of osteoarthritis. *Int. J. Mol. Sci.* **2013**, *14*, 23063–23085. [CrossRef]
91. Largo, R.; Alvarez-Soria, M.A.; Díez-Ortego, I.; Calvo, E.; Sánchez-Pernaute, O.; Egido, J.; Herrero-Beaumont, G. Glucosamine inhibits IL-1beta-induced NFkappaB activation in human osteoarthritic chondrocytes. *Osteoarthr. Cartil.* **2003**, *11*, 290–298. [CrossRef]
92. Chan, P.S.; Caron, J.P.; Orth, M.W. Short-term gene expression changes in cartilage explants stimulated with interleukin beta plus glucosamine and chondroitin sulfate. *J. Rheumatol.* **2006**, *33*, 1329–1340. [PubMed]
93. Wen, Z.H.; Tang, C.C.; Chang, Y.C.; Huang, S.Y.; Hsieh, S.P.; Lee, C.H.; Huang, G.S.; Ng, H.F.; Neoh, C.A.; Hsieh, C.S.; et al. Glucosamine sulfate reduces experimental osteoarthritis and nociception in rats: Association with changes of mitogen-activated protein kinase in chondrocytes. *Osteoarthr. Cartil.* **2010**, *18*, 1192–1202. [CrossRef]
94. Imagawa, K.; de Andrés, M.C.; Hashimoto, K.; Pitt, D.; Itoi, E.; Goldring, M.B.; Roach, H.I.; Oreffo, R.O. The epigenetic effect of glucosamine and a nuclear factor-kappa B (NF-kB) inhibitor on primary human chondrocytes–implications for osteoarthritis. *Biochem. Biophys. Res. Commun.* **2011**, *405*, 362–367. [CrossRef] [PubMed]
95. Waly, N.E.; Refaiy, A.; Aborehab, N.M. IL-10 and TGF-β: Roles in chondroprotective effects of Glucosamine in experimental Osteoarthritis? *Pathophysiology* **2017**, *24*, 45–49. [CrossRef] [PubMed]
96. Li, Y.; Chen, L.; Liu, Y.; Zhang, Y.; Liang, Y.; Mei, Y. Anti-inflammatory effects in a mouse osteoarthritis model of a mixture of glucosamine and chitooligosaccharides produced by bi-enzyme single-step hydrolysis. *Sci. Rep.* **2018**, *8*, 5624. [CrossRef]
97. Kuptniratsaikul, V.; Dajpratham, P.; Taechaarpornkul, W.; Buntragulpoontawee, M.; Lukkanapichonchut, P.; Chootip, C.; Saengsuwan, J.; Tantayakom, K.; Laongpech, S. Efficacy and safety of Curcuma domestica extracts compared with ibuprofen in patients with knee osteoarthritis: A multicenter study. *Clin. Interv. Aging* **2014**, *9*, 451–458. [CrossRef]
98. Lo, Y.Y.; Wong, J.M.; Cruz, T.F. Reactive oxygen species mediate cytokine activation of c-Jun NH2-terminal kinases. *J. Biol. Chem.* **1996**, *271*, 15703–15707. [CrossRef]
99. Chan, P.S.; Caron, J.P.; Orth, M.W. Effect of glucosamine and chondroitin sulfate on regulation of gene expression of proteolytic enzymes and their inhibitors in interleukin-1-challenged bovine articular cartilage explants. *Am. J. Vet. Res.* **2005**, *66*, 1870–1876. [CrossRef] [PubMed]
100. Neil, K.M.; Orth, M.W.; Coussens, P.M.; Chan, P.S.; Caron, J.P. Effects of glucosamine and chondroitin sulfate on mediators of osteoarthritis in cultured equine chondrocytes stimulated by use of recombinant equine interleukin-1beta. *Am. J. Vet. Res.* **2005**, *66*, 1861–1869. [CrossRef] [PubMed]
101. Oesser, S.; Seifert, J. Stimulation of type II collagen biosynthesis and secretion in bovine chondrocytes cultured with degraded collagen. *Cell Tissue Res* **2003**, *311*, 393–399. [CrossRef] [PubMed]
102. Isaka, S.; Someya, A.; Nakamura, S.; Naito, K.; Nozawa, M.; Inoue, N.; Sugihara, F.; Nagaoka, I.; Kaneko, K. Evaluation of the effect of oral administration of collagen peptides on an experimental rat osteoarthritis model. *Exp. Ther. Med.* **2017**, *13*, 2699–2706. [CrossRef]
103. Bourdon, B.; Contentin, R.; Cassé, F.; Maspimby, C.; Oddoux, S.; Noël, A.; Legendre, F.; Gruchy, N.; Galéra, P. Marine Collagen Hydrolysates Downregulate the Synthesis of Pro-Catabolic and Pro-Inflammatory Markers of Osteoarthritis and Favor Collagen Production and Metabolic Activity in Equine Articular Chondrocyte Organoids. *Int. J. Mol. Sci.* **2021**, *22*, 580. [CrossRef]
104. Tong, T.; Zhao, W.; Wu, Y.-Q.; Chang, Y.; Wang, Q.-T.; Zhang, L.-L.; Wei, W. Chicken type II collagen induced immune balance of main subtype of helper T cells in mesenteric lymph node lymphocytes in rats with collagen-induced arthritis. *Inflamm. Res.* **2010**, *59*, 369–377. [CrossRef] [PubMed]
105. Zhu, P.; Li, X.Y.; Wang, H.K.; Jia, J.F.; Zheng, Z.H.; Ding, J.; Fan, C.M. Oral administration of type-II collagen peptide 250-270 suppresses specific cellular and humoral immune response in collagen-induced arthritis. *Clin. Immunol.* **2007**, *122*, 75–84. [CrossRef] [PubMed]
106. Park, K.S.; Park, M.J.; Cho, M.L.; Kwok, S.K.; Ju, J.H.; Ko, H.J.; Park, S.H.; Kim, H.Y. Type II collagen oral tolerance; mechanism and role in collagen-induced arthritis and rheumatoid arthritis. *Mod. Rheumatol.* **2009**, *19*, 581–589. [CrossRef] [PubMed]

107. Jabbari, M.; Barati, M.; Khodaei, M.; Babashahi, M.; Kalhori, A.; Tahmassian, A.H.; Mosharkesh, E.; Arzhang, P.; Eini-Zinab, H. Is collagen supplementation friend or foe in rheumatoid arthritis and osteoarthritis? A comprehensive systematic review. *Int. J. Rheum. Dis.* **2022**, *25*, 973–981. [CrossRef]
108. Zainal, Z.; Longman, A.J.; Hurst, S.; Duggan, K.; Caterson, B.; Hughes, C.E.; Harwood, J.L. Relative efficacies of omega-3 polyunsaturated fatty acids in reducing expression of key proteins in a model system for studying osteoarthritis. *Osteoarthr. Cartil.* **2009**, *17*, 896–905. [CrossRef]
109. Zhang, L.-Y.; Jia, M.-R.; Sun, T. The roles of special proresolving mediators in pain relief. *Rev. Neurosci.* **2018**, *29*, 645–660. [CrossRef]
110. Fattori, V.; Pinho-Ribeiro, F.A.; Staurengo-Ferrari, L.; Borghi, S.M.; Rossaneis, A.C.; Casagrande, R.; Verri, W.A., Jr. The specialised pro-resolving lipid mediator maresin 1 reduces inflammatory pain with a long-lasting analgesic effect. *Br. J. Pharmacol.* **2019**, *176*, 1728–1744. [CrossRef]
111. Schmitz, G.; Ecker, J. The opposing effects of n-3 and n-6 fatty acids. *Prog. Lipid Res.* **2008**, *47*, 147–155. [CrossRef]
112. Sakata, S.; Hayashi, S.; Fujishiro, T.; Kawakita, K.; Kanzaki, N.; Hashimoto, S.; Iwasa, K.; Chinzei, N.; Kihara, S.; Haneda, M.; et al. Oxidative stress-induced apoptosis and matrix loss of chondrocytes is inhibited by eicosapentaenoic acid. *J. Orthop. Res.* **2015**, *33*, 359–365. [CrossRef]
113. Wang, Z.; Guo, A.; Ma, L.; Yu, H.; Zhang, L.; Meng, H.; Cui, Y.; Yu, F.; Yang, B. Docosahexenoic acid treatment ameliorates cartilage degeneration via a p38 MAPK-dependent mechanism. *Int. J. Mol. Med.* **2016**, *37*, 1542–1550. [CrossRef]
114. Matta, J.A.; Miyares, R.L.; Ahern, G.P. TRPV1 is a novel target for omega-3 polyunsaturated fatty acids. *J. Physiol.* **2007**, *578*, 397–411. [CrossRef]
115. Kelly, S.; Chapman, R.J.; Woodhams, S.; Sagar, D.R.; Turner, J.; Burston, J.J.; Bullock, C.; Paton, K.; Huang, J.; Wong, A.; et al. Increased function of pronociceptive TRPV1 at the level of the joint in a rat model of osteoarthritis pain. *Ann. Rheum. Dis.* **2015**, *74*, 252–259. [CrossRef]
116. Kalogerou, M.; Ioannou, S.; Kolovos, P.; Prokopiou, E.; Potamiti, L.; Kyriacou, K.; Panagiotidis, M.; Ioannou, M.; Fella, E.; Worth, E.P.; et al. Omega-3 fatty acids promote neuroprotection, decreased apoptosis and reduced glial cell activation in the retina of a mouse model of OPA1-related autosomal dominant optic atrophy. *Exp. Eye Res.* **2022**, *215*, 108901. [CrossRef]
117. Vučković, S.; Srebro, D.; Vujović, K.S.; Vučetić, Č.; Prostran, M. Cannabinoids and Pain: New Insights From Old Molecules. *Front. Pharmacol.* **2018**, *9*, 1259. [CrossRef]
118. Peng, J.; Fan, M.; An, C.; Ni, F.; Huang, W.; Luo, J. A narrative review of molecular mechanism and therapeutic effect of cannabidiol (CBD). *Basic Clin. Pharmacol. Toxicol.* **2022**, *130*, 439–456. [CrossRef]
119. Fahmi, H.; Martel-Pelletier, J.; Pelletier, J.P.; Kapoor, M. Peroxisome proliferator-activated receptor gamma in osteoarthritis. *Mod. Rheumatol.* **2011**, *21*, 1–9. [CrossRef]
120. Malan, T.P.; Ibrahim, M.M.; Lai, J.; Vanderah, T.W.; Makriyannis, A.; Porreca, F. CB2 cannabinoid receptor agonists: Pain relief without psychoactive effects? *Curr. Opin. Pharmacol.* **2003**, *3*, 62–67. [CrossRef]
121. Manzanares, J.; Julian, M.; Carrascosa, A. Role of the cannabinoid system in pain control and therapeutic implications for the management of acute and chronic pain episodes. *Curr. Neuropharmacol.* **2006**, *4*, 239–257. [CrossRef]
122. Starowicz, K.; Malek, N.; Przewlocka, B. Cannabinoid receptors and pain. *Wiley Interdiscip. Rev. Membr. Transp. Signal.* **2013**, *2*, 121–132. [CrossRef]
123. D'Adamo, S.; Cetrullo, S.; Panichi, V.; Mariani, E.; Flamigni, F.; Borzì, R.M. Nutraceutical Activity in Osteoarthritis Biology: A Focus on the Nutrigenomic Role. *Cells* **2020**, *9*, 1232. [CrossRef]
124. Dwyer, J.T.; Coates, P.M.; Smith, M.J. Dietary Supplements: Regulatory Challenges and Research Resources. *Nutrients* **2018**, *10*, 41. [CrossRef]
125. Klinck, M.P.; Mogil, J.S.; Moreau, M.; Lascelles, B.D.X.; Flecknell, P.A.; Poitte, T.; Troncy, E. Translational pain assessment: Could natural animal models be the missing link? *Pain* **2017**, *158*, 1633–1646. [CrossRef]
126. Adebowale, A.; Du, J.; Liang, Z.; Leslie, J.L.; Eddington, N.D. The bioavailability and pharmacokinetics of glucosamine hydrochloride and low molecular weight chondroitin sulfate after single and multiple doses to beagle dogs. *Biopharm. Drug Dispos.* **2002**, *23*, 217–225. [CrossRef]
127. Wang, L.; Wang, Q.; Qian, J.; Liang, Q.; Wang, Z.; Xu, J.; He, S.; Ma, H. Bioavailability and Bioavailable Forms of Collagen after Oral Administration to Rats. *J. Agric. Food Chem.* **2015**, *63*, 3752–3756. [CrossRef]
128. Paul-Murphy, J.; Ludders, J.W.; Robertson, S.A.; Gaynor, J.S.; Hellyer, P.W.; Wong, P.L. The need for a cross-species approach to the study of pain in animals. *J. Am. Vet. Med. Assoc.* **2004**, *224*, 692–697. [CrossRef]
129. Epstein, M.E.; Rodanm, I.; Griffenhagen, G.; Kadrlik, J.; Petty, M.C.; Robertson, S.A.; Simpson, W. 2015 AAHA/AAFP pain management guidelines for dogs and cats. *J. Feline Med. Surg.* **2015**, *17*, 251–272. [CrossRef]
130. Rialland, P.; Bichot, S.; Moreau, M.; Guillot, M.; Lussier, B.; Gauvin, D.; Martel-Pelletier, J.; Pelletier, J.P.; Troncy, E. Clinical validity of outcome pain measures in naturally occurring canine osteoarthritis. *BMC Vet. Res.* **2012**, *8*, 162. [CrossRef]
131. Caldwell, J.; Gardner, I.; Swales, N. An introduction to drug disposition: The basic principles of absorption, distribution, metabolism, and excretion. *Toxicol. Pathol.* **1995**, *23*, 102–114. [CrossRef]

132. Johnston, S.A. Osteoarthritis. Joint anatomy, physiology, and pathobiology. *Vet. Clin. N. Am. Small Anim. Pract.* **1997**, *27*, 699–723. [CrossRef]
133. Martinez, N.; McDonald, B. A study into the fatty acid content of selected veterinary diets, supplements and fish oil capsules in Australia. *Vet. Dermatol.* **2021**, *32*, 256-e69. [CrossRef]
134. Moreau, M.; Troncy, E. Review of Fortified Foods and Natural Medicinal Products in Companion Animals Afflicted by Naturally Occurring Osteoarthritis. In *Nutritional Modulators of Pain in the Aging Population*, 1st ed.; Watson, R., Zibadi, S., Eds.; Academic press: London, UK, 2017; pp. 281–291. [CrossRef]
135. Williams, P.; Pettitt, R. Nutraceutical use in osteoarthritic canines: A review. *Companion Anim.* **2021**, *26*, 1–5. [CrossRef]

International Journal of
Molecular Sciences

MDPI

Review

Mechanisms of Action and Efficacy of Hyaluronic Acid, Corticosteroids and Platelet-Rich Plasma in the Treatment of Temporomandibular Joint Osteoarthritis—A Systematic Review

Marcin Derwich [1,*], Maria Mitus-Kenig [2] and Elzbieta Pawlowska [3]

1 ORTODENT, Specialist Orthodontic Private Practice in Grudziadz, 86-300 Grudziadz, Poland
2 Department of Experimental Dentistry and Prophylaxis, Medical College, Jagiellonian University in Krakow, 31-008 Krakow, Poland; maria.mitus@interia.pl
3 Department of Orthodontics, Medical University of Lodz, 90-419 Lodz, Poland; elzbieta.pawlowska@umed.lodz.pl
* Correspondence: derwichm@tlen.pl; Tel.: +48-660-723-164

Abstract: Temporomandibular joint osteoarthritis (TMJ OA) is a low-inflammatory disorder with multifactorial etiology. The aim of this review was to present the current state of knowledge regarding the mechanisms of action and the efficacy of hyaluronic acid (HA), corticosteroids (CS) and platelet-rich plasma (PRP) in the treatment of TMJ OA.: The PubMed database was analyzed with the keywords: "(temporomandibular joint) AND ((osteoarthritis) OR (dysfunction) OR (disorders) OR (pain)) AND ((treatment) OR (arthrocentesis) OR (arthroscopy) OR (injection)) AND ((hyaluronic acid) OR (corticosteroid) OR (platelet rich plasma))". After screening of 363 results, 16 studies were included in this review. Arthrocentesis alone effectively reduces pain and improves jaw function in patients diagnosed with TMJ OA. Additional injections of HA, either low-molecular-weight (LMW) HA or high-molecular-weight (HMW) HA, or CS at the end of the arthrocentesis do not improve the final clinical outcomes. CS present several negative effects on the articular cartilage. Results related to additional PRP injections are not consistent and are rather questionable. Further studies should be multicenter, based on a larger group of patients and should answer the question of whether other methods of TMJ OA treatment are more beneficial for the patients than simple arthrocentesis.

Keywords: temporomandibular joint osteoarthritis; hyaluronic acid; corticosteroids; platelet-rich plasma; temporomandibular joint disorders; arthrocentesis; intraarticular injections

Citation: Derwich, M.; Mitus-Kenig, M.; Pawlowska, E. Mechanisms of Action and Efficacy of Hyaluronic Acid, Corticosteroids and Platelet-Rich Plasma in the Treatment of Temporomandibular Joint Osteoarthritis—A Systematic Review. *Int. J. Mol. Sci.* **2021**, *22*, 7405. https://doi.org/10.3390/ijms22147405

Academic Editor: Chih-Hsin Tang

Received: 28 June 2021
Accepted: 8 July 2021
Published: 9 July 2021

1. Introduction

According to the Diagnostic Criteria for Temporomandibular Disorders (DC/TMD), there have been listed twelve different types of temporomandibular disorders (TMD), including: myalgia, local myalgia, myofascial pain, myofascial pain with referral, arthralgia, headache attributed to TMD, disc displacement with reduction, disc displacement with reduction with intermittent locking, disc displacement without reduction with limited opening, disc displacement without reduction without limited opening, degenerative joint disease and subluxation [1].

TMJ arthritic conditions have been subdivided into two groups, namely low-inflammatory and high-inflammatory disorders [2]. Osteoarthritis (OA) and post-traumatic arthritis have been classified as low-inflammatory disorders, whereas rheumatoid arthritis, metabolic arthritic diseases (i.e., gout, pseudogout, lupus erythematosus) and infectious arthritis have been classified as high-inflammatory disorders [2]. The general characteristics for low-inflammatory disorders encompass: the involvement of one or both TMJs, the presence of localized pain and the presence of TMJ crepitation. TMJ clicking and the presence of the rheumatological factor are rare, the erythrocyte sedimentation rate (ESR) is often normal, and the cyclic citrullinated peptide antibody (CPP) is normal; however, the concentration of the C-reactive protein (CRP) may be elevated [2]. Contrary to the low-inflammatory disorders, the high-inflammatory disorders are characterized by bilateral involvement of TMJs, diffused pain, lack of clicking, rare occurrence of crepitation, presence of rheumatoid factor, elevated ESR, CPP and CRP [2].

Temporomandibular joint osteoarthritis (TMJ OA) is considered to be a combination of degenerative joint disease and joint pain [1]. It is a disease involving an entire joint [3,4]. The etiology of TMJ OA is multifactorial [5,6]. We have described it thoroughly in our previous manuscripts [7,8]. Because of the fact that the TMJ OA etiological factors are very complex, the treatment of TMJ OA requires a multidisciplinary approach [7–9]. There have been listed three major aims for the treatment of the TMJ OA, namely TMJ pain reduction, reestablishment of the normal mandibular movements, as well as the improvement of the patients' quality of life [10]. Although there are several different methods of treatment of TMJ OA, none of them is unequivocally the most effective one [10]. The most popular are noninvasive, conservative methods of treatment, including physiotherapy, occlusal splint therapy and pharmacotherapy. Less invasive surgical procedures used in the treatment of the TMJ OA encompass intraarticular injections of HA, CS or growth factors, arthrocentesis alone and finally the combination of arthrocentesis and intraarticular injections. Finally, the invasive surgical procedures comprise arthroscopy and open joint surgeries, including, among others, discectomy, high condylectomy and arthroplasty [7–10].

The aim of this review was to present the current state of knowledge regarding the efficacy of HA, CS and PRP in the treatment of TMJ OA on the basis of the literature.

2. Materials and Methods

2.1. Clinical Question

What is the efficacy of hyaluronic acid (HA), corticosteroids (CS) and platelet-rich plasma (PRP) in the treatment of TMJ OA in humans on the basis of the literature?

2.2. Inclusion and Exclusion Criteria

Table 1 presents inclusion and exclusion criteria for the systematic review.

Table 1. Inclusion and exclusion criteria for the systematic review.

Criteria	List of Specific Criteria
Inclusion criteria	- randomized controlled trials - randomized clinical trials - study population: adolescents (aged: 16 years old or more) and adults diagnosed with TMJ OA - methods of treatment: arthrocentesis or arthroscopy with an additional injection of HA, CS and PRP or intraarticular injections of HA, CS and PRP - papers written in English
Exclusion criteria	- case–control studies - case reports - comments - systematic reviews and metanalyses - usage of animal models - study population: children under 16 years old and patients diagnosed with other types of TMD without concomitant TMJ OA - methods of treatment: conservative methods of treatment (including physiotherapy, occlusal splint therapy and pharmacotherapy) and invasive surgical procedures (open joint surgery) - papers written in languages other than English

TMJ OA—temporomandibular joint osteoarthritis, HA—hyaluronic acid, CS—corticosteroids, PRP—platelet-rich plasma, TMD—temporomandibular joint disorder.

2.3. The PICO Approach

We used the PICO approach to properly develop literature search strategies for this review:

Population:

Adolescents (aged: 16 years old or more) and adult patients who were diagnosed with TMJ OA.

Intervention:

Temporomandibular joint arthrocentesis or arthroscopy with an additional injection of HA, CS and PRP or intraarticular injections of HA, CS and PRP in patients diagnosed with TMJ OA.

Comparison:

Intraarticular injection of HA, CS or PRP, arthrocentesis or arthroscopy with an additional injection of HA, CS or PRP, arthrocentesis or arthroscopy alone, placebo; randomized controlled trials (RCTs) and randomized clinical trials were included in the review.

Outcome:

Decreased pain in the temporomandibular joint area and increased maximum mouth opening.

2.4. Search Strategy

The PubMed database was analyzed with the following keywords: (temporomandibular joint) AND ((osteoarthritis) OR (dysfunction) OR (disorders) OR (pain)) AND ((treatment) OR (arthrocentesis) OR (arthroscopy) OR (injection)) AND ((hyaluronic acid) OR (corticosteroid) OR (platelet rich plasma)). After screening of 363 results, 16 studies were included in this review. We included RCTs and randomized clinical trials in this review.

Figure 1 presents the PRISMA flow diagram for a review of the literature.

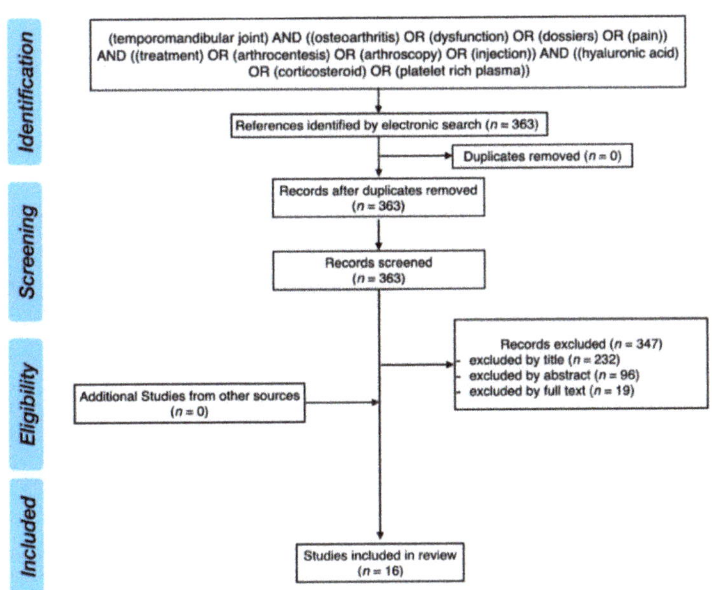

Figure 1. PRISMA flow diagram for review of the literature.

2.5. Cohen's Kappa Coefficient

Cohen's kappa coefficient between the reviewers was of 1.00.

3. Results and Discussion

3.1. Hyaluronic Acid (HA)

HA is a nonsulfated glycosaminoglycan, a polysaccharide, made up of repeated units of D-glucuronic acid and N-acetylglucosamine with alternating beta (1–3) glucuronide and beta (1–4) glucosaminidic bonds. HA physiologically occurs within the articular cartilage and the synovial fluid [11–16]. It is synthesized by fibroblast-like cells, known as the synoviocytes type B [14,17]. There exist three isoforms of hyaluronan synthases in humans, namely HAS1, HAS2 and HAS3 [18,19]. They are integral membrane proteins [19]. HAS1 and HAS2 are responsible for the polymerization of HA chains up to 2000 kDa, whereas HAS3 polymerizes shorter HA chains of the length of 200–300 kDa [20].

HA forms a layer which not only covers but also penetrates the articular surfaces. It is combined with different proteins, coming from the synovial fluid [14]. There are two conformations in which HA occurs: the linear and the spheroidal ones [14]. It has been proven that HA plays a significant role in the nutrition and lubrication of the TMJ articular surfaces [13,14,16]. This role is directly related to the value of the intraarticular pressure, which makes the HA change its conformation. When the intraarticular pressure reaches subatmospheric values, the proteins lose contact with the articular surfaces and the HA assumes a spheroidal conformation, allowing sliding movements within the TMJ. When the intraarticular pressure exceeds atmospheric values, the HA occurs in the linear form and penetrates the fibrocartilage, which is necessary for TMJ nutrition [14]. Moreover, HA is found to stabilize all of the TMJ components [14]. Figure 2 presents the schematic relationship between the TMJ intraarticular pressure and HA conformations on the basis of the literature [14].

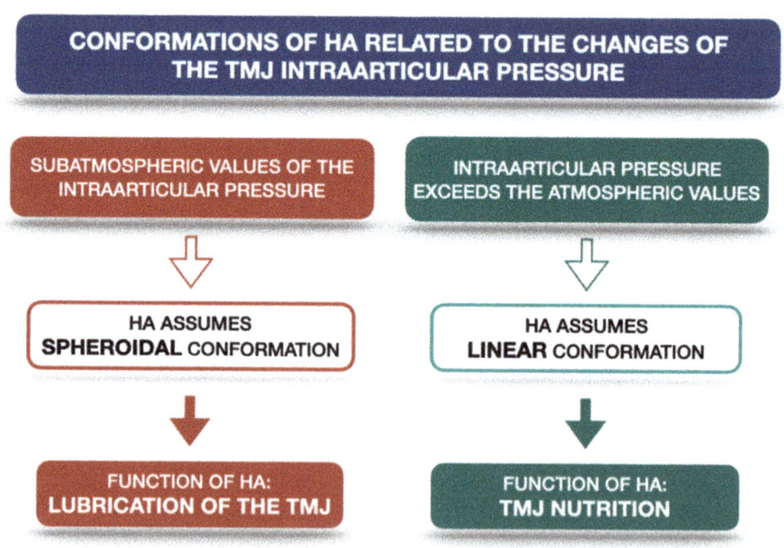

Figure 2. Schematic relationship between the TMJ intraarticular pressure and HA conformations on the basis of the literature [14]. HA—hyaluronic acid, TMJ—temporomandibular joint.

Although the HA lubricates the TMJ articular surfaces, it must be emphasized that HA by itself does not reduce the intraarticular friction satisfactorily (coefficient of friction ca. $\mu \approx 0.3$) [11,21–23]. There are three molecules, HA, lubricin (proteoglycan) and phosphatidylcholine lipids (phospholipids), that form a boundary lubrication layer, which leads to a significant reduction in friction within the joint (coefficient of friction down to $\mu \approx 0.001$ at pressures over 100 atm) [21]. It has been found that lubricin, localized in the superficial zone, anchors the HA chains at the outer surface of the articular cartilage. Therefore, HA becomes attached to the surface and consequently complexes with phosphatidylcholines. Highly hydrated phosphocholine groups become exposed between the opposite cartilage surfaces. This connection forms a boundary lubrication layer [21]. It is also possible for the HA from the synovial fluid to attach simultaneously to the lipids localized on the opposite cartilage surfaces. Surprisingly, these polymer bridges do not increase the friction between the articular surfaces [11]. Lin et al. [11] presented two possible mechanisms which could have explained the observed data. First of all, there are lipid multilayers on each articular surface. The HA polymer bridges are localized on the midplane. Therefore, to eliminate the increased friction, the slip plane is moved from the midplane (which is full of HA bridges) to the interface within one of the lipid multilayers (free of HA). Secondly, lipids from the synovial fluid do interact with the free HA. As a consequence, the number of HA polymer bridges between the articular surfaces becomes reduced [11].

The HA molecular weight influences the viscoelastic properties of the synovial fluid. High-molecular-weight HA (HMW HA), which is more than 1000 kDa, contributes to the viscoelasticity of the synovial fluid [20]. Iturriaga et al. [24] distinguished three different categories of the exogenous HA preparations regarding their molecular weight, namely low-molecular-weight HA (LMW HA) 500–1000 kDa, medium-molecular-weight (MMW HA) 1200–4500 kDa and HMW HA 6000–7000 kDa. HMW HA presents an anti-inflammatory effect [25]. According to the study by Herzog et al. [26], HMW HA controls the hydrodynamics (viscosity, compressive stiffness and elasticity) of the synovial fluid via an entropy-driven excluded volume effect.

Hyaluronidases are the enzymes which are responsible for the degradation of HMW HA into LMW HA [20]. LMW HA presents proinflammatory properties, which are manifested by the induction of macrophage genes' expression [27]. There have been found six different hyaluronidase-like genes within the human genome [28]. However, there are only two major hyaluronidases (HYAL1 and HYAL2) in human somatic tissues [18,28]. The process of HA degradation is associated with aging, inflammation and is also observed in the course of osteoarthritis. It has also been described that the reactive oxidative radical species may inhibit the HA biosynthesis, as well as lead to the depolymerization of the already biosynthesized HA chains [6,29]. The reactive oxidative radical species are released within the TMJ due to the repetitive cycles of temporary hypoxia and re-oxygenation [6]. TMJ mechanical overloading affects the HA metabolism, leading to condylar cartilage degradation [18]. The increased amount of LMW HA is the direct cause of decreased synovial fluid viscosity. As a consequence, the friction between the articular surfaces increases and the articular surfaces become progressively damaged [20]. Takahashi et al. [30] found that a group of patients diagnosed with TMD (internal derangements and OA) presented HA of a significantly lower molecular weight in synovial fluid compared to healthy controls. Guo et al. [31] performed a study in a group of growing rats and confirmed that TMJ mechanical overloading affects the HA metabolism. They found that the functional lateral shift of the mandible stimulated the expression of HYAL1 and HYAL2 in both TMJs. Therefore, the functional lateral shift of the mandible changed the lubrication of the TMJs [31].

According to the recent research, there has been confirmed a relationship between chronic hypoxia, increased HYAL-1 plasma concentration and increased HMW HA degradation. These changes may enhance systemic inflammation in the course of obstructive sleep apnea [32].

Because of the increased amount of LMW HA within osteoarthritic TMJs, some have suggested the use of HMW HA in the treatment of TMJ OA. Tolba et al. [33] observed that intraarticular injections of HMW HA led to a satisfactory reduction in osteoarthritic changes within the TMJs. Similar observations were presented by Duygu et al. [34]. Lemos et al. [35] concluded that HMW HA may have a positive impact on osteoarthritic TMJs, because in individuals treated with HMW HA, the authors observed, among others, limited histologic changes, lower activity of metalloproteinases (MMP-2 and MMP-9), as well as a greater arrangement of collagenous fibers. Contrary to the previously mentioned studies, Iturriaga et al. [24] compared the efficacy of LMW HA and HMW HA intraarticular injections in the treatment of TMJ OA. The authors noticed that better results regarding the repairing processes of the cartilage and the articular disc were obtained with the usage of the LMW HA. Although the results presented by the above-listed authors [24,33–35] seem very promising, it must be emphasized that all of these studies were performed on different animal models, namely rats [33,35] and rabbits [24,34].

3.2. Corticosteroids (CS)

CS are hormones naturally occurring within the human body, which are biosynthesized by the adrenal cortex [36–38]. CS encompass both the glucocorticoids (i.e., cortisol) and mineralocorticoids (i.e., aldosterone) [36]. Glucocorticoids present principally anti-inflammatory and immunosuppressive effects, whereas mineralocorticoids regulate the ionic balance by stimulation of sodium reabsorption and potassium excretion [36,37].

There are several different methods to administer CS, including oral administration, aerosol for inhalation, topical administration, intravenous, intramuscular and finally intraarticular injections [36]. CS intraarticular injections have been used to treat different arthritic diseases (i.e., rheumatoid arthritis, osteoarthritis, gout) since 1951 [39].

There have been described different molecular models of glucocorticoid action [40–45]. The most common one, known as a genomic pathway, is associated with the activity of the glucocorticoid receptor (GR). The GR is localized within the cytoplasm and is part of the multiprotein complex. It is coupled with chaperone proteins and immunophilins. Glucocorticoids become bound to GRs and translocated to the nucleus. Within the nucleus, the GR directly affects (either activates or suppresses) the transcription of different genes by binding glucocorticoid response elements (GREs), by tethering itself to other transcription factors and affecting its activity, or in a composite manner (GR binds to half the GRE, which is near the binding site of another transcription factor) [40–44]. It is also possible for the GR to interact with different transcription factors, preventing their binding to DNA (transcription factor sequestration); to compete with other transcription factors for binding to DNA (competitive binding); and to compete with other transcription factors for cofactors necessary for transcription (co-factor competition) [43,44]. Figure 3 presents a schematic of the genomic action of the glucocorticoid receptor on the basis of the literature [40,41].

The second group of molecular mechanisms of glucocorticoid actions is known as the non-genomic pathway. Non-genomic action does not regulate gene expression; neither does it involve transcriptional processes or protein biosynthesis. Non-genomic action activates signal transduction pathways. It is based on the interactions between the glucocorticoids and the cell membrane (nonspecific interactions), as well as between the glucocorticoids and either cytosolic GRs or membrane-bound GRs [45]. There are four different mechanisms, described as non-genomic pathways, namely non-specific physicochemical interactions with membranes, chaperone protein signaling, mechanism via cell membrane receptors and finally a mechanism based on the competition for phosphoinositide 3-kinase. These mechanisms are not related to the direct combination of the glucocorticoid–GR complex with DNA [46].

Glucocorticoids stimulate the expression of annexin-1 (also known as lipcortin-1), which is the phospholipase A_2 inhibitor. As a consequence, the biosynthesis of lipid mediators becomes inhibited, including the biosynthesis of prostaglandins, prostacyclin and leukotriene. Annexin-1 was also found to regulate, among others, cell proliferation and maturation, as well as neuroendocrine secretion [41,42]. Glucocorticoids also inhibit the transcription of many proinflammatory cytokines, including IL-1β, IL-6 and TNF-α. Therefore, glucocorticoids significantly suppress the inflammatory response [41,42].

There are several different formulations of CS to be injected intraarticularly, which have been accepted by the Food and Drug Administration (FDA) [38]. They can be allocated into one of the two subgroups, depending on the water solubility. Ester (acetate/acetonide) preparations are insoluble in water. They form microcrystalline particulates. Moreover, they present slower release and last longer at the site of injection [37,38]. Exemplary non-soluble CS are: methylprednisolone acetate, betamethasone acetate, hydrocortisone acetate and triamcinolone acetonide [37,38]. Contrary to the previously described group, non-ester preparation (sodium phosphate) formulations are nonparticulate and soluble in water. They begin working rapidly and, at the same time, the duration of their action is shorter. They do not form aggregates within the joint. Exemplary soluble CS are dexamethasone sodium phosphate and betamethasone sodium phosphate [37,38].

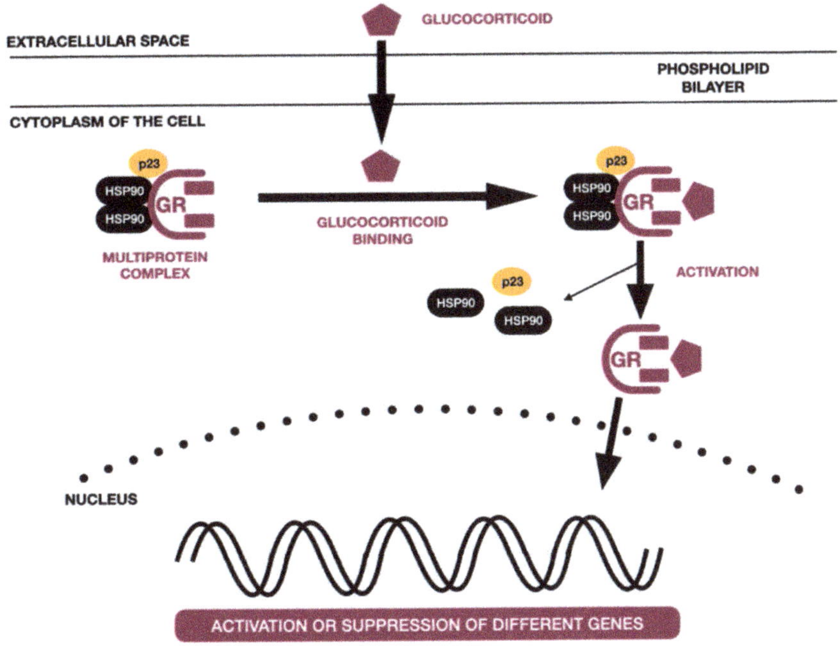

Figure 3. Schematic genomic action of glucocorticoid receptor on the basis of the literature [40,41]. GR—glucocorticoid receptor, hsp90 and p23—chaperone proteins.

Table 2 presents examples of CS injected intraarticularly on the basis of the literature [37,38].

Table 2. Examples of CS injected intraarticularly on the basis of the literature [37,38].

Ester Preparations (Insoluble in Water)	Non-Ester Preparations (Soluble in Water)
Methylprednisolone acetate Betamethasone acetate Triamcinolone acetonide Hydrocortisone acetate	Dexamethasone sodium phosphate Betamethasone sodium phosphate

Intraarticular CS injections may cause several different types of local and systemic side effects. There have been listed the following local side effects: post-injection flare (the most common side effect), pain in the area of injection, subcutaneous trophy, skin depigmentation and soft tissue calcifications. Among the systemic adverse effects of intraarticular CS injection, there have been mentioned: facial flushing (related to the histamine-mediated response), hyperglycemic effects in patients suffering from diabetes (CS leads to insulin resistance), adrenal suppression and menstrual disturbances [36–38]. Moreover, the long-term use of CS leads to osteoporosis, due to the presence of bone catabolism and limited bone formation, associated with osteoblasts hypofunction and apoptosis [36,47].

Monseau et al. [48] presented a list of absolute and relative contraindications to musculoskeletal injections (including both the CS and HA injections) on the basis of the literature. The absolute contraindications to intraarticular injections are: hypersensitivity to CS or any other type of injectable substance, systemic infection or infection in the area of the planned injection (cellulitis, septic arthritis, septic bursitis, osteomyelitis), uncontrolled bleeding disorder, prosthetic or unstable joint and finally intraarticular fracture [48]. The relative contraindications to intraarticular injections are: treated bleeding disorder, hemarthrosis, anticoagulants, immunosuppression, diabetes, increased risk of tendon rupture and pain of psychogenic origin [48].

CS are known to cause several effects on articular cartilage. They alter cartilage matrix metabolism [49], change the mechanical properties of articular cartilage [50] and lead to chondrotoxicity [51]. CS intraarticular injections should not be repeated more than four times per year due to the increased risk of articular cartilage destruction. CS injections simultaneously reduce the pain within the joint and remove effusions around the joint. Although the joint pain reduction appears quickly, it does not last long [36].

3.3. Platelet-Rich Plasma (PRP)

PRP is an autologous concentrate of platelets and growth factors, derived from centrifugated blood [52–54]. There have been listed in the literature two other types of platelet concentrates, namely platelet-rich fibrin (PRF) and plasma rich in growth factors (PRGF) [55]. PRP may be obtained only from the liquid blood. It is impossible to obtain PRP from serum or clotted blood [56].

There are several different commercial protocols to collect blood and to obtain PRP. The differences among them include: the required amount of blood to be taken from the patients, the isolation method, the speed of centrifugation, the amount of obtained concentrated volume after centrifugation, processing time, increase in platelets and platelet capture efficiency [57]. Moreover, it has also been found that different methods of blood centrifugation affect the leukocyte ratios [58].

The number of platelets in 1 μL of blood in healthy individuals ranges from 150,000 to 300,000 [59]. Platelets are responsible for hemostasis and wound healing [52,59]. There are three types of organelles within the platelets: α-granules, dense granules and lysosomes [59]. Alpha granules are the most common ones (approximately 80 granules per cell) [60]. They contain several different types of proteins, including growth factors (i.e., transforming growth factor β, insulin-like growth factor, epidermal growth factor), chemokines, coagulants, anticoagulants, fibrinolytic proteins, adhesion proteins, integral membrane proteins, immune mediators, angiogenic factors and inhibitors and microbicidal proteins [56,59].

The exact mechanism of PRP action remains unclear and is even sometimes questioned [61,62]. It is speculated that PRP enhances wound healing because of the presence of various cytokines, including growth factors. PRP also presents hemostatic properties. Moreover, it may indirectly activate macrophages via serotonin and histamine release, which increase the capillary permeability, consequently leading to the inflammatory cells' access [56,61,62]. Finally, PRP in in vitro studies has been found to stimulate the chondrocytes to engineer the cartilage and the biosynthesis of collagen and proteoglycans [63].

PRP has been used in various medical specialties, including oral and maxillofacial surgery, dermatology, ophthalmology, cardiothoracic surgery and plastic surgery, but also in the treatment of musculoskeletal disorders, including TMJ OA [61,64,65].

3.4. HA, CS and PRP in the Treatment of TMJ OA

HA, CS and PRP may be injected intraarticularly independently as sole, less invasive, surgical procedures or may be injected at the end of other surgical procedures, including arthrocentesis or arthroscopy [66–81].

Arthrocentesis is a minimally invasive surgical procedure, which aims to eliminate the inflammatory mediators from the inside of the TMJ and to disrupt any adhesions within the TMJ. Either physiological solution or Ringer's solution is used for the arthrocentesis. Arthrocentesis is performed most often under local anesthesia [8,66].

Arthroscopy, compared to arthrocentesis, is a more invasive surgical procedure, which is predominantly performed under general anesthesia. Arthroscopy requires at least two different ports. This technique is used not only for the intraarticular operations, but also for the real-time visualization of the TMJ [8,80]. Fernández Sanromán et al. [80] used arthroscopy to record, among others, hypervascularization of retrodiscal tissues, articular disc perforations, synovitis, intraarticular areas of hyperemia, presence of intraarticular adhesions and finally areas of bone exposure.

Although there have been published many studies related to the intraarticular supplementation of HA, CS or PRP, only a few of them are randomized clinical trials (RCTs) that have been performed among patients diagnosed with TMJ OA.

Bergstrand et al. [66] compared the effectiveness of arthrocentesis alone with arthrocentesis combined with an additional injection of HA in the treatment of TMJ OA. The authors presented the most long-term observations (almost 4 years) compared to other RCTs. Bergstrand et al. assessed pain symptoms and jaw function on the basis of the maximum incisor opening, both-side lateral function and mandibular protrusive movement. The authors also analyzed the presence of joint sounds. Both methods led to a significant improvement in jaw function and significant reduction in pain intensity. None of the methods significantly improved joint sound. Both methods were equally effective in the treatment of TMJ OA. Therefore, supplementary injection of HA at the end of arthrocentesis did not improve the final outcome.

Guarda-Nardini et al. [67] compared the efficacy of cycle of 5 single-needle arthrocenteses combined with HA of different molecular weights. The authors injected intraarticularly either LMW HA (Hyalgan) or MMW HA (Sinovial). There were no significant differences between the examined groups, regarding pain at chewing, pain at rest, chewing efficiency, mouth opening and functional limitation. These results indicate that the molecular weight of HA does not affect the efficacy of the TMJ OA treatment.

Contrary to the previously presented studies, Tang et al. [68] did not combine intraarticular injections of HA with arthrocentesis. They compared the results obtained after five intraarticular injections of either HA or physiologic saline solution. The authors found that only patients treated with HA injections presented significant pain reduction in the area of the TMJs. This study indicates that HA may be effective in pain reduction in the treatment of TMJ OA, when arthrocentesis has not been performed and therefore inflammatory mediators have not been flushed out of the joint.

Bouloux et al. [69,70] compared three groups of patients with TMJ OA treated with arthrocentesis combined with the supplementary injection of HA, CS or Ringer's solution. The authors assessed efficiency in pain reduction, changes in quality of life, jaw function and maximum incisal opening. Despite the fact that the group which was supplemented with CS presented the lowest improvement in pain reduction, the obtained results were still statistically significant. Furthermore, there were no significant changes between the examined groups regarding jaw function, as well as maximum incisal opening with and without pain. The authors concluded that all three methods of treatment are equally effective in pain reduction, improving jaw function and maximum incisal opening in patients diagnosed with TMJ OA and that additional CS or HA injection does not provide any benefits. Moreover, none of the presented methods led to a significant improvement in patients' quality of life.

Huddleston Slater et al. [71] assessed the differences in clinical results between arthrocentesis with an additional single-dose injection of isotonic saline 1 cc and arthrocentesis with an additional single-dose injection of CS 1cc. There were no significant differences between the examined groups regarding pain complaints, maximal interincisal opening, as well as functional impairment.

Manfredini et al. [72] compared six different protocols of arthrocentesis with or without supplementary drugs, namely single-session two-needle arthrocentesis, single-session two-needle arthrocentesis plus CS, single-session two-needle arthrocentesis plus LMW HA, single-session two-needle arthrocentesis plus HMW HA, five-weekly two-needle arthrocenteses plus LMW HA and five-weekly single-needle arthrocenteses plus LMW HA. The group of patients treated with single-session two-needle arthrocentesis plus HMW HA was withdrawn from the study because of the severe side effects occurring in two patients. The authors did not find any significant differences among the examined groups regarding changes in the pain at rest, pain at chewing, chewing efficiency and mouth opening.

Bjørnland et al. [73] and Møystad et al. [74] compared the efficacy of two intraarticular injections of either HA or CS in patients diagnosed with TMJ OA. The injections were performed 14 days apart. Bjørnland et al. [73] noticed that only patients treated with HA presented: significantly less pain intensity after 6-month observation and significantly fewer joints with crepitation after first injection. However, there were no significant differences in the improvement of the jaw function, as well as in the presence of the TMJ sounds between the examined groups. Results by Bjørnland et al. [73] support the observations described by Tang et al. [68] regarding the changes in pain intensity after the intraarticular HA injection without simultaneous arthrocentesis. Contrary to Bjørnland, Møystad et al. [74] assessed the presence of the radiographic signs of OA and the progression or regression of osseous changes in the TMJs. The authors did not find any significant radiographic changes between the examined groups.

Isacsson et al. [75] determined the efficacy of a single-dose intraarticular injection of methylprednisolone (CS) and the efficacy of a single-dose intraarticular injection of sodium chloride. There were no statistically significant differences between the examined groups regarding the pain reduction and the function of the mandible. Both groups presented significant pain release and significant improvement in jaw function. However, patients treated with CS developed adverse events related to the treatment more often compared to the patients treated with sodium chloride. Moreover, the injection of methylprednisolone caused increased pain during the first few days after the intervention.

Cömert Kiliç et al. [76] assessed the differences between the clinical outcomes of arthrocentesis performed alone and arthrocentesis with an additional injection of CS. Both methods of treatment led to a statistically significant pain reduction and significant reduction in joint sounds. Only patients who received an additional CS injection presented a statistically significant increase in painless interincisal opening. Comparison of both groups regarding masticatory efficiency, pain complaints, joint sound, painless mouth opening, maximum mouth opening, lateral motion and protrusive motion revealed no statistically significant differences. An additional CS injection did not improve the clinical results.

Apart from the previously described study, Cömert Kiliç et al. [77] compared other methods of treatment of TMJ OA, namely arthrocentesis with lavage and an additional injection of HA and arthrocentesis with lavage and an additional injection of PRP with four consecutive PRP injections (1 per month). The authors found no significant differences between the clinical results obtained in both examined groups. According to the presented study, arthrocentesis with multiple PRP injections was not superior to arthrocentesis with a single HA injection. Finally, Cömert Kiliç et al. [78] also compared the results of arthrocentesis alone with the clinical outcomes of arthrocentesis with lavage and an additional injection of PRP with four consecutive PRP injections (1 per month). Both groups presented a significant reduction in general pain and joint sounds. Moreover, only patients treated with PRP presented significantly increased masticatory efficiency, painless mouth opening and lateral movements after the end of the treatment. However, the only significant difference in clinical outcomes between the groups was related to the masticatory efficiency; specifically, masticatory efficiency was significantly higher in the PRP group. In the authors' opinion, arthrocentesis with PRP is superior compared to arthrocentesis alone.

Hegab et al. [79] also assessed the clinical outcomes after two different combinations of arthrocentesis with either PRP or HA injections. They treated the patients with either three autologous intraarticular injections of 1 mL of PRP once per week for three consecutive weeks after arthrocentesis with 50 mL of lactated Ringer's solution or with three intraarticular injections of 1 mL of LMW HA once per week for three consecutive weeks after arthrocentesis was performed in the same way. After 12-month follow-up, patients treated with PRP presented better clinical outcomes in terms of pain reduction and increased interincisal distance than those who had been treated with LMW HA. However, up to 6 months after the end of the treatment, the PRP group presented significantly increased pain and significantly decreased maximum mouth opening compared to the LMW HA group. The authors found that between the 6th and 12th month after the end of the treatment, the LMW HA group presented a significant decrease in median maximum mouth opening and significant increase in the median pain score. The authors concluded that PRP injections lead to better clinical outcomes than HA. However, they also noticed that patients treated with PRP intraarticular injections presented significantly more complications, including pain during injection, as well as postoperative discomfort.

Finally, there have been published two articles related to arthroscopy [80,81]. Fernández Sanromán et al. [80] performed either arthroscopy with PRGF injection 2 mL or arthroscopy with 5% sodium chloride injection 5 mL in patients diagnosed with Wilkes stage IV internal derangement. Patients treated with an additional PRGF injection presented significantly lower pain scores only 6 and 12 months after the end of the treatment compared to the control group. There were no significant differences between the examined groups regarding pain complaints and maximum mouth opening after 2-year follow-up. The authors indicated that additional PRGF supplementation did not improve the final outcomes. Fernández-Ferro et al. [81] also compared arthroscopy with PRGF injection 5 mL (not 2 mL, as performed by Fernández Sanromán et al. [80]) and arthroscopy with HMW HA injection. Despite the fact that both groups presented a progressive increase in mouth opening, there were no significant differences between the groups. However, PRGF following arthroscopy was more effective than the injection of HA regarding pain control.

Table 3 presents the effectiveness of HA, CS and PRP in the treatment of TMJ OA on the basis of the literature [66–81].

Table 3. Effectiveness of HA, CS and PRP used in the treatment of the TMJ OA on the basis of the literature [66–81].

References	Study Design	Participants and Intervention	Endpoint and Results
Bergstrand et al. (2019) [66]	Randomized, double-blind study	37 patients (30 women, 7 men, aged 23–83 years): - arthrocentesis with lavage alone (17 patients) - arthrocentesis with lavage and an additional injection of HA (20 patients) - all of the patients received conservative therapies before enrollment in the study (education, non-steroidal anti-inflammatory drugs, physiotherapy, occlusal splints)	Endpoint: 47 months (range: 25–79 months) No significant differences regarding maximum incisor opening and pain reduction between the examined groups. Additional HA injection did not improve the final outcome.
Guarda-Nardini et al. (2012) [67]	Randomized, double-blind study	35 patients (30 women, 5 men, mean age—group A: 47.7 ± 15.0 years; group B: 52.9 ± 16.1 years): - group A: arthrocentesis + 1 mL of medium-molecular-weight HA (17 patients) - group B: arthrocentesis + 1 mL of low-molecular-weight HA (18 patients) - all of the patients underwent a cycle of 5 single-needle arthrocenteses with injection of 1 mL of HA (1x/week)	Endpoint: 3 months No significant differences between the examined groups regarding the effectiveness of both methods of treatment.

Table 3. *Cont.*

References	Study Design	Participants and Intervention	Endpoint and Results
Tang et al. (2010) [68]	Randomized, double-blind study	40 patients (21 women, 19 men, aged: 25–63 years): - SH group: 5 injections of sodium hyaluronate 1 mL once a week for 5 weeks (20 patients) - control: 5 injections of physiologic saline solution 1 mL once a week for 5 weeks (20 patients)	Endpoint: after 5-week treatment Only patients treated with SH presented significant pain reduction.
Bouloux et al. (2017) [69,70]	Randomized, double-blind study	102 patients (89 women, 13 men, mean age—group CS: 39.6 ± 18.4 years; group HA: 44.3 ± 17.2 years; group Ringer: 51.8 ± 17.2 years): - arthrocentesis with lavage and an additional injection of CS 1 mL (35 patients) - arthrocentesis with lavage and an additional injection of HA 1 mL (36 patients) - arthrocentesis with lavage and an additional injection of Ringer's solution 1 mL (31 patients)	Endpoint: 3 months No significant differences among the examined groups regarding pain levels, maximum incisal opening, jaw function and quality of life.
Huddleston Slater et al. (2012) [71]	Randomized, double-blind study	28 patients (23 women, 5 men, mean age—control group: 33.9; group CS: 32.6): - control: arthrocentesis with an additional single-dose injection of isotonic saline 1 cc (14 patients) - CS group: arthrocentesis with an additional single-dose injection of CS 1 cc (14 patients)	Endpoint: 24 weeks No significant differences between the examined groups regarding pain complaints, maximal interincisal opening, as well as functional impairment.
Manfredini et al. (2012) [72]	Randomized, single-blind study	60 patients (51 women, 9 men, mean age 50.1 years) - protocol A: single-session two-needle arthrocentesis (11 patients) - protocol B: single-session two-needle arthrocentesis plus CS (9 patients) - protocol C: single-session two-needle arthrocentesis plus LMW HA (11 patients) - protocol D: single-session two-needle arthrocentesis plus HMW HA (5 patients) because of the severe side effects occurring in two patients, the group was withdrawn from the study - protocol E: 5 weekly two-needle arthrocenteses plus LMW HA (12 patients) - protocol F: 5 weekly single-needle arthrocenteses plus LMW HA (12 patients)	Endpoint: 6 weeks No significant differences among the examined groups regarding the pain at rest, pain at chewing, chewing efficiency and mouth opening.
Bjørnland et al. (2007) [73]	Randomized, double-blind study	40 patients (34 women, 6 men, mean age—group HA: 53.4 ± 12.9 years; group CS: 50.0 ± 13.3 years) - S-group: two intraarticular injections 14 days apart with 0.7–1 mL of HA (20 patients) - C-group: two intraarticular injections 14 days apart with 0.7–1 mL of CS (20 patients)	Endpoint: 6 months Patients treated with HA presented: - significantly less pain intensity after 6 months - significantly fewer joints with crepitation after first injection - There were no significant differences in the improvement of jaw function or in the presence of TMJ clicking between the examined groups.

Table 3. *Cont.*

References	Study Design	Participants and Intervention	Endpoint and Results
Møystad et al. (2008) [74]	Randomized, double-blind study	36 patients (31 women, 5 men, mean age—group HA: 51.5 ± 12.9 years; group CS: 48.3 ± 13.5 years) - S-group: two intraarticular injections 14 days apart with HA (17 patients) - C-group: two intraarticular injections 14 days apart with CS (19 patients)	Endpoint: 6 months No significant differences between the examined groups regarding the presence of the radiographic signs of osteoarthritis or regarding the progression or regression of osseous changes in the TMJs.
Isacsson et al. (2019) [75]	Randomized, double-blind study	54 patients (44 women, 10 men, mean age—group A: 48 ± 18.6 years; group B: 56 ± 14.7 years): - group A: 1 mL intraarticular injection of methylprednisolone 40 mg/mL (27 patients) - group B: 1 mL intraarticular injection of sodium chloride (27 patients) - all of the patients received a single-dose intraarticular injection	Endpoint: 4 weeks No significant differences between the examined groups regarding TMJ arthralgia pain reduction. Methylprednisolone led to increased pain following the intervention compared to saline.
Cömert Kiliç et al. (2016) [76]	Randomized clinical trial	24 patients (21 women, 3 men, mean age—control group: 35.08 ± 14.84 years; group CS: 32.58 ± 9.58 years): - control: arthrocentesis (12 patients) - CS group: arthrocentesis with an additional single-dose injection of CS 1 mL (12 patients)	Endpoint: 12 months No significant differences between the examined groups regarding pain complaints or range of motion.
Cömert Kiliç et al. (2016) [77]	Randomized clinical trial	31 patients (26 women, 5 men, mean age: 30.48 ± 13.04 years): - PRP group: arthrocentesis with lavage and an additional injection of PRP 1 mL + 4 consecutive PRP injections (1 per month) (18 patients) - HA group: arthrocentesis with lavage and an additional injection of HA 1 mL (13 patients)	Endpoint: 12 months No significant differences between the examined groups regarding masticatory efficiency, pain complaints, joint sounds, painless mouth opening, maximum mouth opening, lateral and protrusive movement.
Cömert Kiliç et al. (2015) [78]	Randomized clinical trial	30 patients (27 women, 3 men, mean age—control group: 35.08 ± 14.84 years; group PRP: 32.22 ± 14.33 years): - control: arthrocentesis (12 patients) - PRP group: arthrocentesis with lavage and an additional injection of PRP 1 mL + 4 consecutive PRP injections (1 per month) (18 patients)	Endpoint: 12 months No significant differences between the examined groups regarding pain complaints, joint sounds, painless mouth opening, maximum mouth opening, lateral and protrusive movement. Only masticatory efficiency was significantly higher in PRP group.
Hegab et al. (2015) [79]	Randomized single-blind study	50 patients (29 women, 21 men, aged 31–49 years): - PRP group: 3 autologous intraarticular injections of 1 mL of PRP once per week for 3 consecutive weeks after arthrocentesis with 50 mL of lactated Ringer's solution (25 patients) - HA group: 3 intraarticular injections of 1 mL of LMW HA once per week for 3 consecutive weeks after arthrocentesis with 50 mL of lactated Ringer's solution (25 patients)	Endpoint: 12 months PRP performed better than LMW HA during long-term follow-up (12 months) in terms of pain reduction and increased interincisal distance (up to 6 months better results were obtained with LMW HA).

Table 3. *Cont.*

References	Study Design	Participants and Intervention	Endpoint and Results
Fernández Sanromán et al. (2016) [80]	Randomized single-blind study	92 patients (87 women, 5 men, aged 17–67 years): - PRGF group: arthroscopy + PRGF injection 2 mL (42 patients) - control group: arthroscopy + 5% sodium chloride injection 5 mL (50 patients)	Endpoint: 2 years No significant differences between the examined groups regarding pain complaints and maximum mouth opening.
Fernández-Ferro et al. (2017) [81]	Randomized single-blind study	100 patients (94 women, 6 men, aged 18–77 years): - PRGF group: arthroscopy + PRGF injection 5 mL (50 patients) - control group: arthroscopy + HMW HA injection (50 patients)	Endpoint: 18 months No significant differences between the examined groups regarding maximum mouth opening. PRGF following arthroscopy was more effective than the injection of HA regarding pain control.

TMJ—temporomandibular joint, HA—hyaluronic acid, SH—sodium hyaluronate, CS—corticosteroids, PRP—platelet-rich plasma, PRGF—plasma rich in growth factors, LMW HA—low-molecular-weight hyaluronic acid, HMW HA—high-molecular-weight hyaluronic acid.

The above-listed studies differ in methodology, endpoints and obtained results. Many of these studies do compare different protocols of the TMJ OA treatment with the usage of additional intraarticular injections, but at the same they do not compare the obtained results to control groups, which should involve arthrocentesis performed alone. Although the authors find different methods effective, they should also state if the observed methods of treatment are in fact superior to arthrocentesis performed alone. This is important not only for clinical reasons but also for economic ones. The studies that compared different methods of treatment to arthrocentesis alone showed no significant differences regarding the obtained results.

4. Conclusions

Arthrocentesis alone effectively reduces pain and improves jaw function in patients diagnosed with TMJ OA. Additional injections of HA (either LMW HA or HMW HA) or CS at the end of the arthrocentesis do not improve the final clinical outcomes. When arthrocentesis is not performed, the intraarticular injection of HA is more effective in pain reduction compared to injections of either CS or physiologic saline solution. Moreover, it seems that intraarticular injections should be repeated more than once to achieve satisfactory clinical outcomes and therefore the number of intraarticular injections should be further evaluated.

However, it should also be noted that CS directly affect the articular cartilage by altering cartilage matrix metabolism, changing the mechanical properties of the articular cartilage and by leading to chondrotoxicity. Because of the fact that CS do not present any superior effects compared to HA or arthrocentesis either alone or combined with HA, the usage of CS in the treatment of TMJ OA should not be recommended and should be further examined.

Results related to additional PRP injections are not consistent and are rather questionable. It seems that PRP injections do not add any significant improvements to maximum mouth opening, but they may effectively reduce pain. The studies regarding the efficacy of intraarticular injections of PRP should be further evaluated. The amount of PRP injected intraarticularly and the number of injections seem to have an impact on the final clinical outcomes.

It is recommended for further studies to include always the control group of patients treated with arthrocentesis alone. It seems that this minimally invasive surgical procedure is enough to reduce the TMJ pain and to satisfactorily increase the maximum mouth opening by flushing out the inflammatory mediators from the inside of the TMJ. Further studies should be multicenter, based on a larger group of patients and should definitively answer the question of whether other methods of TMJ OA treatment, especially those which require the usage of additional intraarticular supplements, are in fact more beneficial for the patients than simple arthrocentesis.

Author Contributions: Conceptualization, M.D.; methodology, M.D.; validation, M.D., M.M.-K. and E.P.; formal analysis, M.D.; investigation, M.D.; resources, M.D.; writing—original draft preparation, M.D.; writing—review and editing, M.M.-K. and E.P.; visualization, M.D.; supervision, E.P.; project administration, M.D., M.M.-K. and E.P. All authors have read and agreed to the published version of the manuscript.

Funding: This research received no external funding.

Institutional Review Board Statement: Not applicable.

Informed Consent Statement: Not applicable.

Data Availability Statement: The data underlying this article are available in the article.

Conflicts of Interest: The authors declare no conflict of interest.

References

1. Schiffman, E.; Ohrbach, R.; Truelove, E.; Look, J.; Anderson, G.; Goulet, J.-P.; List, T.; Svensson, P.; Gonzalez, Y.; Lobbezoo, F.; et al. Diagnostic Criteria for Temporomandibular Disorders (DC/TMD) for Clinical and Research Applications: Recommendations of the International RDC/TMD Consortium Network* and Orofacial Pain Special Interest Group. *J. Oral Facial Pain Headache* **2014**, *28*, 6–27. [CrossRef] [PubMed]
2. Mercuri, L.G.; Abramowicz, S. Arthritic Conditions Affecting the Temporomandibular Joint. In *Contemporary Oral Medicine*; Farah, C., Balasubramaniam, R., McCullough, M., Eds.; Springer: Cham, Switzerland, 2017. [CrossRef]
3. Glyn-Jones, S.; Palmer, A.J.; Agricola, R.; Price, A.J.; Vincent, T.L.; Weinans, H.; Carr, A.J. Osteoarthritis. *Lancet* **2015**, *386*, 376–387. [CrossRef]
4. Hunter, D.J.; Bierma-Zeinstra, S. Osteoarthritis. *Lancet* **2019**, *393*, 1745–1759. [CrossRef]
5. Wang, X.D.; Zhang, J.N.; Gan, Y.H.; Zhou, Y.H. Current understanding of pathogenesis and treatment of TMJ osteoarthritis. *J. Dent. Res.* **2015**, *94*, 666–673. [CrossRef] [PubMed]
6. Tanaka, E.; Detamore, M.S.; Mercuri, L.G. Degenerative disorders of the temporomandibular joint: Etiology, diagnosis, and treatment. *J. Dent. Res.* **2008**, *87*, 296–307. [CrossRef]
7. Derwich, M.; Mitus-Kenig, M.; Pawlowska, E. Orally Administered NSAIDs-General Characteristics and Usage in the Treatment of Temporomandibular Joint Osteoarthritis-A Narrative Review. *Pharmaceuticals* **2021**, *14*, 219. [CrossRef]
8. Derwich, M.; Mitus-Kenig, M.; Pawlowska, E. Interdisciplinary Approach to the Temporomandibular Joint Osteoarthritis-Review of the Literature. *Medicina* **2020**, *56*, 225. [CrossRef]
9. Gauer, R.L.; Semidey, M.J. Diagnosis and treatment of temporomandibular disorders. *Am. Fam. Physician* **2015**, *91*, 378–386.
10. Al-Moraissi, E.A.; Wolford, L.M.; Ellis E 3rd Neff, A. The hierarchy of different treatments for arthrogenous temporomandibular disorders: A network meta-analysis of randomized clinical trials. *J. Craniomaxillofac. Surg.* **2020**, *48*, 9–23. [CrossRef]
11. Lin, W.; Liu, Z.; Kampf, N.; Klein, J. The Role of Hyaluronic Acid in Cartilage Boundary Lubrication. *Cells* **2020**, *9*, 1606. [CrossRef]
12. Seror, J.; Merkherm, Y.; Kampf, N.; Collinson, L.; Day, A.J.; Maroudas, A.; Klein, J. Articular cartilage proteoglycans as boundary lubricants: Structure and frictional interaction of surface-attached hyaluronan and hyaluronan—Aggrecan complexes. *Biomacromolecules* **2011**, *12*, 3432–3443. [CrossRef]
13. Guarda-Nardini, L.; Masiero, S.; Marioni, G. Conservative treatment of temporomandibular joint osteoarthrosis: Intra-articular injection of sodium hyaluronate. *J. Oral Rehabil.* **2005**, *32*, 729–734. [CrossRef]
14. Cascone, P.; Fonzi Dagger, L.; Aboh, I.V. Hyaluronic acid's biomechanical stabilization function in the temporomandibular joint. *J. Craniofac. Surg.* **2002**, *13*, 751–754. [CrossRef]
15. Manfredini, D.; Piccotti, F.; Guarda-Nardini, L. Hyaluronic acid in the treatment of TMJ disorders: A systematic review of the literature. *Cranio* **2010**, *28*, 166–176. [CrossRef]
16. Ferreira, N.; Masterson, D.; Lopes de Lima, R.; de Souza Moura, B.; Oliveira, A.T.; Kelly da Silva Fidalgo, T.; Carvalho, A.C.P.; DosSantos, M.F.; Grossmann, E. Efficacy of viscosupplementation with hyaluronic acid in temporomandibular disorders: A systematic review. *J. Craniomaxillofac. Surg.* **2018**, *46*, 1943–1952. [CrossRef]
17. Iwanaga, T.; Shikichi, M.; Kitamura, H.; Yanase, H.; Nozawa-Inoue, K. Morphology and functional roles of synoviocytes in the joint. *Arch. Histol. Cytol.* **2000**, *63*, 17–31. [CrossRef]
18. Shinohara, T.; Izawa, T.; Mino-Oka, A.; Mori, H.; Iwasa, A.; Inubushi, T.; Yamaguchi, Y.; Tanaka, E. Hyaluronan metabolism in overloaded temporomandibular joint. *J. Oral Rehabil.* **2016**, *43*, 921–928. [CrossRef]
19. Siiskonen, H.; Oikari, S.; Pasonen-Seppänen, S.; Rilla, K. Hyaluronan synthase 1: A mysterious enzyme with unexpected functions. *Front. Immunol.* **2015**, *6*, 43. [CrossRef]

20. Faust, H.J.; Sommerfeld, S.D.; Rathod, S.; Rittenbach, A.; Ray Banerjee, S.; Tsui, B.M.W.; Pomper, M.; Amzel, M.L.; Singh, A.; Elisseeff, J.H. A hyaluronic acid binding peptide-polymer system for treating osteoarthritis. *Biomaterials* **2018**, *183*, 93–101. [CrossRef]
21. Seror, J.; Zhu, L.; Goldberg, R.; Day, A.J.; Klein, J. Supramolecular synergy in the boundary lubrication of synovial joints. *Nat. Commun.* **2015**, *6*, 6497. [CrossRef]
22. Zhu, L.; Seror, J.; Day, A.J.; Kampf, N.; Klein, J. Ultra-low friction between boundary layers of hyaluronan-phosphatidylcholine complexes. *Acta Biomater.* **2017**, *59*, 283–292. [CrossRef]
23. Das, S.; Banquy, X.; Zappone, B.; Greene, G.W.; Jay, G.D.; Israelachvili, J.N. Synergistic interactions between grafted hyaluronic acid and lubricin provide enhanced wear protection and lubrication. *Biomacromolecules* **2013**, *14*, 1669–1677. [CrossRef]
24. Iturriaga, V.; Vásquez, B.; Bornhardt, T.; Del Sol, M. Effects of low and high molecular weight hyaluronic acid on the osteoarthritic temporomandibular joint in rabbit. *Clin. Oral Investig.* **2021**. [CrossRef]
25. Campo, G.M.; Avenoso, A.; Nastasi, G.; Micali, A.; Prestipino, V.; Vaccaro, M.; D'Ascola, A.; Calatroni, A.; Campo, S. Hyaluronan reduces inflammation in experimental arthritis by modulating TLR-2 and TLR-4 cartilage expression. *Biochim. Biophys. Acta* **2011**, *1812*, 1170–1181. [CrossRef]
26. Herzog, M.; Li, L.; Galla, H.J.; Winter, R. Effect of hyaluronic acid on phospholipid model membranes. *Colloids Surf. B Biointerfaces* **2019**, *173*, 327–334. [CrossRef]
27. McKee, C.M.; Penno, M.B.; Cowman, M.; Burdick, M.D.; Strieter, R.M.; Bao, C.; Noble, P.W. Hyaluronan (HA) fragments induce chemokine gene expression in alveolar macrophages. The role of HA size and CD44. *J. Clin. Investig.* **1996**, *98*, 2403–2413. [CrossRef]
28. Csoka, A.B.; Frost, G.I.; Stern, R. The six hyaluronidase-like genes in the human and mouse genomes. *Matrix Biol.* **2001**, *20*, 499–508. [CrossRef]
29. Greenwald, R.A.; Moy, W.W. Effect of oxygen-derived free radicals on hyaluronic acid. *Arthritis Rheum.* **1980**, *23*, 455–463. [CrossRef]
30. Takahashi, T.; Tominaga, K.; Takano, H.; Ariyoshi, W.; Habu, M.; Fukuda, J.; Maeda, H. A decrease in the molecular weight of hyaluronic acid in synovial fluid from patients with temporomandibular disorders. *J. Oral Pathol. Med.* **2004**, *33*, 224–229. [CrossRef]
31. Guo, X.; Watari, I.; Ikeda, Y.; Yang, W.; Ono, T. Effect of functional lateral shift of the mandible on hyaluronic acid metabolism related to lubrication of temporomandibular joint in growing rats. *Eur. J. Orthod.* **2020**, *42*, 658–663. [CrossRef]
32. Meszaros, M.; Kis, A.; Kunos, L.; Tarnoki, A.D.; Tarnoki, D.L.; Lazar, Z.; Bikov, A. The role of hyaluronic acid and hyaluronidase-1 in obstructive sleep apnoea. *Sci. Rep.* **2020**, *10*, 19484. [CrossRef] [PubMed]
33. Tolba, Y.M.; Omar, S.S.; Nagui, D.A.; Nawwar, M.A. Effect of high molecular weight hyaluronic acid in treatment of osteoarthritic temporomandibular joints of rats. *Arch. Oral Biol.* **2020**, *110*, 104618. [CrossRef] [PubMed]
34. Duygu, G.; Güler, N.; Cam, B.; Kürkçü, M. The effects of high molecular weight hyaluronic acid (Hylan G-F 20) on experimentally induced temporomandibular joint osteoartrosis: Part II. *Int. J. Oral Maxillofac. Surg.* **2011**, *40*, 1406–1413. [CrossRef] [PubMed]
35. Lemos, G.A.; Rissi, R.; Pimentel, E.R.; Palomari, E.T. Effects of high molecular weight hyaluronic acid on induced arthritis of the temporomandibular joint in rats. *Acta Histochem.* **2015**, *117*, 566–575. [CrossRef]
36. Kapugi, M.; Cunningham, K. Corticosteroids. *Orthop. Nurs.* **2019**, *38*, 336–339. [CrossRef]
37. Freire, V.; Bureau, N.J. Injectable Corticosteroids: Take Precautions and Use Caution. *Semin. Musculoskelet. Radiol.* **2016**, *20*, 401–408. [CrossRef]
38. Yaftali, N.A.; Weber, K. Corticosteroids and Hyaluronic Acid Injections. *Clin. Sports Med.* **2019**, *38*, 1–15. [CrossRef]
39. MacMahon, P.J.; Eustace, S.J.; Kavanagh, E.C. Injectable corticosteroid and local anesthetic preparations: A review for radiologists. *Radiology* **2009**, *252*, 647–661. [CrossRef]
40. Ramamoorthy, S.; Cidlowski, J.A. Corticosteroids: Mechanisms of Action in Health and Disease. *Rheum. Dis. Clin. N. Am.* **2016**, *42*, 15–31. [CrossRef]
41. Barnes, P.J. Anti-inflammatory actions of glucocorticoids: Molecular mechanisms. *Clin. Sci. (Lond.)* **1998**, *94*, 557–572. [CrossRef]
42. Ingawale, D.K.; Mandlik, S.K. New insights into the novel anti-inflammatory mode of action of glucocorticoids. *Immunopharmacol. Immunotoxicol.* **2020**, *42*, 59–73. [CrossRef]
43. Quatrini, L.; Ugolini, S. New insights into the cell- and tissue-specificity of glucocorticoid actions. *Cell. Mol. Immunol.* **2021**, *18*, 269–278. [CrossRef]
44. Vandevyver, S.; Dejager, L.; Tuckermann, J.; Libert, C. New insights into the anti-inflammatory mechanisms of glucocorticoids: An emerging role for glucocorticoid-receptor-mediated transactivation. *Endocrinology* **2013**, *154*, 993–1007. [CrossRef]
45. Panettieri, R.A.; Schaafsma, D.; Amrani, Y.; Koziol-White, C.; Ostrom, R.; Tliba, O. Non-genomic Effects of Glucocorticoids: An Updated View. *Trends Pharmacol. Sci.* **2019**, *40*, 38–49. [CrossRef]
46. Buttgereit, F. Glucocorticoids: Surprising new findings on their mechanisms of actions. *Ann. Rheum. Dis.* **2021**, *80*, 137–139. [CrossRef]
47. Kondo, T.; Kitazawa, R.; Yamaguchi, A.; Kitazawa, S. Dexamethasone promotes osteoclastogenesis by inhibiting osteoprotegerin through multiple levels. *J. Cell. Biochem.* **2008**, *103*, 335–345. [CrossRef]
48. Monseau, A.J.; Nizran, P.S. Common injections in musculoskeletal medicine. *Prim. Care* **2013**, *40*, 987–1000. [CrossRef]

49. Céleste, C.; Ionescu, M.; Robin Poole, A.; Laverty, S. Repeated intraarticular injections of triamcinolone acetonide alter cartilage matrix metabolism measured by biomarkers in synovial fluid. *J. Orthop. Res.* **2005**, *23*, 602–610. [CrossRef]
50. Murray, R.C.; DeBowes, R.M.; Gaughan, E.M.; Zhu, C.F.; Athanasiou, K.A. The effects of intra-articular methylprednisolone and exercise on the mechanical properties of articular cartilage in the horse. *Osteoarthr. Cartil.* **1998**, *6*, 106–114. [CrossRef]
51. Dragoo, J.L.; Danial, C.M.; Braun, H.J.; Pouliot, M.A.; Kim, H.J. The chondrotoxicity of single-dose corticosteroids. *Knee Surg Sports Traumatol. Arthrosc.* **2012**, *20*, 1809–1814. [CrossRef]
52. Pietrzak, W.S.; Eppley, B.L. Platelet rich plasma: Biology and new technology. *J. Craniofac. Surg.* **2005**, *16*, 1043–1054. [CrossRef]
53. Chung, P.Y.; Lin, M.T.; Chang, H.P. Effectiveness of platelet-rich plasma injection in patients with temporomandibular joint osteoarthritis: A systematic review and meta-analysis of randomized controlled trials. *Oral Surg. Oral Med. Oral Pathol. Oral Radiol.* **2019**, *127*, 106–116. [CrossRef]
54. Bousnaki, M.; Bakopoulou, A.; Koidis, P. Platelet-rich plasma for the therapeutic management of temporomandibular joint disorders: A systematic review. *Int. J. Oral Maxillofac. Surg.* **2018**, *47*, 188–198. [CrossRef]
55. Al-Hamed, F.S.; Hijazi, A.; Gao, Q.; Badran, Z.; Tamimi, F. Platelet Concentrate Treatments for Temporomandibular Disorders: A Systematic Review and Meta-analysis. *JDR Clin. Trans. Res.* **2021**, *6*, 174–183. [CrossRef]
56. Foster, T.E.; Puskas, B.L.; Mandelbaum, B.R.; Gerhardt, M.B.; Rodeo, S.A. Platelet-rich plasma: From basic science to clinical applications. *Am. J. Sports Med.* **2009**, *37*, 2259–2272. [CrossRef]
57. Le, A.D.K.; Enweze, L.; DeBaun, M.R.; Dragoo, J.L. Current Clinical Recommendations for Use of Platelet-Rich Plasma. *Curr. Rev. Musculoskelet. Med.* **2018**, *11*, 624–634. [CrossRef]
58. Harrison, T.E.; Bowler, J.; Levins, T.N.; Reeves, K.D.; Cheng, A.L. Platelet-Rich Plasma Centrifugation Changes Leukocyte Ratios. *Cureus* **2021**, *13*, e14470. [CrossRef]
59. Gremmel, T.; Frelinger, A.L., 3rd; Michelson, A.D. Platelet Physiology. *Semin. Thromb. Hemost.* **2016**, *42*, 191–204. [CrossRef] [PubMed]
60. King, S.M.; Reed, G.L. Development of platelet secretory granules. *Semin. Cell. Dev. Biol.* **2002**, *13*, 293–302. [CrossRef] [PubMed]
61. Nazaroff, J.; Oyadomari, S.; Brown, N.; Wang, D. Reporting in clinical studies on platelet-rich plasma therapy among all medical specialties: A systematic review of Level I and II studies. *PLoS ONE* **2021**, *16*, e0250007. [CrossRef] [PubMed]
62. Grambart, S.T. Sports medicine and platelet-rich plasma: Nonsurgical therapy. *Clin. Podiatr. Med. Surg.* **2015**, *32*, 99–107. [CrossRef]
63. Akeda, K.; An, H.S.; Okuma, M.; Attawia, M.; Miyamoto, K.; Thonar, E.J.; Lenz, M.E.; Sah, R.L.; Masuda, K. Platelet-rich plasma stimulates porcine articular chondrocyte proliferation and matrix biosynthesis. *Osteoarthr. Cartil.* **2006**, *14*, 1272–1280. [CrossRef]
64. Anitua, E.; Fernández-de-Retana, S.; Alkhraisat, M.H. Platelet rich plasma in oral and maxillofacial surgery from the perspective of composition. *Platelets* **2021**, *32*, 174–182. [CrossRef]
65. Medina-Porqueres, I.; Ortega-Castillo, M.; Muriel-Garcia, A. Effectiveness of platelet-rich plasma in the management of hip osteoarthritis: A systematic review and meta-analysis. *Clin. Rheumatol.* **2021**, *40*, 53–64. [CrossRef]
66. Bergstrand, S.; Ingstad, H.K.; Møystad, A.; Bjørnland, T. Long-term effectiveness of arthrocentesis with and without hyaluronic acid injection for treatment of temporomandibular joint osteoarthritis. *J. Oral Sci.* **2019**, *61*, 82–88. [CrossRef]
67. Guarda-Nardini, L.; Cadorin, C.; Frizziero, A.; Ferronato, G.; Manfredini, D. Comparison of 2 hyaluronic acid drugs for the treatment of temporomandibular joint osteoarthritis. *J. Oral Maxillofac. Surg.* **2012**, *70*, 2522–2530. [CrossRef]
68. Tang, Y.L.; Zhu, G.Q.; Hu, L.; Zheng, M.; Zhang, J.Y.; Shi, Z.D.; Liang, X.H. Effects of intra-articular administration of sodium hyaluronate on plasminogen activator system in temporomandibular joints with osteoarthritis. *Oral Surg. Oral Med. Oral Pathol. Oral Radiol. Endod.* **2010**, *109*, 541–547. [CrossRef]
69. Bouloux, G.F.; Chou, J.; Krishnan, D.; Aghaloo, T.; Kahenasa, N.; Smith, J.A.; Giannakopoulos, H. Is Hyaluronic Acid or Corticosteroid Superior to Lactated Ringer Solution in the Short-Term Reduction of Temporomandibular Joint Pain After Arthrocentesis? Part 1. *J. Oral Maxillofac. Surg.* **2017**, *75*, 52–62. [CrossRef]
70. Bouloux, G.F.; Chou, J.; Krishnan, D.; Aghaloo, T.; Kahenasa, N.; Smith, J.A.; Giannakopoulos, H. Is Hyaluronic Acid or Corticosteroid Superior to Lactated Ringer Solution in the Short Term for Improving Function and Quality of Life After Arthrocentesis? Part 2. *J. Oral Maxillofac. Surg.* **2017**, *75*, 63–72. [CrossRef]
71. Huddleston Slater, J.J.; Vos, L.M.; Story, L.P.; Stegenga, B. Randomized trial on the effectiveness of dexamethasone in TMJ arthrocentesis. *J. Dent. Res.* **2012**, *91*, 173–178. [CrossRef]
72. Manfredini, D.; Rancitelli, D.; Ferronato, G.; Guarda-Nardini, L. Arthrocentesis with or without additional drugs in temporomandibular joint inflammatory-degenerative disease: Comparison of six treatment protocols*. *J. Oral Rehabil.* **2012**, *39*, 245–251. [CrossRef]
73. Bjørnland, T.; Gjaerum, A.A.; Møystad, A. Osteoarthritis of the temporomandibular joint: An evaluation of the effects and complications of corticosteroid injection compared with injection with sodium hyaluronate. *J. Oral Rehabil.* **2007**, *34*, 583–589. [CrossRef]
74. Møystad, A.; Mork-Knutsen, B.B.; Bjørnland, T. Injection of sodium hyaluronate compared to a corticosteroid in the treatment of patients with temporomandibular joint osteoarthritis: A CT evaluation. *Oral Surg. Oral Med. Oral Pathol. Oral Radiol. Endod.* **2008**, *105*, e53–e60. [CrossRef]

75. Isacsson, G.; Schumann, M.; Nohlert, E.; Mejersjö, C.; Tegelberg, Å. Pain relief following a single-dose intra-articular injection of methylprednisolone in the temporomandibular joint arthralgia-A multicentre randomised controlled trial. *J. Oral Rehabil.* **2019**, *46*, 5–13. [CrossRef]
76. Cömert Kiliç, S. Does Injection of Corticosteroid After Arthrocentesis Improve Outcomes of Temporomandibular Joint Osteoarthritis? A Randomized Clinical Trial. *J. Oral Maxillofac. Surg.* **2016**, *74*, 2151–2158. [CrossRef]
77. Cömert Kiliç, S.; Güngörmüş, M. Is arthrocentesis plus platelet-rich plasma superior to arthrocentesis plus hyaluronic acid for the treatment of temporomandibular joint osteoarthritis: A randomized clinical trial. *Int. J. Oral Maxillofac. Surg.* **2016**, *45*, 1538–1544. [CrossRef]
78. Cömert Kiliç, S.; Güngörmüş, M.; Sümbüllü, M.A. Is Arthrocentesis Plus Platelet-Rich Plasma Superior to Arthrocentesis Alone in the Treatment of Temporomandibular Joint Osteoarthritis? A Randomized Clinical Trial. *J. Oral Maxillofac. Surg.* **2015**, *73*, 1473–1483. [CrossRef]
79. Hegab, A.F.; Ali, H.E.; Elmasry, M.; Khallaf, M.G. Platelet-Rich Plasma Injection as an Effective Treatment for Temporomandibular Joint Osteoarthritis. *J. Oral Maxillofac. Surg.* **2015**, *73*, 1706–1713. [CrossRef]
80. Fernández Sanromán, J.; Fernández Ferro, M.; Costas López, A.; Arenaz Bua, J.; López, A. Does injection of plasma rich in growth factors after temporomandibular joint arthroscopy improve outcomes in patients with Wilkes stage IV internal derangement? A randomized prospective clinical study. *Int. J. Oral Maxillofac. Surg.* **2016**, *45*, 828–835. [CrossRef]
81. Fernández-Ferro, M.; Fernández-Sanromán, J.; Blanco-Carrión, A.; Costas-López, A.; López-Betancourt, A.; Arenaz-Bua, J.; Stavaru Marinescu, B. Comparison of intra-articular injection of plasma rich in growth factors versus hyaluronic acid following arthroscopy in the treatment of temporomandibular dysfunction: A randomised prospective study. *J. Craniomaxillofac. Surg.* **2017**, *45*, 449–454. [CrossRef] [PubMed]

International Journal of
Molecular Sciences

MDPI

Review

Ultra-Low Dose Cytokines in Rheumatoid Arthritis, Three Birds with One Stone as the Rationale of the 2LARTH® Micro-Immunotherapy Treatment

Camille Jacques *, Ilaria Floris and Béatrice Lejeune

Preclinical Research Department, Labo'Life France, 1 Rue François Bruneau, 44000 Nantes, France; ilaria.floris@labolife.com (I.F.); beatrice.lejeune@labolife.com (B.L.)
* Correspondence: camille.jacques@labolife.com

Abstract: Tumor necrosis factor-α (TNF-α) and interleukin-1β (IL-1β) are two cytokines involved in the perpetuation of the chronic inflammation state characterizing rheumatoid arthritis (RA). Significant advances in the treatment of this pathology have been made over the past ten years, partially through the development of anti-TNF and anti-IL-1 therapies. However, major side effects still persist and new alternative therapies should be considered. The formulation of the micro-immunotherapy medicine (MIM) 2LARTH® uses ultra-low doses (ULD) of TNF-α, IL-1β, and IL-2, in association with other immune factors, to gently restore the body's homeostasis. The first part of this review aims at delineating the pivotal roles played by IL-1β and TNF-α in RA physiopathology, leading to the development of anti-TNF and anti-IL-1 therapeutic agents. In a second part, an emphasis will be made on explaining the rationale of using multiple therapeutic targets, including both IL-1β and TNF-α in 2LARTH® medicine. Particular attention will be paid to the ULD of those two main pro-inflammatory factors in order to counteract their overexpression through the lens of their molecular implication in RA pathogenesis.

Keywords: rheumatoid arthritis; TNF-α; IL-1β; ultra-low doses; micro-immunotherapy; anti-inflammatory medicines; hormesis; chronic inflammation; inflammatory cytokines

Citation: Jacques, C.; Floris, I.; Lejeune, B. Ultra-Low Dose Cytokines in Rheumatoid Arthritis, Three Birds with One Stone as the Rationale of the 2LARTH® Micro-Immunotherapy Treatment. *Int. J. Mol. Sci.* **2021**, *22*, 6717. https://doi.org/10.3390/ijms22136717

Academic Editor: Chih-Hsin Tang

Received: 20 May 2021
Accepted: 20 June 2021
Published: 23 June 2021

1. An Introduction to Rheumatoid Arthritis and Micro-Immunotherapy

Rheumatoid arthritis (RA) is a widespread systemic autoimmune disease characterized by chronic inflammation of the articular membrane, synovial hyperplasia, and progressive degradation of cartilage and bone, leading to joint destruction. Patients with RA usually experience joint pain, swelling, tenderness, and stiffness, especially in the morning, and they also have to cope with fatigue and depression as the disease represents high personal and social burden [1]. Studies conducted in Northern European and North American areas evaluated RA prevalence at about 0.5–1% [2], whereas it appeared less frequently in low- and middle-income countries, where it is gauged at 0.4% and 0.37% in Southeast Asian and in Eastern Mediterranean regions, respectively [3]. Epidemiologic data reported that RA susceptibility increased with age and that sex was also an important factor to take into account. This debilitating disease affects women at a rate double that in men, and in more aggressive forms [4]. Even if the etiology of RA is still unknown, 50–60% of the cases are hereditary and the human leukocyte antigen (HLA) locus is involved in at least 30% of the overall genetic risk.

As research progresses in delineating the drivers of this pathology, it appears that multiple immune factors, all integrated in a complex network and in a particular temporal frame, are involved in the onset and the progression of the disease. For instance, it is now well-established that numerous pro-inflammatory cytokines and growth factors perpetuate the chronic inflammation state of RA, in particular, interleukin-1β (IL-1β) and tumor necrosis factor-α (TNF-α). Cytokines are typically secreted by immune cells in order to orchestrate diverse cellular functions, such as cell differentiation, activation, migration, survival or proliferation in a paracrine or autocrine manner. As they display pleiotropic effects, can either act synergistically or share redundancy of actions one with the others, a fine-tuned regulation of their interplay is of paramount interest in the proper immune system maintenance and the body's homeostasis. Their perturbation in the development of RA is well-documented, some evidence even showing that a subset of cytokines is already imbalanced before the clinical onset of the disease [5].

Significant advances in the treatment of this pathology have been made over the past ten years and the clinical arsenal mainly encompasses the so-called disease-modifying anti-rheumatic drugs (DMARDs) including methotrexate, sulfasalazine, hydroxychloroquine and leflunomide, the janus-activated kinase 3 (JAK3) inhibitor tofacitinib, glucocorticoids and biologic agents such as infliximab, etanercept, adalimumab, golimumab, and certolizumab pegol. All of them are used in both early and established RA (< or >6 months), depending on patients' values, preferences and comorbidities [6,7]. Regarding the pivotal role played by the resident/immune cells hosted in the synovial tissue in the pathogenesis of the disease, cell-targeted therapies have also been developed. Unfortunately, the parenteral administration required for those therapies is still a limiting factor towards their use. Moreover, some unavoidable issues still persist: (1) most of the therapeutics can only alleviate symptoms without intrinsically treating the root of the problem, ultimately leading to an incomplete remission; (2) regarding the length and the costs of the treatment regimens, some patients struggle with compliance, and (3) side effects are still substantial.

In line with those prerequisites, novel treatments—sequentially able to modulate the expression of multiple immune players over time, as the stage of the pathology evolves—would be of great interest. They would indeed allow to re-establish the body's homeostasis, both at a systemic level and within the injured joint niches. For this purpose, the traditional therapeutic strategy of the micro-immunotherapy medicine (MIM) 2LARTH® has been developed to attenuate the symptoms of rheumatic diseases including RA, within a holistic immunomodulatory approach. Micro-immunotherapy (MI) is a pioneering modulative therapeutic approach that can be employed alone or in association with other therapies, providing clinical benefits while reducing side effects. This strategy combines the use of several immune system mediators such as cytokines, growth factors, hormones, nucleic acids and specific nucleic acids (SNA®), in order to orchestrate both the innate and the adaptive/acquired immune responses. SNA® (European Patent: EP0670164B1) consist of single-stranded DNA molecules of 16–44 bases, specifically designed to target one gene or more, based on sequence complementarity. The active ingredients of the MI medicines are prepared according to repetition series of a two-step process called "sequential kinetic process", consisting of (1) 1/100 dilution of the above-mentioned immune mediator, followed by (2) calibrated vertical shaking, reproduced until the desired dilution is reached. One step of this manufacturing process thus defines 1 CH (centesimal Hahnemannian) dilution, in accordance with the European Pharmacopeia monographs 1038 and 2371, current edition. Low doses (LD) range from 1 CH to 7 CH and are used in MI to boost the immune system, activate or increase protein expression, while ultra-low doses (ULD) aim at modulating (from 8 to 12 CH) and lowering (higher than 12 CH) the expression of protein(s) with upregulated levels. LD and ULD are finally impregnated on lactose-sucrose pillules. MI medicines are based on the principle that a given immune regulator exerts either stimulatory effects when used at LD or displays modulatory/inhibitory features when prepared at ULD.

The first part of this review aims at delineating the pivotal roles played by IL-1β and TNF-α in RA physiopathology, leading to the development of anti-TNF and anti-IL-1 therapeutic agents. In a second part, an emphasis will be made on explaining the rationale of using multiple therapeutic targets, including both IL-1β and TNF-α in 2LARTH® medicine. Particular attention will be paid to the ULD of those two main pro-inflammatory factors in order to counteract their overexpression, through the lens of their molecular implication in RA pathogenesis.

2. IL-1β and TNF-α in the Physiopathology of RA, the Bad and the Ugly

Rheumatoid arthritis, as a form of inflammatory pathology, could be qualified as both (1) a systemic and (2) a localized disease, as the systemic serum cytokine levels are affected over the course of the pathology progression, and also because cytokines crosstalk is intrinsically involved in a complex process that transforms the joint into a site of insistent inflammation-promoting tissue necrosis and degradation. The synovial lining, in normal condition, is mainly made of fibroblastic cells, the so-called "synoviocytes" along with macrophages. During the course of RA onset, the synovial delineation expands dramatically, as the synoviocytes' growth becomes anarchic, finally reaching a point where the synovial membrane is so thick that the joint is completely embedded into a "pannus" structure. In this context, the synovial fibroblasts produce mediators actively participating in the cartilage and joints destruction [8]. Immune cells like B cells, T cells, macrophages, and neutrophils progressively infiltrate the synovial fluids and their crosstalk perpetuates the production of pro-inflammatory cytokines and mediators, such as IL-1β, IL-2, and TNF-α.

2.1. IL-1β, the Bad

Although the IL-1 family originally only encompasses IL-1α and IL-1β, eleven members are currently listed [9]. These cytokines have the ability to bind several kinds of receptors, encoded by nine distinct genes, including coreceptors, decoy receptors, binding proteins and inhibitory receptors. The binding mechanism of both IL-1α and IL-1β is a two-step process starting by the cytokine attachment to the ligand-binding chain, termed type-I receptor (IL-1RI), followed by the recruitment of the coreceptor chain, named the accessory-protein (IL-1RAcP). The transduction of the signal is then mediated by the adaptor protein myeloid and differentiation primary response 88 (MyD88), recruited to the Toll-IL-1 receptor (TIR) domain of IL-1RAcP (Figure 1). A cascade of phosphorylation and ubiquitination events then results in the activation of nuclear factor-κB (NF-κB), leading to the expression of pro-inflammatory genes in the stimulated cells [10]. As IL-1β is mainly produced by myeloid cells upon inflammatory stimulation, this cytokine also plays a major role in immunity and hematopoiesis.

In the RA context, the deleterious effects of the IL-1β within the articular niche are broadly reported, as this cytokine induces cellular responses in the major cells constituting the joint microenvironment (Figure 1). For instance, synovial fibroblasts isolated from RA patients undergoing knee arthroplasty display an increased proliferative capacity in the presence of IL-1β [11]. Stimulation with cytokines at only 1 ng/mL was also shown to induce the expression of matrix metalloproteinases-1 and -3 (MMP-1 and MMP-3), cyclooxygenase-2 (COX-2), and prostaglandin E2 (PGE2), both at RNA and protein levels, through the activation of the MAPKs (mitogen-activated protein kinases) and the NF-κB pathways. Kobayashi et al. confirmed those effects within an osteoarthritis cartilage explant model in which they used the IL-1RA antagonist anakinra to block the IL-1β biologic activity, thus demonstrating the implication of this cytokine in the production of MMPs (MMP-1, MMP-3 and MMP-13) [12]. Moreover, IL-1β also directly acts on chondrocytes in decreasing their viability, as well as inducing their apoptosis, as Chen et al. reported in their in vitro experiments [13]. Interestingly, a distinct pro-inflammatory macrophage subtype characterized by a $CD14^+$ $IL\text{-}1\beta^+$ phenotype was shown to be obviously expanded in RA compared to the non-inflammatory osteoarthritis disease [14].

From a genetic standpoint, some associations have been made between IL-1β mutations and the susceptibility of RA occurrence depending on the population analyzed (Figure 1). A study conducted in Algerian people reported that the (T/T) polymorphism of IL-1B –511 was more frequent in RA patients with anti-citrullinated peptide antibodies (ACPA), compared with the negative ACPA group [15]. This association was confirmed by another study conducted in Indian RA patients, where this polymorphism would tend to be associated with elevated serum anti-CCP (cyclic citrullinated peptides) and high IL-1β levels, both known as inflammatory markers in this context [16]. Furthermore, an ethnicity-specific meta-analysis suggested that the IL-1B −511 C/T polymorphism was associated with RA susceptibility in Caucasians, whereas the IL-1B +3953 C/T polymorphism was associated with susceptibility to RA in Caucasian and in Asian populations [17]. Other studies found that IL-1B +3954 polymorphism was significantly associated with the risk of RA in the overall population and in Asian people [18,19]. Furthermore, an analysis conducted in the Japanese population revealed that individuals affected with both RA and periodontitis may display different distributions of IL-1B +3954 genotypes than healthy controls and subjects with periodontitis only [20]. A British study reported that the IL-1B −1464 C/G allele was less common in RA patients than in healthy individuals, thus suggesting a protective effect of this variant, whereas the statistically significant association between IL-1B −511 A/G and RA was also delineated [21].

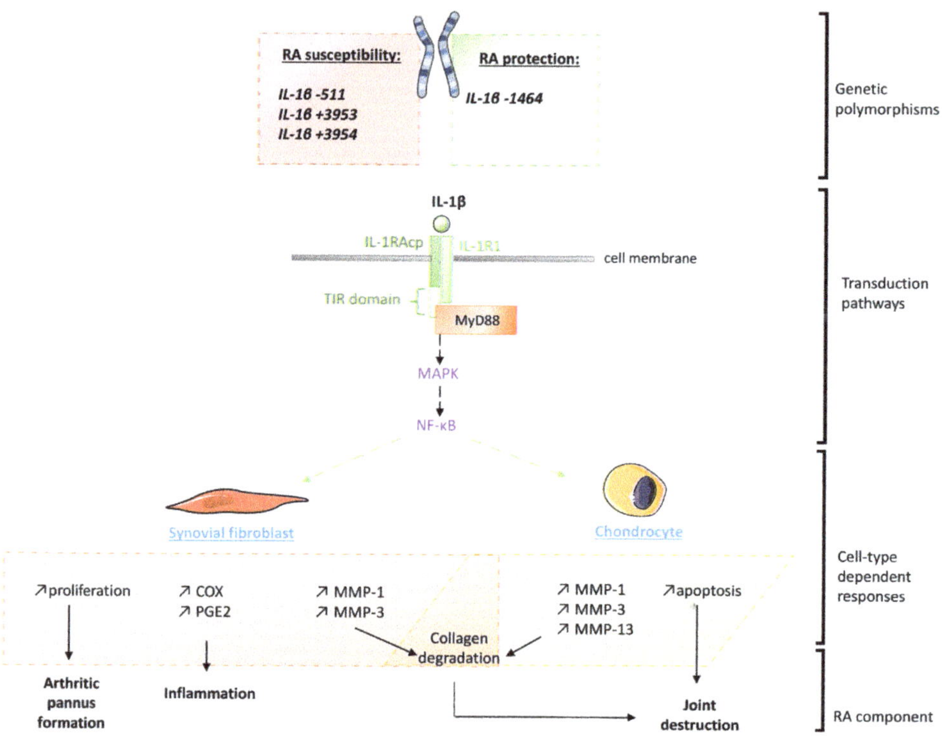

Figure 1. Schematic representation of the different levels of IL-1β's implication in the pathogenesis of rheumatoid arthritis (RA). IL-1R1: Interleukin-1 type-I receptor; IL-1RAcP: IL-1 receptor accessory protein; MAPK: Mitogen-activated protein kinase; MMP: Matrix metalloproteinase; MyD88: Myeloid and differentiation primary response 88; NF-κB: Nuclear factor-κB; PGE2: Prostaglandin E2; TIR: Toll-IL-1 receptor.

2.2. TNF-α, the Ugly

Isolated for the first time in 1975 by Carswell et al., in their endotoxin-mediated tumor necrosis experiments, the body of knowledge about TNF-α has tremendously grown ever since [22]. Many cell types are known to be TNF-α producers, including monocytes and macrophages. Once released, it binds to two different cell-surface receptors, namely, TNF receptor type 1 (TNFR1), also known as p55, which is ubiquitous, and TNFR2, also known as p75, whom the expression is more specific, including immune cells like Tregs for example [23]. As for the IL-1β, TNF-α activates NF-κB signaling by stimulating the proteolytic breakdown of its cytoplasmic inhibitor, IκB (inhibitor of nuclear factor-κB) (Figure 2). This pathway is known to elicit the expression of the TNF-α genes, further inducing various cellular responses including apoptosis, which occurs after the

TNF-α binding to TNFR1, due to the presence of its C-terminal "death domain" [24]. TNF-α's activity blockade through soluble PEGylated TNFR1 was shown to decrease the production of MMP-1, MMP-3 and MMP-13 in femoral condylar cartilage cells cultured from osteoarthritis patients [12]. TNF-α is a major factor of RA development within the synovial niche, as human synovial fibroblasts cultured in presence of TNF-α display increased expression of IL-1β, monocyte chemoattractant protein-1 (MCP1), macrophage inflammatory protein-1 alpha (MIP1α), MMP-1, MMP-3 and receptor activator of nuclear factor-κB ligand (RANKL), an osteoclastogenic cytokine, compared to control cells [25]. In line with these results, TNF-α also induces osteoclast differentiation in macrophages isolated from mouse bone marrow. Anti-TNF was also reported to reduce granulocyte-macrophage colony-stimulating factor (GM-CSF) and vascular endothelial growth factor (VEGF) both in vitro and in patients with RA [26,27].

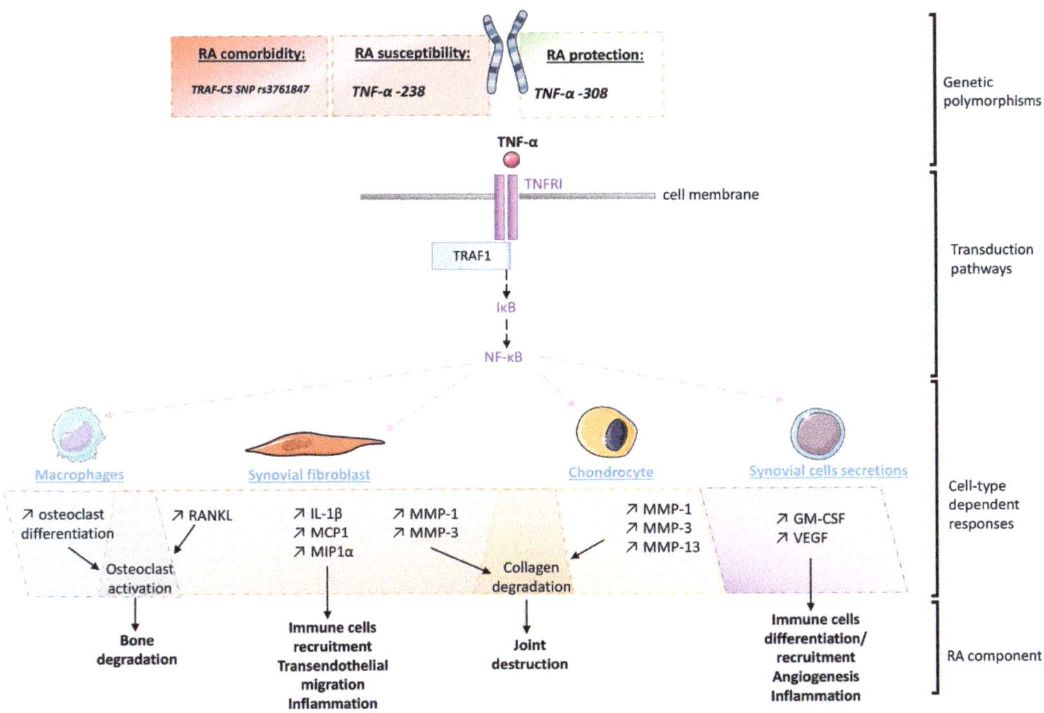

Figure 2. Schematic representation of the different levels of TNF-α's implication in the pathogenesis of rheumatoid arthritis (RA): IL-1β: Interleukin-1β; IκB: Inhibitor of nuclear factor-κB; GM-CSF: Granulocyte-macrophage colony-stimulating factor; MAPK: Mitogen-activated protein kinase; MCP1: Monocyte chemoattractant protein-1; MIP1α: Macrophage inflammatory protein-1 alpha; MMP: Matrix metalloproteinase; NF-κB: Nuclear factor-κB; RANKL: Receptor activator of nuclear factor-κB ligand; SNP: Single nucleotide polymorphism; TIR: Toll-IL-1 receptor; TNFRI: TNF receptor type 1; TRAF1: TNF receptor-associated factor; TRAF-C5: TNF receptor-associated factor 1 and complement component 5; VEGF: Vascular endothelial growth factor.

As for the previously discussed IL-1β, the TNF-α genetic background is linked with RA development (Figure 2). For instance, a study reports that the TNF-α −238 G/A polymorphism contributes to the susceptibility risk to young-onset RA, whereas TNF-α −308 G/A variation may protect against the disease [28]. Interestingly, TNF-α −238 G/A polymorphism was not shown to be an RA susceptibility contributor in the Iranian population [29]. These discrepancies highlight the fact that even if genetics may set up a favorable cellular environment towards the spreading of RA, other regulation aspects should be taken into consideration. Regarding this example, the overall economic and social culture of a population may also be seen as an additional epigenetic layer governing RA occurrence. Moreover, the possible existence of TNF-α gene promoter variants acting as markers for RA severity and treatment response has been reported, reinforcing the role of this growth factor as a key immune player to target in this pathology [30]. Genetic comorbidities involving TNF-α pathway have also been reported, as it was found that RA patients bearing GG homozygosity at the TRAF1-C5 SNP rs3761847 were at a higher risk of death from cancer or sepsis [31]. Indeed, the TNF receptor-associated factor 1 (TRAF1) and complement component 5 (C5) is known to act as a scaffold protein complex and play a direct role in the downstream TNF-α signaling, further reinforcing the link between the TNF-α pathway and the immune escape associated with RA outcome and comorbidities.

3. RA and Cytokines: A TNF-α and IL-1β Crosstalk Modeled Both In Vitro and In Vivo

The synovial niche's crosstalk in RA conditions was studied by Saeki et al., in their in vitro murine arthritis tissue-derived cells model [32]. They recently published that synovial macrophages cultured within conditioned-medium from synovial fibroblasts display changes in genic expression characterized by an upregulation in the expression of inflammatory markers such as Nos2, TNF-α, IL-1β and CD86. Additionally, these macrophages were reported to increase their TNF secretion. Moreover, TNF-α secretion was also found to be induced by DNA stimulation in the RA context, as CpG-rich DNA from blood plasma isolated from an RA patient was shown to stimulate the TLR9-MyD88-NF-kB signaling pathway when added to the culture medium of PBMCs (peripheral blood mononuclear cells) from healthy donors, resulting in a significant increase in the IL-6 and TNF-α secretion [33]. In their study, Schierbeck et al. reported that the TNF-α secretion induced in monocytes stimulated by LPS (lipopolysaccharide) + IFN-γ (interferon-γ) was significantly decreased when the cells were pretreated for one hour with the anti-TNF-α etanercept at either 2 or 8 μg/mL, whereas the anti-IL-1β anakinra (from 2.5 to 20 μg/mL) didn't show any effect on the TNF-α secretion [34]. Furthermore, the gap junction mediator connexin-43 (Cx43) was shown to be involved in both gene expression and secretion of the TNF-α and IL-6 cytokines in a human RA synovial fibroblast model [35]. Matsuki et al. indeed showed that the siRNA-mediated Cx43 inhibition impaired the expression of these cytokines. They also delineated the existence of a retro-control loop, as the TNF-α stimulation of the cells markedly increased their own Cx43 expression. These data even strengthen the fact that TNF-α acts as a key player in the chronicity of the RA disease and its related inflammatory-vicious cycle, as its expression and secretion are induced by a plethora of factors on a broad number of cells from the synovial niche.

The increase of pro-inflammatory cytokines expression such as TNF-α, IL-1β, IL-6 and IL-17, inflammatory mediators like COX-2 and 5-LOX (5-lipoxygenase), as well as the reduction of anti-inflammatory markers such as IL-4 and IL-10 are the hallmark of synovial inflammation and cartilage damages and are extensively monitored parameters in in vivo RA models [36,37]. The CIA (collagen-induced arthritis) model is used as an industry-standard RA model in the evaluation of potential therapeutic agents as it allows for a deep chronic inflammatory process, partially mediated by the induced autoreactivity of T and B cells and reproduces the pannus development, the fibrin deposition, the joint inflammation and its osteo-articular damages characterizing the human disease. In addition, in this model, TNF-α, IL-1β, and IL-6 are also key players in the evolution of the pathology, from its early onset to the chronic phases [38]. In a CIA-induced mice model, it was found that the blockade of IL-1β, TNF-α or a combination of both cytokines delays the start of arthritis [39]. Furthermore, the authors reported that the anti-IL-1β treatment reduced the RA burden to a greater extent than the anti-TNF-α one, both clinically and histologically. Another study performing an in vivo TNF-α inhibition through adalimumab showed that the mRNA expression of IL-2 in the spleen of the treated mice was similar to the one of the healthy control group after daily subcutaneous injections of 1 mg/kg antibody [40]. Moreover, both the IL-1β and the TNF-α protein levels were reduced in the serum as well as in the spleens of the treated animals. In addition, the RANKL mRNA levels were also decreased in the spleens of the treated mice. The study reporting the benefits of using intra-articular injections of the anti-TNF infliximab, loaded onto thermosensitive hydrogel to decrease pro-inflammatory cytokines within the synovial fluids of a rabbit model of RA induced by ovalbumin and complete Freund's adjuvant, is another example illustrating the interplay between TNF-α and IL-1β in vivo [41]. Indeed, two and six weeks after injections, the intra-articular levels of both TNF-α and IL-1β were significantly decreased, compared with the saline-treated control. Altogether, this evidence sustains the therapeutic strategies aiming to individually target these mediators and have already been developed in clinics, whereas they still have to translate into efficient cures devoid of unwanted adverse effects for the patients.

4. Anti-IL-1β and -TNF-α Therapies: Effects and Side Effects of the Conventional Allopathic Doses

IL-1β antagonism has been performed in the context of RA through several options; either targeting the cytokine itself or its receptor. For instance, canakinumab (Ilaris®) is a humanized IgGκ monoclonal antibody against IL-1β, initially developed for the treatment of immune disorders (Figure 3A) [42]. In patients undergoing active RA despite being treated with methotrexate, the addition of subcutaneous injections of 150 mg canakinumab every four weeks over a 12-weeks period improved their therapeutic response regarding the global assessment of disease-related parameters [43]. Kinetic studies and modeling simulations used to extract the dose-response relationships confirmed that 150 mg every four weeks allowed for the capture of the majority of IL-1β, lowering it below an EC_{50} allowing to improve the ACR (American College of Rheumatology) scores in patients with RA [44]. Moreover, canakinumab has been considered as a good option for young patients with severe and/or refractory forms of IL-1-driven RA, in order to avoid joint deformation [45].

Anakinra is a human IL-1R antagonist currently approved for the treatment of RA, leading to significant improvements in disease symptoms and quality of life, regarding pain, Larsen radiographic scores and erythrocytes sedimentation rates, slowing down both radiologic manifestations of joint damages and bone erosion [46,47]. Furthermore, the treatment with this agent was shown to have beneficial effects on inflammatory and metabolic parameters, allowing to discontinue the concomitant use of glucocorticoids and anti-diabetic drugs in patients displaying both RA and type 2 diabetes [48]. Anakinra is mainly used as a second-line treatment in patients previously treated with a failing anti-TNF-α therapy or experiencing cancer or infectious disease such as *Mycobacterium tuberculosis* infections [49].

In parallel with the anti-IL-1β drugs, anti-TNF therapies aim at neutralizing TNF-α, therefore preventing it from exerting its pro-inflammatory role (Figure 3A). In RA, anti-TNF treatment was shown to reduce the production of pro-inflammatory cytokines, including IL-1 and IL-6, thus contributing to the disturbance of the crosstalk between those pathology drivers [50]. To date, several monoclonal antibodies have been developed and are approved by the FDA (Food and Drug Administration) in the United States for clinical use since 1998, such as infliximab, followed by adalimumab, certolizumab or golimumab. Adalimumab is a fully recombinant human monoclonal antibody, while infliximab is a chimeric monoclonal antibody made of about 75% of human-derived amino acids and 25% of mouse-derived amino acids. Certolizumab pegol is the only PEGylated TNF inhibitor, where the PEG (polyethylene glycol) attachment allows to increase its half-life in vivo, while it may also contribute to a better pharmacologic distribution into the inflamed arthritic tissues, compared with non-PEGylated antibodies [51]. Despite their effects in reducing the RA symptoms, those chimeric, human, or humanized antibodies are all associated with more or less severe liver injuries [52]. In addition, according to the European Medicines Agency, adalimumab is very frequently associated with infections and infestations, the more recurrent being the ones related to the respiratory tracts, sepsis, candidiasis and influenza [53]. Other side effects include infections of the skin and the urogenital tract;

hematologic affections, like leukopenia and anemia; metabolism and nutrition defects, like lipids and hepatic enzymes increased levels; nervous system infections, like cephalea; gastrointestinal related disorders, including abdominal pain and nausea; musculo-skeletal pain, and injection-site reactions, like erythema. Anti-TNF drugs can also lead to the development of psoriasis-like skin lesions called paradoxical psoriasis, in about 2–5% of the treated patients, a condition, which, unfortunately, frequently requires the complete cessation of the treatment [54]. Moreover, Rotondo et al. suggested that pharmacologic immunosuppressive therapies such as anti-TNF could modify the immune response to Merkel cell Polyomavirus (MCPyV), thus undermining the outcome for positive MCPyV RA patients and increasing the probability of Merkel cell carcinomas (MCC) development, a rare but aggressive neuroendocrine tumor [55]. A Brazilian study also reported another TNF-α blocker adverse effect, as the use of such therapeutic agents was shown to be associated with high risk of active mycobacterial infections in patients with chronic inflammatory arthritis including RA even if they did not present any evidence of latent tuberculosis infection [56].

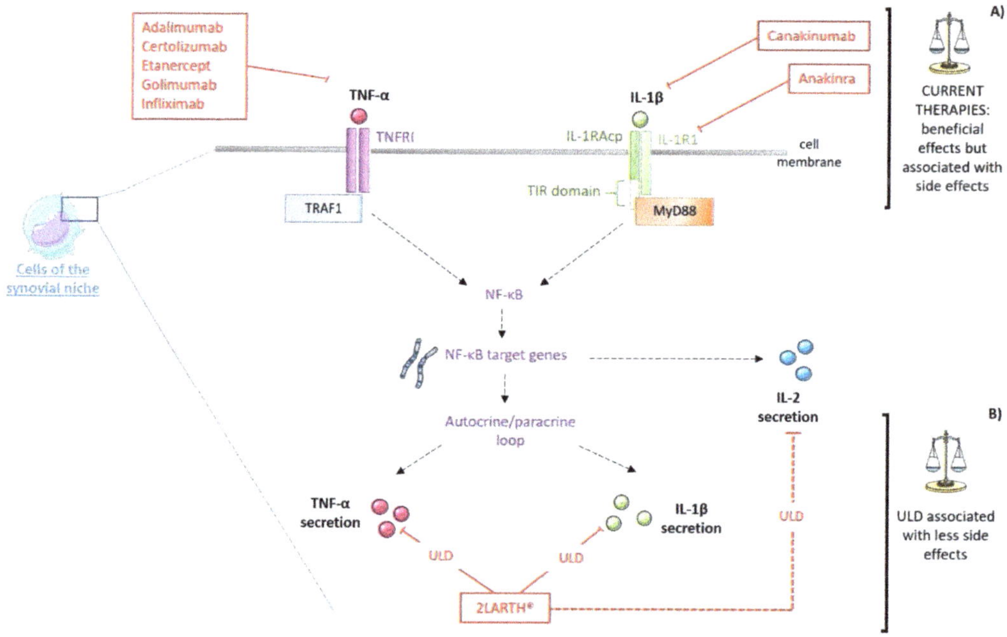

Figure 3. Schematic representation of (**A**) therapeutic targets of current treatments of RA and (**B**) the putative targets of 2LARTH®: IL-1R1: Interleukin-1 type-I receptor; IL-1RAcP: IL-1 receptor accessory protein; MAPK: Mitogen-activated protein kinase; MyD88: Myeloid and differentiation primary response 88; NF-κB: Nuclear factor-κB; TIR: Toll-IL-1 receptor; TNFRI: TNF receptor type 1; TRAF1: TNF receptor-associated factor 1; ULD: Ultra-low dose. Red plain lines represent inhibition mechanisms, red dotted lines represent modulatory mechanisms.

In addition, the TNF-α signalization blockade has also been done by inhibiting the TNF-α binding to its receptor through etanercept, a fully human soluble TNF receptor Fc fusion protein, where a dimer of the extracellular domains of human TNFR2 is fused to the Fc portion of human IgG1. The effectiveness of this drug has been established for the early administration from diagnosis of RA [57,58]. A phase IV study recently assessed the real-world safety and effectiveness of biosimilar etanercept in patients with RA, ankylosing spondylitis or psoriatic arthritis and receiving biosimilar etanercept injections, either 25 mg twice weekly or 50 mg once weekly [59]. The results reported that even if the HAQ (Health

Assessment Questionnaire) scores decreased from 1.32 ± 0.77 at baseline to 0.81 ± 0.61 at 12 months in patients with RA and psoriatic arthritis ($p < 0.01$), some patients still reported adverse effects such as injection-site reactions, abdominal pain and upper respiratory tract infections. The European Medicines Agency reports that the more frequent side effects for this medicine are infections such as bronchitis, cystitis and cutaneous affections, as well as allergic reactions [60].

Interestingly, besides the above-mentioned unwanted side effects, a meta-analysis highlighted that TNF-α antagonists may have a beneficial effect on aortic stiffness, therefore related to cardiovascular risk, which RA patients are more prone to [61].

5. Predictive Markers ... as a New Option towards Personalized Medicine

Along with the development of direct IL-1β and TNF-α inhibition as a therapeutic strategy, attempts were made to use those baseline cytokine levels as predictive biomarkers of RA or markers of treatment responses, allowing for a better stratification of the patients and their clinical care.

IL-1β, IL-2, and TNF-α are undetectable, or at very low levels in human circulation of healthy controls, often under the limit of detection (few pg/mL). Serum levels of IL-1β in healthy subjects were found to be about 3 pg/mL, IL-2 levels of about 14 pg/mL [62,63], and TNF-α levels of about 5 pg/mL [64]. While the circulating levels of those cytokines have been found sometimes higher in RA patients than control groups [64–66], the research is currently still trying to find out the applicability of cytokines as biomarkers in RA [67,68]. In addition, circulating TNF-α and IL-1β levels failed to predict response to rituximab, an anti-CD20 antibody [69]. RA patients with higher basal serum level of several pro-inflammatory cytokines, including IL-1β, IL-2, and TNF-α, were shown to better respond to tocilizumab, an anti-IL-6R treatment [70]. These data highlight the fact that the cytokine profile determination at the time of diagnosis could be used as a tool to orient the treatment strategy. Further in-depth studies are still needed in this area. In line with these results, it has recently been shown that a serum miRNA signature discriminated both RA patients and "at risk individuals" from healthy subjects [71]. The miRNA profiling included eight (miR-126-3p, let-7d-5p, miR-431-3p, miR-221-3p, miR-24-3p, miR130a-3p, miR-339-5p, let-7i-5p) upregulated and one (miR-17-5p) downregulated miRNAs. Interestingly, computational analysis revealed that their predictive targets could be involved in the regulation of inflammatory pathways, including NF-κB signaling, as well as TNF-α and IL-1β.

Regarding their ability to modulate multiple targets at once and to regulate pro-inflammatory pathways and cytokines including TNF-α and IL-1β in autoimmune diseases including RA, miRNAs have also been considered as interesting therapeutic agents on their own [72]. To our knowledge, no direct targeting of IL-1β or TNF-α by such miRNAs have been shown in RA models. Of note, the miR-140-5p has been shown to directly target the 3′UTR region of TNF-α, but this work has been done in a pulmonary arterial hypertension model [73]. Other authors have shown that the simultaneous intra-articular injections of this miRNA with the miR-140-3p ameliorates the RA features [74] and these results are corroborated by the fact that simultaneous overexpression of miR-140-5p and miR-146a in osteoarthritic chondrocytes reduced NF-κb phosphorylation, as well as the expression of TLR4, IL-1β, IL-6, and TNF-α [75]. As an in-depth study of the miRNAs involved in the regulation of these pathways would be worth an entire review, Table 1 provides a non-exhaustive list of some miRNAs which have been shown to be dysregulated in RA, or whom the preclinical data available ultimately lead to a modulation of the TNF-α and/or IL-1β cytokines expression.

Table 1. Non-exhaustive list of miRNAs related to RA pathogenesis and their biological effects on the pro-inflammatory cytokines and factors IL-1β and TNF-α. ND: no data.

miRNA	miRNA Levels in RA	Signaling Pathways/Cytokines Involved or Biological Effects	Authors
126-3-p	up in RA serum	According to the QIAGEN IPA Software, these miRNAs are involved in a network of potential direct and indirect interactions impacting transcription factors and the downstream production of cytokines such as IL-1β and TNF-α.	Cunningham CC et al., 2021 [71]
let-7d-5p	up in RA serum		
431-3p	up in RA serum		
221-3p	up in RA serum		
24-3p	up in RA serum		
130a-3p	up in RA serum		
339-5p	up in RA serum		
let-7i-5p	up in RA serum		
17-5p	down in RA serum		
17-5p	down in erosive RA	MiR-17-5p injections into the paw of arthritic mice induced a reduction of IL-6 and IL-1β, but not TNF-α.	Aurélie Najm et al., 2020 [76]
26b-5p	down in RA serum	MiR-26b-5p mimics treatment alleviated inflammatory responses and reduced Th17 proportion in CIA mice.	Ming-Fei Zhang et al., 2021 [77]
140-5p	ND	Their simultaneous overexpression in Osteoarthritic chondrocytes reduces NF-κb phosphorylation, as well as the expression of TLR4, IL-1β, IL-6 and TNF-α.	Ioanna Papathanasiou et al., 2020 [75]
146a			
140-5p & 140-3p	down in synovial tissues and synovial fibroblasts from RA patients	Intra-articular delivery of these miRNAs ameliorates the clinical and histological features of RA.	Jia-Shiou Peng et al., 2016 [74]
140-5p	ND	The interplay of the miR-140-5p and TNF-α was assessed in a pulmonary arterial hypertension model. The direct targeting of this miRNA towards the TNF-α 3′UTR region was confirmed by Luciferase assays.	Tian-Tian Zhu et al., 2019 [73]
146a	up in CD4+ T cells from RA patients	MiR-146a expression is positively correlated with levels of TNF-α. In vitro studies showed that TNF-α upregulated miR-146a expression in T cells.	Jingyi Li et al., 2010 [78]
363	down in CD4+ T cells from RA patients		
498	down in CD4+ T cells from RA patients		
10a	down in the fibroblast-like synoviocytes of RA patients	MiR-10a downregulation could be triggered by TNF-α and IL-1β and results in the activation of the NF-κB pathway and the promotion of IL-1β, TNF-α, IL-6, IL-8 and MCP-1 expression.	Nan Mu et al., 2016 [79]

Despite the above-mentioned advances in RA treatment and the hope given by a prospective serologic profiling, it is still estimated that about 20–40% of the patients are not good responders to anti-TNF therapies [80]. Such figures reinforce the fact that each therapeutic strategy should be adapted, personalized and open the application field for different cytokine-combining targeting strategies and dosages, such as Micro-Immunotherapy.

6. The Immunotherapy Based on Low Amount of Cytokines

Very few studies reported the use of cytokines at low amounts in clinics. The effect of a low amount IL-2 treatment (1×10^5 IU/3 days) was assessed in vivo and was reported to reduce the severity of vascular and bone lesions in a CIA mice model, when intravenous injections were performed 14 days after the arthritis induction [81]. Moreover, authors showed that the percentage of pro-inflammatory cytokines secreted by spleen cells, such as IFN-γ, IL-17, and TNF-α was significantly reduced by the IL-2 injections. In addition, a prospective clinical study conducted in patients with mild to moderate forms of autoimmune disease, including RA, demonstrated the safety of an injection protocol consisting of a small amount of IL-2 (1×10^6 IU/day) for five days, followed by fortnightly injections for six months [82]. Even if these concentrations are not obtained from centesimal Hahnemannian dilution protocols and a bona-fide sequential kinetic process, their safety for the patients let presume a promising future for the cytokine-based treatment in the context of RA. Regarding the pleiotropic effects of the cytokines and their implication in a broad spectrum of chronic systemic immune-mediated diseases, inhibiting the cell-secretion of such particular mediators through ultra-low delivery of those same exact mediators also seems appealing. Such approaches could be employed either as: (1) therapies on their own, (2) second-line treatments after a first therapy, or (3) scaffold strategies to set up a biological environment allowing a better outcome for future second-line conventional therapies. In the above mentioned (1) context, preliminary clinical, and preclinical studies highlighted the beneficial effects of 2LALERG® as potential preventive MI medicine in patients suffering from allergic airway diseases [83,84]. While in a small number of patients, the double-blind versus placebo study showed that 2LALERG®, when taken two months before the pollinic season, has helped in the management of symptoms, it has worked as well as scaffold therapy (context 3) during the pollinic season, because patients decreased significantly their consumption of antihistamines and intranasal corticosteroids.

The potential effects of MI in the context (1) of chronic infections, such as high-risk human papillomavirus cervical lesions, showed that 2LPAPI®, alone, taken during six months, could induce and/or help in the regression of the cervical lesions, without side effects [85]. In the context (2), a tendency towards a reduced serum level of the cytokine RANTES (regulated upon activation, normal T cells expressed and secreted) was found in patients with systemic immune-mediated diseases undergoing fatty-degenerative osteolysis of the jawbone (FDOJ) surgery and treated with RANTES 27 CH, and no adverse effects were reported by the patients [86]. Surgical removal of FDOJ tissue, highly expressing RANTES, might not be sufficient to recreate the correct immunological environment. By using ULD of that same cytokine after surgery, MI aimed at re-establishing the homeostasis.

Moreover, in the (2) situation, an interesting study reported the positive effects of low dose sequential kinetic activation (SKA) cytokines/antibodies (IL-4, IL-10 and anti-IL-1) orally administered in RA patients who display a low disease activity (LDA) after having been treated with either anti-TNF-α biologic agents and/or DMARDs [87]. Indeed, even if the clinical results were obtained from a small cohort of 34 patients and are not significant, 10 fg/mL/day of the SKA cocktail of cytokines/antibodies allowed a rate of maintenance of LDA of 66.7% versus 42.1% in the DMARD treated group and no side effects were reported.

An in vitro study has been designed to assess the ULD (27 CH) of IL-1β and TNF-α abilities to decrease the TNF-α secretion of human LPS-exposed enriched monocytes after 24 h incubation periods [88]. The results showed a decrease of the TNF-α secretion when the lactose-sucrose pillules impregnated with the 27 CH cytokines, diluted at 11 and 22 mM, were compared with the vehicle-impregnated ones. Interestingly, these results were confirmed in PMA-differentiated THP-1 cells. These anti-inflammatory effects induced by ULD of one cytokine at a time might be explained by the fact that IL-1β and TNF-α are strongly linked by an autocrine positive loop in monocytes after LPS exposure [89]. Taken together, these results support the rationale for the 2LARTH® formula, which was developed to reduce the symptoms of rheumatic pathologies including RA.

7. Micro-Immunotherapy: A Multiple Immune-Targeted Ultra-Low-Dose-Based Strategy to Calm Chronic Inflammation in RA

One of the main challenges of immunotherapy lies in the feasibility of the immune system management by a proper targeting of the immunopathological activity without further affecting the immunosurveillance. Thus, by combining both the advantages of using the immune system players themselves and extremely low dosages, MI could be at a crossroads in the RA treatment too, as the side effects of a conventional treatment would be reduced and/or avoided.

The 2LARTH® is a medicine that was developed to attenuate the symptoms of rheumatic diseases including RA and which is currently notified as a homeopathic medicine under notification number 1507CH36 F1 by the Federal Agency for Medicines and Health Products in Belgium. This medicine consists of different capsules, each one intended to be taken according to the order in which they are packaged in the blister (from 1 to 10), to give daily information to the body. All the capsules are composed of the same cytokines/factors at various ULD depending on the capsule number. Of note, the lactose-sucrose pillules are impregnated with IL-1β at either 10 or 17 CH (i.e., 10–17 CH), TNF-α (10–17 CH), IL-2 (10–12 CH), SNA®-HLA-I (10–16 CH), SNA®-HLA-II (10–16 CH) (conceived to target regions of HLA class I and II genes) and SNA®-ARTH (designed to target the human IL-2 gene at 10–16 CH). The rationale of the HLA-I and HLA-II SNA® targeting relies on the association of RA with key major histocompatibility complexes (MHC) belonging either in type I [90,91], or type II [92,93]. Further studies are still needed to strengthen the knowledge about the effect of these SNA® in the context of RA. The formulation of each capsule of the 2LARTH® is summarized in Table 2.

Table 2. Table summarizing the 2LARTH® formulation and dilutions employed in the different capsules. The dilutions of each cytokine/factor/SNA® at ULD are indicated in CH (Centesimal Hahnemannian). MI medicines are based on the principle that a given immune regulator exerts either stimulatory effects when used at LD or displays modulatory/inhibitory features when prepared at ULD. ULD aim at modulating (from 8 to 12 CH) and lowering (higher than 12 CH) the expression of protein with upregulated levels. HLA: Human Leukocyte Antigen; IL: Interleukin; SNA®: Specific Nucleic Acid; TNF-α: Tumor Necrosis Factor-α; ULD: Ultra-Low Dose.

	2LARTH®	
Ingredients	**Modulatory ULD**	**Inhibitory ULD**
IL-1	10	17
IL-2	10	12
TNF-α	10	17
SNA®-ARTH	10	16
SNA®-HLA-I	10	16
SNA®-HLA-II	10	16

In the same manner as for the evaluation of the anti-inflammatory effects of one single cytokine at a time, IL-1β or TNF-α at 27 CH, Floris et al. reported that 2LARTH® has a significant impact in reducing IL-1β secretion in human enriched monocytes stimulated with LPS [94]. Such effect was noticed at lactose-sucrose concentrations ranging from 5.5 to 22 mM, compared to both untreated and vehicle-LPS stimulated cells. Moreover, the secreted level of TNF-α was also reduced at concentrations ranging from 2.25 to 22 mM in the same conditions, as well as the IL-6 secretion, at 11 and 22 mM. Furthermore, the effects of the treatment have been evaluated in vivo, in a CIA mice model, in which a daily treatment respecting the sequential order of 2LARTH® was administered by oral gavage, starting 30 days after the first immunization [95]. Results showed its efficacy in reducing the clinical score, the degree of edema and the inflammation in treated animals, compared with the control ones. Histological analysis revealed that the synovial hyperplasia was markedly decreased in MI-treated mice, compared to the vehicle group, and the circulating levels of TNF-α decreased too, and were comparable to the healthy control ones.

The "three birds with one stone" strategy of 2LARTH® is illustrated in Figure 3B, as IL-1β, TNF-α, and IL-2 are the principal therapeutic targets, all three used at ULD. We have widely discussed the first two targets, and less dwelt about the third.

Little is known about the genetic background of IL-2 in RA, but it was found that specific diplotypes, meaning the combination of haplotypes from both parents, in occurrence, the IL-2 TG:GG was positively associated with RA in the Turkish population [96]. Interestingly, the implication of this cytokine in joint-related pathologies seems to be dual and its use as a therapeutic target may be approached in a modulatory manner as contradictory data were addressed regarding this cytokine in this particular context. For instance, Paradowska-Gorycka et al. found that patients affected with RA or osteoarthritis have higher serum levels of IL-2 than the healthy controls [97], whereas Wang et al. reported an opposite trend, as the serum level of IL-2 was downregulated in RA patients group compared with healthy one [98].

Beyond the previously discussed mutational background of IL-1β, TNF-α and IL-2 which may predispose to RA development, many epigenetic events also contribute to the fine-tuned regulation of these factors. The plasticity of all these processes ultimately lead to a dynamic panel of pro-inflammatory mediators, highly susceptible to changes over time. A study focused on deciphering if the cytokine profile found in RA patients serum changed over the course of the disease showed that, 3 months after the initial diagnosis, IL-1β was positively correlated with two of the acute phase inflammatory reactants: CRP (C reactive protein) (R^2 = 0.642) and ESR (erythrocyte sedimentation rate) (R^2 = 0.579) [99]. Interestingly, this study also reported that: (i) the levels of IL-1β and IL-2 were both positively correlated (R^2 = 0.829) 6 months post-diagnosis, (ii) IL-1β and TNF levels were not only correlated at the time of the diagnosis (R^2 = 0.956) but also 6 months later (R^2 = 0.847), (iii) IL-2 and TNF showed a positive correlation (R^2 = 0.738) 6 months post-diagnosis too. This study conducted in Poland would need to be generalized to more patients, but it reinforces the fact that a holistic approach to RA treatment, with multiple cytokine targets, could be highly beneficial for patients. These results are in line with the fact that both IL-2 and TNF-α were found to be parts of a specific pro-inflammatory cytokine profile also defined by high levels of CXCL10 and IL-6, characterizing severe outcomes in systemic autoimmune diseases [100].

The wide therapeutic potential of IL-2 in many autoimmune and inflammatory diseases can be illustrated by the fact that, when the dose is high, IL-2 was reported to promote the proliferation of effector T cells, while, when the dose is low, it allowed an activation of the Tregs [101]. In addition, the effect of low dose IL-2 (5 IU/mL) was also shown to inhibit osteoclastogenesis in vitro, a mechanism which is implicated in the bone degradation also occurring in RA [81]. Furthermore, in their study, Yang et al. used the TNF-α-stimulated MH7A cells to show that this stimulation induces both NO and IL-2 production in this "fibroblast-like" synoviocytes, thus reinforcing the modulatory loop existing between TNF-α and IL-2 [102]. As the rationale of using IL-2 in the 2LARTH® is based on its immunomodulatory functions, the 10–12 CH dilution range employed in the sequence of the medicine allows the body's responses to freely adjust by themselves, depending on the organism-specific needs at a particular time (Figure 3B). Moreover, the SNA®-ARTH, which is especially designed to directly target the IL-2 gene, might reinforce and act synergistically with the ULD IL-2.

More preclinical studies are still needed to understand its mode of action, the synergy of its multiple regulators, the benefits of its sequential strategy, and clinical studies are indispensable to confirm and bring out the potential benefit of MI in the context of RA treatment.

8. From the Mouth to the Body: How ULD-Based Medicines Might Act

As the MI delivery route is oromucosal, and the ULD concept is based on a global vision of the body and its internal balance, the crosstalk between the sublingual mucosa cells, the gut tract, and the immune system is a leverage on which this kind of therapy ultimately operates with in order to maintain one's organism inner equilibrium. Moreover, oral immune therapy, as a method of immune systemic modulation, uses the inherited capabilities of the innate system of the gut to readdress both the innate and adaptive immune responses [103]. In line with these considerations, the relationship between TNF-α and the gut epithelium was assessed in transgenic Rag1 mice lacking adaptive T and B cells, in which it was reported that this factor induced enhanced apoptosis in the epithelial cells from the duodenum [104]. In addition, an interesting study correlates the TNF-α serum levels of RA patients with their intestine microbiome [105]. The results showed that *Pelagibacterium* was positively correlated with TNF-α, whereas *Oxalobacter* and *Blautia* were negatively correlated with this factor, suggesting that the gut microflora could be involved in RA progression by altering the cytokine levels. Altogether, these pieces of evidence reinforce the fact that the systemic cytokine modulation occurring in RA could be perpetuated by several integrated factors and that RA treatment could legitimately be considered in a holistic approach, in which the MI has its place.

At cellular levels, MI could be explained by the hormetic dose-specific responses curve characterized by its non-linear shape, when the "stimulus" is tested in a wide range of concentrations. The "hormesis" concept may underpin the cellular adaptation to these ultra-low cell responses, as this notion has been applied to a broad spectrum of independent cellular functions such as proliferation, DNA repair, antioxidant response or autophagy for instance [106]. Hormesis thus characterizes the cellular responses induced by extremely low levels of potentially toxic agents, as adaptive responses of biological systems, in order to improve their functionality and/or tolerance to severe environmental challenges. Hormetic responses are evolutionary-conserved, highly generalizable across phyla and thought to result from multiple integrative signal-transduction processes, thus coordinating a final holistic response. Importantly, hormetic signals originating from a stressed tissue can be transferred to distant tissues or organs, as an overall phenomenon called "remote conditioning" [107]. These manifestations of hormesis have been documented in the context of cardioprotective strategies establishment and pinpointed the remote conditioning as exactly as a systemic response, where (1) the stimulus (chemical substances, electrical signal), (2) the transfer (neuronal and humoral mediators), and (3) the target (receptor activations, transduction pathways within the heart cells) levels were taken into consideration. As RA is also a systemic disease, the hormesis and especially its remote conditioning component could be employed as an explanation of the effectiveness of the ULD used in MI.

9. Conclusions

In conclusion, TNF-α and IL-1β are two key factors involved in the onset and spreading of RA and their increased levels maintain/sustain the chronic inflammation observed both at systemic and articular levels. Their therapeutic targeting is a useful and efficient strategy, as it allows to impair the systemic and synovial-niche cellular crosstalk that they elicit, and which contributes to the pernicious fueling of the pathology. To date, the treatments are still hampered by important side effects and alternative therapies would be of great value for the patients. As a more holistic approach, the MIM claims to restore the body's homeostasis through the use of multiple immunologic agents at ULD (Figure 4). Compared to the single-target approach, MIM 2LARTH® formulation combines together three therapeutic targets: TNF-α, IL-1β, and IL-2, and its ULD-based strategy is promising because it should exert fewer adverse effects. Even if additional preclinical and clinical data are still needed, MIM might be the way to gently intervene, in order to reestablish inner imbalances and to overcome immune diseases such as RA.

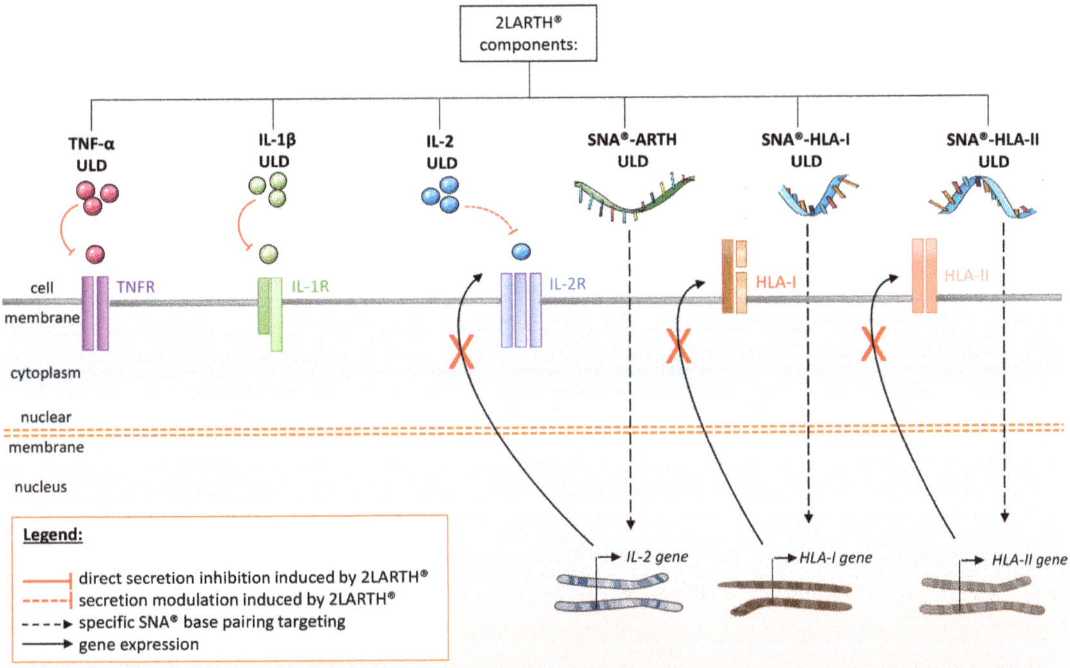

Figure 4. Schematic representation of the multi-targets actions of 2LARTH® within the cells of the synovial niche in rheumatoid arthritis (RA): HLA: Human leukocyte antigen; IL-1R: Interleukin-1 receptor; IL-2R: Interleukin-2 receptor; SNA®: Specific nucleic acid; TNFR: TNF receptor; ULD: Ultra-low dose.

Author Contributions: C.J. wrote the manuscript and prepared the figures. I.F. and B.L. revised the manuscript. All authors have read and agreed to the published version of the manuscript.

Funding: This research received no external funding and was entirely funded by Labo'Life France.

Acknowledgments: The authors thank Paula Carrió for proofreading the final version, and Servier Medical Art (https://smart.servier.com/, accessed date 30 March 2021) for the items used in the figures.

Conflicts of Interest: The authors declare the following potential conflicts of interest with respect to the research, authorship, and/or publication of this article: C.J., I.F. and B.L. work for Labo'Life France, the company service provider of Labo'Life, specialized in preclinical and clinical research, as well as regulatory affairs. This professional relationship does not imply any misconduct on the part of the authors.

Abbreviations

ACPA	Anti-citrullinated peptide antibodies
ACR	American College of Rheumatology
CCP	Cyclic citrullinated peptides
CH	Centesimal Hahnemannian
CIA	Collagen-induced arthritis
COX-2	Cyclooxygenase-2
CRP	C reactive protein
Cx43	Connexin-43
DMARD	Disease-modifying anti-rheumatic drug
ESR	Erythrocyte sedimentation rate
FDA	Food and Drug Administration
FDOJ	Fatty-degenerative osteolysis of the jawbone

GM-CSF	Granulocyte-macrophage colony-stimulating factor
HAQ	Health Assessment Questionnaire
HLA	Human leukocyte antigen
IFN-γ	Interferon-γ
IκB	Inhibitor of nuclear factor-κB
IL-1β	Interleukin-1β
JAK3	Janus-activated kinase 3
LD	Low dose
LDA	Low disease activity
LOX	Lipoxygenase
LPS	Lipopolysaccharide
MAPK	Mitogen-activated protein kinase
MCC	Merkel cell carcinoma
MCPyV	Merkel cell polyomavirus
MHC	Major histocompatibility complex
MI	Micro-immunotherapy
MCP1	Monocyte chemoattractant protein-1
MIM	Micro-immunotherapy medicine
MIP1α	Macrophage inflammatory protein-1 alpha
MMP	Matrix metalloproteinase
MyD88	Myeloid and differentiation primary response 88
NF-κB	Nuclear factor-κB
PBMC	Peripheral blood mononuclear cell
PEG	Polyethylene glycol
PGE2	Prostaglandin E2
RA	Rheumatoid arthritis
RANKL	Receptor activator of nuclear factor-κB ligand
RANTES	Regulated upon activation, normal T cells expressed and secreted
SKA	Sequential kinetic activation
SNA®	Specific nucleic acids
TIR	Toll-IL-1 receptor
TNF-α	Tumor necrosis factor-α
TNFR1	TNF receptor type 1
TRAF1-C5	TNF receptor-associated factor 1 and complement component-5
ULD	Ultra-low dose
VEGF	Vascular endothelial growth factor

References

1. Wolfe, F.; Michaud, K. Predicting depression in rheumatoid arthritis: The signal importance of pain extent and fatigue, and comorbidity. *Arthritis Care Res.* **2009**, *61*, 667–673. [CrossRef] [PubMed]
2. Alamanos, Y.; Drosos, A.A. Epidemiology of adult rheumatoid arthritis. *Autoimmun Rev.* **2005**, *4*, 130–136. [CrossRef] [PubMed]
3. Rudan, I.; Sidhu, S.; Papana, A.; Meng, S.; Xin-Wei, Y.; Wang, W.; Campbell-Page, R.M.; Demaio, A.R.; Nair, H.; Sridhar, D.; et al. Prevalence of rheumatoid arthritis in low- and middle-income countries: A systematic review and analysis. *J. Glob. Health* **2015**, *5*, 010409. [CrossRef] [PubMed]
4. Alamanos, Y.; Voulgari, P.V.; Drosos, A.A. Incidence and prevalence of rheumatoid arthritis, based on the 1987 American College of Rheumatology criteria: A systematic review. *Semin. Arthritis Rheum.* **2006**, *36*, 182–188. [CrossRef] [PubMed]
5. Ridgley, L.A.; Anderson, A.E.; Pratt, A.G. What are the dominant cytokines in early rheumatoid arthritis? *Curr. Opin. Rheumatol.* **2018**, *30*, 207–214. [CrossRef] [PubMed]
6. Singh, J.A.; Saag, K.G.; Bridges, S.L.; Akl, E.A.; Bannuru, R.R.; Sullivan, M.C.; Vaysbrot, E.; McNaughton, C.; Osani, M.; Shmerling, R.H.; et al. 2015 American College of Rheumatology Guideline for the Treatment of Rheumatoid Arthritis. *Arthritis Care Res.* **2016**, *68*, 1–25. [CrossRef]
7. Adis Editorial. *Tofacitinib. Drugs R D* **2010**, *10*, 271–284. [CrossRef]
8. Mousavi, M.J.; Karami, J.; Aslani, S.; Tahmasebi, M.N.; Vaziri, A.S.; Jamshidi, A.; Farhadi, E.; Mahmoudi, M. Transformation of fibroblast-like synoviocytes in rheumatoid arthritis; from a friend to foe. *Autoimmun. Highlights* **2021**, *12*, 3. [CrossRef]
9. Dinarello, C.A. Interleukin-1 in the pathogenesis and treatment of inflammatory diseases. *Blood* **2011**, *117*, 3720–3732. [CrossRef]
10. Weber, A.; Wasiliew, P.; Kracht, M. Interleukin-1 (IL-1) pathway. *Sci. Signal.* **2010**, *3*, cm1. [CrossRef]
11. Lee, E.-G.; Lee, S.; Chae, H.-J.; Park, S.J.; Lee, Y.C.; Yoo, W.-H. Ethyl acetate fraction from Cudrania tricuspidata inhibts IL-1b-induced rheumatoid synovial fibroblast proliferation and MMPs, COX-2 and PGE2 production. *Biol. Res.* **2010**, *43*, 225–231. [CrossRef]

12. Kobayashi, M.; Squires, G.R.; Mousa, A.; Tanzer, M.; Zukor, D.J.; Antoniou, J.; Feige, U.; Poole, A.R. Role of interleukin-1 and tumor necrosis factor α in matrix degradation of human osteoarthritic cartilage. *Arthritis Rheum.* **2005**, *52*, 128–135. [CrossRef]
13. Chen, T.; Zhou, R.; Chen, Y.; Fu, W.; Wei, X.; Ma, G.; Hu, W.; Lu, C. Curcumin ameliorates IL-1β-induced apoptosis by activating autophagy and inhibiting the NF-κB signaling pathway in rat primary articular chondrocytes. *Cell Biol. Int.* **2020**. [CrossRef]
14. Zhang, F.; Wei, K.; Slowikowski, K.; Fonseka, C.Y.; Rao, D.A.; Kelly, S.; Goodman, S.M.; Tabechian, D.; Hughes, L.B.; Salomon-Escoto, K.; et al. Defining inflammatory cell states in rheumatoid arthritis joint synovial tissues by integrating single-cell transcriptomics and mass cytometry. *Nat Immunol.* **2019**, *20*, 928–942. [CrossRef]
15. Allam, I.; Djidjik, R.; Ouikhlef, N.; Louahchi, S.; Raaf, N.; Behaz, N.; Abdessemed, A.; Khaldoun, N.; Tahiat, A.; Bayou, M.; et al. Interleukin-1 and the interleukin-1 receptor antagonist gene polymorphisms study in patients with rheumatoid arthritis. *Pathol. Biol.* **2013**, *61*, 264–268. [CrossRef]
16. Jahid, M.; Rehan-Ul-Haq null Chawla, D.; Avasthi, R.; Ahmed, R.S. Association of polymorphic variants in IL1B gene with secretion of IL-1β protein and inflammatory markers in north Indian rheumatoid arthritis patients. *Gene* **2018**, *641*, 63–67. [CrossRef]
17. Lee, Y.H.; Bae, S.-C. Associations between interleukin-1 and IL-1 receptor antagonist polymorphisms and susceptibility to rheumatoid arthritis: A meta-analysis. *Cell Mol. Biol. (Noisy-le-Grand)* **2015**, *61*, 105–111.
18. Zhu, L.; Chen, P.; Sun, X.; Zhang, S. Associations between Polymorphisms in the IL-1 Gene and the Risk of Rheumatoid Arthritis and Systemic Lupus Erythematosus: Evidence from a Meta-Analysis. *Int. Arch. Allergy Immunol.* **2021**, *182*, 234–242. [CrossRef]
19. Lee, Y.H.; Ji, J.D.; Song, G.G. Association between interleukin 1 polymorphisms and rheumatoid arthritis susceptibility: A metaanalysis. *J. Rheumatol.* **2009**, *36*, 12–15. [CrossRef]
20. Kobayashi, T.; Murasawa, A.; Ito, S.; Yamamoto, K.; Komatsu, Y.; Abe, A.; Sumida, T.; Yoshie, H. Cytokine gene polymorphisms associated with rheumatoid arthritis and periodontitis in Japanese adults. *J. Periodontol.* **2009**, *80*, 792–799. [CrossRef]
21. Harrison, P.; Pointon, J.J.; Chapman, K.; Roddam, A.; Wordsworth, B.P. Interleukin-1 promoter region polymorphism role in rheumatoid arthritis: A meta-analysis of IL-1B-511A/G variant reveals association with rheumatoid arthritis. *Rheumatol. Oxf. Engl.* **2008**, *47*, 1768–1770. [CrossRef]
22. Carswell, E.A.; Old, L.J.; Kassel, R.L.; Green, S.; Fiore, N.; Williamson, B. An endotoxin-induced serum factor that causes necrosis of tumors. *Proc. Natl. Acad. Sci. USA* **1975**, *72*, 3666–3670. [CrossRef]
23. Chen, X.; Bäumel, M.; Männel, D.N.; Zack, O.M.; Oppenheim, J.J. Interaction of TNF with TNF Receptor Type 2 Promotes Expansion and Function of Mouse CD4+CD25+ T Regulatory Cells. *J. Immunol.* **2007**, *179*, 154–161. [CrossRef]
24. Tartaglia, L.A.; Ayres, T.M.; Wong, G.H.W.; Goeddel, D.V. A novel domain within the 55 kd TNF receptor signals cell death. *Cell* **1993**, *74*, 845–853. [CrossRef]
25. Mirza, F.; Lorenzo, J.; Drissi, H.; Lee, F.Y.; Soung, D.Y. Dried plum alleviates symptoms of inflammatory arthritis in TNF transgenic mice. *J. Nutr. Biochem.* **2018**, *52*, 54–61. [CrossRef]
26. Haworth, C.; Brennan, F.M.; Chantry, D.; Turner, M.; Maini, R.N.; Feldmann, M. Expression of granulocyte-macrophage colony-stimulating factor in rheumatoid arthritis: Regulation by tumor necrosis factor-alpha. *Eur. J. Immunol.* **1991**, *21*, 2575–2579. [CrossRef]
27. Paleolog, E.M.; Young, S.; Stark, A.C.; McCloskey, R.V.; Feldmann, M.; Maini, R.N. Modulation of angiogenic vascular endothelial growth factor by tumor necrosis factor alpha and interleukin-1 in rheumatoid arthritis. *Arthritis Rheum.* **1998**, *41*, 1258–1265. [CrossRef]
28. Fatima Rizvi, S.T.; Arif, A.; Azhar, A. TNF gene promoter region polymorphisms and association with young-onset rheumatoid arthritis. *Pak. J. Pharm. Sci.* **2019**, *32*, 2295–2297. [PubMed]
29. Hadinedoushan, H.; Noorbakhsh, P.; Soleymani-Salehabadi, H. Tumor Necrosis Factor Alpha Gene Polymorphism and Association with Its Serum Level in Iranian Population with Rheumatoid Arthritis. *Arch. Rheumatol.* **2016**, *31*, 306–313. [CrossRef] [PubMed]
30. Mohan, V.K.; Ganesan, N.; Gopalakrishnan, R. Association of susceptible genetic markers and autoantibodies in rheumatoid arthritis. *J. Genet.* **2014**, *93*, 597–605. [CrossRef] [PubMed]
31. Panoulas, V.F.; Smith, J.P.; Nightingale, P.; Kitas, G.D. Association of the TRAF1/C5 locus with increased mortality, particularly from malignancy or sepsis, in patients with rheumatoid arthritis. *Arthritis Rheum.* **2009**, *60*, 39–46. [CrossRef]
32. Saeki, N.; Imai, Y. Reprogramming of synovial macrophage metabolism by synovial fibroblasts under inflammatory conditions. *Cell Commun. Signal. CCS* **2020**, *18*. [CrossRef]
33. Speranskii, A.I.; Kostyuk, S.V.; Kalashnikova, E.A.; Veiko, N.N. Enrichment of extracellular DNA from the cultivation medium of human peripheral blood mononuclears with genomic CpG rich fragments results in increased cell production of IL-6 and TNF-a via activation of the NF-kB signaling pathway. *Biomeditsinskaia Khimiia* **2016**, *62*, 331–340. [CrossRef]
34. Schierbeck, H.; Wähämaa, H.; Andersson, U.; Harris, H.E. Immunomodulatory Drugs Regulate HMGB1 Release from Activated Human Monocytes. *Mol. Med.* **2010**, *16*, 343–351. [CrossRef]
35. Matsuki, T.; Arai, Y.; Tsuchida, S.; Terauchi, R.; Oda, R.; Fujiwara, H.; Mazda, O.; Kubo, T. Expression of Connexin 43 in Synovial Tissue of Patients With Rheumatoid Arthritis. *Arch. Rheumatol.* **2015**, *31*, 55–63. [CrossRef]
36. Jing, R.; Ban, Y.; Xu, W.; Nian, H.; Guo, Y.; Geng, Y.; Zang, Y.; Zheng, C. Therapeutic effects of the total lignans from Vitex negundo seeds on collagen-induced arthritis in rats. *Phytomed. Int. J. Phytother. Phytopharm.* **2019**, *58*, 152825. [CrossRef]

37. Lin, B.; Zhang, H.; Zhao, X.-X.; Rahman, K.; Wang, Y.; Ma, X.-Q.; Zheng, C.-J.; Zhang, Q.-Y.; Han, T.; Qin, L.-P. Inhibitory effects of the root extract of Litsea cubeba (lour.) pers. on adjuvant arthritis in rats. *J. Ethnopharmacol.* **2013**, *147*, 327–334. [CrossRef]
38. Rioja, I.; Bush, K.A.; Buckton, J.B.; Dickson, M.C.; Life, P.F. Joint cytokine quantification in two rodent arthritis models: Kinetics of expression, correlation of mRNA and protein levels and response to prednisolone treatment. *Clin. Exp. Immunol.* **2004**, *137*, 65–73. [CrossRef]
39. Williams, R.O.; Marinova-Mutafchieva, L.; Feldmann, M.; Maini, R.N. Evaluation of TNF-α and IL-1 Blockade in Collagen-Induced Arthritis and Comparison with Combined Anti-TNF-α/Anti-CD4 Therapy. *J. Immunol. Am. Assoc. Immunol.* **2000**, *165*, 7240–7245. [CrossRef]
40. Yu, D.; Ye, X.; Che, R.; Wu, Q.; Qi, J.; Song, L.; Guo, X.; Zhang, S.; Wu, H.; Ren, G.; et al. FGF21 exerts comparable pharmacological efficacy with Adalimumab in ameliorating collagen-induced rheumatoid arthritis by regulating systematic inflammatory response. *Biomed. Pharmacother.* **2017**, *89*, 751–760. [CrossRef]
41. Chen, W.; Li, Z.; Wang, Z.; Gao, H.; Ding, J.; He, Z. Intraarticular Injection of Infliximab-Loaded Thermosensitive Hydrogel Alleviates Pain and Protects Cartilage in Rheumatoid Arthritis. *J. Pain Res.* **2020**, *13*, 3315–3329. [CrossRef]
42. Dhimolea, E. Canakinumab. *mAbs.* **2010**, *2*, 3–13. [CrossRef]
43. Alten, R.; Gomez-Reino, J.; Durez, P.; Beaulieu, A.; Sebba, A.; Krammer, G.; Preiss, R.; Arulmani, U.; Widmer, A.; Gitton, X.; et al. Efficacy and safety of the human anti-IL-1beta monoclonal antibody canakinumab in rheumatoid arthritis: Results of a 12-week, phase II, dose-finding study. *BMC Musculoskelet. Disord.* **2011**, *12*, 153. [CrossRef]
44. Ait-Oudhia, S.; Lowe, P.J.; Mager, D.E. Bridging Clinical Outcomes of Canakinumab Treatment in Patients With Rheumatoid Arthritis With a Population Model of IL-1β Kinetics. *CPT Pharmacomet. Syst. Pharmacol.* **2012**, *1*, e5. [CrossRef]
45. Marketos, N.; Bournazos, I.; Ioakimidis, D. Canakinumab for refractory RA: A case report. *Mediterr. J. Rheumatol.* **2018**, *29*, 170–172. [CrossRef]
46. Mertens, M.; Singh, J.A. Anakinra for Rheumatoid Arthritis: A Systematic Review. *J. Rheumatol.* **2009**, *36*, 1118–1125. [CrossRef]
47. Bresnihan, B.; Newmark, R.; Robbins, S.; Genant, H.K. Effects of anakinra monotherapy on joint damage in patients with rheumatoid arthritis. Extension of a 24-week randomized, placebo-controlled trial. *J. Rheumatol.* **2004**, *31*, 1103–1111.
48. Ruscitti, P.; Berardicurti, O.; Cipriani, P.; Giacomelli, R.; TRACK Study Group. Benefits of anakinra versus TNF inhibitors in rheumatoid arthritis and type 2 diabetes: Long-term findings from participants furtherly followed-up in the TRACK study, a multicentre, open-label, randomised, controlled trial. *Clin. Exp. Rheumatol.* **2021**, *39*, 403–406.
49. Cavalli, G.; Dinarello, C.A. Treating rheumatological diseases and co-morbidities with interleukin-1 blocking therapies. *Rheumatol. Oxf. Engl.* **2015**, *54*, 2134–2144. [CrossRef]
50. Charles, P.; Elliott, M.J.; Davis, D.; Potter, A.; Kalden, J.R.; Antoni, C.; Breedveld, F.C.; Smolen, J.S.; Eberl, G.; de Woody, K.; et al. Regulation of cytokines, cytokine inhibitors, and acute-phase proteins following anti-TNF-alpha therapy in rheumatoid arthritis. *J. Immunol.* **1999**, *163*, 1521–1528.
51. Palframan, R.; Airey, M.; Moore, A.; Vugler, A.; Nesbitt, A. Use of biofluorescence imaging to compare the distribution of certolizumab pegol, adalimumab, and infliximab in the inflamed paws of mice with collagen-induced arthritis. *J. Immunol. Methods* **2009**, *348*, 36–41. [CrossRef] [PubMed]
52. Bethesda (MD): National Institute of Diabetes and Digestive and Kidney Diseases. Monoclonal Antibodies. Available online: https://www.ncbi.nlm.nih.gov/books/NBK548844/ (accessed on 30 December 2020).
53. Annexe I Résumé des Caractéristiques du Produit. Available online: https://www.ema.europa.eu/en/documents/product-information/humira-epar-product-information_fr.pdf (accessed on 3 May 2021).
54. Nidegger, A.; Mylonas, A.; Conrad, C. Paradoxical psoriasis induced by anti-TNF—A clinical challenge. *Rev. Med. Suisse* **2019**, *15*, 668–671. [PubMed]
55. Rotondo, J.C.; Bononi, I.; Puozzo, A.; Govoni, M.; Foschi, V.; Lanza, G.; Gafà, R.; Gaboriaud, P.; Touzé, F.A.; Selvatici, R.; et al. Merkel Cell Carcinomas Arising in Autoimmune Disease Affected Patients Treated with Biologic Drugs, Including Anti-TNF. *Clin. Cancer Res. Off. J. Am. Assoc. Cancer Res.* **2017**, *23*, 3929–3934. [CrossRef] [PubMed]
56. Gomes, C.M.F.; Terreri, M.T.; Moraes-Pinto MI de Barbosa, C.; Machado, N.P.; Melo, M.R.; Pinheiro, M.M. Incidence of active mycobacterial infections in Brazilian patients with chronic inflammatory arthritis and negative evaluation for latent tuberculosis infection at baseline–a longitudinal analysis after using TNFa blockers. *Mem. Inst. Oswaldo Cruz.* **2015**, *110*, 921–928. [CrossRef]
57. Moreland, L.W.; Baumgartner, S.W.; Schiff, M.H.; Tindall, E.A.; Fleischmann, R.M.; Weaver, A.L.; Ettlinger, R.E.; Cohen, S.; Koopman, W.J.; Mohler, K.; et al. Treatment of Rheumatoid Arthritis with a Recombinant Human Tumor Necrosis Factor Receptor (p75)–Fc Fusion Protein. *N. Engl. J. Med.* **1997**, *337*, 141–147. [CrossRef]
58. Hayashi, S.; Matsubara, T.; Fukuda, K.; Funahashi, K.; Hashimoto, M.; Maeda, T.; Kamenaga, T.; Takashima, Y.; Matsumoto, T.; Niikura, T.; et al. Predictive factors for effective selection of Interleukin-6 inhibitor and tumor necrosis factor inhibitor in the treatment of rheumatoid arthritis. *Sci. Rep.* **2020**, *10*. [CrossRef]
59. Gharibdoost, F.; Salari, A.-H.; Salesi, M.; Ebrahimi Chaharom, F.; Mottaghi, P.; Hosseini, M.; Sahebari, M.; Nazarinia, M.; Mirfeizi, Z.; Shakibi, M.; et al. Assessment of Treatment Safety and Quality of Life in Patients Receiving Etanercept Biosimilar for Autoimmune Arthritis (ASQA): A Multicenter Post-marketing Surveillance Study. *Adv. Ther.* **2021**, *38*, 1290–1300. [CrossRef]
60. Annexe I Résumé des Caractéristiques du Produit. Available online: https://ec.europa.eu/health/documents/community-register/2019/20191114146217/anx_146217_fr.pdf (accessed on 3 May 2021).

61. Vlachopoulos, C.; Gravos, A.; Georgiopoulos, G.; Terentes-Printzios, D.; Ioakeimidis, N.; Vassilopoulos, D.; Stamatelopoulos, K.; Tousoulis, D. The effect of TNF-a antagonists on aortic stiffness and wave reflections: A meta-analysis. *Clin. Rheumatol.* **2018**, *37*, 515–526. [CrossRef]
62. Kleiner, G.; Marcuzzi, A.; Zanin, V.; Monasta, L.; Zauli, G. Cytokine levels in the serum of healthy subjects. *Mediat. Inflamm.* **2013**, *2013*, 434010. [CrossRef]
63. Italiani, P.; Puxeddu, I.; Napoletano, S.; Scala, E.; Melillo, D.; Manocchio, S.; Angiolillo, A.; Migliorini, P.; Boraschi, D.; Vitale, E.; et al. Circulating levels of IL-1 family cytokines and receptors in Alzheimer's disease: New markers of disease progression? *J. Neuroinflamm.* **2018**, *15*, 342. [CrossRef]
64. Thilagar, S.; Theyagarajan, R.; Sudhakar, U.; Suresh, S.; Saketharaman, P.; Ahamed, N. Comparison of serum tumor necrosis factor-α levels in rheumatoid arthritis individuals with and without chronic periodontitis: A biochemical study. *J. Indian Soc. Periodontol.* **2018**, *22*, 116–121. [CrossRef]
65. Al-Saadany, H.M.; Hussein, M.S.; Gaber, R.A.; Zaytoun, H.A. Th-17 cells and serum IL-17 in rheumatoid arthritis patients: Correlation with disease activity and severity. *Egypt Rheumatol.* **2016**, *38*, 1–7. [CrossRef]
66. Tukaj, S.; Kotlarz, A.; Jóźwik, A.; Smoleńska, Z.; Bryl, E.; Witkowski, J.M.; Lipińska, B. Cytokines of the Th1 and Th2 type in sera of rheumatoid arthritis patients; correlations with anti-Hsp40 immune response and diagnostic markers. *Acta Biochim. Pol.* **2010**, *57*, 327–332. [CrossRef]
67. Dissanayake, K.; Jayasinghe, C.; Wanigasekara, P.; Sominanda, A. Potential applicability of cytokines as biomarkers of disease activity in rheumatoid arthritis: Enzyme-linked immunosorbent spot assay-based evaluation of TNF-α, IL-1β, IL-10 and IL-17A. *PLoS ONE* **2021**, *16*, e0246111. [CrossRef]
68. Centola, M.; Cavet, G.; Shen, Y.; Ramanujan, S.; Knowlton, N.; Swan, K.A.; Turner, M.; Sutton, C.; Smith, D.R.; Haney, D.J.; et al. Development of a multi-biomarker disease activity test for rheumatoid arthritis. *PLoS ONE* **2013**, *8*, e60635. [CrossRef]
69. Fabre, S.; Guisset, C.; Tatem, L.; Dossat, N.; Dupuy, A.M.; Cohen, J.D.; Cristol, J.P.; Daures, J.P.; Jorgensen, C. Protein biochip array technology to monitor rituximab in rheumatoid arthritis. *Clin. Exp. Immunol.* **2009**, *155*, 395–402. [CrossRef]
70. Avdeev, A.S.; Novikov, A.A.; Aleksandrova, E.N.; Panasiuk, E.I.; Nasonov, E.L. The importance of cytokine profile characteristics for evaluating the therapeutic effectiveness of monoclonal antibodies against IL-6 receptors in patients with rheumatoid arthritis. *Klin. Med.* **2014**, *92*, 28–34.
71. Cunningham, C.C.; Wade, S.; Floudas, A.; Orr, C.; McGarry, T.; Wade, S.; Cregan, S.; Fearon, U.; Veale, D.J. Serum miRNA Signature in Rheumatoid Arthritis and "At-Risk Individuals". *Front Immunol.* **2021**, *12*. [CrossRef]
72. Salvi, V.; Gianello, V.; Tiberio, L.; Sozzani, S.; Bosisio, D. Cytokine Targeting by miRNAs in Autoimmune Diseases. *Front. Immunol.* **2019**, *10*, 15. [CrossRef]
73. Zhu, T.-T.; Zhang, W.-F.; Yin, Y.-L.; Liu, Y.-H.; Song, P.; Xu, J.; Zhang, M.-X.; Li, P. MicroRNA-140-5p targeting tumor necrosis factor-α prevents pulmonary arterial hypertension. *J. Cell Physiol.* **2019**, *234*, 9535–9550. [CrossRef]
74. Peng, J.-S.; Chen, S.-Y.; Wu, C.-L.; Chong, H.-E.; Ding, Y.-C.; Shiau, A.-L.; Wang, C.-R. Amelioration of Experimental Autoimmune Arthritis Through Targeting of Synovial Fibroblasts by Intraarticular Delivery of MicroRNAs 140-3p and 140-5p. *Arthritis Rheumatol.* **2016**, *68*, 370–381. [CrossRef] [PubMed]
75. Papathanasiou, I.; Balis, C.; Trachana, V.; Mourmoura, E.; Tsezou, A. The synergistic function of miR-140-5p and miR-146a on TLR4-mediated cytokine secretion in osteoarthritic chondrocytes. *Biochem. Biophys. Res. Commun.* **2020**, *522*, 783–791. [CrossRef] [PubMed]
76. Najm, A.; Masson, F.-M.; Preuss, P.; Georges, S.; Ory, B.; Quillard, T.; Sood, S.; Goodyear, C.S.; Veale, D.J.; Fearon, U.; et al. MicroRNA-17-5p Reduces Inflammation and Bone Erosions in Mice with Collagen-Induced Arthritis and Directly Targets the JAK/STAT Pathway in Rheumatoid Arthritis Fibroblast-like Synoviocytes. *Arthritis Rheumatol.* **2020**, *72*, 2030–2039. [CrossRef] [PubMed]
77. Zhang, M.-F.; Yang, P.; Shen, M.-Y.; Wang, X.; Gao, N.-X.; Zhou, X.-P.; Zhou, L.-L.; Lu, Y. MicroRNA-26b-5p alleviates murine collagen-induced arthritis by modulating Th17 cell plasticity. *Cell Immunol.* **2021**, *365*, 104382. [CrossRef]
78. Li, J.; Wan, Y.; Guo, Q.; Zou, L.; Zhang, J.; Fang, Y.; Zhang, J.; Zhang, J.; Fu, X.; Liu, H.; et al. Altered microRNA expression profile with miR-146a upregulation in CD4+ T cells from patients with rheumatoid arthritis. *Arthritis Res. Ther.* **2010**, *12*, R81. [CrossRef]
79. Mu, N.; Gu, J.; Huang, T.; Zhang, C.; Shu, Z.; Li, M.; Hao, Q.; Li, W.; Zhang, W.; Zhao, J.; et al. A novel NF-κB/YY1/microRNA-10a regulatory circuit in fibroblast-like synoviocytes regulates inflammation in rheumatoid arthritis. *Sci. Rep.* **2016**, *6*. [CrossRef]
80. Fabre, S.; Dupuy, A.M.; Dossat, N.; Guisset, C.; Cohen, J.D.; Cristol, J.P.; Daures, J.P.; Jorgensen, C. Protein biochip array technology for cytokine profiling predicts etanercept responsiveness in rheumatoid arthritis. *Clin. Exp. Immunol.* **2008**, *153*, 188–195. [CrossRef]
81. Sun, H.; Zhao, Y.; Wang, K.; Zhu, L.; Dong, J.; Zhao, J.; Wang, Y.; Li, H.; Sun, X.; Lu, Y. Low dose IL-2 suppress osteoclastogenesis in collagen-induced arthritis via JNK dependent pathway. *Immun. Inflamm. Dis.* **2020**, *8*, 727–735. [CrossRef]
82. Rosenzwajg, M.; Lorenzon, R.; Cacoub, P.; Pham, H.P.; Pitoiset, F.; El Soufi, K.; RIbet, C.; Bernard, C.; Aractingi, S.; Banneville, B.; et al. Immunological and clinical effects of low-dose interleukin-2 across 11 autoimmune diseases in a single, open clinical trial. *Ann. Rheum. Dis.* **2019**, *78*, 209–217. [CrossRef]
83. Van der Brempt, X.; Cumps, J.; Capieaux, E. Efficacité clinique du 2L®ALERG, un nouveau traitement de type immunomodulateur par voie sublinguale dans le rhume des foins: Une étude en double insu contre placebo. *Rev. Fr. Allergol.* **2011**, *51*, 430–436. [CrossRef]

84. Floris, I.; Chenuet, P.; Togbe, D.; Volteau, C.; Lejeune, B. Potential Role of the Micro-Immunotherapy Medicine 2LALERG in the Treatment of Pollen-Induced Allergic Inflammation. *Dose-Response* **2020**, *18*. [CrossRef]
85. Thomas, G.; Cluzel, H.; Lafon, J.; Bruhwyler, J.; Lejeune, B. Efficacy of 2LPAPI®, a micro-immunotherapy drug, in patients with high-risk papillomavirus genital infection. *Adv. Infect. Dis.* **2016**, *06*, 7–14. [CrossRef]
86. Floris, I.; Lechner, J.; Lejeune, B. Follow-up of patients with systemic immunological diseases undergoing fatty-degenerative osteolysis of the jawbone surgery and treated with RANTES 27CH. *J. Biol. Regul. Homeost. Agents* **2018**, *32*, 37–45. Available online: https://www.biolifesas.org/biolife/2018/10/03/follow-up-of-patients-with-systemic-immunological-diseases-undergoing-fatty-degenerative-osteolysis-of-the-jawbone-surgery-and-treated-with-rantes-27ch/ (accessed on 3 March 2021).
87. Martin-Martin, L.; Giovannangeli, F.; Bizzi, E.; Massafra, U.; Ballanti, E.; Cassol, M.; Migliore, A. An open randomized active-controlled clinical trial with low-dose SKA cytokines versus DMARDs evaluating low disease activity maintenance in patients with rheumatoid arthritis. *Drug Des. Dev. Ther.* **2017**, *11*, 985–994. [CrossRef]
88. Floris, I.; Rose, T.; Rojas, J.A.C.; Appel, K.; Roesch, C.; Lejeune, B. Pro-inflammatory cytokines at ultra-low dose exert anti-inflammatory effect in vitro: A possible mode of action involving sub-micron particles? *Dose-Response* **2020**, *18*. [CrossRef]
89. Gane, J.M.; Stockley, R.A.; Sapey, E. TNF-α autocrine feedback loops in human monocytes: The pro- and anti-inflammatory roles of the TNF-α receptors support the concept of selective TNFR1 blockade in vivo. *J. Immunol. Res.* **2016**, *2016*. [CrossRef]
90. Regueiro, C.; Casares-Marfil, D.; Lundberg, K.; Knevel, R.; Acosta-Herrera, M.; Rodriguez-Rodriguez, L.; Lopez-Mejias, R.; Perez-Pampin, E.; Triguero-Martinez, A.; Nuño, L.; et al. HLA-B*08 Identified as the Most Prominently Associated Major Histocompatibility Complex Locus for Anti-Carbamylated Protein Antibody-Positive/Anti-Cyclic Citrullinated Peptide-Negative Rheumatoid Arthritis. *Arthritis Rheumatol.* **2020**. [CrossRef]
91. Aslam, M.M.; John, P.; Fan, K.-H.; Bhatti, A.; Aziz, W.; Ahmed, B.; Feingold, E.; Demirci, F.Y.; Kamboh, M.I. Investigating the GWAS-Implicated Loci for Rheumatoid Arthritis in the Pakistani Population. *Dis. Markers* **2020**. [CrossRef]
92. Huang, Z.; Niu, Q.; Yang, B.; Zhang, J.; Yang, M.; Xu, H.; Cai, B.; Hu, J.; Wu, Y.; Wang, L. Genetic polymorphism of rs9277535 in HLA-DP associated with rheumatoid arthritis and anti-CCP production in a Chinese population. *Clin. Rheumatol.* **2018**, *37*, 1799–1805. [CrossRef]
93. Wan, X.; Wang, Y.; Jin, P.; Zhang, J.; Liu, L.; Wang, Z.; Hu, Y. Influence of HLA Class II Alleles and DRB1-DQB1 Haplotypes on Rheumatoid Arthritis Susceptibility and Autoantibody Status in the Chinese Han Population. *Immunol. Investig.* **2021**, 1–13. [CrossRef]
94. Floris, I.; Appel, K.; Rose, T.; Lejeune, B. 2LARTH®, a micro-immunotherapy medicine, exerts anti-inflammatory effects in vitro and reduces TNF-α and IL-1β secretion. *J. Inflamm. Res.* **2018**, *11*, 397–405. [CrossRef]
95. Floris, I.; García-González, V.; Palomares, B.; Appel, K.; Lejeune, B. The micro-immunotherapy medicine 2LARTH® reduces inflammation and symptoms of rheumatoid arthritis in vivo. *Int. J. Rheumatol.* **2020**, *2020*, 1594573. [CrossRef]
96. Yucel, B.; Sumer, C.; Gok, I.; Karkucak, M.; Alemdaroglu, E.; Ucar, F. Associations between cytokine gene polymorphisms and rheumatoid arthritis in Turkish population. *North. Clin. Istanb.* **2020**, *7*, 563–571. [CrossRef]
97. Paradowska-Gorycka, A.; Wajda, A.; Romanowska-Próchnicka, K.; Walczuk, E.; Kuca-Warnawin, E.; Kmiolek, T.; Stypinska, B.; Rzeszotarska, E.; Majewski, D.; Jagodzinski, P.P.; et al. Th17/Treg-Related Transcriptional Factor Expression and Cytokine Profile in Patients with Rheumatoid Arthritis. *Front. Immunol.* **2020**, *11*. [CrossRef]
98. Wang, P.; Chi, S.; Wang, X.; Cui, Z.; Zhang, Y. Reduction of follicular regulatory T cells is associated with occurrence and development of rheumatoid arthritis. *Xi Bao Yu Fen Zi Mian Yi Xue Za Zhi Chin. J. Cell. Mol. Immunol.* **2021**, *37*, 152–157.
99. Brzustewicz, E.; Henc, I.; Daca, A.; Szarecka, M.; Sochocka-Bykowska, M.; Witkowski, J.; Bryl, E. Autoantibodies, C-reactive protein, erythrocyte sedimentation rate and serum cytokine profiling in monitoring of early treatment. *Cent.-Eur. J. Immunol* **2017**, *42*, 259–268. [CrossRef]
100. Simon, Q.; Grasseau, A.; Boudigou, M.; Le Pottier, L.; Bettachioli, E.; Cornec, D.; Rouvière, B.; Jamin, C.; Le Lann, L.; PRECISESADS Clinical Consortium; et al. A cytokine network profile delineates a common Th1/Be1 pro-inflammatory group of patients in four systemic autoimmune diseases. *Arthritis Rheumatol.* **2021**. [CrossRef]
101. Klatzmann, D.; Abbas, A.K. The promise of low-dose interleukin-2 therapy for autoimmune and inflammatory diseases. *Nat. Rev. Immunol.* **2015**, *15*, 283–294. [CrossRef]
102. Yang, L.; Liu, R.; Fang, Y.; He, J. Anti-inflammatory effect of phenylpropanoids from Dendropanax dentiger in TNF-α-induced MH7A cells via inhibition of NF-κB, Akt and JNK signaling pathways. *Int. Immunopharmacol.* **2021**, *94*, 107463. [CrossRef]
103. Ilan, Y. Oral immune therapy: Targeting the systemic immune system via the gut immune system for the treatment of inflammatory bowel disease. *Clin. Transl. Immunol.* **2016**, *5*, e60. [CrossRef]
104. McGhee, J.R.; Fujihashi, K. Inside the Mucosal Immune System. *PLoS Biol.* **2012**, *5*, e1001397. [CrossRef]
105. Li, Y.; Zhang, S.-X.; Yin, X.-F.; Zhang, M.-X.; Qiao, J.; Xin, X.-H.; Chang, M.-J.; Gao, C.; Li, Y.-F.; Li, X.-F. The Gut Microbiota and Its Relevance to Peripheral Lymphocyte Subpopulations and Cytokines in Patients with Rheumatoid Arthritis. *J. Immunol. Res.* **2021**, *2021*. [CrossRef] [PubMed]
106. Calabrese, E.J.; Mattson, M.P. How does hormesis impact biology, toxicology, and medicine? *NPJ Aging Mech. Dis.* **2017**, *3*. [CrossRef] [PubMed]
107. Kleinbongard, P.; Skyschally, A.; Heusch, G. Cardioprotection by remote ischemic conditioning and its signal transduction. *Pflug. Arch.* **2017**, *469*, 159–181. [CrossRef] [PubMed]

International Journal of
Molecular Sciences

MDPI

Review

Vascular Endothelial Growth Factor Biology and Its Potential as a Therapeutic Target in Rheumatic Diseases

Thi Hong Van Le and Sang-Mo Kwon *

Laboratory for Vascular Medicine and Stem Cell Biology, Convergence Stem Cell Research Center, Medical Research Institute, Department of Physiology, School of Medicine, Pusan National University, Yangsan 50612, Korea; lethihongvan25121978@gmail.com

* Correspondence: smkwon323@pusan.ac.kr; Tel.: +82-51-510-8072

Abstract: Rheumatic diseases constitute a diversified group of diseases distinguished by arthritis and often involve other organs. The affected individual has low quality of life, productivity even life-threatening in some severe conditions. Moreover, they impose significant economic and social burdens. In recent years, the patient outcome has been improved significantly due to clearer comprehension of the pathology of rheumatic diseases and the effectiveness of "treat to target" therapies. However, the high cost and the adverse effects are the concerns and full remissions are not often observed. One of the main processes that contributes to the pathogenesis of rheumatic diseases is angiogenesis. Vascular endothelial growth factor (VEGF), a central mediator that regulates angiogenesis, has different isoforms and functions in various physiological processes. Increasing evidence suggests an association between the VEGF system and rheumatic diseases. Anti-VEGF and VEGF receptor (VEGFR) therapies have been used to treat several cancers and eye diseases. This review summarizes the current understanding of VEGF biology and its role in the context of rheumatic diseases, the contribution of VEGF bioavailability in the pathogenesis of rheumatic diseases, and the potential implications of therapeutic approaches targeting VEGF for these diseases.

Keywords: VEGF; rheumatic diseases; therapeutic target

Citation: Le, T.H.V.; Kwon, S.-M. Vascular Endothelial Growth Factor Biology and Its Potential as a Therapeutic Target in Rheumatic Diseases. *Int. J. Mol. Sci.* **2021**, *22*, 5387. https://doi.org/10.3390/ijms22105387

Academic Editor: Chih-Hsin Tang

Received: 14 April 2021
Accepted: 18 May 2021
Published: 20 May 2021

1. Introduction

The most common rheumatic diseases are characterized by joint inflammation and may involve peri-articular tissues, including tendons, ligaments, bones, and muscles. Other organs, such as the skin, heart, vasculature, eyes, lungs, brain, and intestinal tract may also be affected [1,2]. There are more than 200 degenerative, inflammatory, and autoimmune conditions [3]. Musculoskeletal diseases are one of the top reasons of disability worldwide [4]. The quality of life of affected individuals is lowered significantly. The etiology of rheumatic diseases is often unclear. Additionally, there are many things that need to be clarified in the pathogenesis of rheumatic diseases. So, the therapy treatment in rheumatic diseases has many challenges. Although, in recent decades, the new biologic agents have dramatically changed the prognosis and outcome of some autoimmune arthritis diseases [3]. A clearer understanding of the role of VEGF in skeletal development and growth, also its role of the pathogenesis of rheumatic diseases, may contribute to the development of potentially effective therapies. In this review, we focus on rheumatoid arthritis (RA), osteoarthritis (OA), ankylosing spondyloarthritis (AS), systemic lupus erythematosus (SLE), systemic sclerosis (SSc), and Sjögren syndrome (SS).

Angiogenesis, the development of new vessels from the current ones, is the principal driver of synovitis, the prominent hallmark of rheumatic diseases [5,6]. Nutrients and oxygen supplied via the new vessels augment the inflammatory mass. New vessels forming include several steps. This process occurs when endothelial cells are activated by angiogenic factors that are released during angiogenesis. Subsequently, a series of events happen including proteolytic enzyme secretion, extracellular matrix degradation, endothelial cell migration, and new basement formation, respectively [7].

VEGF participates in almost all steps of angiogenesis [8]. Emerging evidence has shown that VEGF contributes significantly to the pathogenesis of many disorders such as RA, autoimmune diseases because of its role in angiogenesis [5]. Several therapies targeting the VEGF pathway have been used in cancers and diabetic retinopathy treatment [9]. In several rheumatic diseases, anti-VEGF therapies or in the combination with current treatment are experimented in the animal disease model and the results of these studies are promising. We reviewed our present knowledge of VEGF biology and its relationship with the pathogenesis of rheumatic diseases by collecting some data sources, including basic studies, clinical studies, and clinical trials with a particular focus on RA, AS, OA, SLE, SSc, and SS.

2. VEGF Biology and Its Role in Musculoskeletal Physiology

2.1. VEGF Biology

In 1983, Senger et al. first isolated and defined VPF (vascular permeability factor), an original name of VEGF. VEGF is a homodimeric protein with 34–42 kDa in molecular weight [10]. From this, many studies contribute to a clearer understanding of the structure, physiological activities, and its role in pathological conditions. Vascular endothelial growth factor (VEGF, also known as VPF) function as a mitogen specifies in endothelial cells [11]. The role of VEGF in physiological and pathological activities is no doubt. VEGF activity is not limited to the vascular system; VEGF also participates in other physiological activities related to the growth of the fetus, bone, and reproductive system [12,13]. Moreover, VEGF plays an important role in the development of various diseases including tumors forming, hematologic cancer, ocular diseases in diabetes, inflammation, brain edema, and a group of obstetrics and gynecology diseases such as polycystic ovary syndrome, endometriosis, and preeclampsia [12].

In mammals, VEGF-A, -B, -C, -D, and placental growth factor (PlGF) are the members of the VEGF family. VEGF-A has been described as a central regulator of angiogenesis and currently its data are the largest compared to other VEGF members [12]. VEGF121, VEGF165 (VEGF164 in mice), VEGF189, and VEGF206 are its various isoforms, and the major characteristic that differentiates the isoforms is their affinity for heparin [13–15]. VEGF-B strongly expresses in the heart and muscle and contributes to the proliferation of endothelial cells [16], while lymphangiogenesis is regulated by VEGF-C and -D [17].

VEGF receptors consist of distinguished tyrosine kinases (RTKs), VEGFR-1 (Flt-1), VEGFR-2 (KDR/Flk-1), and VEGFR-3 (Flt-4). Their expression varies in various tissues, a pathological condition. There is a difference in the binding position of every isoform. VEGF-A binds to VEGFR-1 and VEGFR-2. VEGF-B and PlGF bind to VEGFR-1. VEGF-C and VEGF-D bind to VEGFR-2 and VEGFR-3 [12]. VEGF-A was initially described as a VPF [10] and shows the role in angiogenesis and mitogenesis [18]. Neuropilin-1 (NRP1) and -2 (NRP2) are co-receptors of VEGFR-1. NRP1 serves as a receptor and binds to the collapsin-semaphorin family, and is required for vascular development [19]. Soker et al. showed that NRP1 is found on endothelial cells and tumor cell surfaces and binds to VEGF165. NRP-1 null mice showed embryonic lethality, suggesting that NRP1 is an essential factor in the growth of the vascular system [20].

VEGF is produced by many types of cells, including fibroblasts [21], macrophages [22], endothelial cells [23], neutrophils [24] and T cells [25]. Various factors regulate VEGF expression including oxygen tension, growth factors, oncogenes, cytokine and cell-bound stimuli, and in turn by VEGF-driven signaling [26–28]. Low oxygen tension induces VEGF mRNA expression in various pathophysiological conditions. Subsequently, HIF-1, a central regulator of hypoxia response, regulates the VEGF expression [29]. Several growth factors provoke VEGF mRNA expression including epidermal growth factor (EGF), transforming growth factor-α, transforming growth factor-β (TGF-β), keratinocyte growth factor, insulin-like growth factor, and cytokines such as interleukin (IL)-1 and IL-6 also contribute to the VEGF regulation [13,26].

The understanding of VEGF has seen significant achievement in recent decades, contributing to the development of new therapies in some special diseases such as cancer or retinopathy. To date, many drugs targeting VEGF pathways have been indicated in a variety of disease conditions with desired effects. In 2004, the first agent approved by the FDA was bevacizumab, a humanized form of anti-VEGF Ab, indicated in metastatic colon cancer [30], and 2 years later, ranibizumab, a recombinant antibody fragment from human, showed the effectiveness in intraocular for age-related macular degeneration treatment [31], Ziv-aflibercept (targets: VEGF-A, VEGF-B, and PlGF), ramucirumab (target: VEGFR-2), and multiple tyrosine kinase inhibitors are indicated in combination with other therapies for various cancers [32]. Pegaptanib, an RNA aptamer, directs against VEGF with a high affinity with the target molecule [33]. In a recent study, faricimab, an antibody that inhibits both VEGF-A and Ang-2, was also shown to be effective and safe in diabetic macular edema in phase II clinical trials [34]. The barrier of anti-VEGF therapies is the concerns about the side effect. The adverse effect of this therapy also reduces considerably by local administration because of the dramatically lower dose compared to systemic administration. Thus, this is a crucial suggestion for various disease studies such as arthritis [30,35]. Currently, several ongoing studies and human clinical trials have focused on VEGF pathways and their combination with other therapies in numerous diseases.

2.2. VEGF in the Musculoskeletal System

Rheumatic diseases are inflammatory diseases that involve various organs and present articular and extra-articular manifestations. Many studies have shown the role of VEGF in various activities of the musculoskeletal system in physiology, pathology condition, and other processes related to the pathogenesis of rheumatic diseases. Besides the uncontroversial role of VEGF in angiogenesis during fetus, organ development, VEGF also showed its crucial role in other aspects of synoviocytes, bone development including endochondral ossification, osteoblast, and osteoclast differentiation. Synovium is a part of the structure of a joint that is a remarkable injury position in rheumatic diseases. VEGF-NRP1 axis regulates the synoviocyte apoptotic process [36]. One of the fundamental processes in the bone development and growth is the process that cartilage is replaced by bone, called endochondral ossification. VEGF also showed the material regulator of this process [37]. In mice, chondrocytes survival and differentiation require the role of VEGF [38]. VEGF expression increases during osteoblast differentiation. VEGF enhances the proliferation of osteoblast [39,40]. Increased bone resorption, one of the characteristics of almost all rheumatic diseases, causes permanent injuries in the bone. VEGF may increase bone resorption by increasing osteoclast activity through its action on VEGFR-1 [41], VEGFR-2 signaling [42,43]. This may be mediated via the interaction of VEGFR and receptor activator of nuclear factor kappa-B ligand [41]. Nakagawa et al. showed that mature osteoclast survival requires the VEGF [43]. Immune cells play an important role in the pathology of autoimmune arthritis, and dysregulation of the immune response is a prominent feature. VEGF directly affects immune cells [44]. VEGF affects inflammatory processes in various ways. In lymphatic endothelial cells, this study observed VEGFR-3 expression and it generates the main signal for lymphangiogenesis. VEGFR1 also exist in the macrophages that produce the cytokine/chemokine. This VEGFR-1-macrophage axis stimulates non-inflammatory and inflammatory responses in arthritis [45]. In RA and OA, synovium showed that HIF-1 and HIF-2, the essential regulators of VEGF signaling, express abundantly [46]. Taken together, VEGF appears to be a considerable factor that contributes to the pathogenesis and various aspects of rheumatic diseases.

3. VEGF in RA

RA is a systemic inflammatory disease characterized by not only chronic synovial membrane (SM) inflammation, cartilage damage, bone erosion, but also other organ damages such as the skin, heart, lungs, and eyes. The incidence of this disease in the general population is about 1% with the highest proportion in middle age. Women have a higher incidence of this disease. The pathogenesis of RA is complicated with the role of many cells including immune cells, fibroblast, chondrocyte, dendritic cells. RA can lead to disability, inferior quality of life, and increased comorbidities. The disease progression and prognosis have been improved considerably by new biologic agents including TNFα inhibitors, IL6 inhibitors, T-cell blockers, Janus kinase inhibitors, in combination with standard therapy [47–49].

The SM is rich in blood vessels [50], and numerous factors have been implicated in increased SM vascularization, including VEGF, TGF-β, and FGF [51]. There is an increase in blood vessel number of synovium and endothelial proliferation in RA. In an early stage of RA, endothelial activation and synovium hyperplasia are detected. Inflammatory cells infiltrate increasingly to SM through new blood vessels during the progression of RA [52]. Taken together, in RA, promoting and maintaining synovial hyperplasia requires angiogenesis. VEGF, a proangiogenic factor, plays an essential role in synovial angiogenesis [53], a key process during the development and progression of RA. Synovial angiogenesis reduces in VEGF knockout mice using antigen-induced models of arthritis [54], which suggests that VEGF contributes to the pathology of RA. VEGF and its receptors are detectable in serum and synovial fluids. VEGF expression is observed in synovial macrophages and fibroblasts of RA patients [55–60]. Moreover, several studies have reported that SM endothelial cells and cells of the lining layer also high express in RA. VEGF regulates the migration and proliferation of endothelial cells in RA [58,59]. In RA synovial tissue, VEGF-A and their receptors express higher compared to normal tissue [60]. Kim et al. showed that VEGF-NRP also prevents synoviocyte apoptosis by inducing Bcl-2 expression and translocation of Bax [36]. This leads to synovial hyperplasia called "pannus", which is a prominent characteristic of RA. Bone erosion is another crucial characteristic of RA disease. Bone destruction depends on the osteoclast differentiation and VEGF also has a role in this process in RA. VEGF impact on osteoclast differentiation both directly regulates osteoclast differentiation from monocytes and induces fibroblast-secreted RANKL (nuclear factor-kappa-B ligand), a central cytokine in osteoclast differentiation [61]. Additionally, VEGF is also associated with disease activity as well as other markers. VEGF concentration was found to be significantly different in various rheumatic diseases, including RA, SLE, antiphospholipid syndrome, and mixed connective tissue disease. VEGF was expressed at the highest concentration among these diseases in that study [62]. VEGF concentration in the serum increases and correlates with disease activity, C-reactive protein level, and radiographic progression [63,64]. In clinical studies, VEGF was used as a marker to assess treatment response. Synovial VEGF expression, as well as synovial vascularization, decrease significantly in RA treatment with infliximab in the combination therapy with methotrexate [65]. High VEGF levels strongly correlate with RA pathogenesis. Another angiogenic cytokine, PlGF, represents the synovitis severity of RA as assessed by ultrasound [66]. Recently, some studies reported that serum VEGF is more valuable than traditional factors such as CRP in determining the treatment response of patients receiving biologic DMARDs [66,67]. In the management of RA, the optimal goal is prevention of permanent injuries in a joint, so the diagnosis in the early stage of the disease is key. Assessment by biomarker may be more sensitive compared to disease activity score in this stage [67]. Additionally, VEGF-C gene polymorphisms may contribute to susceptibility, potential diagnostic markers, and therapeutic targets in patients with RA [68]. Studies have shown that several pathways are related to VEGF in RA. Expression and secretion of VEGF in RA may occur via the IL-6/JAK2/STAT3/VEGF pathway [69]. VEGF/Ang2-induced proangiogenic/inflammatory mechanisms are mediated by Notch signaling pathways in RA [70]. This suggests that the VEGF/Ang2-Notch and IL-6/JAK2/STAT3/VEGF axes may be potential therapeutic targets.

The effect of anti-VEGF therapy or its combination with current therapy was investigated in animal models. In a murine model of collagen-induced arthritis, Miotla et al.

used soluble VEGF receptor for collagen-induced arthritis treatment and showed that the disease severity decreased in this treatment group [71]. Other studies also showed the consistency in the effectiveness of anti-VEGF polyclonal antibodies in collagen-induced arthritis model [72,73]. A study used VEGF blockade monotherapy in the comparison with current monotherapies such as tocilizumab or methotrexate with promising results. This study compared the effect of ranibizumab (anti-VEGF antibody) and tocilizumab (interleukin-6R antagonist) in rat adjuvant-induced arthritis by intra-plantar injection. The effects on inflammatory, angiogenesis, apoptosis inhibition were observed in both groups. Interestingly, anti-VEGF reduces the bone and cartilage destruction compared to methotrexate or tocilizumab treatment [74]. Another anti-VEGF signaling agent, Ramucirumab, is a monoclonal antibody against the VEGFR2, and co-therapy with methotrexate showed synergistic effects in a RA experimental model. Ramucirumab is also used by intra-plantar injection [75]. Recent evidence suggests that anti-VEGF therapy by intra-articular injection may be an option for monotherapy or the combination with standard therapy. Further studies are required to evaluate the effect or anti-VEGF therapy in RA treatment.

4. VEGF in AS

Seronegative spondyloarthritis group consists of AS, reactive arthritis, psoriatic arthritis, enteropathic arthropathy, undifferentiated spondyloarthropathy. AS is the most common of the seronegative spondyloarthritis diseases, with onset at a young age; it may cause disability if undiagnosed and untreated. AS is a chronic progressive disease. Clinical symptoms include low back pain, sacroiliitis, enthesitis, spinal ankylosis, and deformity. Inflammatory bowel disease, acute anterior uveitis, psoriasis, cardiovascular disease, iritis, and pulmonary involvement are other manifestations [76]. Current treatments for spondyloarthritis are anti-inflammation drugs and several biological agents. Targeted therapy includes TNF-α inhibitors (etanercept, infliximab, golimumab, adalimumab, and certolizumab pegol), IL-12/23 inhibitors (ustekinumab), and IL-17 inhibitors (secukinumab and ixekizumab) [77]. Treatment with anti-TNF-α inhibitors has been proven to be an important strategy; however, its effect on the radiographic progression of the disease remains unclear. Therefore, improved understanding of AS pathology will contribute to targeted and combination therapies for AS treatment.

Diagnosis of early inflammatory arthritis significantly improves patient outcomes, because the permanent injuries can be prevented. Besides joint injuries such as bone erosion in synovial joints, AS patients suffer new bone formation and new cartilage was followed by calcification [78,79] that lead to syndesmophytes, anthesophytes, spine ankylosis, these damages cannot recover. The mechanism of this process remains unclear. Angiogenesis is one of the hypotheses to explain about the new bone formation in AS. Not only new bone formation but also sacroiliitis, and enthesitis that are various manifestations of AS, require angiogenesis. VEGF is a central regulator of this process [80]. Fearon et al. observed that VEGF is also expressed in early inflammatory arthritis and is closely related to angiopoietins [81]. It suggests that VEGF may be a potential factor that regulates these events in the pathogenesis of early AS. VEGF may directly regulate osteoblast differentiation from synovial fibroblast that contributes to the new bone formation in AS [82]. Moreover, VEGF may stimulate the COX2 pathway [83]. VEGF also participates in inflammatory in AS [84]. Thus, VEGF may be a target for the treatment of arthritic diseases. Several studies showed that macrophages in SM and entheses of AS secrete VEGF [82,85,86]. Thus, this suggests that VEGF has various functions apart from angiogenesis. VEGF is also a factor to assess the progression, prediction, and susceptibility of this disease in numerous studies. There is a significant increase in serum VEGF levels in AS patients compared to healthy persons [87–89]. VEGF concentration also has a difference in the serum and synovial fluid. In AS patients with peripheral arthritis, VEGF levels are lower considerably in synovial fluid compared to serum levels [88]. Additionally, some evidence showed that VEGF correlates with clinical manifestations such as peripheral arthritis [88] and Bath Ankylosing Spondylitis Disease Activity Index by evaluation the fatigue, spinal pain, joint pain, enthesitis, morning stiffness [84,88,90], other markers of inflammatory [84,91], and duration [89]. However, extra-articular manifestations, syndesmophytes, or the severity of sacroiliitis do not register the association with VEGF [84,89]. Therefore, serum VEGF may be considered a marker of disease activity in AS [84,88,92]. However, another study supported that VEGF only shows a part of the disease progression [93]. Various isoforms of VEGF have also shown inconsistent results. For example, in a study by Bandinelli et al., the levels of VEGF-C did not show a correlation with disease activity [94]. Prediction through spinal radiographic progression serves as the main factor in the prognosis and treatment choice of AS, although it is challenging. VEGF may better predict bone damages in patients with axial spondyloarthritis [88,93,95]. In contrast, Braun et al. did not show any correlation between VEGF and disease activity score based on clinical manifestations and abnormal signs in magnetic resonance imaging. [96]. However, VEGF in combination with other factors such as biomarkers, clinical characteristics, predict better for radiographic progression in axial spondyloarthritis [97]. TNFα inhibitors are the biologic agents that are indicated frequently in AS. VEGF levels also significantly decrease following anti-TNFα therapy [91,98,99]. VEGF also correlates with bone mineral density in AS treatment with infliximab [99]. VEGF levels decrease sharply in AS treated with secukinumab (Anti-IL-17A monoclonal antibody), and decreases in VEGF levels also correlate with inflammatory osteogenic biomarkers [100]. Additionally, VEGF also associates with extra joints and spine manifestations in spondyloarthritis such as subclinical gut inflammation. VEGF and PIGF levels markedly increased in the intestinal mucosa of AS patients without any history of gut inflammation compared to healthy controls [101]. Several studies also support that VEGF is related to AS susceptibility [87], suggesting that VEGF plays a role in the pathogenesis of AS.

A study assessed the effect of anti-VEGF therapy in AS mouse model of proteoglycan-induced arthritis by injection of soluble fms-like tyrosine kinase-1 (sFlt-1), a secretory decoy receptor for VEGF. It supported that disease activity improves significantly in the group treatment compared to the control group [102]. Currently, the main therapies for AS include non-steroid drug and anti-TNFα, both of them target in inflammatory process with limitations remaining in radiograph progression prevention. Lacout et al. suggested that bone homeostasis should be targeted in AS treatment. Anti-VEGF such as bevacizumab may be a potential therapy for severe disease activity and fast progression [103].

5. VEGF in SLE

SLE is the most typical autoimmune disease with various autoantibodies detecting. Other organ damages include skin, hair, blood, nervous system, kidney, vascular, lung, and musculoskeletal manifestations. Women of childbearing age are a high incidence [104]. The etiology of SLE is unclear; many factors are mentioned comprising the gene, ethnic, immune regulatory, hormone, and environment. SLE has many severe complications that lead to life-threatening of patients. In recent decades, the outcome of SLE patients improved considerably because of new immunosuppressant agents [105].

VEGF levels are associated with SLE risk, active SLE risk, lupus nephritis risk [106], and the risk of SLE in a Chinese Han population related to VEGFR1 gene polymorphisms [107]. VEGF is an independent predictor of disease activity [106,108]. In pediatric-onset SLE, VEGF was shown to be one of the six markers of endothelial dysregulation. Therefore, VEGF may be a potent biomarker for pediatric-onset SLE activity as well as organ involvement. It is also helpful for understanding vascular pathogenesis and disease monitoring [109]. VEGF associates with the incidence of clinical manifestations of SLE. Oral ulceration is a common symptom in SLE patients that has a relationship with VEGF [109]. Additionally, VEGF may be contributed to the raised frequency of neuropsychiatric disorders in SLE patients [110]. Female SLE patients in pregnancy often progress more severely with active SLE and various complications to both mother and fetus. Preeclampsia also is an obstetrics disease in pregnancy. To answer the SLE patients in the acute phase of SLE with nephritis or inactive SLE or preeclampsia is challenging to clinicians due to overlapping symptoms. Recent publications showed that there is a significant difference in VEGF level between preeclampsia, inactive SLE, and active lupus nephritis. So, this result suggests that VEGF level may be a useful marker to clinicians [111]. Lupus nephritis is a severe manifestation and prognosis in patients with SLE. VEGF-A participates in the pathogenesis of proliferation lupus nephritis via its impact on the relationship of endothelial cells and epithelial cells [112]. VEGF levels relate to the development of kidney damage [106]. Another study also showed that there is a considerable increase of VEGF in lupus nephritis compared to the non-lupus nephritis and the control group. However, there was no statistically significant relationship between serum VEGF levels and the histological classes of lupus nephritis [113]. Thus, VEGF may be contributing to the pathogenesis of these manifestations. Furthermore, there was a decrease in the level of VEGF-A in SLE patients taking mycophenolate mofetil compared to the non-taking mycophenolate mofetil group [114]. Another study observed that the level of VEGF-R2 significantly decreased in a group of SLE patients treated for a long time compared to the group of newly diagnosed, untreated SLE patients. Various drugs, including prednisone, immunosuppressive drugs were used in this study [115]. VEGF correlates with disease activity [116–118].

6. VEGF in OA

OA is the most common joint disorder in middle age and elderly people. OA affects all parts of joints, including cartilage, subchondral bone, synovium, ligaments, and periarticular muscle. Cartilage degeneration is fundamental damage [119]. OA is the principal cause of disability and pain [120]. Disease-modifying drugs are currently not available, and therapy is mainly aimed at symptom relief [121].

Angiogenesis forms a network of neovascularization in synovium called OA pannus. Angiogenesis associates with osteophytes formation, VEGF promotes this process [122]. Hyperangiogenesis contributes to synovial inflammation and microstructural deterioration during OA [70]. Augmentation of VEGF signaling exacerbates joint OA formation by increasing osteoclast differentiation, metalloproteinase, and chondrocyte apoptosis leads to bone and cartilage destruction [123]. There is increased expression of VEGF in the entire structure of joints, synovial fluid in OA. Its receptors strongly express in OA chondrocytes. Similarly, VEGF also registers the increase in serum and synovial fluid [124–126]. The role of VEGF is observed in various processes of bone homeostasis. VEGF enhances osteoclast differentiation, osteoclast survival, RANKL secretion [123]. There is an increase of VEGF levels in osteoblasts from patients who replaced total hip [127]. VEGF can be used as a marker to monitor the response to OA therapy [128]. Pain is the key symptom of OA and the mechanism of pain in OA is not completely understood; therefore, a clear understanding of the pathogenesis of pain in OA is essential for the development of targeted therapies. Tanako et al. supported that in human knee OA, VEGF experienced a positive correlation with pain score [129] and Galballa et al. also showed that VEGF not only correlates with pain but also in clinical and radiology symptoms [130]. One of the factors that contributes to the mechanism of pain is the growth of sensory nerves. This process is stimulated by proangiogenic factors [131]. Pain hypersensitivity is a phenomenon that is observed in OA. Several studies suggest that VEGF signaling has an association with this condition [132–134]. VEGF also increases the expression of several types of MMP, especially MMP-13, key factor results in cartilage degeneration [123,135]. Moreover, hypoxia, a crucial mediator of the VEGF axis, contributes to temporomandibular joint osteoarthritis and accelerates the angiogenesis of condylar cartilage through the HIF-1-VEGF-Notch signaling pathway. HIF-1α and Notch may be novel therapeutic targets for temporomandibular joint osteoarthritis [136]. The accumulated evidence shows that VEGF signaling participates in various aspects of OA including synovitis, mechanism of pain, bone and cartilage destruction.

In vivo studies have also shown positive results with VEGF-targeted therapy. In a rabbit OA model due to trauma, there is a significant decrease in pain, cartilage destruction, synovium inflammatory in group treatment with bevacizumab, a VEGF blocker by intra-articular injection. Moreover, they do not register any adverse effect [137]. Oral administration of a VEGFR-2 kinase inhibitor attenuated OA progression in a mouse model of post-traumatic human knee OA [38]. Anti VEGF signaling seems to be a potential therapy in OA and using anti-VEGF agents by local administration may show more benefits.

7. VEGF in SSc

SSc is a rare autoimmune disease marked by the fibrosis of the skin, and involvement of internal organs, especially the vascular system, lung, kidney, and gastrointestinal system and is caused by excessive collagen deposition, immunological disturbances, and accompanying vascular changes. Genetic, environmental, vascular, autoimmunological, and microchimeric factors contribute to the pathogenesis of SSc. The cause of this disease is unknown and the limitation in the treatment therapies leads to the poor outcome of SSc patients. Thus, the tools for early diagnosis and effective intervention are required. A better understanding of the pathology of SSc may contribute to potentially effective therapies to improve SSc patient outcomes. Microvascular damage and dysfunction of angiogenesis are identified abnormalities. Tissue fibrosis results from series events including endothelial dysfunction, inflammatory, increased vascular permeability, platelet aggregation [138–140]. Impaired angiogenesis is detected in the digit ulcers of SSc patients [141]. There is a significant increase in serum VEGF levels in both the early and established stages of SSc [142,143]. Jinin et al. suggested that VEGFR-2 level may be an indicator for microangiopathy and helpful for diagnosis in SS [144]. Avouac et al. reported that VEGFR-1 level decreased in SSc patients compared to those in the healthy control. There is a significant increase of VEGF and its receptor expression in skin lesion from SSc patients [144,145].

Pulmonary fibrosis, pulmonary hypertension, and renal involvement are the main causes of mortality. Serum VEGF levels may act as biomarkers for interstitial lung involvement [146]. VEGF does not correlate with intrarenal stiffness and renal function in patients with SSc [147]. VEGF, pigment epithelium-derived factor (PEDF) levels, and the VEGF/PEDF register considerable changes, and they seem to be useful tools for disease activity assessment [148]. However, some studies show that the relationship of VEGF with pulmonary pressure is still unclear [148,149]. VEGF is also used as a marker in combination with other factors to predict disease activity in SSc [143]. VEGF and Ang/Tie2 dysfunction lead to peripheral microvasculopathy in SSc [150]. Nintedanib inhibits simultaneously three types of receptors including the platelet-derived growth factor, fibroblast growth factor, and vascular endothelial growth factor tyrosine kinase, and is approved for idiopathic pulmonary fibrosis. Huang et al. assessed the effect of nintedanib in a mouse model of SSc with promising results. The pulmonary arterial hypertension, microangiopathy destruction, pulmonary, myocardial, and dermal fibrosis are improved in group treatment [151]. Taken together, the inhibitors targeting VEGF signaling may be a potential therapy for SSc treatment.

8. VEGF in SS

Primary SS is an autoimmune disease characterized by chronic inflammation that results in dryness of the eye, mouth, and an increased the size of parotid gland. The incidence rate is 0.2–0.5% of the adult population. SS is the most common in middle-aged women [152]. The risk of dental caries and oral infections results in an inferior quality of life. Angiogenesis represents a novel potential marker for primary SS and may contribute significantly to the pathogenesis [153]. VEGF-C expressed in epithelial cells and inflammatory cells of primary SS. There is a considerable increase in VEGFR-3 expression in lymphatic vessels. In primary SS, this study showed that the increased expression of VEGF-C correlates with immune cells, cytokine, and lymphatic EPC originated from bone marrow [154]. Furthermore, the role of VEGF is also supported by another study that showed that tumor necrosis factor alpha converting enzyme (TACE) in TACE/VEGF-R2/NF-κB dysregulation participates in SS pathogenesis [155]. However, the role of VEGF in SS remains controversial, because another study did not show any change in VEGF levels in SS patients. Detection of serum VEGF is less sensitive than detection of VEGF in saliva but the role of saliva VEGF in pathogenesis of SS is unclear [156]. With the evidence limitation, the function of VEGF in SS remains relatively modest.

9. Summary

Taken together, VEGF shows its role in the pathogenesis of many diseases in rheumatology. VEGF is a marker in disease activity assessment and treatment following. The function of VEGF in rheumatic diseases is summarized in Table 1. VEGF contributes to various aspects of the pathogenesis of joint damage in rheumatic diseases including angiogenesis, synovitis, inflammatory, osteoclast differentiation and cartilage degradation. Interestingly, VEGF reveals the association with the mechanism of pain in OA. The role of VEGF in the development of joint injuries is illustrated in Figure 1.

Table 1. The role of VEGF in rheumatic diseases.

Rheumatic Diseases	Mechanisms	Clinical Results
Rheumatoid arthritis	Regulate the migration, proliferation of endothelial cells Prevent the synoviocyte apoptosis Regulate osteoclast differentiation, induce RANKL secretion IL-6/JAK2/STAT3/VEGF VEGF/Ang2-Notch	High levels Correlate with disease activity, C-reactive protein, radiographic progression VEGF-C contribute to the susceptibility Treatment therapy reduces VEGF expression
Ankylosing spondylitis	Regulate osteoblast differentiation Stimulate COX2 pathway Participate in inflammatory	Correlate with peripheral arthritis, BASDI, inflammatory markers, duration Predict bone damage Correlate with bone mineral density in infliximab treatment Associated with subclinical gut inflammation Anti TNFα, anti-IL-17A decreased serum VEGF levels
Systemic lupus erythematosus	Endothelial dysfunction	High level in lupus nephritis Associated with SLE risk, active SLE, lupus nephritis risk Predictor of disease activity Associated with oral ulceration, neuropsychiatric disorders Correlate with disease activity MMF decreased the VEGF-A levels.
Osteoarthritis	Promote the neovascularization in synovium Increase osteoclast differentiation, osteoclast survival, RANKL secretion Increase metalloproteinase Increase chondrocyte apoptosis Accelerated angiogenesis via HIF-1-VEGF-Notch	Associated with pain, clinical and radiology symptoms
Systemic sclerosis	VEGF/Ang/Tie2 dysfunction	High levels Associated with microangiopathy Biomarker for interstitial lung involvement Combination with other factors to predict disease activity
Sjögren syndrome	TACE/VEGF-R2/NF-κB dysregulation	Remain unclear

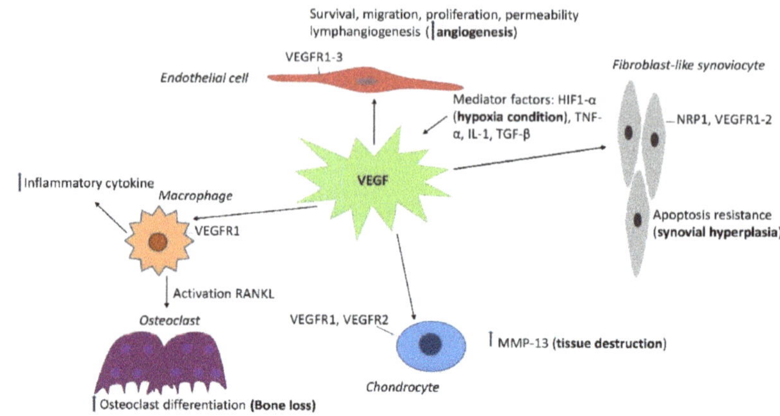

Figure 1. Schematic diagram of the role of VEGF in the development of joint injuries in rheumatic diseases. VEGF plays an important role in angiogenesis, the prominent characteristic of arthritis. VEGF and its receptor strongly express in synovial tissue, fluid. VEGF-NRP1 axis leads to apoptotic resistance of synoviocytes. VEGFR-1 is expressed on the membrane of macrophages. VEGF axis regulates the inflammatory process by cytokine production as well as enhanced bone resorption via increased osteoclast differentiation. In OA, VEGF may increase the expression of MMP-13, leading to tissue destruction.

Targeting angiogenesis via inhibition of VEGF may be a potential therapy in rheumatic diseases. However, to minimize the drawbacks of anti-VEGF therapy, appropriate clinical trials are needed to test its safety, efficacy, cost-effectiveness, and methods need to be developed to control the binding ability of drugs to targeted injuries. Based on current evidence, anti-VEGF therapy may be most likely adjunctive therapy for arthritis. Local administration shows more beneficially because of low dose requirement and adverse effect minimizing. In the SSc mouse model, VEGF inhibitor also shows its effect in the improvement of pulmonary hypertension, skin, and lung fibrosis. More studies are needed to clarify the role of VEGF and the effect of anti-VEGF therapy in rheumatic diseases.

Author Contributions: T.H.V.L. conceptualized the review, performed literature survey, wrote the manuscript, and made the figure, table. S.-M.K. edited and supervised. All authors have read and agreed to the published version of the manuscript.

Funding: The work was supported by a grant from the National Research Foundation (NRF-2020R1A2C2101297, NRF-2015M3A9B4066493, and NRF-2015R1A5A2009656), and the Korean Health Technology R&D Project, Ministry of Health and Welfare (HI18C2459, and HI18C2458) funded by the Korean government.

Conflicts of Interest: The authors declare no conflict of interest.

Abbreviations

VEGF	Vascular Endothelial Growth Factor
RA	Rheumatoid arthritis
OA	Osteoarthritis
AS	Alkylosing spondyloarthritis
SLE	Systemic lupus erythematous
SM	Synovial membrane
SSc	Systemic sclerosis
SS	Sjögren syndrome
PIGF	Placental growth factor
MMPs	Matrix metalloproteinases

VPF	Vascular permeability factor
RANKL	Nuclear factor-kappa-B ligand
RTKs	Receptor tyrosine kinases
NRP	Neuropilin
HIF	Hypoxia-inducible factors
TGF-β	Transforming growth factor-β
EPCs	Endothelial precursor cells
PEDF	Pigment epithelium-derived factor
TACE	Tumor necrosis factor alpha converting enzyme

References

1. Gourley, M.; Miller, F.W. Mechanisms of Disease: Environmental factors in the pathogenesis of rheumatic disease. *Nat. Clin. Pr. Rheumatol.* **2007**, *3*, 172–180. [CrossRef] [PubMed]
2. Goldblatt, F.; O'Neill, S.G. Clinical aspects of autoimmune rheumatic diseases. *Lancet* **2013**, *382*, 797–808. [CrossRef]
3. Heijde, V.D.D.; Daikh, D.I.; Betteridge, N.; Burmester, G.; Hassett, A.L.; Matteson, E.L.; Vollenhoven, R.V.; Lakhanpal, S. Common language description of the term rheumatic and musculoskeletal diseases (RMDs) for use in communication with the lay public, healthcare providers and other stakeholders endorsed by the European League Against Rheumatism (EULAR) and the American College of Rheumatology (ACR). *Ann. Rheum. Dis.* **2018**, *77*, 829–832. [PubMed]
4. Vos, T.; Abajobir, A.A.; Abate, K.H.; Abbafati, C.; Abbas, K.M.; Abd-Allah, F.; Abdulkader, R.S.; Abdulle, A.M.; Abebo, T.A.; Abera, S.F.; et al. Global, regional, and national incidence, prevalence and years lived with disability for 328 diseases and injuries for 195 countries, 1990–2016: A systematic analysis for the Global Burden of Disease Study 2016. *Lancet* **2017**, *390*, 1211–1259. [CrossRef]
5. Carvalho, J.F.; Blank, M.; Shoenfeld, Y. Vascular Endothelial Growth Factor (VEGF) in Autoimmune Diseases. *J. Clin. Immunol.* **2007**, *27*, 246–256. [CrossRef]
6. Walsh, D.A. Angiogenesis and arthritis. *Rheumatology* **1999**, *38*, 103–112. [CrossRef]
7. Risau, W. Mechanisms of angiogenesis. *Nat. Cell Biol.* **1997**, *386*, 671–674. [CrossRef]
8. Distler, J.H.W.; Hirth, A.; Kurowska-Stolarska, M.; Gay, R.E.; Gay, S.; Distler, O. Angiogenic and angiostatic factors in the molecular control of angiogenesis. *Q. J. Nucl. Med. Mol. Imaging* **2003**, *47*, 149.
9. Apte, R.S.; Chen, D.S.; Ferrara, N. VEGF in Signaling and Disease: Beyond Discovery and Development. *Cell* **2019**, *176*, 1248–1264. [CrossRef]
10. Senger, D.R.; Galli, S.J.; Dvorak, A.M.; Perruzzi, C.A.; Harvey, V.S.; Dvorak, H.F. Tumor cells secrete a vascular permeability factor that promotes accumulation of ascites fluid. *Science* **1983**, *219*, 983–985. [CrossRef]
11. Plate, K.H.; Warnke, P.C. Vascular endothelial growth factor. *J. Neuro Oncol.* **1997**, *35*, 363–370. [CrossRef]
12. Ferrara, N.; Gerber, H.-P.; LeCouter, J. The biology of VEGF and its receptors. *Nat. Med.* **2003**, *9*, 669–676. [CrossRef] [PubMed]
13. Ferrara, N.; Davis-Smyth, T. The biology of vascular endothelial growth factor. *Endocr. Rev.* **1997**, *18*, 4–25. [CrossRef]
14. Poltorak, Z.; Cohen, T.; Sivan, R.; Kandelis, Y.; Spira, G.; Vlodavsky, I.; Keshet, E.; Neufeld, G. VEGF145, a Secreted Vascular Endothelial Growth Factor Isoform That Binds to Extracellular Matrix. *J. Biol. Chem.* **1997**, *272*, 7151–7158. [CrossRef]
15. Houck, K.; Leung, D.; Rowland, A.; Winer, J.; Ferrara, N. Dual regulation of vascular endothelial growth factor bioavailability by genetic and proteolytic mechanisms. *J. Biol. Chem.* **1992**, *267*, 26031–26037. [CrossRef]
16. Olofsson, B.; Pajusola, K.; Kaipainen, A.; Von Euler, G.; Joukov, V.; Saksela, O.; Orpana, A.; Pettersson, R.F.; Alitalo, K.; Eriksson, U. Vascular endothelial growth factor B, a novel growth factor for endothelial cells. *Proc. Natl. Acad. Sci. USA* **1996**, *93*, 2576–2581. [CrossRef]
17. Alitalo, K.; Tammela, T.; Petrova, T.V. Lymphangiogenesis in development and human disease. *Nat. Cell Biol.* **2005**, *438*, 946–953. [CrossRef]
18. Leung, D.W.; Cachianes, G.; Kuang, W.J.; Goeddel, D.V.; Ferrara, N. Vascular endothelial growth factor is a secreted angiogenic mitogen. *Science* **1989**, *246*, 1306–1309. [CrossRef]
19. Soker, S.; Fidder, H.; Neufeld, G.; Klagsbrun, M. Characterization of Novel Vascular Endothelial Growth Factor (VEGF) Receptors on Tumor Cells That Bind VEGF165 via Its Exon 7-encoded Domain. *J. Biol. Chem.* **1996**, *271*, 5761–5767. [CrossRef]
20. Kawasaki, T.; Kitsukawa, T.; Bekku, Y.; Matsuda, Y.; Sanbo, M.; Yagi, T.; Fujisawa, H. A requirement for neuropilin-1 in embryonic vessel formation. *Development* **1999**, *126*, 4895–4902. [CrossRef]
21. Pertovaara, L.; Kaipainen, A.; Mustonen, T.; Orpana, A.; Ferrara, N.; Saksela, O.; Alitalo, K.; Pertovaara, L.; Kaipainen, A.; Mustonen, T.; et al. Vascular endothelial growth factor is induced in response to transforming growth factor-beta in fibroblastic and epithelial cells. *J. Biol. Chem.* **1994**, *269*, 6271–6274. [CrossRef]
22. McLaren, J.; Prentice, A.; Charnock-Jones, D.S.; Millican, S.A.; Müller, K.H.; Sharkey, A.M.; Smith, S.K. Vascular endothelial growth factor is produced by peritoneal fluid macrophages in endometriosis and is regulated by ovarian steroids. *J. Clin. Investig.* **1996**, *98*, 482–489. [CrossRef] [PubMed]
23. Namiki, A.; Brogi, E.; Kearney, M.; Kim, E.A.; Wu, T.; Couffinhal, T.; Varticovski, L.; Isner, J.M. Hypoxia Induces Vascular Endothelial Growth Factor in Cultured Human Endothelial Cells. *J. Biol. Chem.* **1995**, *270*, 31189–31195. [CrossRef] [PubMed]

24. Taichman, N.S.; Young, S.; Cruchley, A.T.; Taylor, P.; Paleolog, E. Human neutrophils secrete vascular endothelial growth factor. *J. Leukoc. Biol.* **1997**, *62*, 397–400. [CrossRef]
25. Freeman, M.R.; Schneck, F.X.; Gagnon, M.L.; Corless, C.; Soker, S.; Niknejad, K.; Peoples, G.E.; Klagsbrun, M. Peripheral blood T lymphocytes and lymphocytes infiltrating human cancers express vascular endothelial growth factor: A potential role for T cells in angiogenesis. *Cancer Res.* **1995**, *55*, 4140–4145.
26. Neufeld, G.; Cohen, T.; Gengrinovitch, S.; Poltorak, Z. Vascular endothelial growth factor (VEGF) and its receptors. *FASEB J.* **1999**, *13*, 9–22. [CrossRef]
27. Semenza, G.L. HIF-1: Mediator of physiological and pathophysiological responses to hypoxia. *J. Appl. Physiol.* **2000**, *88*, 1474–1480. [CrossRef]
28. Semenza, G.L. HIF-1: Using Two Hands to Flip the Angiogenic Switch. *Cancer Metastasis Rev.* **2000**, *19*, 59–65. [CrossRef]
29. Dor, Y.; Porat, R.; Keshet, E. Vascular endothelial growth factor and vascular adjustments to perturbations in oxygen homeostasis. *Am. J. Physiol. Physiol.* **2001**, *280*, C1367–C1374. [CrossRef]
30. Ferrara, N.; Hillan, K.J.; Gerber, H.-P.; Novotny, W. Discovery and development of bevacizumab, an anti-VEGF antibody for treating cancer. *Nat. Rev. Drug Discov.* **2004**, *3*, 391–400. [CrossRef]
31. Rosenfeld, P.J.; Brown, D.M.; Heier, J.S.; Boyer, D.S.; Kaiser, P.K.; Chung, C.Y.; Kim, R.Y. Ranibizumab for Neovascular Age-Related Macular Degeneration. *N. Engl. J. Med.* **2006**, *355*, 1419–1431. [CrossRef]
32. Zirlik, K.; Duyster, J. Anti-Angiogenics: Current Situation and Future Perspectives. *Oncol. Res. Treat.* **2017**, *41*, 166–171. [CrossRef]
33. Gragoudas, E.S.; Adamis, A.P.; Cunningham, E.T.; Feinsod, M.; Guyer, D.R. Pegaptanib for Neovascular Age-Related Macular Degeneration. *N. Engl. J. Med.* **2004**, *351*, 2805–2816. [CrossRef]
34. Nicolò, M.; Desideri, L.F.; Vagge, A.; Traverso, C.E. Faricimab: An investigational agent targeting the Tie-2/angiopoietin pathway and VEGF-A for the treatment of retinal diseases. *Expert Opin. Investig. Drugs* **2021**, *30*, 193–200. [CrossRef]
35. Lynch, S.S.; Cheng, C.M. Bevacizumab for Neovascular Ocular Diseases. *Ann. Pharmacother.* **2007**, *41*, 614–625. [CrossRef]
36. Kim, W.-U.; Kang, S.S.; Yoo, S.-A.; Hong, K.-H.; Bae, D.-G.; Lee, M.-S.; Hong, S.W.; Chae, C.-B.; Cho, C.-S. Interaction of vascular endothelial growth factor 165 with neuropilin-1 protects rheumatoid synoviocytes from apoptotic death by regulating Bcl-2 expression and Bax translocation. *J. Immunol.* **2006**, *177*, 5727–5735. [CrossRef]
37. Duan, X.; Murata, Y.; Liu, Y.; Nicolae, C.; Olsen, B.R.; Berendsen, A.D. Vegfa regulates perichondrial vascularity and osteoblast differentiation in bone development. *Development* **2015**, *142*, 1984–1991. [CrossRef]
38. Nagao, M.; Hamilton, J.L.; Kc, R.; Berendsen, A.D.; Duan, X.; Cheong, C.W.; Li, X.; Im, H.-J.; Olsen, B.R. Vascular Endothelial Growth Factor in Cartilage Development and Osteoarthritis. *Sci. Rep.* **2017**, *7*, 1–16. [CrossRef]
39. Fiedler, J.; Leucht, F.; Waltenberger, J.; Dehio, C.; Brenner, R.E. VEGF-A and PlGF-1 stimulate chemotactic migration of human mesenchymal progenitor cells. *Biochem. Biophys. Res. Commun.* **2005**, *334*, 561–568. [CrossRef]
40. Deckers, M.M.L.; Karperien, M.; Bent, C.V.D.; Ymashita, T.; Papapoulos, S.E.; Löwik, C.W.G.M. Expression of vascular endothelial growth factors and their receptors during osteoblast differentiation. *Endocrinology* **2000**, *141*, 1667–1674. [CrossRef]
41. Aldridge, S.; Lennard, T.; Williams, J.; Birch, M. Vascular endothelial growth factor receptors in osteoclast differentiation and function. *Biochem. Biophys. Res. Commun.* **2005**, *335*, 793–798. [CrossRef] [PubMed]
42. Yang, Q.; McHugh, K.P.; Patntirapong, S.; Gu, X.; Wunderlich, L.; Hauschka, P.V. VEGF enhancement of osteoclast survival and bone resorption involves VEGF receptor-2 signaling and β3-integrin. *Matrix Biol.* **2008**, *27*, 589–599. [CrossRef]
43. Nakagawa, M.; Kaneda, T.; Arakawa, T.; Morita, S.; Sato, T.; Yomada, T.; Hanada, K.; Kumegawa, M.; Hakeda, Y. Vascular endothelial growth factor (VEGF) directly enhances osteoclastic bone resorption and survival of mature osteoclasts. *FEBS Lett.* **2000**, *473*, 161–164. [CrossRef]
44. Khan, K.A.; Kerbel, R.S. Improving immunotherapy outcomes with anti-angiogenic treatments and vice versa. *Nat. Rev. Clin. Oncol.* **2018**, *15*, 310–324. [CrossRef] [PubMed]
45. Shibuya, M. VEGF-VEGFR system as a target for suppressing inflammation and other diseases. *Endocr. Metab. Immune Disord. Drug Targets* **2015**, *15*, 135–144. [CrossRef]
46. Giatromanolaki, A.; Sivridis, E.; Maltezos, E.; Athanassou, N.; Papazoglou, D.; Gatter, K.C.; Harris, A.L.; I Koukourakis, M. Upregulated hypoxia inducible factor-1α and -2α pathway in rheumatoid arthritis and osteoarthritis. *Arthritis Res.* **2003**, *5*, R193–R201. [CrossRef]
47. Austen, K.F.; Frank, M.M.; Atkinson, J.P.; Cantor, H. *Rheumatoid Arthitis. Samter's Immunologic Diseases*, 6th ed.; Lippincott Williams & Wilkins: Philadelphia, PA, USA, 2001; pp. 427–463.
48. Hansildaar, R.; Vedder, D.; Baniaamam, M.; Tausche, A.-K.; Gerritsen, M.; Nurmohamed, M.T. Cardiovascular risk in inflammatory arthritis: Rheumatoid arthritis and gout. *Lancet Rheumatol.* **2021**, *3*, e58–e70. [CrossRef]
49. De Cock, D.; Hyrich, K. Malignancy and rheumatoid arthritis: Epidemiology, risk factors and management. *Best Pr. Res. Clin. Rheumatol.* **2018**, *32*, 869–886. [CrossRef]
50. Colville-Nash, P.R.; Scott, D.L. Angiogenesis and rheumatoid arthritis: Pathogenic and therapeutic implications. *Ann. Rheum. Dis.* **1992**, *51*, 919–925. [CrossRef]
51. Koch, A.E. Angiogenesis: Implications for rheumatoid arthritis. *Arthritis Rheum.* **1998**, *41*, 951–962. [CrossRef]
52. Szekanecz, Z.; Koch, A.E. Angiogenesis and its targeting in rheumatoid arthritis. *Vasc. Pharmacol.* **2009**, *51*, 1–7. [CrossRef]

53. Yoo, S.-A.; Bae, D.-G.; Ryoo, J.-W.; Kim, H.-R.; Park, G.-S.; Cho, C.-S.; Chae, C.-B.; Kim, W.-U. Arginine-Rich Anti-Vascular Endothelial Growth Factor (Anti-VEGF) Hexapeptide Inhibits Collagen-Induced Arthritis and VEGF-Stimulated Productions of TNF-α and IL-6 by Human Monocytes. *J. Immunol.* **2005**, *174*, 5846–5855. [CrossRef]
54. Mould, A.W.; Tonks, I.D.; Cahill, M.M.; Pettit, A.R.; Thomas, R.; Hayward, N.K.; Kay, G.F. Vegfb gene knockout mice display reduced pathology and synovial angiogenesis in both antigen-induced and collagen-induced models of arthritis. *Arthritis Rheum.* **2003**, *48*, 2660–2669. [CrossRef]
55. Lee, S.S.; Joo, Y.S.; Kim, W.U.; Min, D.J.; Min, J.K.; Park, S.H.; Cho, C.S.; Kim, H.Y. Vascular endothelial growth factor levels in the serum and synovial fluid of patients with rheumatoid arthritis. *Clin. Exp. Rheumatol.* **2001**, *19*, 321–324.
56. Koch, A.E. Angiogenesis as a target in rheumatoid arthritis. *Ann. Rheum. Dis.* **2003**, *62*, 60–67. [CrossRef]
57. Bottomley, M.; Webb, N.; Watson, C.; Holt, P.; Freemont, A.; Brenchley, P. Peripheral blood mononuclear cells from patients with rheumatoid arthritis spontaneously secrete vascular endothelial growth factor (VEGF): Specific up-regulation by tumour necrosis factor-alpha (TNF-α) in synovial fluid. *Clin. Exp. Immunol.* **1999**, *117*, 171–176. [CrossRef]
58. Fava, R.A.; Olsen, N.J.; Spencer-Green, G.; Yeo, K.T.; Yeo, T.K.; Berse, B.; Jackman, R.W.; Senger, D.R.; Dvorak, H.F.; Brown, L.F. Vascular permeability factor/endothelial growth factor (VPF/VEGF): Accumulation and expression in human synovial fluids and rheumatoid synovial tissue. *J. Exp. Med.* **1994**, *180*, 341–346. [CrossRef]
59. Koch, A.E.; Harlow, L.A.; Haines, G.K.; Amento, E.P.; Unemori, E.N.; Wong, W.L.; Pope, R.M.; Ferrara, N. Vascular endothelial growth factor. A cytokine modulating endothelial function in rheumatoid arthritis. *J. Immunol.* **1994**, *152*, 4149–4156.
60. Ikeda, M.; Hosoda, Y.; Hirose, S.; Okada, Y.; Ikeda, E. Expression of vascular endothelial growth factor isoforms and their receptors Flt-1, KDR, and neuropilin-1 in synovial tissues of rheumatoid arthritis. *J. Pathol.* **2000**, *191*, 426–433. [CrossRef]
61. Kim, H.-R.; Kim, K.-W.; Kim, B.-M.; Cho, M.-L.; Lee, S.-H. The Effect of Vascular Endothelial Growth Factor on Osteoclastogenesis in Rheumatoid Arthritis. *PLOS ONE* **2015**, *10*, e0124909. [CrossRef]
62. Wojdasiewicz, P.; Wajda, A.; Haładyj, E.; Romanowska-Próchnicka, K.; Felis-Giemza, A.; Nałęcz-Janik, J.; Walczyk, M.; Olesinska, M.; Tarnacka, B.; Paradowska-Gorycka, A. IL-35, TNF-α, BAFF, and VEGF serum levels in patients with different rheumatic diseases. *Reumatologia* **2019**, *57*, 145–150. [CrossRef] [PubMed]
63. Paleolog, E.M. Angiogenesis in rheumatoid arthritis. *Arthritis Res. Ther.* **2002**, *4*, S81. [CrossRef] [PubMed]
64. Lee, Y.H.; Bae, S.-C. Correlation between circulating VEGF levels and disease activity in rheumatoid arthritis: A meta-analysis. *Z. Rheumatol.* **2016**, *77*, 240–248. [CrossRef] [PubMed]
65. Kanbe, K.; Inoue, K.; Inoue, Y.; Suzuki, Y. Histological analysis of synovium in cases of effect attenuation associated with infliximab therapy in rheumatoid arthritis. *Clin. Rheumatol.* **2008**, *27*, 777–781. [CrossRef] [PubMed]
66. Kim, J.; Kong, J.-S.; Lee, S.; Yoo, S.-A.; Koh, J.H.; Jin, J.; Kim, W.-U. Angiogenic cytokines can reflect the synovitis severity and treatment response to biologics in rheumatoid arthritis. *Exp. Mol. Med.* **2020**, *52*, 843–853. [CrossRef]
67. Taylor, P.C. VEGF and imaging of vessels in rheumatoid arthritis. *Arthritis Res.* **2002**, *4*, S99–S107. [CrossRef] [PubMed]
68. Dai, C.; Kuo, S.-J.; Hu, S.-L.; Tsai, C.-H.; Huang, Y.-L.; Huang, C.-C.; Wang, L.; Xu, G.; Su, C.-M.; Tang, C.-H. VEGF-C Gene Polymorphisms Increase Susceptibility to Rheumatoid Arthritis. *Int. J. Med Sci.* **2019**, *16*, 1397–1403. [CrossRef]
69. Cheng, W.-X.; Huang, H.; Chen, J.-H.; Zhang, T.-T.; Zhu, G.-Y.; Zheng, Z.-T.; Lin, J.-T.; Hu, Y.-P.; Zhang, Y.; Bai, X.-L.; et al. Genistein inhibits angiogenesis developed during rheumatoid arthritis through the IL-6/JAK2/STAT3/VEGF signalling pathway. *J. Orthop. Transl.* **2020**, *22*, 92–100. [CrossRef]
70. Gao, W.; Sweeney, C.; Walsh, C.A.; Rooney, P.; McCormick, J.; Veale, D.J.; Fearon, U. Notch signalling pathways mediate synovial angiogenesis in response to vascular endothelial growth factor and angiopoietin 2. *Ann. Rheum. Dis.* **2012**, *72*, 1080–1088. [CrossRef]
71. Miotla, J.; Maciewicz, R.; Kendrew, J.; Feldmann, M.; Paleolog, E. Treatment with Soluble VEGF Receptor Reduces Disease Severity in Murine Collagen-Induced Arthritis. *Lab. Investig.* **2000**, *80*, 1195–1205. [CrossRef]
72. Lu, J.; Kasama, T.; Kobayashi, K.; Yoda, Y.; Shiozawa, F.; Hanyuda, M.; Negishi, M.; Ide, H.; Adachi, M. Vascular Endothelial Growth Factor Expression and Regulation of Murine Collagen-Induced Arthritis. *J. Immunol.* **2000**, *164*, 5922–5927. [CrossRef]
73. Sone, H.; Kawakami, Y.; Sakauchi, M.; Nakamura, Y.; Takahashi, A.; Shimano, H.; Okuda, Y.; Segawa, T.; Suzuki, H.; Yamada, N. Neutralization of Vascular Endothelial Growth Factor Prevents Collagen-Induced Arthritis and Ameliorates Established Disease in Mice. *Biochem. Biophys. Res. Commun.* **2001**, *281*, 562–568. [CrossRef]
74. Abdel-Maged, A.E.-S.; Gad, A.M.; Abdel-Aziz, A.K.; Aboulwafa, M.M.; Azab, S.S. Comparative study of anti-VEGF Ranibizumab and Interleukin-6 receptor antagonist Tocilizumab in Adjuvant-induced Arthritis. *Toxicol. Appl. Pharmacol.* **2018**, *356*, 65–75. [CrossRef]
75. Abdel-Maged, A.E.; Gad, A.M.; Wahdan, S.A.; Azab, S.S. Efficacy and safety of Ramucirumab and methotrexate co-therapy in rheumatoid arthritis experimental model: Involvement of angiogenic and immunomodulatory signaling. *Toxicol. Appl. Pharmacol.* **2019**, *380*, 114702. [CrossRef]
76. Poddubnyy, D.; Haibel, H.; Listing, J.; Märker-Hermann, E.; Zeidler, H.; Braun, J.; Sieper, J.; Rudwaleit, M. Baseline radiographic damage, elevated acute-phase reactant levels, and cigarette smoking status predict spinal radiographic progression in early axial spondylarthritis. *Arthritis Rheum.* **2012**, *64*, 1388–1398. [CrossRef]
77. Zhu, W.; He, X.; Cheng, K.; Zhang, L.; Chen, D.; Wang, X.; Qiu, G.; Cao, X.; Weng, X. Ankylosing spondylitis: Etiology, pathogenesis, and treatments. *Bone Res.* **2019**, *7*, 22. [CrossRef]

78. Yu, T.; Zhang, J.; Zhu, W.; Wang, X.; Bai, Y.; Feng, B.; Zhuang, Q.; Han, C.; Wang, S.; Hu, Q.; et al. Chondrogenesis mediates progression of ankylosing spondylitis through heterotopic ossification. *Bone Res.* **2021**, *9*, 1–12. [CrossRef]
79. Sieper, J.; Braun, J.; Rudwaleit, M.; Boonen, A.; Zink, A. Ankylosing spondylitis: An overview. *Ann. Rheum. Dis.* **2002**, *61*, 8–18. [CrossRef] [PubMed]
80. Yamamoto, T. Angiogenic and Inflammatory Properties of Psoriatic Arthritis. *ISRN Dermatol.* **2013**, *2013*, 1–7. [CrossRef]
81. Fearon, U.; Griosios, K.; Fraser, A.; Reece, R.; Emery, P.; Jones, P.F.; Veale, D.J. Angiopoietins, growth factors, and vascular morphology in early arthritis. *J. Rheumatol.* **2003**, *30*, 260–268.
82. Liu, K.; He, Q.; Tan, J.; Liao, G. Expression of TNF-α, VEGF, and MMP-3 mRNAs in synovial tissues and their roles in fibroblast-mediated osteogenesis in ankylosing spondylitis. *Genet. Mol. Res.* **2015**, *14*, 6852–6858. [CrossRef] [PubMed]
83. Kawashima, M.; Fujikawa, Y.; Itonaga, I.; Takita, C.; Tsumura, H. The effect of selective cyclooxygenase-2 inhibitor on human osteoclast precursors to influence osteoclastogenesis In Vitro. *Mod. Rheumatol.* **2009**, *19*, 192–198. [CrossRef] [PubMed]
84. Drouart, M.; Saas, P.; Billot, M.; Cedoz, J.-P.; Tiberghien, P.; Wendling, D.; Toussirot, E. High serum vascular endothelial growth factor correlates with disease activity of spondylarthropathies. *Clin. Exp. Immunol.* **2003**, *132*, 158–162. [CrossRef] [PubMed]
85. Braun, J.; Bollow, M.; Neure, L.; Seipelt, E.; Seyrekbasan, F.; Herbst, H.; Eggens, U.; Distler, A.; Sieper, J. Use of immunohistologic and in situ hybridization techniques in the examination of sacroiliac joint biopsy specimens from patients with ankylosing spondylitis. *Arthritis Rheum.* **1995**, *38*, 499–505. [CrossRef]
86. Laloux, L.; Voisin, M.-C.; Allain, J.; Martin, N.; Kerboull, L.; Chevalier, X.; Claudepierre, P. Immunohistological study of entheses in spondyloarthropathies: Comparison in rheumatoid arthritis and osteoarthritis. *Ann. Rheum. Dis.* **2001**, *60*, 316–321. [CrossRef]
87. Wang, M.; Zhou, X.; Zhang, H.; Liu, R.; Xu, N. Associations of the VEGF level, VEGF rs2010963 G/C gene polymorphism and ankylosing spondylitis risk in a Chinese Han population. *Immunol. Lett.* **2016**, *179*, 56–60. [CrossRef]
88. Lin, T.-T.; Lu, J.; Qi, C.-Y.; Yuan, L.; Li, X.-L.; Xia, L.-P.; Shen, H. Elevated serum level of IL-27 and VEGF in patients with ankylosing spondylitis and associate with disease activity. *Clin. Exp. Med.* **2014**, *15*, 227–231. [CrossRef]
89. Przepiera-Będzak, H.; Fischer, K.; Brzosko, M. Serum VEGF, EGF, basic FGF and acidic FGF levels and their association with disease activity and extra-articular symptoms in ankylosing spondylitis. *Pol. Arch. Intern. Med.* **2016**, *126*, 290–292. [CrossRef]
90. Pedersen, S.J.; Hetland, M.L.; Sørensen, I.J.; Østergaard, M.; Nielsen, H.J.; Johansen, J.S. Circulating levels of interleukin-6, vascular endothelial growth factor, YKL-40, matrix metalloproteinase-3, and total aggrecan in spondyloarthritis patients during 3 years of treatment with TNFα inhibitors. *Clin. Rheumatol.* **2010**, *29*, 1301–1309. [CrossRef]
91. Appel, H.; Janssen, L.; Listing, J.; Heydrich, R.; Rudwaleit, M.; Sieper, J. Serum levels of biomarkers of bone and cartilage destruction and new bone formation in different cohorts of patients with axial spondyloarthritis with and without tumor necrosis factor-alpha blocker treatment. *Arthritis Res. Ther.* **2008**, *10*, R125. [CrossRef]
92. Sakellariou, G.T.; Iliopoulos, A.; Konsta, M.; Kenanidis, E.; Potoupnis, M.; Tsiridis, E.; Gavana, E.; Sayegh, F.E. Serum levels of Dkk-1, sclerostin and VEGF in patients with ankylosing spondylitis and their association with smoking, and clinical, inflammatory and radiographic parameters. *Jt. Bone Spine* **2017**, *84*, 309–315. [CrossRef]
93. Prajzlerová, K.; Grobelná, K.; Pavelka, K.; Šenolt, L.; Filková, M. An update on biomarkers in axial spondyloarthritis. *Autoimmun. Rev.* **2016**, *15*, 501–509. [CrossRef]
94. Bandinelli, F.; Milia, A.F.; Manetti, M.; Lastraioli, E.; Amico, M.D.; Tonelli, P.; Fazi, M.; Arcangeli, A.; Matucci-Cerinic, M.; Ibba-Manneschi, L. Lymphatic endothelial progenitor cells and vascular endothelial growth factor-C in spondyloarthritis and Crohn's disease: Two overlapping diseases? *Clin. Exp. Rheumatol.* **2015**, *33*, 195–200.
95. Poddubnyy, D.; Conrad, K.; Haibel, H.; Syrbe, U.; Appel, H.; Braun, J.; Rudwaleit, M.; Sieper, J. Elevated serum level of the vascular endothelial growth factor predicts radiographic spinal progression in patients with axial spondyloarthritis. *Ann. Rheum. Dis.* **2013**, *73*, 2137–2143. [CrossRef]
96. Braun, J.; Baraliakos, X.; Hermann, K.-G.A.; Xu, S.; Hsu, B. Serum Vascular Endothelial Growth Factor Levels Lack Predictive Value in Patients with Active Ankylosing Spondylitis Treated with Golimumab. *J. Rheumatol.* **2016**, *43*, 901–906. [CrossRef]
97. Rademacher, J.; Tietz, L.M.; Le, L.; Hartl, A.; Hermann, K.-G.A.; Sieper, J.; Mansmann, U.; Rudwaleit, M.; Poddubnyy, D. Added value of biomarkers compared with clinical parameters for the prediction of radiographic spinal progression in axial spondyloarthritis. *Rheumatology* **2019**, *58*, 1556–1564. [CrossRef]
98. Tošovský, M.; Bradna, P.; Andrys, C.; Andrýsová, K.; Cermakova, E.; Soukup, T. The vegf and BMP-2 levels in patients with ankylosing spondylitis and the relationship to treatment with tumour necrosis factor alpha inhibitors. *Acta Med. Hradec Kral.* **2014**, *57*, 56–61. [CrossRef]
99. Visvanathan, S.; Van Der Heijde, D.; Deodhar, A.; Wagner, C.; Baker, D.G.; Han, J.; Braun, J. Effects of infliximab on markers of inflammation and bone turnover and associations with bone mineral density in patients with ankylosing spondylitis. *Ann. Rheum. Dis.* **2008**, *68*, 175–182. [CrossRef]
100. Kaaij, M.H.; Helder, B.; Van Mens, L.J.J.; Van De Sande, M.G.H.; Baeten, D.L.P.; Tas, S.W. Anti-IL-17A treatment reduces serum inflammatory, angiogenic and tissue remodeling biomarkers accompanied by less synovial high endothelial venules in peripheral spondyloarthritis. *Sci. Rep.* **2020**, *10*, 1–11. [CrossRef]
101. Hindryckx, P.; Laukens, D.; Serry, G.; Van Praet, L.; Cuvelier, C.; Mielants, H.; Peeters, H.; Elewaut, D.; De Vos, M. Subclinical gut inflammation in spondyloarthritis is associated with a pro-angiogenic intestinal mucosal phenotype. *Ann. Rheum. Dis.* **2011**, *70*, 2044–2048. [CrossRef]

102. Yu, Z.; Zhang, Y.; Gao, N.; Yong, K. Suppression of Development of Ankylosing Spondylitis Through Soluble Flt-1. *Cell. Physiol. Biochem.* **2015**, *37*, 2135–2142. [CrossRef]
103. Lacout, A.; Carlier, R.Y.; El Hajjam, M.; Marcy, P.Y. VEGF inhibition as possible therapy in spondyloarthritis patients: Targeting bone remodelling. *Med. Hypotheses* **2017**, *101*, 52–54. [CrossRef]
104. Cervera, R.; Khamashta, M.A.; Font, J.; Sebastiani, G.D.; Gil, A.; Lavilla, P.; Doménech, I.; O Aydintug, A.; Jedryka-Góral, A.; De Ramón, E. Systemic lupus erythematosus: Clinical and immunologic patterns of disease expression in a cohort of 1000 patients. The European Working Party on Systemic Lupus Erythematosus. *Medicine* **1993**, *72*, 113–124. [CrossRef]
105. Cooper, G.S.; Dooley, M.A.; Treadwell, E.L.; Clair, E.W.S.; Parks, C.G.; Gilkeson, G.S. Hormonal, environmental, and infectious risk factors for developing systemic lupus erythematosus. *Arthritis Rheum.* **2001**, *41*, 1714–1724. [CrossRef]
106. Tang, W.; Zhou, T.; Zhong, Z.; Zhong, H. Meta-analysis of associations of vascular endothelial growth factor protein levels and -634G/C polymorphism with systemic lupus erythematosus susceptibility. *BMC Med. Genet.* **2019**, *20*, 46. [CrossRef]
107. Yuan, Z.-C.; Xu, W.-D.; Wang, J.-M.; Wu, Q.; Zhou, J.; Huang, A.-F. Gene polymorphisms and serum levels of sVEGFR-1 in patients with systemic lupus erythematosus. *Sci. Rep.* **2020**, *10*, 1–11. [CrossRef] [PubMed]
108. Willis, R.; Smikle, M.; Deceulaer, K.; Romay-Penabad, Z.; Papalardo, E.; Jajoria, P.; Harper, B.; Murthy, V.; Petri, M.; Gonzalez, E.B. Clinical associations of proinflammatory cytokines, oxidative biomarkers and vitamin D levels in systemic lupus erythematosus. *Lupus* **2017**, *26*, 1517–1527. [CrossRef] [PubMed]
109. Aterido, A.; Julià, A.; Carreira, P.; Blanco, R.; López-Longo, J.J.; Venegas, J.J.P.; Olivé, À.; Andreu, J.L.; Aguirre-Zamorano, M.Á.; Vela, P.; et al. Genome-wide pathway analysis identifies VEGF pathway association with oral ulceration in systemic lupus erythematosus. *Arthritis Res.* **2017**, *19*, 138. [CrossRef] [PubMed]
110. Taha, S.; Gamal, S.; Nabil, M.; Naeem, N.; Labib, D.; Siam, I.; Gheita, T.A. Vascular endothelial growth factor G1612A (rs10434) gene polymorphism and neuropsychiatric manifestations in systemic lupus erythematosus patients. *Rev. Bras. Reum.* **2017**, *57*, 149–153. [CrossRef]
111. De Jesús, G.R.; Lacerda, M.I.; Rodrigues, B.C.; Santos, F.C.D.; Nascimento, A.P.D.; Porto, L.C.; Jesús, N.R.D.; Levy, R.A.; Klumb, E.M. VEGF, PlGF and sFlt-1 serum levels allow differentiation between active lupus nephritis during pregnancy and preeclampsia. *Arthritis Care Res.* **2020**, *73*, 717–721. [CrossRef]
112. Yuan, M.; Tan, Y.; Wang, Y.; Wang, S.X.; Yu, F.; Zhao, M.H. The associations of endothelial and podocyte injury in proliferative lupus nephritis: From observational analysis to in vitro study. *Lupus* **2019**, *28*, 347–358. [CrossRef]
113. Ghazali, W.S.W.; Iberahim, R.; Ashari, N.S.M. Serum Vascular Endothelial Growth Factor (VEGF) as a Biomarker for Disease Activity in Lupus Nephritis. *Malays. J. Med. Sci.* **2017**, *24*, 62–72. [CrossRef]
114. Slight-Webb, S.; Guthridge, J.M.; Chakravarty, E.F.; Chen, H.; Lu, R.; Macwana, S.; Bean, K.; Maecker, H.T.; Utz, P.J.; James, J.A. Mycophenolate mofetil reduces STAT3 phosphorylation in systemic lupus erythematosus patients. *JCI Insight* **2019**, *4*, e124575. [CrossRef]
115. Hrycek, A.; Janowska, J.; Cieślik, P. Selected angiogenic cytokines in systemic lupus erythematosus patients. *Autoimmunity* **2009**, *42*, 459–466. [CrossRef]
116. Castejon, R.; Castañeda, A.; Sollet, A.; Mellor-Pita, S.; Tutor-Ureta, P.; Jimenez-Ortiz, C.; Yebra-Bango, M. Short-term atorvastatin therapy improves arterial stiffness of middle-aged systemic lupus erythematosus patients with pathological pulse wave velocity. *Lupus* **2017**, *26*, 355–364. [CrossRef]
117. Robak, E.; Woźniacka, A.; Sysa-Jedrzejowska, A.; Stepień, H.; Robak, T. Serum levels of angiogenic cytokines in systemic lupus erythematosus and their correlation with disease activity. *Eur. Cytokine Netw.* **2001**, *12*, 445–452.
118. Bărbulescu, A.L.; Vreju, A.F.; Bugă, A.M.; Sandu, R.E.; Criveanu, C.; Tudoraşcu, D.R.; Gheonea, I.A.; Ciurea, P.L. Vascular endothelial growth factor in systemic lupus erythematosus-correlations with disease activity and nailfold capillaroscopy changes. *Romanian J. Morphol. Embryol.* **2015**, *56*, 1011–1016.
119. Neogi, T.; Zhang, Y. Epidemiology of Osteoarthritis. *Rheum. Dis. Clin. N. Am.* **2013**, *39*, 1–19. [CrossRef]
120. Lo, J.; Chan, L.; Flynn, S. A Systematic Review of the Incidence, Prevalence, Costs, and Activity and Work Limitations of Amputation, Osteoarthritis, Rheumatoid Arthritis, Back Pain, Multiple Sclerosis, Spinal Cord Injury, Stroke, and Traumatic Brain Injury in the United States: A 2019 Update. *Arch. Phys. Med. Rehabil.* **2021**, *102*, 115–131. [CrossRef]
121. Goldring, M.B.; Berenbaum, F. Emerging targets in osteoarthritis therapy. *Curr. Opin. Pharmacol.* **2015**, *22*, 51–63. [CrossRef]
122. Macdonald, I.J.; Liu, S.-C.; Su, C.-M.; Wang, Y.-H.; Tsai, C.-H.; Tang, C.-H. Implications of Angiogenesis Involvement in Arthritis. *Int. J. Mol. Sci.* **2018**, *19*, 2012. [CrossRef] [PubMed]
123. Shen, P.; Jiao, Z.; Zheng, J.S.; Xu, W.F.; Zhang, S.Y.; Qin, A.; Yang, C. Injecting vascular endothelial growth factor into the temporomandibular joint induces osteoarthritis in mice. *Sci. Rep.* **2015**, *5*, 16244. [CrossRef] [PubMed]
124. Pfander, D.; Körtje, D.; Zimmermann, R.; Weseloh, G.; Kirsch, T.; Gesslein, M.; Cramer, T.; Swoboda, B. Vascular endothelial growth factor in articular cartilage of healthy and osteoarthritic human knee joints. *Ann. Rheum. Dis.* **2001**, *60*, 1070–1073. [CrossRef] [PubMed]
125. Enomoto, H.; Inoki, I.; Komiya, K.; Shiomi, T.; Ikeda, E.; Obata, K.-I.; Matsumoto, H.; Toyama, Y.; Okada, Y. Vascular Endothelial Growth Factor Isoforms and Their Receptors Are Expressed in Human Osteoarthritic Cartilage. *Am. J. Pathol.* **2003**, *162*, 171–181. [CrossRef]
126. Hamilton, J.L.; Nagao, M.; Levine, B.R.; Chen, D.; Olsen, B.R.; Im, H.-J. Targeting VEGF and Its Receptors for the Treatment of Osteoarthritis and Associated Pain. *J. Bone Miner. Res.* **2016**, *31*, 911–924. [CrossRef] [PubMed]

127. Corrado, A.; Neve, A.; Cantatore, F.P. Expression of vascular endothelial growth factor in normal, osteoarthritic and osteoporotic osteoblasts. *Clin. Exp. Med.* **2011**, *13*, 81–84. [CrossRef] [PubMed]
128. Wang, X.; Fang, W.; Li, Y.; Long, X.; Cai, H. Synovial fluid levels of VEGF and FGF-2 before and after intra-articular injection of hyaluronic acid in patients with temporomandibular disorders: A short-term study. *Br. J. Oral Maxillofac. Surg.* **2021**, *59*, 64–69. [CrossRef]
129. Takano, S.; Uchida, K.; Inoue, G.; Matsumoto, T.; Aikawa, J.; Iwase, D.; Mukai, M.; Miyagi, M.; Takaso, M. Vascular endothelial growth factor expression and their action in the synovial membranes of patients with painful knee osteoarthritis. *BMC Musculoskelet. Disord.* **2018**, *19*, 1–8. [CrossRef]
130. Gaballah, A.; Hussein, N.A.; Risk, M.; Elsawy, N.; Elabasiry, S. Correlation between synovial vascular endothelial growth factor, clinical, functional and radiological manifestations in knee osteoarthritis. *Egypt. Rheumatol.* **2016**, *38*, 29–34. [CrossRef]
131. Suri, S.; Gill, S.E.; De Camin, S.M.; McWilliams, D.F.; Wilson, D.; Walsh, D.A. Neurovascular invasion at the osteochondral junction and in osteophytes in osteoarthritis. *Ann. Rheum. Dis.* **2007**, *66*, 1423–1428. [CrossRef]
132. Mapp, P.I.; Walsh, D.A. Mechanisms and targets of angiogenesis and nerve growth in osteoarthritis. *Nat. Rev. Rheumatol.* **2012**, *8*, 390–398. [CrossRef]
133. Kiguchi, N.; Kobayashi, Y.; Kadowaki, Y.; Fukazawa, Y.; Saika, F.; Kishioka, S. Vascular endothelial growth factor signaling in injured nerves underlies peripheral sensitization in neuropathic pain. *J. Neurochem.* **2014**, *129*, 169–178. [CrossRef]
134. Selvaraj, D.; Gangadharan, V.; Michalski, C.W.; Kurejova, M.; Stösser, S.; Srivastava, K.; Schweizerhof, M.; Waltenberger, J.; Ferrara, N.; Heppenstall, P.; et al. A Functional Role for VEGFR1 Expressed in Peripheral Sensory Neurons in Cancer Pain. *Cancer Cell* **2015**, *27*, 780–796. [CrossRef]
135. Wu, Y.; Li, M.; Zeng, J.; Feng, Z.; Yang, J.; Shen, B.; Zeng, Y. Differential Expression of Renin-Angiotensin System-related Components in Patients with Rheumatoid Arthritis and Osteoarthritis. *Am. J. Med. Sci.* **2020**, *359*, 17–26. [CrossRef] [PubMed]
136. Chen, Y.; Zhao, B.; Zhu, Y.; Zhao, H.; Ma, C. HIF-1-VEGF-Notch mediates angiogenesis in temporomandibular joint osteoarthritis. *Am. J. Transl. Res.* **2019**, *11*, 2969–2982.
137. Nagai, T.; Sato, M.; Kobayashi, M.; Yokoyama, M.; Tani, Y.; Mochida, J. Bevacizumab, an anti-vascular endothelial growth factor antibody, inhibits osteoarthritis. *Arthritis Res. Ther.* **2014**, *16*, 427. [CrossRef]
138. Roumm, A.D.; Whiteside, T.L.; Medsger, T.A.; Rodnan, G.P. Lymphocytes in the skin of patients with progressive systemic sclerosis. *Arthritis Rheum.* **1984**, *27*, 645–653. [CrossRef] [PubMed]
139. Freemont, A.J.; Hoyland, J.; Fielding, P.; Hodson, N.; Jayson, M.I.V. Studies of the microvascular endothelium in uninvolved skin of patients with systemic sclerosis: Direct evidence for a generalized microangiopathy. *Br. J. Dermatol.* **2008**, *126*, 561–568. [CrossRef]
140. Prescott, R.J.; Freemont, A.J.; Jones, C.J.P.; Hoyland, J.; Fielding, P. Sequential dermal microvascular and perivascular changes in the development of scleroderma. *J. Pathol.* **1992**, *166*, 255–263. [CrossRef]
141. Silva, I.; Almeida, C.; Teixeira, A.; Oliveira, J.; Vasconcelos, C. Impaired angiogenesis as a feature of digital ulcers in systemic sclerosis. *Clin. Rheumatol.* **2016**, *35*, 1743–1751. [CrossRef]
142. Distler, O.; Del Rosso, A.; Giacomelli, R.; Cipriani, P.; Conforti, M.L.; Guiducci, S.; Gay, R.E.; Michel, B.A.; Brühlmann, P.; Müller-Ladner, U.; et al. Angiogenic and angiostatic factors in systemic sclerosis: Increased levels of vascular endothelial growth factor are a feature of the earliest disease stages and are associated with the absence of fingertip ulcers. *Arthritis Res. Ther.* **2002**, *4*, 1–10. [CrossRef]
143. Gigante, A.; Gasperini, M.L.; Rosato, E.; Navarini, L.; Margiotta, D.; Afeltra, A.; Muscaritoli, M. Phase angle could be a marker of microvascular damage in systemic sclerosis. *Nutrition* **2020**, *73*, 110730. [CrossRef] [PubMed]
144. Jinnin, M.; Makino, T.; Kajihara, I.; Honda, N.; Makino, K.; Ogata, A.; Ihn, H. Serum levels of soluble vascular endothelial growth factor receptor-2 in patients with systemic sclerosis. *Br. J. Dermatol.* **2009**, *162*, 751–758. [CrossRef]
145. Distler, O.; Distler, J.H.W.; Scheid, A.; Acker, T.; Hirth, A.; Rethage, J.; Michel, B.A.; Gay, R.E.; Müller-Ladner, U.; Matucci-Cerinic, M.; et al. Uncontrolled Expression of Vascular Endothelial Growth Factor and Its Receptors Leads to Insufficient Skin Angiogenesis in Patients With Systemic Sclerosis. *Circ. Res.* **2004**, *95*, 109–116. [CrossRef]
146. De Santis, M.; Ceribelli, A.; Cavaciocchi, F.; Crotti, C.; Massarotti, M.; Belloli, L.; Marasini, B.; Isailovic, N.; Generali, E.; Selmi, C. Nailfold videocapillaroscopy and serum VEGF levels in scleroderma are associated with internal organ involvement. *Autoimmun. Highlights* **2016**, *7*, 5. [CrossRef]
147. Gigante, A.; Navarini, L.; Margiotta, D.; Amoroso, A.; Barbano, B.; Cianci, R.; Afeltra, A.; Rosato, E. Angiogenic and angiostatic factors in renal scleroderma-associated vasculopathy. *Microvasc. Res.* **2017**, *114*, 41–45. [CrossRef]
148. Głodkowska-Mrówka, E.; Górska, E.; Ciurzyński, M.; Stelmaszczyk-Emmel, A.; Bienias, P.; Irzyk, K.; Siwicka, M.; Lipińska, A.; Ciepiela, O.; Pruszczyk, P.; et al. Pro- and antiangiogenic markers in patients with pulmonary complications of systemic scleroderma. *Respir. Physiol. Neurobiol.* **2015**, *209*, 69–75. [CrossRef]
149. Mcmahan, Z.; Schoenhoff, F.; Van Eyk, J.E.; Wigley, F.M.; Hummers, L.K. Biomarkers of pulmonary hypertension in patients with scleroderma: A case–control study. *Arthritis Res. Ther.* **2015**, *17*, 201. [CrossRef]
150. Moritz, F.; Schniering, J.; Distler, J.H.W.; Gay, R.E.; Gay, S.; Distler, O.; Maurer, B. Tie2 as a novel key factor of microangiopathy in systemic sclerosis. *Arthritis Res. Ther.* **2017**, *19*, 105. [CrossRef]

151. Huang, J.; Maier, C.; Zhang, Y.; Soare, A.; Dees, C.; Beyer, C.; Harre, U.; Chen, C.-W.; Distler, O.; Schett, G.; et al. Nintedanib inhibits macrophage activation and ameliorates vascular and fibrotic manifestations in the Fra2 mouse model of systemic sclerosis. *Ann. Rheum. Dis.* **2017**, *76*, 1941–1948. [CrossRef]
152. Kvarnström, M.; Ottosson, V.; Nordmark, B.; Wahren-Herlenius, M. Incident cases of primary Sjögren's syndrome during a 5-year period in Stockholm County: A descriptive study of the patients and their characteristics. *Scand. J. Rheumatol.* **2014**, *44*, 135–142. [CrossRef]
153. Sisto, M.; Lisi, S.; Ingravallo, G.; Lofrumento, D.D.; D'Amore, M.; Ribatti, D. Neovascularization is prominent in the chronic inflammatory lesions of Sjögren's syndrome. *Int. J. Exp. Pathol.* **2014**, *95*, 131–137. [CrossRef]
154. Alunno, A.; Ibba-Manneschi, L.; Bistoni, O.; Rosa, I.; Caterbi, S.; Gerli, R.; Manetti, M. Mobilization of lymphatic endothelial precursor cells and lymphatic neovascularization in primary Sjögren's syndrome. *J. Cell. Mol. Med.* **2016**, *20*, 613–622. [CrossRef]
155. Sisto, M.; Lisi, S.; Lofrumento, D.D.; D'Amore, M.; Frassanito, M.A.; Ribatti, D. Sjögren's syndrome pathological neovascularization is regulated by VEGF-A-stimulated TACE-dependent crosstalk between VEGFR2 and NF-κB. *Genes Immun.* **2012**, *13*, 411–420. [CrossRef] [PubMed]
156. Błochowiak, K.J.; Trzybulska, D.; Olewicz-Gawlik, A.; Sikora, J.J.; Nowak-Gabryel, M.; Kociecki, J.; Witmanowski, H.; Sokalski, J. Levels of EGF and VEGF in patients with primary and secondary Sjögren's syndrome. *Adv. Clin. Exp. Med.* **2018**, *27*, 455–461. [CrossRef]

International Journal of
Molecular Sciences

MDPI

Review

Targeting CCN Proteins in Rheumatoid Arthritis and Osteoarthritis

Iona J. MacDonald [1], Chien-Chung Huang [2,3], Shan-Chi Liu [4], Yen-You Lin [1] and Chih-Hsin Tang [1,2,5,6,7,*]

1 Graduate Institute of Basic Medical Science, Collage of Medicine, China Medical University, Taichung 40402, Taiwan; ionamac@gmail.com (I.J.M.); chas6119@gmail.com (Y.-Y.L.)
2 School of Medicine, Collage of Medicine, China Medical University, Taichung 406040, Taiwan; u104054003@cmu.edu.tw
3 Division of Immunology and Rheumatology, Department of Internal Medicine, China Medical University Hospital, Taichung 404332, Taiwan
4 Department of Medical Education and Research, China Medical University Beigang Hospital, Yunlin 65152, Taiwan; sdsaw.tw@yahoo.com.tw
5 Graduate Institute of Biomedical Sciences, Collage of Medicine, China Medical University, Taichung 406040, Taiwan
6 Chinese Medicine Research Center, China Medical University, Taichung 406040, Taiwan
7 Department of Biotechnology, College of Health Science, Asia University, Taichung 413305, Taiwan
* Correspondence: chtang@mail.cmu.edu.tw

Abstract: The CCN family of matricellular proteins (CYR61/CCN1, CTGF/CCN2, NOV/CCN3 and WISP1-2-3/CCN4-5-6) are essential players in the key pathophysiological processes of angiogenesis, wound healing and inflammation. These proteins are well recognized for their important roles in many cellular processes, including cell proliferation, adhesion, migration and differentiation, as well as the regulation of extracellular matrix differentiation. Substantial evidence implicates four of the proteins (CCN1, CCN2, CCN3 and CCN4) in the inflammatory pathologies of rheumatoid arthritis (RA) and osteoarthritis (OA). A smaller evidence base supports the involvement of CCN5 and CCN6 in the development of these diseases. This review focuses on evidence providing insights into the involvement of the CCN family in RA and OA, as well as the potential of the CCN proteins as therapeutic targets in these diseases.

Keywords: CCN proteins; CCN family; rheumatoid arthritis; osteoarthritis; juvenile idiopathic arthritis

Citation: MacDonald, I.J.; Huang, C.-C.; Liu, S.-C.; Lin, Y.-Y.; Tang, C.-H. Targeting CCN Proteins in Rheumatoid Arthritis and Osteoarthritis. *Int. J. Mol. Sci.* **2021**, 22, 4340. https://doi.org/10.3390/ijms22094340

Academic Editor: Yousef Abu-Amer

Received: 24 March 2021
Accepted: 20 April 2021
Published: 21 April 2021

1. Introduction

Of the more than 100 different types of arthritis, rheumatoid arthritis (RA) and osteoarthritis (OA) are two of the most common [1]. The chronic inflammation and autoimmunity associated with RA disease principally targets the synovium, provoking the membrane lining to produce synovial fluid that causes synovitis and joint pain, and ultimately chronic and progressive joint erosion [2]. OA is a whole-joint disease involving the increased remodeling of the articular cartilage, subchondral bone and bone marrow compartments, as well as the synovium, during its onset and progression [3]. Although these are two distinct arthritis diseases, some similar clinical and pathological manifestations exist, such as joint stiffness, synovial inflammation, destruction of the articular cartilage and bone erosion [4]. Treatment remains a significant clinical challenge in these diseases. In spite of the recent emergence of targeted therapies and immune-modulating agents for RA, a sizeable proportion remain treatment-refractory and experience increasing clinical impairment and even premature mortality [5–7]. Moreover, no disease-modifying treatments exist as yet for OA [8]. Enhancing our understanding about the ways in which CCN proteins affect the pathophysiological processes of these forms of arthritis may lead to future treatment strategies that target the functions and mechanisms of action of these proteins, and effectively alleviate patients' suffering.

The CCN family consists of six matricellular proteins, cysteine-rich 61 (CYR61/CCN1), connective tissue growth factor (CTGF/CCN2), nephroblastoma-overexpressed (NOV/CCN3), Wnt-1 induced secreted protein-1 (WISP1/CCN4), Wnt-1 induced secreted protein-2 (WISP2/CCN5) and Wnt-1 induced secreted protein-3 (WISP3/CCN6), all of which are essential players in the key pathophysiological processes of angiogenesis, wound healing and inflammation [9]. They are well recognized for their important roles in many cellular processes including cell proliferation, adhesion, migration and differentiation, and the regulation of extracellular matrix (ECM) differentiation [9]. Much evidence has implicated four of the proteins (CCN1, CCN2, CCN3 and CCN4) in the inflammatory pathologies of RA [10–13] and OA [14–20]; the evidence base is smaller for CCN5 and CCN6 in these diseases [21–24]. Interestingly, although much similarity exists among the primary structures of the CCN proteins, the considerable differences identified in their three-dimensional structures result in distinctly different protein interactions and known binding partners that result in distinctly different functions [25]. Moreover, interactions between CCNs enable the regulation of cellular function and various receptors including insulin-like growth factors, heparan sulfate proteoglycans and integrins, among others [25]. Finally, the CCN proteins are vital contributors to the biological processes mentioned above (angiogenesis, adhesion, migration and differentiation, ECM remodeling, cartilage growth and maintenance, wound healing and inflammation) [25].

This review discusses the evidence regarding the involvement of CCN proteins in RA and OA (see Table 1 and Figure 1).

Table 1. Evidence regarding the involvement of CCN proteins in RA and OA.

CCN Protein	Disease	Targets	Target Factors		Results	References
CCN1	OA	osteoblast	IL-6, oncostatin M	↑	inflammation	[26]
	OA	cartilage	ADAMTS-4	↓	chondrocyte cloning	[15,27,28]
	RA	synovial fluid	CCL2	↑	inflammation	[11]
	RA	RA FLS	IL-1β, IL-6, IL-17	↑	inflammation	[29–31]
	RA	osteoblast	VEGF	↑	angiogenesis	[32]
	RA	RA FLS	MMP-3	↑	inflammation	[33]
CCN2	OA	OASF	CCL2/MCP-1	↑	inflammation	[34]
	OA	cartilage	Wnt-β-catenin	↑	chondroprotective	[35]
	RA	RASF	M-CSF, RANKL	↑	osteoclastogenesis	[36]
	RA	RA FLS	VEGF	↑	angiogenesis	[37]
CCN3	OA	cartilage	IL-1β	↓	protective effect	[38]
Other CCNs						
CCN4	OA	OASF	VCAM-1	↑	monocyte adhesion	[39]
	OA	synovium, cartilage	MMPs	↑	synovium & cartilage damage	[40]
CCN6	normal	chondrocyte	collagen II, aggrecan, SOD	↑	cartilage growth	[41]
	OA	chondrocyte	ADAMTS-4, ADAMTS-5	↓	anticatabolic effects	[42]
			MMP-1, MMP-10	↑		

RA, rheumatoid arthritis; OA, osteoarthritis; IL-6, interleukin 6; ADAMTS-4, a disintegrin and metalloproteinase with thrombospondin motif 4; CCL2, chemokine ligand 2; FLS, fibroblast-like synoviocyte; VEGF, vascular endothelial growth factor; MMP, matrix metallopeptidase; OASF, osteoarthritis synovial fibroblast; MCP-1, monocyte chemoattractant protein-1; RASF, rheumatoid arthritis synovial fibroblast; M-CSF, macrophage colony-stimulating factor; RANKL, receptor activator of nuclear factor-kappa B ligand; VCAM-1, vascular cell adhesion molecule-1; SOD, superoxide dismutase.

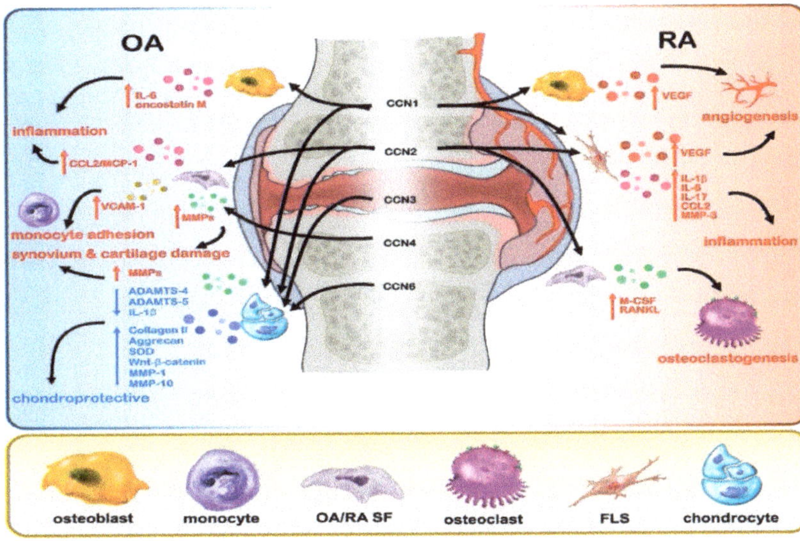

Figure 1. Graphical representation of the effects of CCN proteins 1–6 in RA and OA disease.

2. CCN1 in RA and OA

CCN1 can play an important and harmful role in OA disease by promoting the production of inflammatory cytokines such as interleukin 6 (IL-6) and oncostatin M in human osteoblasts through integrin-dependent signaling [26]. Furthermore, CCN1 overexpression accelerates inflammation and matrix degradation in human OA cartilage [28]. *Ccn1* messenger RNA (mRNA) and *ADAMTS-4* (a disintegrin and metalloproteinase with thrombospondin motif 4) mRNA is significantly upregulated in human OA cartilage tissue compared with normal, non-OA cartilage [15,27]. Moreover, *Ccn1* and *ADAMTS-4* mRNA expression is positively correlated in OA cartilage tissue, while levels of CCN1 and ADAMTS-4 protein expression are markedly upregulated in OA chondrocytes, compared with those in normal chondrocytes [27]. CCN1 stimulates the proliferation of OA chondrocytes through ADAMTS-4 [27]. Intriguingly, CCN1 activities can also be beneficial in OA. The binding of CCN1 with ADAMTS-4 enables CCN1 to suppress ADAMTS-4 aggrecanase activities, which are critical to the development of OA disease [15,27]. Notably, IL-1β promotes ADAMTS-4 and inhibits CCN1 expression [27]. CCN1 expression in OA chondrocytes is also inhibited by IL-1α [15] and upregulated by transforming growth factor beta (TGF-β) [27]. Interestingly, TGF-β-treated human OA chondrocytes have demonstrated aggrecanase activity after knockdown of CCN1 expression, which suggests that modulating CCN1 and TGF-β activity may promote the repair of OA cartilage [27]. Thus, the evidence appears to be conflicting as to the effects of CCN in OA. Further studies are needed to fully understand the relationships.

Chronic synovitis in RA joints results from the persistent production of proinflammatory cytokines IL-1 and tumor necrosis factor alpha (TNF-α) from activated mononuclear cells, inducing cartilage degradation [43]. The chemotaxis, survival and proliferation pathways in mononuclear cells can be activated by chemokines [44], including chemokine ligand 2 (CCL2, also known as monocyte chemoattractant protein-1 (MCP-1), a critical regulator in the process of monocyte migration and infiltration to the site of RA inflammation, as CCL2/MCP-1 is produced at significantly higher levels in blood, synovial fluid and synovial tissue from patients with RA compared with samples from non-RA controls [45,46]. High levels of CCN1 expression are also found in RA synovial fluid compared with synovial fluid from patients without RA [11], while CCN1 expression is minimal in RA hip and knee cartilage and absent in normal hip cartilage [47].

Several lines of evidence demonstrate that CCN1 is a key contributor to the RA disease process. CCN1 induces upregulation of CCL2/MCP-1 expression in osteoblasts, and subsequently, promotes monocyte migration by inhibiting microRNA (miR)-518-5p [11]. As a component of the ECM, CCN1 plays a role in endothelial cell adhesion, migration, proliferation, and differentiation [48]. CCN1 interacts with IL-17 to promote fibroblast-like synoviocyte (FLS) proliferation in RA synovial fluid and inhibits FLS apoptosis, contributing to the hyperplasia of synovial lining cells [29]. Attacks by FLS on RA synovial tissue and cartilage implicates CCN1 as a key contributor to the joint erosion and destruction seen in RA disease [29], which is emphasized by subsequent research revealing that CCN1 promotes IL-17 production in RA by upregulating IL-6 in human RA FLS [30]. CCN1 also increases synthesis of the precursor IL-1β (pro-IL-1β) in human RA FLS [31] and upregulates vascular endothelial growth factor (VEGF) expression in osteoblasts, inducing endothelial progenitor cell (EPC)-angiogenesis in RA disease [32].

Much cellular and preclinical evidence has suggested that modulating CCN1 expression in RA disease has therapeutic potential [49]. Promising experimental findings suggest the feasibility of designing peptide-based vaccination against RA. The murine monoclonal antibody (mAb) 093G9 specifically targets CCN1 and effectively antagonizes its effects on the production of pro-IL-1β and matrix metallopeptidase (MMP)-3 expression by FLS [33], while in mice with collagen-induced arthritis (CIA), mAb 093G9 treatment reduces inflammatory reactions and ameliorates joint disease [30]. Structural and functional investigations have delineated the CCN1 epitope that is recognized by 093G9 and defined its epitope specificity, opening up the possibilities for developing mAb drugs and peptide vaccines targeting CCN1 [33].

In summary, CCN1 is both beneficial and harmful for OA and harmful in RA. CCN1 increases the expression of oncostatin M in human osteoblastic cells [26], synthesizes pro-IL-1β and enhances the expression of MMP-3 in human RA FLS [31], promotes FLS proliferation and participates in RA pathogenesis via the IL-17-dependent pathway [49] and also promotes the expression of CCL2 and monocyte migration by inhibiting miR-518-5p expression in osteoblasts via mitogen-activated protein kinase (MAPK) signaling [11].

3. The Role of CCN2 in RA and OA

All layers of normal cartilage express CCN2 protein and mRNA in a small percentage of chondrocytes, whereas OA cartilage is characterized by markedly increased numbers of CCN2-positive chondrocytes that correlate with increasingly severe OA disease [50]. Our laboratory has previously described finding high levels of CCL2/MCP-1 expression in OA synovial fibroblasts (OASFs) compared with normal synovial fibroblasts, and we have observed that treating OASFs with CCN2 increases CCL2/MCP-1 expression [34]. OASFs and supernatants from CCN2-treated OASFs promote the migration of monocyte cells via the αvβ5 integrin, focal adhesion kinase (FAK), mitogen-activated protein (MEK), extracellular signal-regulated kinase (ERK), and nuclear factor-kappa B (NF-κB)/AP-1 signaling transduction pathway [34].

Intriguingly, CCN2 can promote proliferation and differentiation of articular chondrocytes without inducing their hypertrophic calcification [51]. Thus, it has been hypothesized that articular chondrocytes promote CCN2 production in OA cartilage, and thereby, increase the cell number and compensate for the deficiency in the ECM [51]. This is supported by research showing that in rats with monoiodoacetic acid (MIA)-induced OA, a single injection of recombinant CCN2 into the joint cavity effectively repaired articular cartilage and ameliorated OA disease, which suggests that CCN2 may help to regenerate articular cartilage [52]. Likewise, transgenic mice that overexpress *Ccn2* in articular cartilage appear to be protected against OA-like degenerative changes in aged knee joint cartilage, which may mean that CCN2 stabilizes articular cartilage [53]. The idea that CCN2 plays a chondroprotective role is supported by findings showing significantly accelerated degeneration of lumbar intervertebral discs (IVDs) in *Ccn2*-knockout mice [35]. An analysis of CCN2 expression in rat IVD cells found that Wnt-β-catenin signaling regulates the *Ccn2* gene and protein via the MAPK pathway, raising the possibility that it could be worth targeting Wnt-β-catenin signaling in preclinical treatment of IVD degeneration [54]. Interestingly, some research has reported that the deletion of *Ccn2* in mice increases articular cartilage thickness and prevents the development of OA in cut cartilage [55], whereas other researchers have found that *Ccn2* deletion in articular chondrocytes of male transgenic mice fails to protect them from developing post-traumatic osteoarthritis [56]. In brief, most research supports the potential beneficial role of CCN2 in OA.

In regard to RA disease, CCN2 is strongly expressed in the matrix and perivascular cells in RA human hip and knee synovium samples, as well as in chondrocytes from RA hip and knee cartilage [47]. In normal human hip synovium, CCN2 is moderately expressed in the superficial layers, matrix and perivascular cells, and weakly expressed in normal hip cartilage [47]. The wide-ranging biological activity of CCN2 is characterized by inflammatory, wound healing and profibrotic activity [57,58], proangiogenic activity [57], protumorigenic activity [59] and the promotion of endochondral ossification [60]. In relation to RA, serum CCN2 concentration has shown significant discriminative ability and superior diagnostic performance compared with the rheumatoid factor (RF) and anti-citrullinated protein antibodies (ACPA) assays, which lack sensitivity and specificity [61]. Serum CCN2 discriminates RA from other rheumatic diseases, such as ankylosing spondylitis, gout, systemic lupus erythematosus and OA [61]. Serum CCN2 concentrations are higher in patients with active RA compared with CCN2 concentrations in normal healthy controls and patients with inactive RA disease; CCN2 also promotes articular destruction in RA by increasing osteoclastogenesis [36] and FLS proliferation in RA [62]. Investigations suggest that CCN2 acts synergistically with macrophage colony-stimulating factor (M-CSF) and receptor activator of nuclear factor-kappa B ligand (RANKL) to promote osteoclastogenesis and that excessive CCN2 production by RA synovial fibroblasts (RASFs) enhances osteoclastic function through integrin αVβ3-mediated pathways such as FAK and ERK1/2 phosphorylation [36]. CCN2 contains four distinct modules that are connected in tandem-insulin-like growth factor-binding protein (IGFBP)-like, von Willebrand factor (vWF) type C repeat, thrombospondin type 1 (TSP-1) repeat and carboxyl-terminal (CT) modules [63]. Inhibiting each of these modules with mAbs neutralizes the effect of CCN2 in human RA synovial cells [63]. In vivo investigations suggest that targeting CCN2 function may be beneficial in RA, as arthritis was significantly ameliorated in CIA mice administered neutralizing anti-CTGF mAb, which effectively suppressed pathologic proliferation of T lymphocytes and restored aberrant osteoclastogenesis [64].

A proteomics analysis has confirmed the importance of angiogenesis in RA progression, by demonstrating the upregulation of CCN2 and other vasculature development-related proteins in cultures of FLS from patients with RA compared with FLS from healthy normal controls [37]. Furthermore, *Ccn2* and *VEGF* mRNA and protein expression are markedly downregulated in RA FLS transfected with CCN2 knockdown, while recombinant human CCN2 significantly enhances the proliferation and migration of human umbilical vein endothelial cells (HUVECs) in Transwell assays [37]. Interestingly, cellular studies have implicated CCN2 in the regulation of MMP expression in RASFs [65]. After subjecting RASFs to 24 h of 10-hydroxy-2-decenoic acid (10H2DA) treatment, CCN2 expression was downregulated and subsequent investigations found that as CCN2 expression decreased in RASFs, so did levels of MMP expression [65]. Notably, several endogenous anti-inflammatory/proresolution lipid mediators are capable of accelerating the resolution of inflammation [66]. These proresolving mediators include resolvins, which are derived from the polyunsaturated omega-3 fatty acids docosahexanoic acid (DHA) or eicosapentanoic acid (EPA) [66]. The D- and E-series resolvins exhibit potent anti-inflammatory/proresolution effects in animal models of inflammation [66]. In particular, one study has demonstrated that resolvin D1 (RvD1) effectively decreases pannus formation and reduces cartilage damage in CIA mice by suppressing concentrations of CCN2 and proinflammatory cytokines in serum and RA FLS, through the upregulation of miR-146a-5p [67]. The above studies mostly confirm the aggravating character of CCN2 in RA.

In summary, CCN2 is beneficial for OA, but possibly harmful for RA. For instance, CCN2 may regenerate OA articular cartilage [52] and help to stabilize the matrix, since *Ccn2* overexpression in articular cartilage seems to protect against OA-like degenerative changes in transgenic mice [53]. CCN2 may also be chondroprotective, as IVD degeneration is significantly accelerated in *Ccn2*-knockout mice [35]. Research indicating that CCN2 expression in rat IVD cells is regulated by Wnt-β-catenin signaling suggests that targeting Wnt-β-catenin signaling may be worth considering in the treatment of IVD degeneration [54]. In contrast, it appears that the less CCN2 the better in RA, as the downregulation of CCN expression in RASFs is accompanied by decreasing levels of MMP expression [65].

4. The Role of CCN3 in RA and OA

Several studies demonstrate the benefits of CCN3 in OA pathogenesis. Investigations into CCN3 functioning in adult mice have revealed that loss of normal CCN3 function impairs the homeostasis of articular cartilage cells in the adult knee joint and leads to severe OA-like pathology in all tissues of the joint, accompanied by high Osteoarthritis Research Society International (OARSI) scores [68]. These investigations are supported by later research showing that CCN3 is present in epiphyseal chondrocytes of newborn rats and in normal articular cartilage of young mice and rats, but is rapidly downregulated in rat knees with MIA-induced OA [69]. The researchers described protective implications of exogenous CCN3 in rats with MIA-induced OA, as CCN3-treated OA knees exhibited less cartilage degeneration according to tidemark integrity scoring and had higher lubricin expression in the articular cartilage compared with untreated knees [69]. Investigations using human and rat OA articular cartilage, as well as an anterior cruciate ligament transection (ACLT) rat model of OA, have demonstrated that recombinant CCN3 or CCN3 overexpression is protective in OA by suppressing IL-1β-induced activation of the PI3K/AKT/mTOR signaling pathway [38]. In another investigation, treating rat IVD nucleus pulposus cells with increasing doses of recombinant CCN3 dose-dependently reduced antiproliferative activity, while TGF-β treatment increased nucleus pulposus cell proliferation, which was not blocked by the addition of CCN3, indicating that TGF-β overrides the antiproliferative function of CCN3 [70]. The trend towards increased TGF-β expression during disc degeneration and reduction in CCN3 expression, accompanied by a simultaneous increase in CCN2 expression, may reflect a reparative response that enhances matrix synthesis and promotes changes in cell numbers [70]. However, in experiments involving cartilage-specific CCN3-overexpressing transgenic mice, researchers have described CCN3-driven degradative changes in aging articular cartilage [71]. In those studies, CCN3-overexpressing articular cartilage was characterized by severe degenerative changes that increased with aging and the increased accumulation of CCN3 appeared to promote chondrocyte senescence [71].

The exact role of CCN3 in RA is uncertain. Expression patterns of CCN3 in human joints confirm the absence of CCN3 in normal hip synovium and cartilage, RA hip or RA knee cartilage and OA hip and OA knee cartilage, while CCN3 is weakly expressed in the superficial layers and matrix of RA knee and OA hip synovium samples [47]. Some researchers have suggested that CCN3 could serve as a disease activity biomarker for RA, with significant positive correlations observed between CCN3 levels and 28-joint Disease Activity Score (DAS28, whether characterized by erythrocyte sedimentation rate [ESR] or C-reactive protein [CRP]), with higher DAS28 scores reflecting worsening disease [13]. Significant positive correlations have also been recorded between CCN3 levels and titers of RA-specific anti-cyclic citrullinated peptide antibody (anti-CCP Ab), and between CCN3 and IL-6 expression; no such associations have been observed between CCN3 and RF, or CCN3 and TNF-α [13].

In summary, CCN3 is beneficial for OA and plays an important role in the development of RA disease. CCN3 levels decrease rapidly after MIA injection in rat OA knees and exogenous CCN3 treatment is associated with less articular cartilage damage in rat OA knees compared with untreated knees [69]. Interestingly, some researchers have reported finding that during degenerative disc disease, TGF-β suppresses CCN3 activity and upregulates CCN2 expression, a phenomenon that may be associated with a reparative response [70]. In RA, higher serum CCN3 correlates with higher DAS28 scores, inflammatory markers and greater disease severity [13].

5. The Role of CCN4 in RA and OA

WISP1 may be a useful molecular target in OA. A genetic variation at the *WISP1* gene locus appears to influence spinal OA, with one study reporting that postmenopausal Japanese women with the AA genotype (without the G allele) at the *WISP1* 2364A/G single nucleotide polymorphism (SNP) had significantly higher spinal endplate sclerosis scores compared with women carrying the G allele [72]. The study researchers suggested that performing *WISP1* genotyping could be beneficial in the prevention and management of spinal OA. This notion is supported by a later analysis of differential gene expression profiles in OA cartilage that identified several novel genes implicated in OA pathophysiology [73]. When the researchers combined a mill-based RNA isolation technique with high-density oligonucleotide array analysis to examine differential gene expression patterns of chondrocytes in damaged and intact human cartilage within the same knee OA joints, six genes (including *WISP1*) were found to be upregulated in the lesional cartilage area (not in nonlesional areas) of all patients [73]. None of the six genes had previously been identified as playing a role in the damaging effects of OA joint destruction [73].

Investigations into intracellular signaling pathways have helped to clarify important ways in which CCN4 contributes to OA pathophysiology. In one study, CCN4 stimulation of human OASFs upregulated vascular cell adhesion molecule-1 (VCAM-1) expression via the Syk, PKCδ, JNK, c-Jun and AP-1 signaling pathways, which promoted monocyte adhesion to the OASFs [39]. In another study, expression profiling of Wnt signaling molecules confirmed marked increases in CCN4 expression in human and murine OA cartilage and synovium, and the researchers found that recombinant WISP1 stimulation of macrophages and chondrocytes upregulated MMPs and aggrecanase, apparently independently of IL-1 [40]. They also reported that inoculating the articular joints of naïve mice with WISP1 adenovirus enhanced MMP expression in the synovium and cartilage extracellular matrix damage, independently of IL-1α and IL-1β [40]. In contrast, other researchers suggest that stimulating OASFs with CCN4 induces time- and concentration-dependent increases in IL-6 production via the $\alpha v\beta 5$ integrin, PI3K, Akt and NF-κB signaling pathways, emphasizing an important role for IL-6 during OA pathogenesis [74].

A series of investigations by a research group from the Netherlands has examined the implications of Wnt signaling and WISP1 expression in OA pathology [17–20]. Intra-articular injection of Wnt8a and Wnt16 into murine knee joints increased protease activity in the joint and induced cartilage damage, which was significantly decreased after inhibiting the canonical Wnt signaling pathway with the selective inhibitor Dickkopf-1 (DKK-1) [17]. Moreover, the study evidence linked overexpression of WISP1, a downstream protein of canonical Wnt signaling, to OA-like damage in the cartilage that was similar to that of Wnt8a and Wnt16 overexpression [17]. Interestingly, canonical Wnt signaling did not appear to involve IL-1 [17]. In their 2016 review of evidence implicating the Wnt signaling pathway in OA disease, van den Bosch and colleagues concluded that the complexity of this pathway and its multilayered crosstalk with TGF-β signaling (an important contributor to joint homeostasis) makes it difficult to determine the risk of undesired side effects [18]. Targeting WISP1 for OA therapy seems more feasible, which is supported by study findings showing that it is possible to regulate various aspects of OA pathology without interfering with normal processes in mice lacking *Wisp1*, an experimental model of OA [19]. Subsequent in vitro research by the same study group has confirmed that increased expression of *WISP1* is detrimental for cartilage integrity [20].

Whereas CCN4 is not expressed in normal hip synovium samples and is undetectable in normal hip, RA knee and RA hip cartilage obtained from patients undergoing joint replacement, weak-to-moderate CCN4 expression has been found in the superficial layers, matrix and perivascular cells of OA hip, RA knee and OA knee synovium samples from patients with advanced RA or OA disease [47]. Associations between several *WISP1* SNPs and RA susceptibility in Han Chinese warrant the use of CCN4 as a diagnostic marker to stratify individuals at risk of developing RA, and CCN4 might serve as a potential target in RA disease [12]. Meanwhile, another study demonstrates that miR-515-5p could inhibit *WISP1* gene expression in human RA FLS [75], but the function of CCN4 in RA is not well understood yet.

In summary, CCN4 is harmful for OA, and *Ccn4* genetic polymorphisms are associated with RA susceptibility. A genetic variation in the *WISP1* gene locus is associated with spinal OA [72] and certain genes have been implicated in OA pathophysiology [73]. CCN4 stimulation of human OASFs increases VCAM-1 expression [39] and increases IL-6 production [74], while increases in Wnt signaling and WISP1 expression are linked to OA pathology [17,19,20]. In RA, *WISP-1* polymorphisms have been linked to RA susceptibility in Han Chinese [12], while miR-515-5p inhibits *WISP-1* gene expression in human RA FLS [75].

6. The Role of CCN5 in RA and OA

In normal human hip synovium samples, CCN5 is moderately expressed in the superficial layers, matrix and perivascular cells, whereas in samples taken from patients with advanced RA or OA, CCN5 expression is strong in RA and OA knee and hip synovium, but minimal in RA and OA cartilage [47]. Interestingly, real-time quantitative-polymerase chain reaction (qPCR) analysis of *WISP2* expression in arthritic synovial tissues by Tanaka and colleagues detected preferential expression of *WISP2* mRNA in all five human RA synovial tissue samples, compared with just one of four human OA synovial tissues [22], whereas a later qPCR analysis found *WISP2* mRNA and protein expression in human OA synovial synovium, infrapatellar fat pad tissues and human primary chondrocytes, as well as significantly higher *WISP2* mRNA expression in OA infrapatellar fat pads compared with samples from healthy controls [76]. Tanaka and colleagues also observed dose- and time-dependent upregulation of *WISP2* by estrogen in RASFs, which was substantially increased when RASFs were activated by Wnt signaling in the presence of estrogen [22]. In an examination of bone phenotype of adult CCN5/WISP5 knockout ($Ccn5^{LacZ/LacZ}$) mice, loss of *Ccn5* did not appear to affect trabecular bone mineral density (BMD), bone volume fraction (BV/TV) or cortical bone thickness [24]. However, the study researchers noted that while these mice do not exhibit a discernable phenotype, it does not necessarily mean that *Ccn5* is unimportant in bone homeostasis; for instance, *Ccn3/Nov* knockout mice do not show an overt skeletal phenotype, but their bone healing is accelerated after injury [24]. In view of the limited reports, more research is needed to fully characterize how *Ccn5* affects synovitis in OA and RA.

In summary, CCN5 expression is increased in OA and RA disease. *WISP2* mRNA expression is significantly increased in human OA infrapatellar fat pad samples compared with healthy tissue samples [76]. Interestingly, an investigation into the biological role of CCN5 has reported that CCN5 is not required for normal bone formation, although it is necessarily unimportant in bone biology, since *Ccn3/Nov* knockout mice lack an overt skeletal phenotype but exhibit accelerated bone healing after injury; this might also be the case for *Ccn5* [24]. In RA, *WISP2* is synergistically upregulated in RASFs by estrogen and WNT pathways, which suggests that WISP2 is involved in the pathology of the disease [22].

7. The Role of CCN6 in RA and OA

Investigations into the mode of action of WISP3 and its function during cartilage growth and maintenance have ascertained that WISP3 is an important structural component of cartilage [41]. WISP3 is secreted from chondrocyte lines, while pure recombinant WISP3 protein appears to function as a ligand and signals via autocrine and/or paracrine modes [41]. Besides regulating collagen II and aggrecan expression, WISP3 may also contribute to cartilage growth and maintenance by promoting superoxide dismutase (SOD) expression and activity in chondrocytes [41]; such activity is very important for sustaining tissue homeostasis under conditions of cellular hypertrophy that may contribute to cartilage degeneration and the development of degenerative joint disease [77]. Interestingly, Lamb and colleagues have speculated that the functional consequences of WISP3 secretion could be impaired by disruption of the signal peptide that flanks the associated WISP3*84AA SNP within intron 1 [23]. More clarification is needed on this aspect.

CCN6 expression is generally undetectable in hip and knee joint tissues from patients with advanced RA or OA, and is minimal in the multilayered synovial cells from RA and OA knees [47], although evidence of high WISP3/CCN6 expression in end-stage OA cartilage suggests that CCN6 has a role in cartilage homeostasis [42]. It is speculated that the high expression of WISP3/CCN6 in end-stage OA cartilage may reflect attempts by cartilage to inhibit aggrecan breakdown and prevent further cartilage damage [42]. Moreover, the overexpression of WISP3/CCN6 in immortalized chondrocyte C-28/I2 cells is associated with substantially reduced levels of ADAMTS-4 and ADAMTS-5 expression, whereas MMP-1 and MMP-10 expression is increased, while gene silencing of WISP3/CCN6 in cytokine-stimulated primary chondrocytes enhances ADAMTS-5 expression and suppresses MMP-10 expression, suggesting that CCN6 has anticatabolic effects [42].

Higher levels of *WISP3* mRNA have been observed in RA synovium and FLS compared with OA and normal synovial tissue, and proinflammatory cytokines can further increase *WISP3* mRNA expression in RA FLS [21]. Intriguingly, similar levels of WISP3 protein expression in RA, OA and normal synovium suggest a lack of coordinated regulation between WISP3 protein and mRNA [21]. Interestingly, WISP3 appears to have an important role in the development of juvenile idiopathic arthritis (JIA), a group of chronic inflammatory arthropathies of childhood with onset before the age of 16 years [78]. Much research has explored the genetic basis of JIA, but the etiology of this disease is still not well understood [79,80]. Early initiation of disease-modifying antirheumatic drugs (DMARDs) is advised by the American College of Rheumatology (ACR) for pediatric patients with JIA [81]. One analysis of *WISP3* SNPs in blood samples obtained from two independent cohorts of patients with polyarticular-course JIA (≥5 joints involved) that included diagnoses of extended oligoarthritis, RF-negative polyarthritis and RF-positive polyarthritis, found replication of a positive association with an SNP within the first intron of the *WISP3* gene (WISP3*G84A) [23]. Individuals homozygous (AA) for G84A had a two-fold higher risk for polyarticular-course JIA compared with those who were not AA homozygous [23].

In summary, CCN6 is possibly beneficial for OA. High WISP3/CCN6 expression in end-stage OA cartilage suggests that CCN6 contributes to cartilage homeostasis [42]. Moreover, CCN6 is involved in complex context-dependent roles in cartilage biology, according to the evidence showing that WISP3/CCN6 mediates metalloproteinase expression through different pathways and modulates various signaling cascades [42]. Not only is *WISP3* gene expression in RA synovium and FLS markedly higher than that in OA and normal synovial tissue, but WISP3 mRNA expression is significantly increased in RA FLS when stimulated by proinflammatory cytokines [21]. Finally, replication of a positive association with a polymorphism within the first intron of the *WISP3* gene increases the risk of developing polyarticular-course JIA [23].

8. Conclusions

Several lines of evidence suggest that it is worthwhile to target the different members of the CCN family in both OA and RA disease. However, because of different effects of CCN proteins in RA and OA, an individualized approach with these CCN proteins for the management of these arthritis disorders should be considered in future applications.

Funding: This study was supported by China Medical University Hospital (DMR-110-022; Approval date: 1 November 2020 and DMR-110-157; Approval date: 1 November 2020) and China Medical University Beigang Hospital (CMUBHR 109-007; Approval date: 1 August 2020 and CMUBHR109-011; Approval date: 1 August 2020).

Institutional Review Board Statement: Not applicable.

Informed Consent Statement: Not applicable.

Data Availability Statement: Not applicable.

Conflicts of Interest: The authors declare no conflict of interest. The funders had no role in the writing of this manuscript, or in the selection of research papers referred to in this manuscript.

References

1. Senthelal, S.; Li, J.; Goyal, A.; Bansal, P.; Thomas, M.A. *Arthritis*; StatPearls: Treasure Island, FL, USA, 2021.
2. Imas, J.J.; Zamarreño, C.R.; Zubiate, P.; Sanchez-Martín, L.; Campión, J.; Matías, I.R. Optical Biosensors for the Detection of Rheumatoid Arthritis (RA) Biomarkers: A Comprehensive Review. *Sensors* **2020**, *20*, 6289. [CrossRef] [PubMed]
3. Hügle, T.; Geurts, J. What drives osteoarthritis?—synovial *versus* subchondral bone pathology. *Rheumatology* **2016**, *56*, 1461–1471. [CrossRef] [PubMed]
4. Tang, C.-H. Research of Pathogenesis and Novel Therapeutics in Arthritis. *Int. J. Mol. Sci.* **2019**, *20*, 1646. [CrossRef] [PubMed]
5. Lim, H.; Lee, S.H.; Lee, H.T.; Lee, J.U.; Son, J.Y.; Shin, W.; Heo, Y.-S. Structural Biology of the TNFα Antagonists Used in the Treatment of Rheumatoid Arthritis. *Int. J. Mol. Sci.* **2018**, *19*, 768. [CrossRef] [PubMed]
6. Buch, M.H. Defining refractory rheumatoid arthritis. *Ann. Rheum. Dis.* **2018**, *77*, 966–969. [CrossRef] [PubMed]
7. Chen, S.-J.; Lin, G.-J.; Chen, J.-W.; Wang, K.-C.; Tien, C.-H.; Hu, C.-F.; Chang, C.-N.; Hsu, W.-F.; Fan, H.-C.; Sytwu, H.-K. Immunopathogenic Mechanisms and Novel Immune-Modulated Therapies in Rheumatoid Arthritis. *Int. J. Mol. Sci.* **2019**, *20*, 1332. [CrossRef]
8. Ghouri, A.; Conaghan, P.G. Update on novel pharmacological therapies for osteoarthritis. *Ther. Adv. Musculoskelet. Dis.* **2019**, *11*. [CrossRef]
9. Henrot, P.; Truchetet, M.-E.; Fisher, G.; Taïeb, A.; Cario, M. CCN proteins as potential actionable targets in scleroderma. *Exp. Dermatol.* **2018**, *28*, 11–18. [CrossRef] [PubMed]
10. Jun, J.-I.; Lau, L.F. Taking aim at the extracellular matrix: CCN proteins as emerging therapeutic targets. *Nat. Rev. Drug Discov.* **2011**, *10*, 945–963. [CrossRef] [PubMed]
11. Chen, C.-Y.; Fuh, L.-J.; Huang, C.-C.; Hsu, C.-J.; Su, C.-M.; Liu, S.-C.; Lin, Y.-M.; Tang, C.-H. Enhancement of CCL2 expression and monocyte migration by CCN1 in osteoblasts through inhibiting miR-518a-5p: Implication of rheumatoid arthritis therapy. *Sci. Rep.* **2017**, *7*, 1–11. [CrossRef]
12. Kuo, S.-J.; Hsua, P.-W.; Chien, S.-Y.; Huang, C.-C.; Hu, S.-L.; Tsai, C.-H.; Su, C.-M.; Tang, C.-H. Associations between WNT1-inducible signaling pathway protein-1 (WISP-1) genetic polymorphisms and clinical aspects of rheumatoid arthritis among Chinese Han subjects. *Medicine* **2019**, *98*, e17604. [CrossRef] [PubMed]
13. Wei, Y.; Peng, L.; Li, Y.; Zhang, N.; Shang, K.; Duan, L.; Zhong, J.; Chen, J. Higher Serum CCN3 Is Associated with Disease Activity and Inflammatory Markers in Rheumatoid Arthritis. *J. Immunol. Res.* **2020**, *2020*, 1–7. [CrossRef]
14. Kular, L.; Pakradouni, J.; Kitabgi, P.; Laurent, M.; Martinerie, C. The CCN family: A new class of inflammation modulators? *Biochimie* **2011**, *93*, 377–388. [CrossRef] [PubMed]
15. Chijiiwa, M.; Mochizuki, S.; Kimura, T.; Abe, H.; Tanaka, Y.; Fujii, Y.; Shimizu, H.; Enomoto, H.; Toyama, Y.; Okada, Y. CCN1 (Cyr61) Is Overexpressed in Human Osteoarthritic Cartilage and Inhibits ADAMTS-4 (Aggrecanase 1) Activity. *Arthritis Rheumatol.* **2015**, *67*, 1557–1567. [CrossRef] [PubMed]
16. Tu, M.; Yao, Y.; Qiao, F.H.H.; Wang, L. The pathogenic role of connective tissue growth factor in osteoarthritis. *Biosci. Rep.* **2019**, *39*. [CrossRef] [PubMed]
17. Bosch, M.H.V.D.; Blom, A.B.; Sloetjes, A.W.; Koenders, M.I.; Van De Loo, F.A.; Berg, W.B.V.D.; Van Lent, P.L.; Van Der Kraan, P.M. Induction of Canonical Wnt Signaling by Synovial Overexpression of Selected Wnts Leads to Protease Activity and Early Osteoarthritis-Like Cartilage Damage. *Am. J. Pathol.* **2015**, *185*, 1970–1980. [CrossRef] [PubMed]
18. Bosch, M.H.V.D.; Gleissl, T.A.; Blom, A.B.; Berg, W.B.V.D.; Van Lent, P.L.; Van Der Kraan, P.M. Wnts talking with the TGF-β superfamily: WISPers about modulation of osteoarthritis. *Rheumatology* **2015**, *55*, 1536–1547. [CrossRef] [PubMed]
19. Bosch, M.V.D.; Blom, A.; Kram, V.; Maeda, A.; Sikka, S.; Gabet, Y.; Kilts, T.; Berg, W.V.D.; van Lent, P.; van der Kraan, P.; et al. WISP1/CCN4 aggravates cartilage degeneration in experimental osteoarthritis. *Osteoarthr. Cartil.* **2017**, *25*, 1900–1911. [CrossRef] [PubMed]
20. Bosch, M.H.J.V.D.; Ramos, Y.F.M.; Hollander, W.D.; Bomer, N.; Nelissen, R.G.H.H.; Bovée, J.V.M.G.; Berg, W.B.V.D.; Lent, P.L.E.M.V.; Blom, A.B.; Van Der Kraan, P.M.; et al. Increased WISP1 expression in human osteoarthritic articular cartilage is epigenetically regulated and decreases cartilage matrix production. *Rheumatology* **2019**, *58*, 1065–1074. [CrossRef]
21. Cheon, H.; Boyle, D.L.; Firestein, G.S. Wnt1 inducible signaling pathway protein-3 regulation and microsatellite structure in arthritis. *J. Rheumatol.* **2004**, *31*, 2106–2114. [PubMed]
22. Tanaka, I.; Morikawa, M.; Okuse, T.; Shirakawa, M.; Imai, K. Expression and regulation of WISP2 in rheumatoid arthritic synovium. *Biochem. Biophys. Res. Commun.* **2005**, *334*, 973–978. [CrossRef]
23. Lamb, R.; Thomson, W.; Ogilvie, E.; Donn, R.; Rheumatology, T.B.S.O.P.A.A. Wnt-1-inducible signaling pathway protein 3 and susceptibility to juvenile idiopathic arthritis. *Arthritis Rheum.* **2005**, *52*, 3548–3553. [CrossRef]
24. Jiang, J.; Zhao, G.; Lyons, K.M. Characterization of bone morphology in CCN5/WISP5 knockout mice. *J. Cell Commun. Signal.* **2018**, *12*, 265–270. [CrossRef] [PubMed]

25. Sun, C.; Zhang, H.; Liu, X. Emerging role of CCN family proteins in fibrosis. *J. Cell. Physiol.* **2021**, *236*, 4195–4206. [CrossRef] [PubMed]
26. Chen, C.-Y.; Su, C.-M.; Huang, Y.-L.; Tsai, C.-H.; Fuh, L.-J.; Tang, C.-H. CCN1 Induces Oncostatin M Production in Osteoblasts via Integrin-Dependent Signal Pathways. *PLoS ONE* **2014**, *9*, e106632. [CrossRef] [PubMed]
27. Yang, B.; Ni, J.; Long, H.; Huang, J.; Yang, C.; Huang, X. IL-1β-induced miR-34a up-regulation inhibits Cyr61 to modulate osteoarthritis chondrocyte proliferation through ADAMTS-4. *J. Cell. Biochem.* **2018**, *119*, 7959–7970. [CrossRef]
28. Feng, M.; Peng, H.; Yao, R.; Zhang, Z.; Mao, G.; Yu, H.; Qiu, Y. Inhibition of cellular communication network factor 1 (CCN1)-driven senescence slows down cartilage inflammaging and osteoarthritis. *Bone* **2020**, *139*, 115522. [CrossRef] [PubMed]
29. Zhang, Q.; Wu, J.; Cao, Q.; Xiao, L.; Wang, L.; He, D.; Ouyang, G.; Lin, J.; Shen, B.; Shi, Y.; et al. A critical role of Cyr61 in interleukin-17-dependent proliferation of fibroblast-like synoviocytes in rheumatoid arthritis. *Arthritis Rheum.* **2009**, *60*, 3602–3612. [CrossRef] [PubMed]
30. Lin, J.; Zhou, Z.; Huo, R.; Xiao, L.; Ouyang, G.; Wang, L.; Sun, Y.; Shen, B.; Li, D.; Li, N. Cyr61 Induces IL-6 Production by Fibroblast-like Synoviocytes Promoting Th17 Differentiation in Rheumatoid Arthritis. *J. Immunol.* **2012**, *188*, 5776–5784. [CrossRef] [PubMed]
31. Zhu, X.; Song, Y.; Huo, R.; Zhang, J.; Sun, S.; He, Y.; Gao, H.; Zhang, M.; Sun, X.; Zhai, T.; et al. Cyr61 participates in the pathogenesis of rheumatoid arthritis by promoting proIL-1β production by fibroblast-like synoviocytes through an AKT-dependent NF-κB signaling pathway. *Clin. Immunol.* **2015**, *157*, 187–197. [CrossRef]
32. Chen, C.-Y.; Su, C.-M.; Hsu, C.-J.; Huang, C.-C.; Wang, S.-W.; Liu, S.-C.; Chen, W.-C.; Fuh, L.-J.; Tang, C.-H. CCN1 Promotes VEGF Production in Osteoblasts and Induces Endothelial Progenitor Cell Angiogenesis by Inhibiting miR-126 Expression in Rheumatoid Arthritis. *J. Bone Miner. Res.* **2016**, *32*, 34–45. [CrossRef]
33. Zhong, C.; Huo, R.; Hu, K.; Shen, J.; Li, D.; Li, N.; Ding, J. Molecular basis for the recognition of CCN1 by monoclonal antibody 093G9. *J. Mol. Recognit.* **2017**, *30*, e2645. [CrossRef]
34. Liu, S.-C.; Hsu, C.-J.; Fong, Y.-C.; Chuang, S.-M.; Tang, C.-H. CTGF induces monocyte chemoattractant protein-1 expression to enhance monocyte migration in human synovial fibroblasts. *Biochim. Biophys. Acta BBA Bioenerg.* **2013**, *1833*, 1114–1124. [CrossRef]
35. Bedore, J.; Sha, W.; McCann, M.R.; Liu, S.; Leask, A.; Séguin, C.A. Loss of notochord-derived CCN2 results in impaired intervertebral disc development and premature disc degeneration in mice with notochord-specific deletion of CCN. *Arthritis Rheum.* **2013**, *65*, 2634–2644. [CrossRef] [PubMed]
36. Nozawa, K.; Fujishiro, M.; Kawasaki, M.; Kaneko, H.; Iwabuchi, K.; Yanagida, M.; Suzuki, F.; Miyazawa, K.; Takasaki, Y.; Ogawa, H.; et al. Connective tissue growth factor promotes articular damage by increased osteoclastogenesis in patients with rheumatoid arthritis. *Arthritis Res. Ther.* **2009**, *11*, R174. [CrossRef] [PubMed]
37. Wang, J.-G.; Xu, W.-D.; Zhai, W.-T.; Li, Y.; Hu, J.-W.; Hu, B.; Li, M.; Zhang, L.; Guo, W.; Zhang, J.-P.; et al. Disorders in angiogenesis and redox pathways are main factors contributing to the progression of rheumatoid arthritis: A comparative proteomics study. *Arthritis Rheum.* **2012**, *64*, 993–1004. [CrossRef] [PubMed]
38. Huang, X.; Ni, B.; Mao, Z.; Xi, Y.; Chu, X.; Zhang, R.; Ma, X.; You, H. NOV/CCN3 induces cartilage protection by inhibiting PI3K/AKT/mTOR pathway. *J. Cell. Mol. Med.* **2019**, *23*, 7525–7534. [CrossRef] [PubMed]
39. Liu, J.-F.; Hou, S.-M.; Tsai, C.-H.; Huang, C.-Y.; Hsu, C.-J.; Tang, C.-H. CCN4 induces vascular cell adhesion molecule-1 expression in human synovial fibroblasts and promotes monocyte adhesion. *Biochim. Biophys. Acta BBA Bioenerg.* **2013**, *1833*, 966–975. [CrossRef] [PubMed]
40. Blom, A.B.; Brockbank, S.M.; Van Lent, P.L.; Van Beuningen, H.M.; Geurts, J.; Takahashi, N.; Van Der Kraan, P.M.; Van De Loo, F.A.; Schreurs, B.W.; Clements, K.; et al. Involvement of the Wnt signaling pathway in experimental and human osteoarthritis: Prominent role of Wnt-induced signaling protein 1. *Arthritis Rheum.* **2009**, *60*, 501–512. [CrossRef] [PubMed]
41. Davis, L.; Chen, Y.; Sen, M. WISP-3 functions as a ligand and promotes superoxide dismutase activity. *Biochem. Biophys. Res. Commun.* **2006**, *342*, 259–265. [CrossRef] [PubMed]
42. Baker, N.; Sharpe, P.; Culley, K.; Otero, M.; Bevan, D.; Newham, P.; Barker, W.; Clements, K.M.; Langham, C.J.; Goldring, M.B.; et al. Dual regulation of metalloproteinase expression in chondrocytes by Wnt-1-inducible signaling pathway protein 3/CCN6. *Arthritis Rheum.* **2012**, *64*, 2289–2299. [CrossRef]
43. Van Roon, J.A.G.; Van Roy, J.L.A.M.; Lafeber, F.P.J.G.; Bijlsma, J.W.J.; Gmelig-Meyling, F.H.J. Prevention and reversal of cartilage degradation in rheumatoid arthritis by interleukin-10 and interleukin-4. *Arthritis Rheum.* **1996**, *39*, 829–835. [CrossRef] [PubMed]
44. O'Hayre, M.; Salanga, C.L.; Handel, T.M.; Allen, S.J. Chemokines and cancer: Migration, intracellular signalling and intercellular communication in the microenvironment. *Biochem. J.* **2008**, *409*, 635–649. [CrossRef] [PubMed]
45. Koch, A.E.; Kunkel, S.L.; Harlow, L.A.; Johnson, B.; Evanoff, H.L.; Haines, G.K.; Burdick, M.D.; Pope, R.M.; Strieter, R.M. Enhanced production of monocyte chemoattractant protein-1 in rheumatoid arthritis. *J. Clin. Investig.* **1992**, *90*, 772–779. [CrossRef] [PubMed]
46. Akahoshi, T.; Wada, C.; Endo, H.; Hirota, K.; Hosaka, S.; Takagishi, K.; Kondo, H.; Kashiwazaki, S.; Matsushima, K. Expression of monocyte chemotactic and activating factor in rheumatoid arthritis. regulation of its production in synovial cells by interleukin-1 and tumor necrosis factor. *Arthritis Rheum.* **1993**, *36*, 762–771. [CrossRef] [PubMed]
47. Komatsu, M.; Nakamura, Y.; Maruyama, M.; Abe, K.; Watanapokasin, R.; Kato, H. Expression profles of human CCN genes in patients with osteoarthritis or rheumatoid arthritis. *J. Orthop. Sci.* **2015**, *20*, 708–716. [CrossRef]

48. Lau, L.F. CCN1/CYR61: The very model of a modern matricellular protein. *Cell. Mol. Life Sci.* **2011**, *68*, 3149–3163. [CrossRef] [PubMed]
49. Xu, T.; He, Y.-H.; Wang, M.-Q.; Yao, H.-W.; Ni, M.-M.; Zhang, L.; Meng, X.-M.; Huang, C.; Ge, Y.-X.; Li, J. Therapeutic potential of cysteine-rich protein 61 in rheumatoid arthritis. *Gene* **2016**, *592*, 179–185. [CrossRef]
50. Omoto, S.; Nishida, K.; Yamaai, Y.; Shibahara, M.; Nishida, T.; Doi, T.; Asahara, H.; Nakanishi, T.; Inoue, H.; Takigawa, M. Expression and localization of connective tissue growth factor (CTGF/Hcs24/CCN2) in osteoarthritic cartilage. *Osteoarthr. Cartil.* **2004**, *12*, 771–778. [CrossRef] [PubMed]
51. Kubota, S.; Takigawa, M. The role of CCN2 in cartilage and bone development. *J. Cell Commun. Signal.* **2011**, *5*, 209–217. [CrossRef] [PubMed]
52. Nishida, T.; Kubota, S.; Kojima, S.; Kuboki, T.; Nakao, K.; Kushibiki, T.; Tabata, Y.; Takigawa, M. Regeneration of Defects in Articular Cartilage in Rat Knee Joints by CCN2 (Connective Tissue Growth Factor). *J. Bone Miner. Res.* **2004**, *19*, 1308–1319. [CrossRef]
53. Itoh, S.; Hattori, T.; Tomita, N.; Aoyama, E.; Yutani, Y.; Yamashiro, T.; Takigawa, M. CCN Family Member 2/Connective Tissue Growth Factor (CCN2/CTGF) Has Anti-Aging Effects That Protect Articular Cartilage from Age-Related Degenerative Changes. *PLoS ONE* **2013**, *8*, e71156. [CrossRef] [PubMed]
54. Hiyama, A.; Morita, K.; Sakai, D.; Watanabe, M. CCN family member 2/connective tissue growth factor (CCN2/CTGF) is regulated by Wnt–β-catenin signaling in nucleus pulposus cells. *Arthritis Res.* **2018**, *20*, 217. [CrossRef] [PubMed]
55. Tang, X.; Muhammad, H.; McLean, C.; Miotla-Zarebska, J.; Fleming, J.; Didangelos, A.; Önnerfjord, P.; Leask, A.; Saklatvala, J.; Vincent, T.L. Connective tissue growth factor contributes to joint homeostasis and osteoarthritis severity by controlling the matrix sequestration and activation of latent TGFβ. *Ann. Rheum. Dis.* **2018**, *77*, 1372–1380. [CrossRef] [PubMed]
56. Keenan, C.M.; Ramos-Mucci, L.; Kanakis, I.; Milner, P.I.; Leask, A.; Abraham, D.; Bou-Gharios, G.; Poulet, B. Post-traumatic osteoarthritis development is not modified by postnatal chondrocyte deletion of Ccn2. *Dis. Model. Mech.* **2020**, *13*. [CrossRef]
57. Perbal, B. CCN proteins: Multifunctional signalling regulators. *Lancet* **2004**, *363*, 62–64. [CrossRef]
58. Kubota, S.; Takigawa, M. Cellular and molecular actions of CCN2/CTGF and its role under physiological and pathological conditions. *Clin. Sci.* **2015**, *128*, 181–196. [CrossRef]
59. Planque, N.; Perbal, B. A structural approach to the role of CCN (CYR61/CTGF/NOV) proteins in tumourigenesis. *Cancer Cell Int.* **2003**, *3*, 15. [CrossRef] [PubMed]
60. Takigawa, M.; Nakanishi, T.; Kubota, S.; Nishida, T. Role of CTGF/HCS24/ecogenin in skeletal growth control. *J. Cell. Physiol.* **2003**, *194*, 256–266. [CrossRef] [PubMed]
61. Yang, X.; Lin, K.; Ni, S.; Wang, J.; Tian, Q.; Chen, H.; Brown, M.A.; Zheng, K.; Zhai, W.; Sun, L.; et al. Serum connective tissue growth factor is a highly discriminatory biomarker for the diagnosis of rheumatoid arthritis. *Arthritis Res.* **2017**, *19*, 257. [CrossRef] [PubMed]
62. Ding, S.; Duan, H.; Fang, F.; Shen, H.; Xiao, W. CTGF promotes articular damage by increased proliferation of fibroblast-like synoviocytes in rheumatoid arthritis. *Scand. J. Rheumatol.* **2016**, *45*, 282–287. [CrossRef] [PubMed]
63. Miyashita, T.; Morimoto, S.; Fujishiro, M.; Hayakawa, K.; Suzuki, S.; Ikeda, K.; Miyazawa, K.; Morioka, M.; Takamori, K.; Ogawa, H.; et al. Inhibition of each module of connective tissue growth factor as a potential therapeutic target for rheumatoid arthritis. *Autoimmunity* **2016**, *49*, 109–114. [CrossRef] [PubMed]
64. Nozawa, K.; Fujishiro, M.; Kawasaki, M.; Yamaguchi, A.; Ikeda, K.; Morimoto, S.; Iwabuchi, K.; Yanagida, M.; Ichinose, S.; Morioka, M.; et al. Inhibition of Connective Tissue Growth Factor Ameliorates Disease in a Murine Model of Rheumatoid Arthritis. *Arthritis Rheum.* **2013**, *65*, 1477–1486. [CrossRef]
65. Wang, J.-G.; Ruan, J.; Li, C.-Y.; Li, Y.; Zhai, W.-T.; Zhang, W.; Ye, H.; Shen, N.-H.; Lei, K.-F.; Chen, X.-F.; et al. Connective tissue growth factor, a regulator related with 10-hydroxy-2-decenoic acid down-regulate MMPs in rheumatoid arthritis. *Rheumatol. Int.* **2012**, *32*, 2791–2799. [CrossRef] [PubMed]
66. Stopka-Farooqui, U.H.O. Proresolving mediators: New therapies to treat inflammatory diseases. *Clin. Lipidol.* **2015**, *10*, 8. [CrossRef]
67. Sun, W.; Ma, J.; Zhao, H.; Xiao, C.; Zhong, H.; Ling, H.; Xie, Z.; Tian, Q.; Chen, H.; Zhang, T.; et al. Resolvin D1 suppresses pannus formation via decreasing connective tissue growth factor caused by upregulation of miRNA-146a-5p in rheumatoid arthritis. *Arthritis Res.* **2020**, *22*, 1–14. [CrossRef]
68. Roddy, K.; Boulter, C. Targeted mutation of NOV/CCN3 in mice disrupts joint homeostasis and causes osteoarthritis-like disease. *Osteoarthr. Cartil.* **2015**, *23*, 607–615. [CrossRef] [PubMed]
69. Janune, D.; El Kader, T.A.; Aoyama, E.; Nishida, T.; Tabata, Y.; Kubota, S.; Takigawa, M. Novel role of CCN3 that maintains the differentiated phenotype of articular cartilage. *J. Bone Miner. Metab.* **2016**, *35*, 582–597. [CrossRef] [PubMed]
70. Tran, C.M.; Smith, H.E.; Symes, A.J.; Rittié, L.; Perbal, B.; Shapiro, I.M.; Risbud, M.V. Transforming growth factor β controls CCN3 expression in nucleus pulposus cells of the intervertebral disc. *Arthritis Rheum.* **2011**, *63*, 3022–3031. [CrossRef]
71. Kuwahara, M.; Kadoya, K.; Kondo, S.; Fu, S.; Miyake, Y.; Ogo, A.; Ono, M.; Furumatsu, T.; Nakata, E.; Sasaki, T.; et al. CCN3 (NOV) Drives Degradative Changes in Aging Articular Cartilage. *Int. J. Mol. Sci.* **2020**, *21*, 7556. [CrossRef]
72. Urano, T.; Narusawa, K.; Shiraki, M.; Usui, T.; Sasaki, N.; Hosoi, T.; Ouchi, Y.; Nakamura, T.; Inoue, S. Association of a single nucleotide polymorphism in the WISP1 gene with spinal osteoarthritis in postmenopausal Japanese women. *J. Bone Miner. Metab.* **2007**, *25*, 253–258. [CrossRef] [PubMed]

73. Geyer, M.; Grassel, S.; Straub, R.H.; Schett, G.; Dinser, R.; Grifka, J.; Gay, S.; Neumann, E.; Müller-Ladner, U. Differential transcriptome analysis of intraarticular lesional vs intact cartilage reveals new candidate genes in osteoarthritis pathophysiology. *Osteoarthr. Cartil.* **2009**, *17*, 328–335. [CrossRef]
74. Hou, C.-H.; Tang, C.-H.; Hsu, C.-J.; Hou, S.-M.; Liu, J.-F. CCN4 induces IL-6 production through $\alpha v\beta 5$ receptor, PI3K, Akt, and NF-κB singling pathway in human synovial fibroblasts. *Arthritis Res. Ther.* **2013**, *15*, R19. [CrossRef] [PubMed]
75. Cai, D.; Hong, S.; Yang, J.; San, P. The Effects of microRNA-515-5p on the Toll-Like Receptor 4 (TLR4)/JNK Signaling Pathway and WNT1-Inducible-Signaling Pathway Protein 1 (WISP-1) Expression in Rheumatoid Arthritis Fibroblast-Like Synovial (RAFLS) Cells Following Treatment with Receptor Activator of Nuclear Factor-kappa-B Ligand (RANKL). *Med. Sci. Monit.* **2020**, *26*. [CrossRef]
76. Conde, J.; Scotece, M.; Abella, V.; Gómez, R.; López, V.; Villar, R.; Hermida, M.; Pino, J.; Gómez-Reino, J.J.; Gualillo, O. Identification of Novel Adipokines in the Joint. Differential Expression in Healthy and Osteoarthritis Tissues. *PLoS ONE* **2015**, *10*, e0123601. [CrossRef] [PubMed]
77. Jallali, N.; Ridha, H.; Thrasivoulou, C.; Underwood, C.; Butler, P.; Cowen, T. Vulnerability to ROS-induced cell death in ageing articular cartilage: The role of antioxidant enzyme activity. *Osteoarthr. Cartil.* **2005**, *13*, 614–622. [CrossRef]
78. Martini, A.; Lovell, D.J. Juvenile idiopathic arthritis: State of the art and future perspectives. *Ann. Rheum. Dis.* **2010**, *69*, 1260–1263. [CrossRef]
79. Goettel, A.M.; DeClercq, J.; Choi, L.; Graham, T.B.; Mitchell, A.A. Efficacy and Safety of Abatacept, Adalimumab, and Etanercept in Pediatric Patients with Juvenile Idiopathic Arthritis. *J. Pediatr. Pharmacol. Ther.* **2021**, *26*, 157–162. [CrossRef]
80. Leong, J.Y.; Guan, Y.J.; Albani, S.; Arkachaisri, T. Recent advances in our understanding of the pathogenesis of juvenile idiopathic arthritis and their potential clinical implications. *Expert Rev. Clin. Immunol.* **2018**, *14*, 933–944. [CrossRef] [PubMed]
81. Ringold, S.; Angeles-Han, S.T.; Beukelman, T.; Lovell, D.J.; Cuello, C.A.; Becker, M.L.; Colbert, R.A.; Feldman, B.M.; Ferguson, P.J.; Gewanter, H.L.; et al. 2019 American College of Rheumatology/Arthritis Foundation Guideline for the Treatment of Juvenile Idiopathic Arthritis: Therapeutic Approaches for Non-Systemic Polyarthritis, Sacroiliitis, and Enthesitis. *Arthritis Rheum.* **2019**, *71*, 717–734. [CrossRef] [PubMed]

MDPI
St. Alban-Anlage 66
4052 Basel
Switzerland
Tel. +41 61 683 77 34
Fax +41 61 302 89 18
www.mdpi.com

International Journal of Molecular Sciences Editorial Office
E-mail: ijms@mdpi.com
www.mdpi.com/journal/ijms

www.ingramcontent.com/pod-product-compliance
Lightning Source LLC
Chambersburg PA
CBHW061804210926
51850CB00006B/610

* 9 7 8 3 0 3 6 5 8 0 8 4 5 *